Principles and Practice
of Pediatric Optometry

Principles and Practice of Pediatric Optometry

Edited by

Alfred A. Rosenbloom, O.D., M.A.

Meredith W. Morgan, O.D., Ph.D.

With 32 Contributors

J. B. Lippincott Company   Philadelphia
Grand Rapids   New York   St. Louis   San Francisco
London   Sydney   Tokyo

Acquisitions Editor: Nancy Mullins
Project Coordinator: Lori J. Bainbridge
Compositor: Bi-Comp. Inc.
Printer/Binder: R. R. Donnelley & Sons
Production: Spectrum Publisher Services, Inc.

6 5 4 3 2 1

Library of Congress Cataloging-in-Publication Data

Principles and practice of pediatric optometry/edited by Alfred A.
   Rosenbloom and Meredith Morgan.
      p.   cm.
      Includes bibilographical references.
      Includes index.
      ISBN 0-397-50917-0
      1. Vision disorders in children—Diagnosis. 2. Optometry.
I. Rosenbloom, Alfred A. II. Morgan, Meredith W.
      [DNLM: 1. Optometry. 2. Vision Disorders—diagnosis, 3. Vision
Disorders—in infancy & childhood. 4. Vision Disorders—therapy.]
RE48.2.C5P75   1990
618.92'09775—dc20
DLC
for Library of Congress   90-6079
                                                               CIP

To our grandchildren and to all children—may they enjoy the blessings inherent in the priceless gift of vision

Contributors

Leonard Apt, M.D., is professor of ophthalmology at the University of California, Los Angeles, School of Medicine, and Director Emeritus of the division of pediatric ophthalmology at the Jules Stein Eye Institute at UCLA. He established the first full-time division of pediatric ophthalmology at a medical school in the United States at UCLA in 1961. Dr. Apt is board-certified in both pediatrics and ophthalmology. His book *Diagnostic Procedures in Pediatric Ophthalmology* was one of the first texts devoted to the new subspecialty. In addition to his research and numerous contributions in the ophthalmology literature, with emphasis in the areas of pediatric pharmacology and ocular motility, he has authored chapters on the eye in widely used pediatric reference texts.

William R. Baldwin, O.D., Ph.D., is dean, College of Optometry, University of Houston. His distinguished career in optometric education includes serving as president, New England College of Optometry, and dean, Pacific University College of Optometry. He has been instrumental in starting schools of optometry through the world. In 1991, he will assume the presidency of River Blindness Foundation, Houston, Texas. A major research and publication interest is myopia in children.

Ross Beauchamp, Ph.D, received his Ph.D. degree in Psychology from Brown University in 1970 under the direction of Lorrin Riggs. He did postdoctoral work in neurophysiology of vision with C. C. Hunt and Nigel Daw in the Department of Physiology and Biophysics at Washington Medical School. Then in 1971, he joined the faculty of the School of Optometry at the University of Waterloo where he remains to the present. Dr. Beauchamp's teaching and research interests include the neurophysiology and neuroanatomy of vision, especially the neural mechanisms responsible for color vision and ocular accommodation.

William R. Bobier, O.D., M.Sc., Ph.D., is an assistant professor in the School of Optometry at the University of Waterloo. His interest is in binocular vision particularly the identification of factors which may impair the development of accommodation and vergence functions in the early years of life. This research has involved the design and application of photorefractive techniques in order to facilitate the measure of refraction and accommodation in infants and young children.

Emilio Campos, M.D., is professor of pediatric ophthalmology at the University of Modena Medical School, Modena, Italy. He was trained both in Trieste and Modena by Professor Bruno Bagolini who is well known for his studies in pediatric ophthalmology. Campos completed postdoctoral studies with Professor Jay M. Enoch in Florida and initiated a pediatric service at Louisiana State University Department of Ophthalmology. He later returned to the University of Modena and has worked for many years both there and at the University of Bologna in many phases of ophthalmology, but generally concentrating upon pediatric care. Both he and Enoch have maintained an interest in optimizing vision in neonates born with various form of sensory deprivation.

Michael H. Cho, O.D., is assistant professor of optometry and chief of Ophthalmic Materials Services at the University of Alabama at Birmingham School of Optometry. He is the first appointed contributing editor of the *Journal of the American Optometric Association* in the field of oph-

thalmic materials. Cho has done research and has authored many articles in ophthalmic materials with emphasis in progressive addition lenses.

Paul B. Donzis, M.D., is clinical instructor of ophthalmology at UCLA School of Medicine and the Jules Stein Eye Institute. He is past recipient of a National Eye Institute research training grant and a grant from the Heed Ophthalmic Foundation. His research interests include diseases of the cornea and complications of contact lenses. He is the author of numerous articles in these areas as well as the growth and development of the human eye.

Leland W. Carr, O.D., is the director of clinics for the College of Optometry, Northeastern State University, Tahlequah, Oklahoma. He received the Doctor of Optometry degree in 1981 from Ferris State College. He is an associate professor of optometry at Northeastern State University. Dr. Carr previously served in the capacity of director of Pathology Services and remains active in both the didactic and clinical portions of the program. He has published and lectured extensively at the local, state, and national levels.

Jay M. Enoch, O.D., Ph.D., professor and dean at the School of Optometry, University of California, Berkeley, and professor of Physiological Optics in Ophthalmology, University of California, San Francisco. He served for over 17 years as head of the contact lens clinic in the Department of Ophthalmology, Washington University, Saint Louis and later as head of a special clinic for problem cases at the Department of Ophthalmology at the University of Florida in Gainesville before joining the faculty at the University of California. In each of these institutions he has had opportunity to participate in the early correction of newborn and young children who have had developmental abnormalities of the eye, including cataracts and a variety of other conditions. Emilio Campos, his co-author, at one time served at postdoctoral fellow in Enoch's laboratory (at the University of Florida). Since then, they have worked extensively on neonatal populations.

Enoch has also been active in studies of photoreceptor optics and function, experimental perimetry, and several studies linking basic vision science to clinical applications.

Merton C. Flom, O.D., Ph.D., is professor and associate dean (graduate studies and research) at the College of Optometry, University of Houston. He is a past president of the American Academy of Optometry and former editor of the *American Journal of Optmetry and Physiological Optics*. Flom's research interest is binocular vision, amblyopia, and strabismus. He now serves on the Vision Research Review Committee of the National Eye Institute and on the Committee on Vision of the National Academy of Sciences/National Research Council.

John R. Griffin, O.D., M.S. Ed., is professor of optometry and chairman of the Department of Optometric Practice, Southern California College of Optometry, Fullerton, California. Among his contributions are more than a hundred publications in professional journals and several textbooks including co-authoring of *Genetics for Primary Eye Care Practitioners*. His research interests are in the fields of binocular vision, dyslexia, and genetics.

David Grisham, O.D., M.S., F.A.A.D., is chief of the Binocular Vision Clinic at the University of California Berkeley, School of Optometry and teaches courses in optometric case analysis, vision therapy, reading disabilities, and pediatric optometry. He coordinates and instructs in a masters degree program in reading disabilities at UC Berkeley specifically designed for optometrists. His research and publications focus on the efficacy of vision therapy and the relationships between vision and reading. He also participates in international vision service programs.

Gunilla Haegerström-Portnoy, O.D., Ph.D., is associate professor of optometry and physiological optics at the School of Optometry, University of California, Berkeley. Her primary research interest is in color vision and the application of psychophysics to clinical populations. Examples include the effects of long-term radiation exposure on vision of the older adult and the characteristics of residual color vision in congenital achromats. In addition, she is clinically active in a special program designed to evaluate vision function in multihandicapped children with low vision.

Siret D. Jaanus, Ph.D., M.S., is professor of pharmacology at the Southern California College of Optometry, Fullerton, California. She is the associate editor and a contributor to *Clinical Ocular Pharmacology*, a widely acclaimed text on ocular drug utilization for students and practitioners, now in its second edition. A recipient of the Paul Yarwood Award, she presently serves on the editorial board for *Ophthalmic Drug Facts*, a practical and comprehensive ophthalmic drug information compendium.

Randall T. Jose, O.D., a Diplomate Fellow in Low Vision (of which he was the first chairman) of the American Academy of Optometry and a member of its Executive Council, received his doctorate in optometry from the University of California, Berkeley. He served as a tenured associate professor in the College of Optometry at the University of Houston and director of the Houston Vision Rehabilitation from 1980 to 1989. In addition to his participation in, and design of, a multitude of workshops on low vision, he has authored more than fifty articles on the subjects related to low vision. He has also written a book on low vision, *Understanding Low Vision*, and contributed to three others, organized and developed a series of low vision articles for *Optometric Weekly*, worked as technical editor for the *Review of Optometry*, and served as founding editor and publisher of a low vision specialty journal which is now published by Media Publications as the *Journal of Vision Rehabilitation*. Jose is currently the director of clinical services for the Low Vision Center of Tulsa, and adjunct clinical professor at Northeastern State University–College of Optometry.

David G. Kirschen, O.D., Ph.D., is the chief of binocular vision and orthoptic services at the Jules Stein Eye Institute, UCLA School of Medicine, and an associate professor of vision science and optometry at the Southern California College of Optometry. He also maintains a private practice in Brea, California specializing in pediatric optometry and adult strabismus. His research interests and publications have been in the areas of amblyopia, strabismus, and infant acuity assessment. He received the Teacher of the Year award in 1989 from SCCO and he is currently the chairman of the Program Committee of the American Academy of Optometry.

Meredith W. Morgan, O.D., Ph.D., is professor and dean emeritus of the School of Optometry, University of California, Berkeley. Morgan's primary interest is binocular vision and clinical optometry. His contributions to optometry and visual science have been recognized by the Apollo Award of the American Optometric Association, the Prentice Medal of the American Academy of Optometry, the Berkeley Citation of the University of California, and four honorary degrees. He is the author of *The Optics of Ophthalmic Lenses* and co-editor of *Vision and Aging, General and Clinical Perspectives*.

Alfred A. Rosenbloom, O.D., M.A., D.O.S., is an educator and administrator whose primary academic and research interests are in the fields of clinical optometry, low vision, and optometric gerontology. He is director of the Low Vision Service, Chicago Lighthouse for the Blind. For 25 years, Rosenbloom served as dean and then president of the Illinois College of Optometry. He is an adjunct professor, College of Optometry, University of Houston, a Diplomate in Low Vision of the American Academy of Optometry, and serves as chairman, Low Vision Section of the American Optometric Association. Rosenbloom is a contributing author to seven textbooks, as well as a writer in the fields of optometry, vision rehabilitation, and professional education.

Michael W. Rouse, O.D., M.S.Ed., is an associate professor at the Southern California College of Optometry, chief of the Vision Therapy Service at the Optometric Center of Fullerton, and a Diplomate in the Binocular Vision and Perception Section of the American Academy of Optometry. In addition to clinical teaching responsibilities, he currently lectures in the binocular vision tract. His research interests are binocular vision, vision perception, pediatric optometry, and optometric education. He has published numerous articles and research papers, and has presented over 50 continuing education courses and presentations in the area of binocular vision and perception.

Julie B. Ryan, O.D., M.S., is an associate professor at the Southern California College of Optometry, Fullerton, California. Ryan lectures in Pediatric Optometry and teaches in vision therapy at the college where she served as chief, Pediatric Optometry Services. Currently, she is in private practice in Irvine, California specializing in pediatric optometry and vision therapy. Ryan is a Diplomate in Binocular Vision and Perception of the American Academy of Optometry.

Mitchell Scheiman, O.D., F.A.A.O., F.C.O.V.D., is chief of the Pediatric/Binocular Vision Service at the Pennsylvania College of Optometry, and an associate professor of Optometry at the college. His primary interest is binocular vision. Scheiman has written numerous papers on binocular vision disorders, vision therapy, and pediatric optometry.

Paulette P. Schmidt, O.D., M.S., is an assistant professor of optometry and physiological optics and chief of the Exceptional Child and Infant Vision Testing Laboratory, Orthoptic/Strabismus and Pediatric Services at The Ohio State University College of Optometry, Columbus, Ohio. Schmidt's primary research and teaching interest is in the vision of the developing human visual system.

Geraldine T. Scholl, Ph.D., M. Ed., B. Mus., is professor emeritus, School of Education, The University of Michigan, Ann Arbor, Michigan. She has a B. Mus. degree from Marygrove College (Detroit), an M. Ed. from Wayne State University and a Ph.D. from the University of Michigan. She is a former teacher of visually handicapped children and of emotionally disturbed children; and elementary principal of a residential school for blind children. She has been a member of the Board of Trustees of the American Foundation for the Blind for a number of years and has served as secretary, president, and is currently vice-chair of the Board. In 1985 she received the Migel Medal from the American Foundation for the Blind for her outstanding service to blind and visually impaired persons. She has published numerous articles in professional journals related to blind and visually handicapped persons, has contributed chapters to many books, and has edited several books, the most recent of which is *Foundations of Education for Blind and Visually Handicapped Children and Youth: Theory and Practice*.

Clifton M. Schor, O.D., Ph.D., is full professor, graduate advisor in physiological optics and optometric residencies, and former acting associate dean of the University of California School of Optometry. Schor's primary interests are sensory and motor aspects of binocular vision. These interests include both normal and anomalous states. Schor is co-editor of *Vergence Eye Movements: Basic and Clinical Aspects*. His work has been recognized by the Glenn Fry Award and the Garland Clay Award of the American Optometric Association and American Academy of Optometry. Research topics include investigation of stereopsis, sensory fusion and binocular rivalry, vergence eye movements, accommodation, optokinetic nystagmus, VOR, and Hering's law of equal and symmetrical eye movements.

Herbert D. Simons, Ed.M. O.D., Ed.D., is associate professor of education at the University of California, Berkeley and director of the M.A.

program in reading disability, which provides optometrists with advanced training in the diagnosis and treatment of reading disabilities. Simons' primary interest is in the reading process and the relationship of vision to reading. In addition to his publications in educational journals he has contributed to the optometric literature on the relationship of vision anomalies to reading problems.

Jacob G. Sivak, L.Sc.O., O.D., Ph.D., is a professor in the School of Optometry and in the Department of Biology at the University of Waterloo. He is currently the director of the School of Optometry and the associate dean of Science for Optometry. He has published widely on topics dealing with the anatomy, physiology, and optical performance of the eye. In 1984 he was awarded the Glenn Fry Award of the American Optometric Association.

Harold A. Solan, O.D., M.A., is professor of optometry and director of the Learning Disabilities Unit at the State College of Optometry/State University of New York. After completing his optometry degree, Solan was awarded an M.A. degree in reading in 1951 and in developmental psychology in 1970 at Teachers College, Columbia University. Solan has more than 50 publications to his credit, which include several monographs and three books, dealing with visual training, eye movements, and learning related visual and perceptual disorders. He has lectured throughout the United States and in Canada, Europe, and Australia. Solan has been the recipient of numerous awards. He is a Fellow of the American Academy of Optometry and a Diplomate in Visual Training and Perception. He also was chairman of the Section of Binocular Vision and Perception. In addition, he is a Fellow in the COVD, a Diplomate of the Multidisciplinary Academy of Clinical Education, and a member of the International Academy for Research in Learning Disabilities.

Lesley L. Walls, O.D., M.D., is the dean of the College of Optometry at Northeastern State University in Tahlequah, Oklahoma. He attended optometry school at the University of California at Berkeley and medical school at the University of California at Davis. He is also clinical professor of Family Practice at the University of Oklahoma Health Sciences Center at Tulsa, Oklahoma. Walls has lectured widely to both optometric and medical groups on various primary care subjects. He continues to be active in patient care as both a family physician and as an optometrist.

Barry A. Weissman, O.D., Ph.D., was educated at the School of Optometry, University of California, Berkeley, receiving his O.D. in 1972 and Ph.D. in physiological optics in 1979. He has experience in private practice, and was also a member of the Contact Lens Service of Hadassah-Hebrew University Hospital, Jerusalem, Israel for over a year. Weissman is currently a professor of ophthalmology at the Jules Stein Eye Institute, UCLA School of Medicine, and chief of Contact Lens Service there. He is a Diplomate in the Cornea-Contact Lens Section of the American Academy of Optometry, and a Fellow, a member of the editorial review board of the *Journal of the American Optometric Association* for cornea and contact lens topics, and a member of the International Society for Contact Lens Research. Current research interests include oxygen delivery to the cornea, mathematical modeling of hydrogel flexure, and complications (especially infection) associated with contact lens wear. He is also co-editor of a textbook in contact lens care with Edward S. Bennett, due to be published in late 1990.

Bruce C. Wick, O.D., is an associate professor of Optometry at the College of Optometry, University of Houston. Wick's primary teaching and research interests are binocular vision, pediatrics, and aniseikonia. He is a Diplomate in Binocular Vision and Perception of the American Academy of Optometry and has served on the review board of the *Journal of the American Optometric Association* and the editorial council of the *American Journal of Optometry and Physiological Optics*.

Bradford W. Wild, O.D., Ph.D., is professor and dean of the School of Optometry, University of Alabama at Birmingham. His primary interest is optics, especially ophthalmic optics. He has served as the president of the Ohio Optometric Association and as the president of the American Academy of Optometry. He has also served as the chairman of the Council on Optometric Education.

Alana M. Zambone, Ph.D., has recently assumed the position of coordinator of International Outreach Services, Hilton/Perkins International Program, Perkins School for the Blind. Prior to assuming this position she was the national consultant in Multiple Disabilities and Early Childhood for the American Foundation for the Blind. For the past 16 years, she has taught and directed programs for children and adults with visual impairments and additional disabilities, and their families; coordinated and taught in graduate programs for special educators in the areas of visual impairments, severe multiple disabilities, and early childhood; coordinated multidisciplinary educational diagnostic programs for children with a variety of disabling conditions and their families; and consulted and published in areas related to service coordination, child and family services, and assessment and intervention planning for children and adults with visual and severe multiple disabilities. She is currently working on a book and several monographs on assessment of children with severe multiple disabilities and visual impairment, and coordination among teachers serving this population of students.

Foreword

The profession of optometry has grown significantly in knowledge, skill, and organization in a remarkably short time. The educational preparation of optometrists for public service has doubled in three decades. In addition, the profession has developed sophisticated research and graduate programs resulting in an increasing number of Ph.D.'s in various aspects of vision science. The scope and volume of this vision research is illustrated at the papers and poster sessions of the American Academy of Optometry each year.

The profession and its educators have learned to utilize this flow of new information in the classroom and clinic as well as in extensive continuing education programs. Remarkably, too, the profession has learned to encompass the research of other disciplines as that knowledge contributes to the development of optometry as a primary care health profession. The combination of these two major developments has lead to an exciting mix of basic vision science and clinical application.

In studying its newly acquired clinical skills, the profession began to look at the societal needs for vision care and to take responsibility for the community's vision welfare. Studies of the epidemiology of vision problems identified the young and the elderly to be the groups at greatest risk.

In 1986 Drs. Morgan and Rosenbloom addressed the vision problems of the elderly through their publication of *Vision and Aging: General and Clinical Perspectives*, a contribution of general and clinical information which made a quantum leap from the landmark *Vision of the Aging Patient* of Hirsch and Wick published in 1960. *Vision and Aging* has brought the subject of optometric gerontology up to date with the inclusion of a great deal of new material and a careful review of controversial issues. It has met with significant acclaim and has already established itself as a required textbook in optometric gerontology.

Principles and Practice of Pediatric Optometry by Morgan and Rosenbloom utilizes the technique so successfully employed in *Vision and Aging*. The editors identified the scope and content of the book and sought experts to prepare chapters reflecting their expertise. This organizational structure reflects the broad knowledge and deep concern of these two great senior authors. Surveying research literature from the perspective of the 1990s, *Principles and Practice of Pediatric Optometry* brings up to date *Vision of Children* by Hirsch and Wick published in 1963.

The editors are to be congratulated on their wise choice of contributing authors. Each one is a recognized authority in a particular field of the growth, development, and care of children. They bring a holistic perspective on pediatric patient care, viewing children as unique and diverse individuals.

This text not only deals with the identification, assessment, and management of vision problems that occur in young children but it also places the technical issues of visual function of children within a developmental, psychological, and social context. The contributing authors provide the scope and depth of knowledge that sharpens this text's focus and makes it a truly significant contribution to the optometric and ophthalmological literature.

Although the book is not a "how to" text, it has a definite clinical orientation with a major emphasis on primary optometric care. An obvious deep concern for children and their welfare is a theme common to every chapter. In addition to the text, the references at the end of each chapter are another timely, important resource.

Principles and Practice of Pediatric Optometry is indeed a welcome volume of material of immediate use to the primary care optometrist, the optometry student, and faculty of optometry schools. The profession of optometry owes a debt of gratitude to Meredith W. Morgan and Alfred A. Rosenbloom for the monumental effort and sterling achievement of bringing this volume to us at this most propitious time.

HENRY B. PETERS, O.D., M.A.
Dean Emeritus
School of Optometry, The Medical Center
University of Alabama at Birmingham

Preface

It has been 25 years since the publication of *Vision of Children* by Monroe J. Hirsch and Ralph E. Wick (2). Since that time, there have been many new and exciting advances in electronics, electroneurophysiology, genetics, and pharmacology. All of these have led to an enormous increase in our knowledge of the visual processes and to the development of new and accurate techniques for measuring visual functions in infants who unlike adults can neither fixate on demand nor respond verbally to questions about how and what they see. These advances have also led to an increased understanding of the nature of comprehensive vision care.

An extensive literature concerning the neurological development and organization of the visual system of animals, particularly cats and monkeys, has also become available. While it may be questionable whether we can at the present time use an animal model to explain the development of vision in humans (4), the information is intriguing and all optometrists dealing with children should be aware of it and its possible implications. In addition to this great increase in knowledge about visual processes, there has been a change in the nature and scope of optometry as it has moved from its sole focus upon the process of vision to a concern with total vision care. Today, most optometric graduates consider themselves to be the primary health care practitioner in the field of vision care. As a primary health care practitioner, it is imperative that optometrists have expert, up-to-date knowledge about infants and children and the development of vision. It is also necessary that they are fully aware of the role and services of other professions serving this age group.

The growth in scientific knowledge and the

emergence of optometry as a primary care health profession are probably sufficient to justify a new, multiauthored book on pediatric vision. There are, however, other considerations which have led the editors to organize this book. While it is obviously true that seeing is not essential to learning and even to the perception of space since blind persons do learn and do orient themselves in a three-dimensional world, ordinarily, seeing and learning develop together and are mutually supportive and interrelated. It is this mutually interrelated development involving growth, seeing, maturation, and learning which is the central concept of *vision* in this text. It was clear to the editors then that in organizing a book on pediatric optometry there must be a concern with the processes of growth, development, maturation, learning, and behavior. Indeed, discussing vision as a process sets this book apart from most recent ophthalmological texts on this same subject. A review of eight recent ophthalmological books reveals their primary aim is to provide an understanding of diagnosis, treatment, and management of children's eye disorders. A few have chapters on visually impaired children and the subjects of reading and learning but the major emphasis is clearly on diagnosis and treatment of disease and on surgery. This text is not meant to duplicate or supplant these excellent publications but rather to supplement them by an emphasis on vision as a process, primarily from the optometric point of view.

Infants and young children are unable to communicate completely and specifically. Their experience is limited and consequently they have no real way of knowing if anything is amiss in their visual experiences. Children, however, do communicate by their behavior but unfortunately there may not be a specific behavior associated with a specific defect or problem. Optometrists caring for infants and toddlers must be aware of normal and aberrant behavior in order to make valid clinical judgments as to whether vision development is proceeding as it should. The optometrist must also appreciate the importance of the interdisciplinary nature of vision care, requiring a close working relationship between optometrists, parents, pediatricians, and teachers.

Early optometric care is essential to the welfare of every child. Animal experiments indicate that there are critical periods in the development of the visual system (5). There is also evidence of a sensitive period in the development of human vision (1, 3). In general, the evidence indicates that the developmental anomalies which occur can most easily be prevented in the first 5–7 years of life; therefore, the most significant corrective or preventive care should occur during this period. Animal data indicate that sensory deprivation during the critical period leads to poor visual performance of various kinds including amblyopia, strabismus, and myopia depending on the nature and degree of deprivation. It may be possible to enhance visual perception while preventing the development of amblyopia, anisometropia, squint, or myopia. If there is a period in which performance can be most easily enhanced, it is logical to conclude that it occurs sometimes during the first 5–7 years.

The data reported by Mohindra and her associates (6) indicate that the refractive anomalies, particularly the magnitude of astigmatism, frequently change radically and rapidly during the first few years of life. The evidence also seems to indicate that "emmetropization" and the development and retention of normal binocular acuity and vision are somehow dependent on good retinal images. These two facts seem to indicate that different criteria for the correction of refractive anomalies should be used for infants than those normally used for adults. It would also seem apparent that monitoring should be frequent. Prudence would indicate that frequent monitoring should occur whenever any therapy is used. Indeed, as Scholl has stated, "The process of growth and development is at the same time similar for all children and unique for each child. It is similar in that there are identifiable stages through which all children progress; it is unique in that the rate of progression differs for each child" (7).

It is evident that different techniques of detection, measurement, and correction of vision anomalies must be used for infants and young children than that normally used for mature patients. The actual age at which normal clinical procedures may be used efficiently and accurately varies with each child but it is usually between the ages of 4 and 8. In order to obtain accurate information, and to make correct judgments, an optometrist who wishes to serve children younger than age 4 must be familiar with the many special techniques available. This is essential in order to obtain accurate information and to make correct judgments.

In view of the complex interrelationship of factors stated above, the editors have concluded that a book dealing with infant vision care is warranted and that such a book should include information concerning the vision care of children and adolescents with a major emphasis on the first 6 years of life. This is the age range usually designated by the word "pediatrics" hence, *Principles and Practice of Pediatric Optometry*. After consultation with knowledgeable colleagues, the editors decided upon the general outline designating the subject matter to be included. Limitations of space prohibit making this book all-inclusive; consequently, many topics the editors wished to include are omitted and many knowledgeable writers are consequently not represented. We have also concluded that the subject matter is so complex that no one individual could be sufficiently knowledgeable to encompass all facets of this subject and therefore the editors have decided that each chapter should be written by a different individual with special knowledge in the chosen subject areas.

The material in each chapter is the work of the writer of that particular chapter. There are three major divisions within this text. The first six chapters cover basic background information on growth and development, both general and specific. The next eight chapters are essentially clinical in nature covering the diagnosis and management of the anomalies of vision in the provision of primary vision care to infants and children. The final nine chapters cover specific aspects of comprehensive vision care.

The scope and content/emphasis of the book has been planned for the advanced optometric student and the practicing optometrist. The writers have assumed that the reader has basic knowledge of anatomy, physiology, and pathology as well as skills in essential clinical methods, procedures, and management. This text is neither a procedural manual nor a recipe book. Moreover, it is not intended as a substitute for subject matter texts such as those on growth and development, optics, refractive procedures, and ocular disease. This text is patient-oriented and emphasizes vision care during the first 6 years of life. If it truly serves its purpose, this text will be a significant resource for "hands on" training and experience in this most important and satisfying phase of vision care. The editors' goal is to engender an understanding of the complex processes involved in pediatric vision care. Although new techniques and understandings may be developed in the future, it is our expectation that the information and knowledge which the reader derives from this text will continue to be valid and practical.

REFERENCES

1. Banks, M. S., R. N. Aslin, R. D. Letson (1975) Sensitive period for development of human binocular vision, Science 190:675–677.

2. Hirsch, M. J. and R. Wick, eds. (1963) Vision of Children, Chilton Co., Philadelphia.

3. Hohman, A. and O. D. Creutzfeldt (1975) Squint and development of binocularity in humans, Nature 254:613–614.

4. Marg, E. (1982) Prentice Memorial Lecture: Is the animal model for stimulus deprivation amblyopia in children valid or useful? Amer. J. Optom. & Physiol. Optics 59:451–461.

5. Mitchell, D. E. (1981) Sensitive period in visual development. In Aslin, R., ed., Development of Perception: Physiological Perspectives, Vol. 2, The Visual Systems, Academic Press, N.Y., pp. 3–43.

6. Mohindra, I., R. Held, J. Siviazda, and S. Bull (1978) Astigmatism in infants, Science 202:329.

7. Scholl, G. T. (1986) Growth and development, In G. Scholl, ed., Foundations of Education for Blind and Visually Handicapped Children and Youth: Theory and Practice, Amer. Found. Blind, N.Y., p. 65.

Contents

Introduction

PART ONE: GROWTH AND DEVELOPMENT

Part One includes information about the nature of growth and the developmental characteristics of infants and children. Such knowledge is essential background for understanding visual development and function.

The first chapter by Dr. Geraldine Scholl summarizes normal growth and development of children in the physical/motor, mental/cognitive, and social/emotional areas. Research findings related to variations in the growth and development of children are cited and selected theories of child development are summarized and evaluated by their conceptional orientation.

Drs. Jacob Sivak and William Bobier (Chapter 2) discuss the optical components of the eye in terms of their embryology and postnatal growth

during the early years of life. While the mechanisms which coordinate this development are not fully understood, the authors' comment that only when such processes become understood can the practitioner confidently define clinical models involving diagnosis and management.

In the next chapter, Dr. Ross Beauchamp describes the normal development of the retina and visual pathways in humans noting that gaps in our knowledge about the human nervous system must often be extrapolated from research data gathered from monkey or cat. He emphasizes that the characteristics of the adult visual system are established before birth and several years thereafter as the neurons of the retina and visual pathways differentiate and make their permanent synaptic connections.

Dr. Clifton Schor's chapter on visuomotor development describes the nature of oculomotor development and evaluates relevant research that defines the components of oculomotor performance. He notes that many of the characteristically immature oculomotor functions observed in infants resemble the abnormal oculomotor behavior that characterizes developmental disorders such as strabismus and amblyopia, as well as disorders of the central nervous system, such as Parkinson's disease.

In "Genetics and Congenital Ocular Disorders," Dr. John Griffin summarizes ocular genetics by describing common congenital ocular diseases, modes of genetic transmission, commonly observed genetic problems, and "rules" for effective genetic counseling by the primary eye care optometrist.

In "Refractive Status in Infants and Children," Dr. William R. Baldwin organizes the subject into three major topical units: (1) ametropia expressed as the spherical equivalent refraction with expected prevalences and changes from infancy to young adulthood; (2) astigmatism, anisometropia and other refractive variants outside the range of normal biological variation; and (3) changes in refractive status involving optical and axial properties from birth through adolescence. A concluding section considers ethnic differences, cultural differences, and refractive abnormalities associated with congenital disease and birth defects.

PART TWO: GENERAL DIAGNOSIS AND MANAGEMENT

The chapters in Part Two describe essential considerations in the examination, diagnosis and management of the normal child. The influence of factors described in the preceding part is related to aspects of diagnosis and management of children.

Drs. Michael Rouse and Julie Ryan's chapter on "The Optometric Examination and Management of Children" describes the clinical management of children by age group—infants and toddlers, preschoolers, and school-age children. A visual examination strategy is stated by the use of the problem-oriented record approach to optometric procedures, analysis, and management. Pediatric testing sequences appropriate to age and developmental level are thoroughly pre-

sented from a primary optometric care orientation.

In "Spectacles for Children," Drs. Michael Cho and Bradford Wild present guidelines for the selection of frame types, lens materials, adjustments and modifications, and psychosocial considerations in prescribing eyewear for children.

In "Contact Lenses for Children," Drs. Barry Weissman and Paul Donzis describe the refractive applications, prosthetic uses, lens design considerations, evaluation, and lens care procedures for contact lenses for children under 5 years of age.

In "Issues in the Clinical Management of Binocular Anomalies," Dr. Merton Flom focuses on the central issue of whether or not to treat a child's binocular anomaly—which includes strabismus and heterophoria, and their associated conditions such as suppression and amblyopia. The problems of strabismics (abnormal binocular vision and a conspicuous deviation) and of phoria patients (ocular discomfort and impaired vision performance) are discussed and compared. Criteria for functional and cosmetic correction of strabismus as well as successful treatment of phorias are presented. A step-by-step analysis is made of numerous factors believed to influence the prognosis for functional correction of strabismus, the result of which is a prognosis model that allows the optometrist to estimate the probability of obtaining a functional correction of a child's strabismus based on the type of squint and presence or absence of certain, but not all, associated conditions.

In "A Model for Treating Binocular Anomalies," Drs. Merton Flom and Bruce Wick start from the premise that an informed decision has been made to treat the child's binocular anomaly. They discuss in logical order the various treatment options available for the management of binocular anomalies, which culminates in a model for treating strabismics and another for treating phoria patients. The models provide a sequence, that is, the order in which different treatment options should be considered, for each of the main kinds of strabismus and phorias.

In "Vision Therapy for Preschool Children," Dr. Bruce Wick provides details on vision therapy management, presents different strategies of vision therapy, and describes modifications of vision therapy programs that are necessary when working with preschoolers. Contrary to the common view that children cannot actively participate in vision training until they are about 5 years old. Dr. Wick shows, with descriptions and case reports, how vision therapy can be effective for toddlers and even infants.

The chapter "Ocular Pharmacology" by Dr. Siret Jaanus is a guide for the application of diagnostic pharmaceutical agents in the optometric evaluation of the young child. The author also considers ocular side effects and/or toxicity of commonly used drugs and management considerations in selected ocular conditions.

The concluding chapter in this part by Drs. Leonard Apt and David Kirschen is an inclusive summary of *Ocular and Systemic Diseases of Infants and Children.* Their discussions of pediatric eye diseases are presented by clinical manifestations, etiological factors, clinical course, and available treatment modalities.

PART THREE: SPECIFIC CONDITIONS IN DIAGNOSIS AND MANAGEMENT

The chapters in Part Three describe essential considerations in the detection, examination, diagnosis, and management of specific problems associated with visual dysfunction in children. Drs. Randy Jose and Alfred Rosenbloom describe optometric care of "The Visually Impaired Child" including developmental characteristics, common causes of visual impairment, low vision assessment/management, and referral considerations. Unique aspects of diagnostic testing are described and selected low-vision devices are presented in relation to the unique developmental and learning needs of these children.

Another dimension of exceptionality is the "Assessment and Management of the Exceptional Child" by Dr. Mitchell Scheiman. He stresses the special needs of different MMH children and the importance of early identification and intervention by the primary care optometrist. This population group assumes greater significance since a large percentage of children with handicapping conditions also may have one or more vision anomalies such as refractive anomalies,

strabismus, amblyopia, nystagmus, accommodative disorders, visual perceptual anomalies, and ocular disease.

The special needs of the aphakic neonate is presented by Drs. Emilio C. Campos and Jay M. Enoch. In their chapter "The Management of the Aphakic Neonate," the authors note that the surgery and postsurgical care of neonates with developmental and traumatic cataracts presents complex management considerations including advanced contact lens fitting, correction of aniseikonia, and in some cases, strabismological complications.

Although few statistics are available regarding ocular trauma in children, it is a major public health problem. In "Ocular Trauma and Emergencies," Drs. Leland Carr and Lesley Walls discuss various aspects of the child's response to ocular injury, examination techniques, and management approaches. Prevention is emphasized especially during sports or play activities.

In her chapter entitled "Color Vision," Dr. Gunilla Haegerström-Portnoy comments on the reasons for testing color vision in children: (1) to identify at an early age those children who have congenital color vision defects primarily for educational planning purposes; and (2) to determine the presence and severity of acquired color vision defects for the purpose of diagnosis and for functional recommendations regarding the capabilities of the affected child. Reliability and validity of color vision tests for children and recommendations for test batteries for different age groups are presented.

In "Vision Screening," Dr. Paulette Schmidt considers the rationale for vision screening, surveys and evaluates the large number of vision screening techniques, and comments on the limitations and comparative effectiveness of various vision screening procedures in correctly identifying children with vision problems.

The chapters "Learning Disabilities" by Dr. Harold Solan and "Perspectives on Reading Disabilities" by Drs. J. David Grisham and Herbert D. Simons present comprehensive surveys of relevant literature and the role of vision function in therapeutic approaches aimed at mediating the disability. Both chapters present in-depth knowledge of the various complex aspects of reading and learning disabilities in children. The primary care optometrist should not only diagnose and manage vision disorders competently but also serve as an important member of the interdisciplinary team caring for children with learning and reading disabilities.

The concluding chapter by Dr. Alana Zambone based on legislation impacting children emphasizes the optometrists role as an important member of a team of professionals, parents, and other caregivers. Each professional as a team member has specific responsibilities for meeting the educational needs of children with severe vision dysfunction. This presentation could serve as a model for dealing with less severe vision dysfunctions.

PART ONE

Growth and Development

Chapter 1

Growth and Development

Geraldine T. Scholl

Relationships in the helping professions are facilitated by the professional's knowledge of developmental and behavioral characteristics of the patient and of what might be expected of persons of comparable status, age, and other demographic and cultural characteristics. Such background information enhances the helping relationship.[1]

The focal point in the practice of optometry is a person, for our purposes, a child.

Knowledge of normal child growth and development will help the practitioner to assess what can be expected in responses during the examination, what variations from the normal pattern some children might display, and how to assess and manage these variations appropriately and effectively. Knowledge of how children learn can help the practitioner determine the best methods for motivating patients at various growth and developmental levels in order to maximize the child's cooperation.

This chapter presents an overview of characteristics of normal growth and development from birth through adolescence; outlines briefly some theories regarding growth and development; and summarizes for each area of growth and development the normal progression, determinants of variations and

---

[1] Portions of this chapter are reprinted with permission from Scholl GT: Growth and Development and portions are adapted from Scholl, GT: Multicultural Considerations and Scholl, GT: Visual Impairments and Other Exceptionalities. In Scholl GT (ed.): Foundations of Education for Blind and Visually Handicapped Children and Youth: Theory and Practice. New York, American Foundation for the Blind, 1986.

informal assessment procedures. The final section of the chapter summarizes how learning occurs and offers suggestions to help the practitioner apply these principles in the practice of optometry with children. The content of this chapter provides a foundation for the remaining chapters in this book. The primary focus is the early years, but developmental characteristics and needs during infancy and adolescence are also discussed.

NORMAL GROWTH AND DEVELOPMENT

Characteristics

Several basic concepts should be noted that relate to children's growth and development: What is "normal"? How does growth occur? In speaking of children's growth and development, the concept of normal is usually equated with what is average, or in statistical terms, the mean. By definition, when any variable is measured in a population, half of all persons' values fall above this hypothetical point and half fall below it. Usually we consider variations around the mean, both above and below, as being within a normal range for any particular characteristic. Statistically the normal range usually includes about two thirds of the total population. Thus, about two thirds of children are normal for any characteristic or behavior, although in any aspect of children's growth and development, there can be a wide variation between a child at the upper limit of the two thirds and one at the lower limit.

The development of most characteristics and behaviors occurs in a predictable sequence common to all children, but the rate of development is unique for each individual. Some persons achieve their full potential earlier and some later than others, so chronological age may not always be relevant when assessing the developmental level. For some characteristics, such as height, when the limit is reached development stops (although later, height may diminish somewhat due to the aging process). For other characteristics, such as weight, there can be a wide fluctuation

over the life span of the individual, and a person rarely maintains a constant weight for long periods. The limit of some characteristics may never be reached, as the process of refining that behavior continues throughout life. Maturity is an example. Does any person achieve complete maturity? The process of maturing continues throughout life. With children, we often describe maturity in terms of a chronological age, such as 2-year-old behavior, meaning that the behavior is normal or average for a 2-year-old but is not appropriate for a younger or an older child. When such descriptions are applied to behavior they imply that the person is behaving either in an immature fashion or like a much older child.

Although many behaviors develop in a sequential pattern, there may be variations. Some steps in the sequence leading to learning to skip might be outlined as follows: holding up the head, sitting, creeping, standing, walking, running, hopping, skipping. But some children may never creep, and some may skip before they can hop on one foot. Typically, before learning to write, a child must understand language, speak, and read, but some handicapped children, such as those with hearing impairments, delayed speech, or cerebral palsy, may not speak but may learn to read and often learn to write simultaneously in order to express themselves. Usually it is not possible to teach a behavior out of sequence (for example, to teach a child to skip before he or she has mastered walking). However, in children with a hearing impairment, delayed language, or cerebral palsy, the development of an unspoken inner language enables the child to skip the speaking stage in the sequence. While the sequence is similar for all children, the rate of progression through the sequence is unique for each child and any child's rate of progression may differ from area to area. A 2-year-old may function at the chronological age level physically but lag behind in cognitive development.

In spite of such variations, there is a commonality to human development that allows us to describe norms for various levels and to predict future development on the basis of the present status. The following section describes the normal or average developmental progression in the psychomotor, cognitive, and affective areas of growth and development.

Aspects

The literature typically delineates three areas of growth and development: psychomotor (including physical and sensory-perceptual skills), cognitive (including language), and affective development. In this section each will be treated separately, but in reality they are unitary and so closely interrelated that they cannot easily be separated. Each part describes briefly the normal patterns of growth and development. The next section will discuss selected theoretical positions related to these areas including developmental milestones.

Although we usually think of growth and development as beginning at birth, during the 9 months of life that typically precede that event, there are significant changes in the fetus. By 8 weeks after conception the nervous and muscular systems are becoming organized, and the gender of the fetus is recognizable. Environmental factors are critical in determining whether the infant will be healthy at birth.

Psychomotor Development

Beginning at conception and continuing through the first few years of life, physical growth predominates, setting the stage for later cognitive and affective development. For example, during the first year of life, the infant increases in length by 50 percent and in weight by 200 percent (19). After the first year, growth slows down until the minor spurt at puberty. Physical control is gained in a head-to-foot, or cephalocaudal, sequence (e.g., the infant must be able to hold the head steady before he or she can sit); from trunk to extremities (e.g., control of the trunk is gained before control of arms and legs); and from large muscle to small muscle control (e.g., control of arms and hands before control

of fingers). Concurrently with physical development, sensory perceptual development is progressing. By 2 months an infant can follow an object with the eyes and by 6 months can grasp an object. This ability to track and then to reach and grasp marks the beginning of learning to control arms, hands, and finally fingers.

Infants prepare for walking in a similar sequence. First they hold up their heads and view the world from an eyes-front position. Then they learn to sit without support. As the object world outside catches their interest, they attempt to reach and grasp and begin to propel themselves toward objects by crawling or creeping. Further exploration stimulates them to stand, first by holding on to an object and later alone. Soon they are walking, usually by 12 to 15 months, and running, jumping, and skipping by 5 years. Preschool and early elementary age children are usually in constant motion as they attempt to satisfy their basic need for movement. Some children who are more active might be labeled hyperactive when in reality their behavior is within the normal range.

During adolescence girls and boys experience a physical growth spurt: girls on the average at about age 12 and boys 2 years later. This completes the general physical growth and development cycle. While this is taking place the adolescent may have difficulty controlling a rapidly growing body, may be awkward, and may have poor coordination. Other important changes take place simultaneously: the development of the reproductive system and the attendant secondary sex characteristics with the attainment of sexual maturity. Following the adolescent growth spurt height does not increase but the young person continues to refine muscle coordination and the ability to use the body in physical activities.

Cognitive Development

Early psychomotor development lays the foundation for the development of cognition and the expanding mental abilities in the child. Early sensory exploration of the object world by the infant and toddler enhances perceptual development and leads to the formation of concepts upon which abstractions are based. Concepts grow out of the perceptual process and are enriched as the child develops language. The breadth of perceptual experiences determines in large measure the breadth of conceptual development. To be meaningful, concepts must be based on sensory experiences. There are several theories of human cognitive development, but Piaget's stages of intellectual development will be outlined here.

Cognition Piaget describes the first 2 years of life as the sensorimotor stage, during which time infants progress from reflex activities to more systematic and organized behavior. They learn that they have control over the object world and will search visually for a lost toy. They will reach for toys and grasp them. They learn that objects are independent of them. They learn to imitate and to respond to people through imitative behavior. Finally, they take the first steps toward establishing verbal communication.

At approximately 2 years of age, children enter the symbolic, or preconceptual, phase, when the imitative behavior of the previous period becomes internal imitation (which Piaget calls accommodation) and provides them with symbols that acquire meaning through assimilation. They apply symbols in a playful make-believe fashion to other situations as they test out their appropriateness.

At about 4 years, children enter the phase of intuitive thought. This stage and the preceding preconceptual phase are sometimes called the preoperational stage. During this period children employ imitation more or less consciously as they identify with those around them. This leads to their expanded social horizons and interest in the world.

Children pass through the stage of concrete operations from approximately 7 to 11 years of age. They acquire the ability to order and to relate experiences into a *gestalt*, or an organized whole. They establish systems of classification and move from inductive to deductive thinking. They begin to look beyond the family for models to imitate.

At about age 12, children enter the stage of formal operations, Piaget's final period of cognitive development. During this stage, adolescents move from the concrete to the abstract. They enter the world of ideas; formulate hypotheses concerning various results of actions and consider what might occur; they reach an understanding of the world and where they fit into it.

Communication Speech is defined as the vocal-motor channel of language performance and is the means by which language is communicated. Language is the code whereby concepts about the world are represented through a system of arbitrary signals for communication (2). Language binds and creates relationships among persons, events, and situations. Speech and language are usually referred to as communication.

The acquisition of speech begins with cooing at about 16 weeks. Infants begin to babble at about 28 weeks and put sounds together at about 40 weeks. Language development proceeds in a similar sequential fashion. At 28 weeks, infants attend to voices and by 40 weeks they respond to simple commands. By 15 months they say single words to express ideas, and by 2 years they put words together to form simple sentences.

At about 4 years of age language becomes repetition, monologue, and collective monologue, which Piaget describes as egocentric, because the child is not interested in what others are saying. During the stage of concrete operations, children begin to use speech and language as means of sharing and relaying information, particularly as they become more interested in social interactions. During the period of formal operations, speech and language become means of communicating thoughts and ideas.

Affective Development

It is difficult to separate cognitive and affective development, as they are interrelated and exert reciprocal influences on each other. Piaget (26) suggests that the cognitive area is the development of behaviors as they relate to objects whereas the affective area is the development of behaviors as they relate to people. In addition, emotional, social, personality, and moral development overlap, so they are grouped under the rubric of affective development.

Affective development begins when the mother and father hold the newborn infant for the first time. This closeness initiates bonding and the beginning of a long period of affective development that should produce an independent self-confident adult. Parental fondling and cuddling mark the beginning of learning to love and be loved; bonding provides a base of security from which the infant can move into the external world.

As infants grow older, eye contact with the parents or primary caregivers initiates a social relationship. Visual contact seems to be an essential element in this early process of building relationships.

During this time, children are also developing a self-concept, that is, a perception of what is self and what is not self in the physical and social environment. The initial development of the self-concept begins in infancy and continues throughout life, undergoing constant modification in response to the environment and experience.

Vision provides infants with the first experience in recognizing self as distinct from the environment. As they observe the mother moving away from and toward them, they learn that she is an object distinct from them. Through visual exploration they discover their fingers and hands, toes and feet, often spending hours visually exploring their relationship to themselves. Gradually they learn that they are a part of themselves, unlike other people and their toys, which can be separated from their bodies. This process of developing a body image, an aspect of self-concept, continues through visual exploration of other parts of the body, through mimicry of parents and siblings, and later through observation and study of themselves in a mirror.

From the parents, infants expand their world to include other family members, including siblings. From the security gained through meaningful family attachments and relationships and with increased physical maturation that permits them to move about more freely in the environment, children reach out to people outside the family and build social and emotional relationships with them. Acceptance comes from compatibility and correspondence with peer group norms. Again, visual contacts with others supply the necessary feedback for children to initiate relationships and to know when they are acceptable and accepted. Through vision they learn which behaviors are accepted in a particular setting and imitate those that will make them acceptable.

The recognition of self as an individual is facilitated by parents and family. In the home, love and acceptance, opportunities to move from a protected to a semiprotected position outside the family, and communicated expectations of success help children develop a positive view of themselves.

The self-concept continues to evolve throughout childhood as experiences with success and failure form the basis for evaluating oneself and one's capabilities. The peer group provides further feedback and reinforcement necessary to learn about the self, giving approval or disapproval, encouragement or discouragement for actions and behavior. Such give and take is often nonverbal, such as frowns or smiles.

During adolescence the socialization process continues in the peer group, which now provides the base of security that the family provided previously. A peer group gives adolescents an opportunity to define themselves as group members, to gain an understanding of relationships, to interact with their equals, and to realize that they are of value to others. Difficulties may arise when peer group norms conflict with family norms. At this point adolescents must develop their own set of behavioral norms, drawing from peers and family.

During adolescence, a perception of the self as male or female emerges as the result of prior experiences such as the opportunity to identify with an appropriate gender model and to imitate the dress, mannerisms, and behavior of that model.

Puberty, the onset of the ability to procreate, presents adolescents with a dilemma. Their bodies are mature enough to reproduce, but society views them as too immature to meet the consequences of their procreative efforts. A system of values becomes incorporated into the self during this period that is based primarily on family and peer relationships and experiences. This moral development is the core component of human adaptation and the key to survival in our society. The formation of a personal value system has been cited as a criterion marking the end of adolescence (28).

To accept oneself as a person of worth and as a contributing member of society is the ultimate objective of adolescence. The self-concept is responsive to the environment throughout life, and it changes constantly in response to environmental changes (15).

Preparing for a vocation is another task of adolescence. Assuming productive employment is a valued aspect of American society, and adolescents spend time during their secondary school years exploring careers, discussing vocational possibilities with family, peers, and school personnel, and finally arriving at a decision of the most appropriate vocational goal as they prepare to move into adulthood.

This brief overview of the normal progression in the three areas of growth and development furnishes a framework for reviewing the selected group of theoretical positions related to growth and development.

Theories

Several theories of growth and development have evolved over the years that place varying emphasis on the nature of the human being, the nature-nurture controversy, and what is it that develops. It should be noted that no one theory presents a view of the total child; each has strengths and weaknesses; and each asks different questions about development. This section presents eight theories: two address physical and sensory-perceptual development; two, cognitive development; three, social and emotional aspects, and the last, moral development. Table 1.1 presents a brief summary of these eight stages by chronological age. It should be noted that these ages are approximate. Further, not all the specific details and components are included. The reader will find more detailed information in the references listed at the top of each column.

Physical

On first meeting a child physical development is easiest to observe, and developmental levels are probably best assessed informally by the optometrist. The developmental milestones in the first column of Table 1.1 are gathered from several sources.

Sensory-Perceptual

Learning begins with the sensory system. The senses are stimulated by sights, sounds, touches, tastes, and smells around us. The nerves transmit sensory stimulation messages to the brain, which gradually gives meaning to the sensations as they become perceptions. When perceptions group themselves into patterns, concepts are formed, which are the basis for thinking and for communicating abstract ideas (1). Much more is known about the visual and auditory sensory systems than the tactile, kinesthetic, and olfactory ones, partly because the latter three contribute minimally to the process of learning in our particular culture.

A good selection of puzzles, coloring books, drawing materials, books, blocks and other manipulative toys of varying complexity in the waiting room can help the optometrist observe which are selected by a particular child and what developmental level that selection indicates.

Communication

After age 6 years, communication skills are elaborations of the earlier milestones in speech and language. Communication is another area that can be assessed informally by the optometrist. Initiating a conversation and noting the child's use of words, asking the child to count or tell a story, instructing the child to perform one or two simple tasks, or

Table 1.1 SELECTED THEORIES OF CHILD DEVELOPMENT

Year	Physical (6, 14, 16, 31)	Sensory/Perceptual (1, 31)	Communication (2, 14, 31)	Cognitive (7, 22)	Psychosexual (10, 25, 29)	Psychosocial (4, 5)	Development Tasks (12, 13)	Moral Development (3, 19)
0	Controls head Turns over Sits unaided Crawls, scoots Stands alone Walks alone	Startle reflex Attends to light Turns head to sounds Eyes follow moving objects Reaches and grasps Pincer grasp	Understands first words Coos, babbles Puts sounds together Understands about 100 words	*Early sensorimotor* Reflexes modified Primary circular reactions (trial-and-error learning involving own body) Systematic imitation	*Oral stage* Successful feeding leads to security Mouth is source of gratification Needs sucking experiences	*Basic trust vs. basic mistrust* Dependence on caregivers Trust results from having basic needs met	*Stage 1* Learns to take solid food Learns to walk Learns to talk	*Completely egocentric* No moral concepts Fear of punishment
1	Walks up and down stairs holding on "Rides" wagon Basic control of body complete Pulls toys Seats self in chair	Fits objects together Matches objects Points to objects in books Scribbles Imitates actions Draws crude circles	Understands simple instructions Speaks 200 words and two-word sentences Uses the word "no" Uses words for requests Repeats two numbers	*Later sensorimotor* Invents meanings Object concept begins Begins problem solving	*Anal stage* Problems with toilet training lead to conflicts about compliance with external demands Retention and expulsion of feces chief source of pleasure	*Autonomy vs. shame* Need to adjust to socialization demands in toilet training and conforming to household routines, at the same time preserving independence		
2	Runs Jumps in place Stands on one foot Walks on tiptoe Kicks ball	Matches colors/forms Imitates other's movements Puts two puzzle pieces together Puts pegs in holes	Uses question words Uses present & past tense of verbs Repeats three numbers Uses pronouns	*Preoperational* Egocentrism Uses signifiers (symbols, signs) Rigidity of thought Thinking nonverbal Semilogical reasoning			*Stage 2* Learns to control elimination of body wastes Begins to learn sex differences and sexual modesty	

Table 1.1 (Continued)

Year	Physical (6, 14, 16, 31)	Sensory/Perceptual (1, 31)	Communication (2, 14, 31)	Cognitive (7, 22)	Psychosexual (10, 25, 29)	Psychosocial (4, 5)	Development Tasks (12, 13)	Moral Development (3, 19)
3	Rides simple tricycle Hops on one foot Walks on a line Balances on one foot Throws ball overhand Catches bounced ball	Matches identical-shaped objects Can copy a cross Discriminates most basic forms Builds tower of nine blocks	Counts to three Understands and uses verbs, pronouns, adjectives Sometimes uses complete sentences		*Phallic stage* Pride in body and skills Penis and clitoris centers of erotic pleasure Oedipal conflict	*Initiative vs. guilt* Need to adjust to rules Desire to explore Developing sense of right and wrong	Forms concepts and learns language to describe social and physical reality Gets ready to read Learns to distinguish between right and wrong Begins to develop a conscience	*Preconventional* Punishment and obedience orientation subject to caretakers' demands for regulation or interactions
4	Walks backward Jumps forward Walks up and down stairs alone Turns somersault	Colors, cuts, pastes Draws square Perceives details in objects/pictures Prints some letters	Gives account of events Carries out a sequence of two simple directions Conversation is egocentric monologue					Instrumental relativist orientation: parties have favors each one wants
5	Skips Skates Walks on balance beam Can hop 6 feet Jumps rope	Perceives relationships in pictures, abstract figures, symbols Copies first name Matches letters/words Prints numbers 1 to 5	Intelligible speech Carries on a conversation Uses pronouns correctly Grammar resembles that of adults in his family					
6	Carts things in wagon Active stage Climbs trees Likes stunts Tries broad jump	Explores all materials Handedness established Pastes and glues Likes tinkertoys Holds pencil	Begins to read Begins to write Takes turns in conversation	*Concrete operations* Develops concept of conservation Recognizes relationships Organizes and relates experiences into organized whole Temporal-spatial representations Establishes systems of classification Moves from inductive to deductive thinking	*Latency stage* Sexual interests reduced Repression of childhood sexuality Free to concentrate on developmental tasks of childhood	*Industry vs. inferiority* Facing and meeting expectations of others Developing sense of self Coping with frustration and failure	*Stage 3* Learns physical skills necessary for ordinary games Builds wholesome attitudes toward oneself as a growing organism Learns to get along with age mates Learns an appropriate masculine/feminine role Develops fundamental skills of reading, writing, and calculating	
7	Can ride bicycle Repeats activities Bats a ball Exhibits extremes in activities	Touches and manipulates everything	Uses language to share information					
8	Body movements more graceful Enjoys games	Increased speed/smoothness of fine coordination Draws in perspective						

Age	Physical / Motor	Writing & Language	Cognitive (Piaget)	Psychosexual	Psychosocial	Developmental Tasks	Moral Development (Kohlberg)
9	More skilled in motor performance; Interested in competitive sports	In writing: uniform spaces between letters; Drawings more detailed	Learns reversibility; Can reverse direction in thinking			Develops a conscience; Achieves personal independence; Develops attitudes toward social groups and institutions; Develops concepts necessary for everyday living	*Conventional level*; Interpersonal concordance or Good Boy–Nice Girl orientation, each party committed to other's welfare; Society system and conscience maintenance—equality under the law; society-wide system of cooperation
10	Movements more relaxed and casual						
11							
12	Growth spurt in girls	Uses language to communicate ideas	*Formal operations*; Advanced logical and mathematical schema; Comprehension of abstract or symbolic content; Reduced need of objects for thinking; Moves from concrete to abstract; Mentally performs transformations; Possibility dominates reality; Cognitive structures attain high level of equilibrium; Develops hypotheses of what might be; Thought becomes flexible	*Genital stage*; New, more mature personality develops; More mature sexual and intimacy relationships	*Identity vs. role confusion*; Needs to question old values to achieve mature sense of identity; Overidentifies with heroes; "Falling in love"; Clannish, cruel to those who are different; Idealistic outlook on society	*Stage 4*; Achieves new and more mature relations with age-mates, both sexes; Achieves a masculine/feminine social role; Accepts one's physique; Achieves emotional independence from parents; Prepares for marriage and family life; Prepares for a career; Acquires set of values and ethical system to guide behavior	*Postconventional*; Social contract orientation; Universal ethical principle orientation
13	Development of reproductive system in girls—pubic hair, breasts, menstrual cycle						
14	Growth spurt in boys; Development of reproductive system and secondary sex characteristics in boys						
15	Boys: increased muscle strength, coordination						

Expanded with permission from Chart 4.1: Selected theories of child development. Scholl GT: Growth and Development. In Scholl GT (ed): Foundations of Education for Blind and Visually Handicapped Children and Youth: Theory and Practice, pp. 68–70. New York, American Foundation for the Blind, 1986.

asking the child to describe what happened on the way to the office are ways to do this.

Cognitive

Piaget's theory of cognitive development (see above) is perhaps the most widely known. The milestones are summarized in Table 1.1 (Cognitive).

Psychosexual

The focus of the psychosexual developmental perspective is on the dynamic interaction of three abstract concepts: the id, or innate drives; the ego, the reality mediator; and the superego, the conscience (22). Freud described the interplay and relative importance of these constructs during various stages and their contributions to personality development.

It should be noted that Freud developed his theories from work with patients, most of whom had some degree of neurosis. His treatment was historical, that is, he helped the patient return to the origin of the problem, which was typically during infancy or early childhood. Through free association and analysis of dreams, early memories, and drawings, he helped the patient resolve the problem. His observation that the origin of most of the patients' problems was in the early years shaped his theories. Freud's contributions lie in his abilities as a meticulous observer and an original thinker and in his focus on individual differences.

Psychosocial

Erikson, one of the neo-Freudians, moved away from Freud's biological approach and expanded on the influence of social factors on development (22, 23). He focused on the development of identity, his name for the ego, in eight psychosocial stages of the entire life span. (Table 1.1 includes the first five stages.) He viewed each stage as a conflict between two opposing forces that needed to be resolved before the person could move on to the next level.

Erickson's contribution was his emphasis on the social influences on development,

which derived from studies of various social settings and cultures, and on his emphasis on life as a quest for identity (22). His own writings (4, 5) are an excellent source for further exploration of his theories.

Developmental Tasks

Havighurst was influenced by Erikson and his theory of psychosocial development. Consequently, he identified developmental tasks that would balance needs of the individual with society's demands (12). He viewed nature as providing the possibilities for human development, which are realized through learning within the cultural frame. The mastery of the developmental tasks leads to happiness and to later success, whereas absence of mastery leads to personal unhappiness, disapproval from society, and difficulty in mastering subsequent tasks.

Moral Development

Kohlberg and his associates elaborated on Piaget's work on moral development and focused on the evolution of morals and values in the individual (3). He based his work on studies of American adolescents who were presented with moral dilemmas. On the basis of his studies, he defined three levels of moral thinking, each with two related stages. Children under age four are viewed as egocentric and amoral.

Assessing Developmental Levels Informally

The preceding descriptions and Table 1.1 describe what normal children are like in various aspects of their development at particular ages. The descriptions of the characteristics for age level and aspect of development might be used in several ways for informal assessment of the developmental level of a young patient. Each aspect can be evaluated by inspection of a specific column. For example, a rough idea of the child's physical development relative to chronological age may be gained by looking down the Physical column at each item and comparing the child's physical development and movement ability, to the age norm in the Year column. This will indicate whether the child is behind, on target, or advanced for age. Another approach is to read the items horizontally for the child's age to determine the expected behaviors. The optometrist might do this in advance of meeting the child, in preparation for the interview or examination, in order to know roughly what to expect.

Knowledge and understanding of the child's developmental level and possible behaviors help the optometrist select techniques that might be useful in the course of the interview and examination, but it is important to remember that a child who is in the upper part of the normal range and one in the lower part on any developmental or behavioral characteristic may be very different.

In order to facilitate observation, the waiting room should have appropriate children's furniture and toys, books, and games that appeal to various ages. Coloring books and blank paper for drawings with a supply of crayons, chalk and a board, and pencils are also valuable. Manipulative toys such as blocks keep younger children busy and more occupied if they must wait. The child's selection and use of toys provide an excellent opportunity for the practitioner to observe children and how they play and their relationship to the mother or other caregiver. The waiting room can provide a natural setting for initiating rapport with the child prior to the examination.

In order to maximize the opportunity for observation on the initial visit, the optometrist may wish to go to the waiting room for the child rather than having the office assistant or technician bring the child to the examining room. Beginning with the chronological age of the patient, the practitioner can form an idea of what the developmental level might be. It takes years of study and observation to refine these skills. Table 1.2 lists some points to observe and questions to ask the child in order to make an informal assessment. Suggestions for the initial meeting with the child are included in Chapter 7.

Table 1.2 POINTS TO OBSERVE AND QUESTIONS TO ASK WHEN MEETING A 5-YEAR-OLD PATIENT

Physical/psychomotor characteristics
 Is the child large or small for the chronological age?
 Does the child look well-fed?
 How would movement be characterized (e.g., smooth, jerky)?
 Can the child skip?
 Can the child manipulate small objects (e.g., pick up a pin)?
 Is the child quiet or in constant motion?
Cognitive/language
 Is the child attending school? What grade or school?
 Can the child carry on a simple conversation?
 Is speech understandable?
 How well-developed is the sentence structure?
 What kind of toy or book did the child select while waiting?
 How far can the child count?
 In counting five objects such as blocks, does the child match the object to his saying the number?
Social/emotional
 Does the child cling to the mother or go far away from her?
 Is the child interested in other children in the waiting room?
 How well does the child relate to you initially?
 How willing is the child to leave the parent or caregiver?
 Does the child take your hand or walk independently to the office?

Determinants of variations and formal and informal assessments useful in determining developmental levels are described in the next section.

Suggested Readings

Barraga NC: Sensory Perceptual Development. In Scholl GT (ed): Foundations of Education for Blind and Visually Handicapped Children and Youth. New York, American Foundation for the Blind, 1986.

Hendrick J: The Whole Child: Early Education for the Eighties. St. Louis, Times Mirror/Mosby, 1984.

Mussen PH, Conger JJ, Kagan J: Child Development and Personality, 5th ed. New York, Harper & Row, 1979.

Peters DL, Neisworth JT, Yawkey TD: Early Childhood Education: From Theory to Practice. Monterey CA, Brooks/Cole, 1985.

Scholl GT: Growth and Development. In Scholl GT (ed): Foundations of Education for Blind and Visually Handicapped Children and Youth. New York, American Foundation for the Blind, 1986.

Determinants of Variations in Growth and Development

In this section I consider some variations that may be attributed to heredity and environment, and particularly those that might classify the child as exceptional.

Hereditary and Environment

There is little that can be done to alter hereditary characteristics such as eye or hair color without some type of environmental intervention, such as using tinted contact lenses or coloring the hair. There are some medical interventions that can be used during the prenatal period for certain hereditary conditions. For example, when Rh factors of fetus and mother are incompatible, blood transfusions can be performed to prevent damage to the neonate. Other conditions can be modified postnatally through medical intervention such as surgical repair for spina bifida or cleft palate or increasing height with hormone therapy. (For a discussion of genetic and nongenetic disorders of the eye, modes of genetic transmission of eye conditions, and genetic counseling see Chapter 5.)

In general, we say that heredity sets the limits or capacities of the individual and determines the framework for development. The environment provides the setting, which can prevent or discourage full development of those capabilities or provide an enriched and optimal setting in which to reach full potential. Such environmental factors may be prenatal, perinatal, or postnatal. The optometrist will want to inquire about any such problems because of their possible effects on growth and development and on the presence of vision problems. Guidelines for taking a case history are presented in Chapter 7.

Table 1.3 lists some of the pre-, peri-, and postnatal factors. We sometimes fail to think about the environment as having an impact

Table 1.3   POTENTIAL SOURCES OF DEVELOPMENTAL DELAYS DURING THE PRENATAL, PERINATAL, AND POSTNATAL PERIODS

Prenatal
  Age of the mother at the time of the pregnancy
  Health of the mother and father at the time of conception
  Chromosomal abnormalities
  Nutrition and general health during pregnancy
  Substance abuse during pregnancy—how often, how much, what kind (tobacco, alcohol, drugs)
  History of accidents or injuries
  History of abuse by the spouse
  Illness during pregnancy, especially viral diseases, particularly German measles; venereal diseases
  Rh factor–incompatability of maternal and fetal blood types
  Acquired immunodeficiency syndrome (AIDS)
  Human immunodeficiency virus (HIV)
Perinatal
  Premature delivery: how early, weight of infant, time in a perinatal intensive care unit
  Long and difficult delivery
  Breech presentation
  Respiratory distress after birth
  Difficulties sucking when nursing
  Allergy to mother's milk
Postnatal
  Feeding and sucking problems
  Allergies to food
  Lead poisoning
  History of illnesses during the first year, especially high-fever viral illnesses and infectious diseases
  History of abuse to the child
  Accidents, particularly head trauma: cause, treatment, effect
  Hospitalizations: reasons, length of stay, surgical procedures

on the development of the fetus. Fetal life is, in reality, one of the most critical and vulnerable times in human existence. The age, behavior, nutrition, and physical condition of the mother during pregnancy can have profound effects on the developing fetus: very young mothers and those nearing menopause are particularly at risk; poor nutrition and any types of substance abuse, a history of accidents or injuries, and illness during pregnancy, particularly such viral illnesses as German measles, may also damage the growing fetus. Any one of these factors may cause delayed or defective development, and some may cause visual impairment. Knowing the early history may help the optometrist understand and work with a child's physical or mental problems. Numerous factors at the time of birth can also contribute to delayed or defective development. Prematurity is probably one of the more significant ones.

In addition to the postnatal factors (e.g., difficulty sucking, feeding problems, allergies to foods, high fevers, childhood diseases) insufficient environmental stimulation may retard development. The home environment must provide new experiences and adequate sensory stimulation to enhance the child's expanding knowledge of the world, which is critically important in communication and cognitive development. A child who lives in an intellectually impoverished environment frequently has problems in school because of an inadequate experiential background.

Of special concern in recent years is the growing prevalence of child abuse. Infants and young children with developmental problems seem to be particularly vulnerable to abuse. All persons who work with children should know the signs of abuse. Table 1.4 lists some of the common ones. Although the optometrist may not be in a position to observe some of these signs, a child's behavior may suggest a discussion of the situation with the child's teacher.

Signs of sexual and emotional abuse are especially difficult to identify. Children, especially very young ones, have difficulty understanding these forms of abuse and communicating with adults about them. The optometrist who suspects such abuse will need to develop rapport and gain the child's confidence before such information will be forthcoming.

All states now mandate reporting of child abuse. Optometrists should know the law in their state, particularly their legal obligation to report. Most communities have one or more designated agencies that provide information about referral procedures and advice on how to handle such situations. The Social Services section of the telephone directory usually includes such information.

Cultural Background

The United States is a nation of diverse racial and ethnic backgrounds, religious affiliations, socioeconomic levels, and regional differences. Although early in our history there was a movement toward cultural amalgamation—the melting pot phenomenon—some minority groups continue to experience discrimination from the majority culture. Increasing concern is currently directed toward providing those with different cultural backgrounds equal opportunity to participate in all aspects of our society.

Although the impact of these differences is greater in school, social service, and rehabilitation settings, some problems may arise in the practice of optometry—customs which may be foreign to the optometrist, the patient's attitudes particularly toward authority figures, and language differences that may interfere with communication.

In the United States the typical mode of greeting someone, including children, is a handshake and eye contact. This is not true in all cultures: in some the norm is a kiss on each cheek, an embrace, a bow. It may be proper to minimize eye contact, especially when greeting or speaking with a person of higher status, an elder, or, in some cultures, of the opposite sex. Social distance is also important. In some cultures people stand at some distance away when speaking and in others they stand close and bring their faces together. In cultures where the extended family is emphasized, the entire family may

Table 1.4 PHYSICAL AND BEHAVIORAL INDICATORS OF CHILD ABUSE AND NEGLECT

Type of Abuse or Neglect	Physical Indicators	Behavioral Indicators
Physical abuse	Unexplained bruises and welts —on face, lips, mouth —on torso, back, buttocks, thighs —in various stages of healing —clustered, forming regular patterns —reflecting shape of article used to inflict (electrical cord, belt buckle) —on several different surface areas —regularly appear after absence, weekend, or vacation Unexplained burns: —cigar, cigarette burns, especially on soles, palms, back, or buttocks —immersion burns (socklike, glovelike, doughnut-shaped on buttocks or genitalia) —patterned like electric burner, iron, etc. —rope burns on arms, legs, neck, or torso Unexplained fractures: —to skull, nose, facial structure —in various stages of healing —multiple or spiral fractures Unexplained lacerations or abrasions: —to mouth, lips, gums, eyes —to external genitalia	Wary of adult contacts Apprehensive when other children cry Behavioral extremes: —aggressiveness or withdrawal Frightened of parents Afraid to go home Reports injury by parents
Physical neglect	Consistent hunger, poor hygiene, inappropriate dress Consistent lack of supervision, especially in dangerous activities or long periods Unattended physical problems or medical needs Abandonment	Begging, stealing food Extended stays at school (early arrival and late departure) Constant fatigue, listlessness, or falling asleep in class Alcohol or drug abuse Delinquency (e.g., thefts) States there is no caretaker
Sexual abuse	Difficulty in walking or sitting Torn, stained, or bloody underclothing Pain or itching in genital area Bruises or bleeding in external genitalia, vaginal, or anal areas Pregnancy	Unwilling to change for gym or participate in PE class Withdrawal, fantasy, or infantile behavior Bizarre, sophisticated, or unusual sexual behavior or knowledge Poor peer relationships Delinquent or runaway Reports sexual assault by caretaker

Table 1.4   (*Continued*)

Type of Abuse or Neglect	Physical Indicators	Behavioral Indicators
Emotional Maltreatment	Speech disorders Lags in physical development Failure to thrive	Habit disorders (sucking, biting, rocking, etc.) Conduct disorders (antisocial, destructive, etc.) Neurotic traits (sleep disorders, inhibition of play) Psychoneurotic reactions (hysteria, obsession, compulsion, phobias, hypochondria)

From: Broadhurst DD: The Educator's Role in the Prevention and Treatment of Child Abuse and Neglect. Washington DC, National Center for Child Abuse and Neglect, Children's Bureau, Administration of Children, Youth, and Families. U.S. Dept. of Health, Education & Welfare, 1979.

accompany the patient to the doctor's office. In cultures where time and being on time are not important, misunderstandings may arise when the patient is told to be at the office at a particular time.

The optometrist should keep in mind that some communities have different customs and there is a need to accept them and work within the framework of the culture of the individual patient. If the optometrist is having difficulty understanding a cultural group within the community, it is often possible to speak with the community leader of that group for interpretation and better understanding of the patient's point of view. It is better to seek help in understanding the individual than to risk offending a patient or misunderstanding a particular behavior.

EXCEPTIONALITIES

Sometimes variations in growth and development are so great that special education is necessary to enable a child to gain maximum benefit from school. When these variations have an impact on the learning process, special programs and services may be required by federal and state legislation. Other variations without educational implications can usually be managed in the regular classroom.

Variations That Require Special Education Programs or Services

P.L. 94-142, The Education of All Handicapped Children Act passed in 1975, was a landmark piece of legislation in the history of education. It was amended and expanded in 1983 (P.L. 98-199) and again in 1987 (P.L. 99-457). The provisions of P.L. 94-142 and its amendments require states to provide handicapped children with a full range of programs and services that will enable them to receive a free appropriate education in the least restrictive environment. Eleven categories of exceptionality were defined (Table 1.5). Each handicapped child must be assessed in the areas of suspected disability to determine whether the disability is sufficiently severe

Table 1.5   P.L. 94-142–RECOGNIZED CATEGORIES OF HANDICAPS

Deaf	Seriously emotionally disturbed
Deaf–blind	
Hard of hearing	Specific learning disability
Mentally retarded	
Multihandicapped	Speech impaired
Orthopedically impaired	Visually handicapped
Other health impaired	

to adversely affect educational performance. The decision for eligibility for special education programs and services and for placement must be made by a multidisciplinary team. Placement must be in the least restrictive environment for a particular child. Each school district must have available a continuum of alternative programs ranging from regular classes to institutional or residential placements, in order to meet the educational needs of persons with all types and degrees of disability. The rules and regulations accompanying the legislation include detailed definitions of what children are to be served; descriptions of the full range of services to be provided; information about assessment procedures, and other details about the administration of the programs. Each state must submit a plan to the U.S. Department of Education detailing how the legislation will be implemented in that particular state. These state and local plans are available from the state departments of education (30). It should be noted that labeling terminology varies among the states. The optometrist should find out what the appropriate terms are in any particular state from the State Department of Education or from the local special education office in the public school system.

Each child must have a complete assessment in the areas of educational need by specialists recognized in the child's disability area, evaluation by a multidisciplinary team, and an individualized educational program listing goals and objectives developed by the team, including the parents and the child, if appropriate. A more complete description of the most pertinent legislative provisions for the practice of optometry, particularly this team approach and its specific functions, is included in Chapter 23. Relevant components for the comprehensive assessment (listed in Table 1.6) are selected based on the suspected disability and the child's educational needs.

Definitions, etiology, impact on the three areas of growth and development, assessment, and resources for the eleven categories of handicaps provide an overview for optometrists who may meet various types of handi-

Table 1.6 COMPONENTS IN THE COMPREHENSIVE ASSESSMENT

Vision/hearing
  Examination by an optometrist or the appropriate medical specialist
  Functional assessment of the sensory loss
  Assessment of efficiency of use of remaining vision/hearing
  Sensory devices evaluation (hearing and vision)
Intelligence/aptitude
  Cognitive development
  Intellectual functioning
  Communication skills
Sensory/motor skills
  Gross and fine motor development
  Perceptual learning
Academic skills/concept development
  Achievement in reading, writing, spelling, mathematics
  Language development
  Listening and auditory discrimination skills
  Concepts: temporal, quantitative, positional, directional, and sequential
  Study skills
Social/emotional/affective
  Behavioral control
  Social and affective learning
  Adaptive living skills
  Recreation and leisure skills
Functional living skills
  Daily living skills/activities of daily living
  Orientation and mobility skills
  Community travel and use
  Career and prevocational skills

Source: Reprinted from Hall A, Scholl GT, Swallow R-M: Psychoeducational Assessment. In Scholl GT (ed): Foundations of Education for Blind and Visually Handicapped Children and Youth: Theory and Practice, p 192. New York, American Foundation for the Blind, 1986.

capped children. Definitions are derived from those included in P.L. 94-142. Care should be observed regarding the assessment portion for each disability area; results of tests standardized for a normal population must be interpreted cautiously. Further, it should be noted that these descriptions assume there is no other accompanying impairment, that the impairment was present at birth (congenital), and that exceptions are to be anticipated when the general descriptions are applied to a particular individual. Any text used in introductory special education courses can be a good source of additional information about these categories.

Deaf/Hard of Hearing

Definition Deaf and hard-of-hearing children possess a hearing impairment that adversely affects their educational performance. Deaf children have such a severe impairment that they cannot understand speech through hearing alone, even with a hearing aid; hard of hearing children have a less severe hearing impairment such that amplification usually enables them to understand speech.

Etiology About 12 percent of hearing impairments in children can be attributed to heredity (18). Other prenatal factors include rubella, maternal viral infections, and Rh factor incompatibility. Perinatal factors include prematurity and prolonged lack of oxygen immediately after birth. Postnatal conditions include meningitis, otitis media, high fevers, infections, and brain concussions.

Impact on Growth and Development A hearing impairment in and of itself usually has little effect on physical and psychomotor development. Hearing-impaired children make good use of visual imitation and have few problems with coordination. The absence of hearing does have a profound effect on cognitive development, particularly in communication skills where inability to hear, and so thus to imitate speech, places them at a distinct disadvantage. There may be some problems in social and emotional development, partly because of the isolating nature of the disability (26).

Assessment The primary diagnostician for hearing impairments is the otologist, a medical specialist in the ear and hearing, who will determine the cause of the hearing impairment and whether any treatment will improve it; closely allied is the audiologist, who measures the type and extent of the hearing loss and recommends a hearing aid to maximize residual hearing.

Administering and interpreting any assessment instruments standardized on a normal population to persons with sensory deficits must be done with caution. To assess intelligence, individually administered nonverbal and performance tests are usually recommended. Standardized achievement tests are frequently used to measure educational progress. The difficulty in employing such instruments for hearing-impaired children lies in the disadvantage they have in reading; whereas deaf children in the lower grades may read at grade level, when the materials in the upper grades introduce more difficult vocabulary and abstractions, the deaf child is placed at a distinct disadvantage because of his limited communication skills. Zieziula (32) presents a good overview and description of formal instruments that can be used with hearing-impaired children and adults.

Resources For more detailed information about hearing-impaired children, in addition to that included in introductory college texts in special education, the following books are recommended:

Furth HG: Deafness and Learning. Belmont, CA, Wadsworth, 1973.
Quigley SP, Kretschmer RE: The Education of Deaf Children. Baltimore, University Park Press, 1982.

The following agencies supply additional information about hearing impairments:

Alexander Graham Bell Association for the Deaf, 3417 Volta Place NW, Washington, DC 20017.
National Information Center on Deafness, Gallaudet College, Kendall Green, Washington, DC 20002.

Mentally Retarded

Definition The American Association on Mental Deficiency defines mental retardation as "significantly subaverage general intellectual functioning existing concurrently with deficits in adaptive behavior and manifested during the developmental period" (9, p. 1).

Because of the many different levels of ability among children in this category, three major subgroups have been identified according to approximate IQ scores:

Mild/Educable—IQ 50–55 to about 70
Moderate/Trainable—IQ 35–40 to 50–55
Severe/Profound/Custodial—
 IQ below 20 to 35–40

Etiology There are numerous contributing factors for mental retardation, in fact, almost every one included in Table 1.3. Some of the major prenatal factors include rubella, Rh factor incompatibility, chromosomal abnormalities (e.g., Down's syndrome, Turner's syndrome), genetic abnormalities (e.g., phenylketonuria), maternal alcoholism (e.g., fetal alcohol syndrome), syphilis, herpes simplex II, toxoplasmosis, and malnutrition. Perinatal factors include premature birth, oxygen deprivation, and long and difficult labor. Postnatal factors include lead poisoning, high fevers, viral illnesses (e.g., encephalitis, meningitis), infectious diseases (e.g., Reyes' syndrome), and head trauma. Many of these factors are relevant for multiple impairments as well.

Impact on Growth and Development Physical development is likely to be significantly below normal, particularly in moderately and severely retarded children. Poor coordination and retarded psychomotor development are characteristic of all groups. Needless to say, retarded cognitive development and poor communication skills are the major deficiencies, and maximum attainment is usually no higher than Piaget's stage of concrete operations. In the affective aspect, social and emotional development are frequently delayed, although educational remediation can enhance these abilities.

Assessment With their many problems, children in this group should receive a comprehensive assessment including all components included in Table 1.6. Of special importance are instruments to assess intellectual abilities and adaptive behavior, as these are the two major determinants of eligibility for special education services and assessment of sensory functions (vision and hearing). (See also Chapter 16.)

Resources The following books will supplement the material in introductory special education texts:

MacMillan DL: Mental Retardation in School and Society. Boston, Little, Brown, 1982.
Neisworth JT, Smith RM: Retardation: Issues, Assessment and Intervention. New York, McGraw-Hill, 1978.

These organizations are good sources of information:

American Association on Mental Deficiency, 5201 Connecticut Ave NW, Washington, DC 20015.
National Association for Retarded Citizens, 2709 Ave E East, Arlington, TX 76011.

Orthopedically Impaired/Other Health Impaired

Definition The number of children affected by orthopedic and medical conditions is small and the population very diverse. I will refer to the group as "physically impaired," because many do not have orthopedic impairments, that is, impairments of the musculoskeletal system. A more appropriate classification divides physical impairments according to the body system involved: cardiopulmonary (asthma, cystic fibrosis, heart defects); musculoskeletal (amputations, arthritis, arthrogryposis, burns, muscular dystrophy, scoliosis); and neurologic (cerebral palsy, epilepsy, traumatic brain injury, spinal cord injury, myelomeningocele) (18). Except for those with cerebral palsy, and, in certain instances to a more limited extent, muscular dystrophy, myelomeningocele, and brain injury, most children with these conditions are not eligible for special education programs and services because their disabilities do not usually affect their educational performance adversely.

Etiology Each of these conditions can be the result of factors related to the prenatal, perinatal, and postnatal conditions in Table 1.3.

Impact on Growth and Development Only conditions that have special education implications are included here. Cerebral palsy can affect all areas of growth and development, depending on its severity. Psychomotor function is most frequently affected, and many children are unable to walk independently and must use crutches, walkers, or a wheel chair for mobility. Depending on the area of the brain affected, cognitive development, and particularly communication, can be seriously affected. Affective function can be disturbed if adjustment to the disability is a problem.

Mental retardation frequently accompanies myelomeningocele and muscular dystrophy, and that condition, rather than the physical impairment, is the major handicap of these children. Visual and auditory impairments are often present as well.

Assessment Medical and paramedical personnel are typically involved in a major way in the assessment of these children. Physical and occupational therapists are usually on the assessment team and take an active role in remedial and educational programs. Speech therapists are involved if there is a communication problem. The skills of the school psychologist and school social worker are also used in assessment, remediation, and particularly work with parents. Because of the multiplicity of the presenting problems, these children's problems require a team approach.

Resources Supplemental material to introductory special education texts include:

Bigge J: Teaching Individuals with Physical and Multiple Disabilities, 2nd ed. Columbus OH, Charles E Merrill, 1982.
Blackman JA: Medical Aspects of Developmental Disabilities in Children Birth to Three. Iowa City, The University of Iowa, 1983.
Bleck EE, Nagel DA (eds): Physically Handicapped Children—A Medical Atlas for Teachers, 2nd ed. New York, Grune & Stratton, 1983.
Campbell H: Measuring Abilities of Severely Handicapped Students. Springfield IL, Charles C Thomas, 1981.

Additional information may be obtained from:

National Easter Seal Society for Crippled Children and Adults, 2012 West Ogden Ave, Chicago, IL 60612.
United Cerebral Palsy Association, 66 East 34th St, New York, NY 10016.

Seriously Emotionally Disturbed

This category contains a large heterogeneous group of disorders that have many labels, according to each state's regulations. Definitions likewise vary, and there is little agreement about what constitutes appropriate assessment and what remedial procedures should be used in school programs.

Definition Emotional problems of children have a wide range of behavioral manifestations, many of which can be managed in a regular classroom with some modifications. Some emotional disturbances may be temporary, as when illness or a divorce in the family may require the child to make adjustments in life style. Children with more serious problems are referred for special education services. To qualify, one or more of the following characteristics that can adversely affect school performance must be evident over a long period and to a marked degree: inability to learn not explained by intellectual, sensory, or health factors; inability to form or maintain satisfactory interpersonal relationships; inappropriate behavior or feelings; generally pervasive mood of unhappiness or depression; tendency to develop physical symptoms or fears.

Autism is usually classified in this group of problems, although in some states it is a separate category or is included with physical handicaps. Autism is defined as "a severely incapacitating lifelong developmental disability that usually appears during the first 3 years of life" (18, p. 423). Assessment and remedial techniques are controversial; a wide variety of both are used, with varying degrees of success.

Etiology No single etiological factor can account for all emotional disturbances. In many cases a mismatch between the child's environment and needs will contribute to the development of emotional and behavioral problems. There is some evidence for the presence of genetic factors in autism.

Impact on Growth and Development There is little evidence that physical or cognitive growth is affected by an emotional disturbance. Poor school performance may be attributed to inability to learn or to lack of motivation to learn, but actual native intellectual or cognitive growth usually is not retarded. It is social and emotional growth and development that are delayed, since they are the principal areas affected by emotional disturbances.

Assessment The diagnostic specialists for this category of disorders include psychiatrists, psychologists, and school social workers. Most assessment is informal observation of behavior to look at the developmental milestones described in Table 1.1.

Resources Many books are available on emotional disturbances and the management of emotionally disturbed children. The following ones are illustrative.

Paul J, Epanchin B (eds): Emotional Disturbance in Children. Columbus, OH, Charles E Merrill, 1982.
Knoblock P: Teaching Emotionally Disturbed Children. Boston, Houghton Mifflin, 1983.
Morse WC: The Education and Treatment of Socio-emotionally Impaired Children and Youth. Syracuse, Syracuse University Press, 1985.

Many communities and states have organizations that provide information and support groups for parents and their emotionally disturbed children. A listing is usually available from the State Department of Education, the local school district, or the telephone directory.

The largest professional organization is:

American Orthopsychiatric Association, 1790 Broadway, New York, NY 10019.

A national parent group is:

National Society for Autistic Children, 306 31st St, Huntington, WV 10016.

Specific Learning Disability

Learning disability is probably the most controversial area of special education. Educators disagree about definition, appropriate assessment procedures, and effective methods of remediation. It also receives the largest portion of reimbursement funding under the provisions of P.L. 94-142 and its subsequent amendments.

Definition To qualify for special education programs and services for a learning disability, a child must demonstrate a disorder in one or more of the basic processes of understanding or using spoken or written language (that is, the ability to listen, think, speak, read, write, spell, or do mathematical calculations). Learning problems due to visual, auditory, or motor handicaps; mental retardation; or environmental, cultural, or economic disadvantage are not included in this definition. The implementation and interpretation of the criteria for eligibility included in this definition vary among the states, and it is not uncommon for a child who is eligible for special education in one state to be ineligible in another.

Kirk and Chalfont (17) divide learning disabilities into two broad categories: developmental (attention disorders, memory disorders, visual perception and perceptual-motor disorders, thinking disorders, and language disorders) and academic learning disabilities (reading, spelling, writing, and arithmetic).

Etiology For many children etiological factors include brain or central nervous system dysfunction, although this diagnosis is often made on the basis of "soft" neurologic signs; heredity; environmental deprivation and malnutrition; and biochemical imbalances (18).

Impact on Growth and Development Physical growth and development typically are normal, except that frequently motor coordination is poor. In earlier times this problem was sometimes labeled the clumsy child syndrome. Intellectual and cognitive abilities typically are within the normal range, although underachievement (a significant discrepancy between IQ and achievement level) is frequently used as a criterion for identification and eligibility for services. Although learning disabilities do not have a direct impact on social and emotional growth and development, indirect effects may contribute to the development of emotional and behavior problems. These factors include poor self-concept, frustration at the inability to compete with peers, frequent failure, and lack of motivation.

Assessment Usually, standardized tests of achievement and intelligence are used to determine eligibility. Diagnostic tests in reading and arithmetic help to pinpoint the specific problem and to plan an appropriate remedial program. Chapter 21 provides more detailed information on learning disabilities.

Resources Two of the many references on learning disabilities are:

Kirk SA, Chalfont JC: Academic and Developmental Learning Disabilities. Denver, Love Publishing Company, 1984.
Lerner J: Learning Disabilities: Theories, Diagnosis, and Teaching Strategies, 4th ed. Boston, Houghton Mifflin, 1985.

Most states have one or more organizations related to this area. Frequently, they are chapters of the national organization:

Association for Children with Learning Disabilities, 4156 Library Rd, Pittsburgh, PA 15234.

Speech Impaired

Speech-impaired children typically are enrolled in regular classes and speech therapy is provided by a speech therapist. Children with severe language problems may be enrolled in special classes; those with moderate and mild impairments attend regular classes and receive speech and language therapy regularly.

Definition The federal definition of speech-impaired does include language disorders although the two are really separate entities. Communication disorder is probably a more accurate term. Communication disorders include speech impairments (stuttering, impaired articulation or voice) and language impairments.

Etiology Communication problems can result from a variety of etiologies. Some speech problems, such as cleft palate, are the result of genetic prenatal factors; others, such as stuttering, may arise from a variety of causes, including emotional problems; still others, such as poor articulation, can result from slight to moderate hearing impairments or from poor models of speech in the environment. Severe language problems, such as aphasia, and communication problems associated with cerebral palsy, may result from brain injury; others, such as delayed language development, may be related to the environment, as when there is inadequate stimulation to develop language.

Impact on Growth and Development Communication problems have little impact on physical and psychomotor growth, but children with neurological impairments may have poor motor coordination. Cognitive and intellectual development tend to be within normal ranges but language development may be retarded or even defective, depending upon the severity of the communication problem. Disturbed social and emotional development are probably more the results of environmental reactions and attitudes than of the disability itself.

Assessment The major diagnostic specialist is the speech, hearing, and language therapist. A variety of formal and informal instruments is available.

Resources The following references are helpful for additional information:

Bloom L, Lahey M: Language Development and Language Disorders. New York, John Wiley, 1978.

Hixon T, Shriberg L, Saxman J (eds): Introduction to Communication Disorders. Englewood Cliffs NJ, Prentice-Hall, 1980.

Van Riper C: Speech Correction: Principles and Methods, 6th ed. Englewood Cliffs NJ, Prentice-Hall, 1978.

The major professional organization is:

American Speech, Hearing and Language Association, 9030 Old Georgetown Rd, Washington, DC 20014.

Visually Handicapped

Definition   Visually handicapped children are those whose visual impairment, even with the best possible optical correction, adversely affects school performance.

Etiology and Impact on Growth and Development   These are discussed in Chapter 15.

Assessment   The major diagnosticians of visual impairment are the optometrist and ophthalmologist. Procedures for vision assessment are described in Chapter 7. Relevant components from the comprehensive assessment (Table 1.6) typically are administered by school personnel.

Resources   The major resource for educational programs is:

Scholl GT (ed): Foundations of Education for Blind and Visually Handicapped Children and Youth: Theory and Practice. New York, American Foundation for the Blind, 1986.

The national agency for information and referral is:

The American Foundation for the Blind, 15 West 16th St, New York, NY 10011.

Deaf-Blind/Multihandicapped

These two categories are considered together because of their similarities. Deaf-blind children have severe hearing and vision impairments that prevent them from receiving an appropriate education in programs for either deaf and hearing-impaired or visually handicapped children. Multihandicapped children have concomitant impairments, the combination of which precludes their being educated in programs designed for children with one impairment. The variety of combinations of impairments is almost infinite, which tends to complicate educational planning and remediation.

The reader is referred to the preceding sections for definitions, etiology, impact on growth and development, and assessment for information on each impairment. It should be noted that a multihandicapped child cannot be viewed as one with two or more impairments, each one of which is to be remediated as though in isolation but rather as having two or more impairments which interact on all aspects of their development and thereby complicate the educational planning process.

Resources   The advent of P.L. 94-142 stimulated the development of programs and services for severely and multiply handicapped children. The following references are of help in this area:

Doyle P, Goodman J, Grotsky J, Mann L: Helping the Severely Handicapped Child: A Guide for Parents and Teachers. New York, Crowell, 1979.

Sailor W, Guess D: Severely Handicapped Students: An Instructional Design. Boston, Houghton Mifflin, 1983.

Other Variations Usually Found in Regular Classes

Several conditions may have implications in areas of life other than education, but children having such conditions are not eligible for special education programs and services. Children with such problems typically attend regular classes. Some conditions are more problematic for adolescents and adults, especially because of discriminatory employment practices.

Physical Problems

A wide variety of conditions affect all three systems, as outlined earlier, but usually have minimal impact on school progress. Table 1.7 lists some of the more common conditions, their typical cause, and their effects on the child's functioning. The *definition* and *etiology* of physical handicaps were discussed under Orthopedically Impaired/Other Health Impaired, above.

Impact on Growth and Development The impact on growth and development of these conditions depends on several variables: type of onset (gradual or traumatic) prior to diagnosis; age of onset; severity and type of condition; and body system affected. If the impairment is present from birth and is due to either a prenatal or a perinatal factor, the impact on growth and development, particularly physical growth, can be considerable. On the other hand, if it is acquired and the child's earlier development had been normal, the problem may affect only subsequent growth and development. Many of these conditions are disabling and may foster dependency that can lead to immature social and emotional adjustment. Parents' and community attitudes may enhance or undermine a child's self-concept and adjustment.

Assessment The major diagnostician typically is the appropriate medical specialist.

Communication with this specialist is essential to determine the amount and type of physical activity that the child can tolerate without incurring further damage or exacerbating the condition. Psychological and educational assessment are usually the same as for nonhandicapped children at similar intellectual and maturity levels.

Resources The references listed above in Orthopedically Impaired/Other Health Impaired are useful for this group of disorders as well. In addition to the National Easter Seal Society for Crippled Children and Adults, agencies and organizations for most of the major health problems provide additional information.

American Diabetes Association, 1 West 48th St, New York, NY 10020.
Epilepsy Foundation of America, 1828 L St NW, Washington, DC 20036.

Underachievement and Reading Disabilities
Some children have difficulty achieving in school but have no evidence of a disability, even a mild one. Often the reasons for underachievement are related to the school or to society. School may not be meaningful or relevant for children from lower socioeconomic groups: school programs are frequently

Table 1.7   SELECTED PHYSICAL PROBLEMS THAT ARE NOT CLASSIFIED AS ELIGIBLE FOR SPECIAL EDUCATION PROGRAMS AND SERVICES

Condition	Description	Etiology	Impact
Amputations	Absence or loss of all or part of upper or lower limbs	Congenital or acquired	No impact on cognition; mobility may require prosthesis; hands and fingers may require prosthetic devices
Arthritis (juvenile rheumatoid or Still's disease)	Inflammation of joints causing aches and pains; chronic condition; may become progressive	Unknown, but may be autoimmune reaction	No impact on cognition; mobility and dexterity may be affected
Asthma	Chronic disease that involves coughing, wheezing, breathing difficulty	Unknown; may be due to allergies	Severe attacks require immediate medical care; no impact on learning

Table 1.7 (*Continued*)

Condition	Description	Etiology	Impact
Brittle bone disease	Defect in bone protein that causes bones to break easily; distinctive blue sclera characteristic	Hereditary	Hearing and vision losses common; physical activities restricted
Cancer	Malignant tumor or carcinoma that can affect any part of the body	No one cause; may be multiple	Early diagnosis essential to initiate treatment
Cystic fibrosis	Hypersecretion of mucus in lungs, pancreas, and other organs	Hereditary	Life expectancy about 14 years; physical activities restricted
Juvenile diabetes mellitus	Inability to metabolize food because body cannot make insulin	Hereditary	Special diet and insulin necessary; energy level may be reduced
Epilepsy	Brain disorder characterized by recurring excessive neuronal discharge resulting in seizures	Multiple causes	First aid for seizures necessary; medications can control frequency of seizures
Fetal alcohol syndrome	Retarded physical and mental development	Heavy drinking by mother during pregnancy	Characteristic facial features, flattened appearance
Heart defects	Shortness of breath, pain, cyanosis	Acquired; most are congenital	Easily fatigued; physical activities restricted
Hemophilia	Blood does not clot or clots slowly	Hereditary	Very restricted physical activity
Marfan's syndrome	Disorder of connective tissue resulting in skeletal changes	Hereditary	Vision problems common
Myelomeningocele (spina bifida)	Open defect in bones of spine; surgery needed to close the opening	Congenital; tends to occur in families	May be mentally retarded; incontinence common
Scoliosis	Lateral curvature of spine; may be corrected by surgery or braces	Congenital but cause unknown	Physical activities may need restriction
Sickle cell anemia	Defect in which hemoglobin is sensitive to decreases in oxygen so round red cells become sickle shaped; incurable at present	Hereditary, found primarily in blacks	May require medical care for swelling, pain, and fever
Tourette's syndrome	Progressively violent jerks of face, shoulders, and extremities	Unknown	Needs understanding; does not usually affect development

Data from Goldenson RM (ed): Disability and Rehabilitation Handbook. New York, McGraw-Hill, 1978; Kirk SA, Gallagher JJ: Educating Exceptional Children, pp. 463–471. Boston, Houghton-Mifflin, 1986; Osol A (ed): Blakiston's Gould Medical Dictionary. New York, McGraw-Hill, 1972.

geared to middle class children. The degree of parental support and interest appear to affect school achievement; in a society with a high rate of single-parent families, where earning a living is the highest priority, some parents may not have time or energy to help the child with school work. Some parents were themselves alienated by their school experiences and by the system; their children have no role models to follow. Underachievement related to these causes must be resolved through concerted efforts to bring alienated persons into the mainstream of the school and to supply remedial assistance that will enable children to profit from the educational program.

Reading problems are common in many school districts. Sometimes they result from long-term truancy or slower development that prevents children from learning to read at the usual age. In Chapter 22 this area is discussed in greater detail.

Suggested Readings

Most introductory texts for special education courses are useful sources of additional information.

Kirk SA, Gallagher JJ: Educating Exceptional Children, 6th ed. Boston, Houghton Mifflin, 1989.

Scholl GT (ed): The School Psychologist and the Exceptional Child. Reston VA, Council for Exceptional Children, 1985.

HOW LEARNING OCCURS

Learning must be considered in the context of the learner and of his or her interrelationship with the environment. The preceding sections described the physical and psychomotor; cognitive, intellectual, and communicative; and social and affective growth and development of the normal child. Variations were identified in growth patterns of children who are eligible for special education programs and services and in those of children enrolled in regular classes. Differences among children are based on their individual growth and development patterns and the ex-

tent to which their environment provides optimal opportunities for growth and learning. Typically, the environment expands as children grow and develop, particularly in the social and emotional areas. First, they learn their particular place in both the immediate and extended family, develop their self-concepts, and learn acceptable behaviors. Their world then expands to peers through experiences in nursery school and later in school. The world continues to expand from the immediate community to the larger world— city, state, nation, world. For some children the environment does not provide such support. A cognitively impoverished environment, a disoriented family constellation, the influence of poorly adjusted peers, or cognitive and emotional impoverishment may inhibit adjustment to the adult world. On entering school, such children may not have reached the stage of readiness for learning or they may not be sufficiently motivated to take advantage of schooling. The "teachable moment" may not have arrived or it may have passed. In their teaching role optometrists must be aware of both the developmental and the experiential levels of children in order to present themselves most effectively and apply their skills for the children's benefit.

Every adult has had some experience with learning and with teaching someone something. In the process he or she applied several theories of learning without being aware of them. The value of learning theories is that they help us analyze our beliefs, why particular methods work or don't work in certain situations and with certain people, and how we can teach more effectively. The following section summarizes some principles of learning derived from two major theoretical approaches.

Conditioning or Reinforcement

We all use principles of conditioning every time we tell someone they did well or did poorly, or punish or reward a child or a pet, or pamper ourselves with some treat. There are two principal kinds of conditioning: classical and instrumental. Most persons are familiar with the experiments of Ivan Pavlov with his dogs. They illustrate classical or respondent conditioning in which a new stimulus (in this case, the sound of a bell) is paired with a stimulus (food) that produces a response (salivation). The subject connects the two stimuli or "learns" and will respond to the bell by salivating even when no food is presented.

This form of conditioning, pairing two stimuli, characterizes many of our learning experiences, both positive and negative. For example, if a child finds the first visit to the optometrist's office unpleasant (long wait, no toys, chairs not comfortable, mother scolds for not sitting still), the child may react to subsequent visits with apprehension, fear, and reluctance to enter the office. On the other hand, the child who finds the first visit fun (new toys to play with, happy playtime with mother, lots of things to explore, interested adults) will look forward to subsequent visits with pleasure. Thus the neutral stimulus (the office) can come to be viewed either positively or negatively by the child depending on the circumstances of that first visit.

Instrumental or operant conditioning relies on reinforcement to shape or mold behavior. A behavior that is rewarded (positive reinforcement) is likely to be repeated; a behavior that avoids something painful or unpleasant (negative reinforcement) is also likely to be repeated. Negative reinforcement that immediately follows a behavior will tend to discourage repetition of the behavior. For example, if the mother in the optometrist's office praises the child when he is behaving well or offers a cookie, the good behavior will tend to continue. On the other hand, if the mother gives a fussy child a cookie, the child will resort to fussing to get another cookie. Scolding or spanking a fussy child may work if it is done while the child is misbehaving and if the child understands the reason for the scolding or spanking.

In using instrumental conditioning certain conditions must be met. First, it is important that a child's developmental level is compatible with the response being sought, that is, the act or behavior is part of the child's response repertoire. For example, in

an eye examination using the Snellen Chart, the optometrist cannot elicit a letter name from a child who doesn't know the alphabet. He must either be taught his letters, or the optometrist must use another response mode, such as pictures. It is also important to know what is a reinforcer or reward for a particular child. A child who is not interested in food may not respond when offered a cookie but may when given a ball to play with. For this particular child, the ball is a stronger reinforcer.

Reinforcers can be positive—something the child likes, such as the ball in the illustration above—or negative—something the child wants to avoid, such as a spanking. In either case the reinforcer must be given at the moment when the act or behavior occurs; if given early, a positive reinforcer can become a bribe (giving the ball on condition that the act or behavior be performed), or if given later, a negative reinforcer can become a punishment (having Daddy give a spanking when he comes home from work).

Both positive and negative reinforcement encourage continuation of behaviors that are already occurring. Behaviors that are not occurring naturally must be taught. For example, even very young children can be taught names of letters on the eye chart provided they can see them, that the differences between the letters are easily recognizable (A and B are better than C and O); that the entire alphabet is not used; and that sufficient time is allowed for them to learn the letters. In order to help their child learn a sufficient number of letters to read the eye chart, parents can be encouraged to use positive reinforcement (yes, you are right) or negative reinforcement (no, try again), like that used in some recognition-type computer learning games.

Shaping (successive approximation) is another way of teaching something new. The task is broken down into very small segments that will accrete into the target behavior. Some initial step in this progression can usually be identified in current behavior. By beginning there with positive reinforcement and adding subsequent steps that are in turn reinforced and dropping reinforcement for earlier steps, this method frequently works in behavior management. An example would be to seize a moment or situation when a hyperactive child is quiet and to give immediate positive reinforcement (food or praise). Subsequent hyperactive behavior is ignored until the child is quiet again. By using positive reinforcement only during periods of quiet, no matter how brief they are at first, you can build up to a reasonable period of quiet during which to accomplish your goal. Applications of behavioral management techniques to the practice of optometry are discussed in Chapter 7.

Gestalt, Field, or Cognitive Approaches

The behavior modification approach has been criticized by some learning theorists for changing small bits of behavior through reinforced practice on parts. Sometimes the "whole" is lost in this process. These theorists view learning as beginning with the whole and then analyzing the parts and placing emphasis on the whole rather than on parts or details. Several theories emphasize this approach. The gestaltists view learning as taking place through insight. The learner looks at the entire field and extracts from it those elements that have meaning for him or her and that can be organized into a meaningful whole. In doing this the learner has arrived at an insightful conclusion on his or her own. The field theorists view the person as operating in a field of forces where internal forces (attitudes, feelings, needs of the individual) are interacting with external forces (the environment as perceived by the individual). The challenge to the optometrist in applying this theory is to learn the nature of both the internal and the external forces for any individual child so that the most appropriate elements can be emphasized or modified to facilitate learning. Finally, the cognitive theorists view learning as an exercise in problem solving, in which the optometrist must structure the environment so that the child has a problem to solve (21).

For optometrists who usually work with children on a short-term basis, these theories may have limited relevance. The most important point, however, is the emphasis on the child operating in a total environment. If any changes are to be affected for the good of the child, it is critical to view the child as functioning in a variety of settings (fields): home, school, playground, optometrist's office, community, each of which must be taken into account when attempting to modify an undesirable behavior. Some easily distracted children are drawn to irrelevant stimuli in their fields (they are field dependent). Others ignore irrelevant stimuli (they are field independent). For field-dependent children, the optometrist must restructure the field to reduce the number of irrelevant stimuli so that they can focus on the elements that enable learning to take place or behavior to change.

Suggested Readings

Any introductory text on educational psychology provides more detailed information. The following include an illustrative text and a reference written in interesting lay language.

Lindgren HC: Educational Psychology in the Classroom, 6th ed. New York, Oxford University Press, 1980.
Pryor K: Don't Shoot the Dog! The New Art of Teaching and Training. New York, Bantam Books, 1985.

REFERENCES

1. Barraga N: Visual Handicaps and Learning. Austin TX, Educational Resources, 1983.
2. Bloom L, Lahey M: Language Development and Language Disorders. New York, John Wiley, 1978.
3. Carroll JL, Rest JR: Moral Development. In Wolman BB, Striker G (eds): Handbook of Developmental Psychology. Englewood Cliffs NJ, Prentice-Hall, 1982.
4. Erikson EH: Childhood and Society, 2nd ed. New York, WW Norton, 1963.

5. Erikson EH: Identity: Youth and Crisis. New York, WW Norton, 1968.

6. Gesell A, Ilg FL: The Child from Five to Ten. New York, Harper & Brothers, 1946.

7. Ginsburg H, Opper S: Piaget's Theory of Intellectual Development: An Introduction. Englewood Cliffs NJ, Prentice-Hall, 1969.

8. Goldenson RM, Dunham JR, Dunham CS: Disability and Rehabilitation Handbook. New York, McGraw-Hill, 1978.

9. Grossman HJ (ed): Manual on Terminology and Classification in Mental Retardation. Washington, American Association on Mental Deficiency, 1983.

10. Hall CS: A Primer of Freudian Psychology. New York, World, 1954.

11. Hall A, Scholl G, Swallow R-M: Psychoeducational Assessment. In Scholl G (ed): Foundations of Education for Blind and Visually Handicapped Children and Youth: Theory and Practice. New York, American Foundation for the Blind, 1986.

12. Havighurst RJ: Human Development and Education. New York, David McKay, 1953.

13. Havighurst RJ: Developmental Tasks and Education. New York, David McKay, 1972.

14. Hendrick J: The Whole Child: Early Education for the Eighties, 3rd ed. St. Louis, Times Mirror/Mosby, 1984.

15. Kagan J: The Nature of the Child. New York, Basic Books, 1984.

16. Kagan J, Coles R (ed): Twelve to Sixteen: Early Adolescence. New York, WW Norton, 1971.

17. Kirk S, Chalfont J: Academic and Developmental Learning Disabilities. Denver, Love, 1984.

18. Kirk SA, Gallagher JJ: Educating Exceptional Children. Boston, Houghton Mifflin, 1986.

19. Kohlberg L: The Philosophy of Moral Development: Moral Stages and the Idea of Justice. New York, Harper & Row, 1981.

20. Krogman WM: Child Growth. Ann Arbor, University of Michigan Press, 1972.

21. Lindgren HC: Educational Psychology in the Classroom, 6th ed. New York, Oxford University Press, 1980.

22. Miller PH: Theories of Developmental Psychology. San Francisco, WH Freeman, 1983.

23. Noam GG, Higgins RC, Goethals GW: Psychoanalytic Approaches to Developmental Psychology. In Wolman BB, Striker G (eds): Handbook of Developmental Psychology. Englewood Cliffs NJ, Prentice-Hall, 1982.

24. Osol A (ed): Blakiston's Gould Medical Dictionary, 3rd ed. New York, McGraw-Hill, 1972.

25. Pearson GHJ: Psychoanalysis and the Education of the Child. New York, WW Norton, 1954.

26. Piaget J: Intelligence and Affectivity: Their Relationship during Child Development. Palo Alto, CA, Annual Reviews, 1981.

27. Quigley SP, Kretschmer RE: The Education of Deaf Children. Baltimore, University Park Press, 1982.

28. Siegel O: Personality Development in Adolescence. In Wolman BB, Stricker BB (eds): Handbook of Developmental Psychology. Englewood Cliffs NJ, Prentice-Hall, 1982.

29. Thompson C: Psychoanalysis: Evolution and Development. New York, Hermitage House, 1950.

30. US Department of Health, Education, and Welfare: Federal Register: Education of Handicapped Children. Washington, USDHEW, August 23, 1977.

31. White BL: The First Three Years of Life. New York, Prentice-Hall Press, 1985.

32. Zieziula FR: Assessment of Hearing-Impaired People: A Guide for Selecting Psychological, Educational, and Vocational Tests. Washington, Gallaudet College Press, 1982.

Chapter 2

Optical Components of the Eye: Embryology and Postnatal Development

Jacob G. Sivak

William R. Bobier

This chapter discusses the optical components of the eye in terms of embryology and growth during the early years of life. The mechanisms that coordinate this development are not fully understood, and only when they are can we confidently define our clinical models. For example, optical correction to prevent strabismus and amblyopia reflects the need of the visual system to receive clear and balanced retinal images early during its development (see Chap. 3); yet it may not be desirable to prescribe full correction at this stage, as some problems could self-correct through emmetropization (see below). Only with an understanding of these fundamental processes can the appropriate clinical trials be conducted to determine when and by how much early refractive errors should be corrected.

OCULAR EMBRYOLOGY OF THE HUMAN EYE AND ITS RELEVANCE TO OPTICAL FUNCTION

Embryonic Development of the Human Eye

Two of the three main germinal tissues (ectoderm and mesoderm) form the human eye (8, 27). This includes both the surface and neural ectoderm. The ectodermal structures of the eye are formed through a common process of differential growth that is exemplified by early separation of the neural ectoderm from its surface relation. Here we see the rapid growth of surface tissue along the two sides of the upper embryonic midline. Two bulges—the neural crests—form a groove, which later becomes a tube as the crests grow toward each other. Finally, the tube (the dorsal hollow nerve cord) is separated from the surface (Fig. 2.1).

Formation of a neural tube leads to the formation of the earliest components of the brain, the forebrain, midbrain, and hindbrain. The neural ectoderm components of the eye develop from the bilateral outgrowths of the forebrain. Even before the neural tube is completely closed, two depressions (the optic pits) are visible in the developing forebrain. With further rapid growth, these pits become vesicles (pouches). Later, with still more growth, the outer wall of each vesicle collapses inward, or invaginates, to form the optic cup. This is the first indication of the spherical eye shape that we are accustomed to seeing. The embryonic eye is at this stage connected to the forebrain by way of an optic stalk. The invagination of the optic vesicle to form the cup results in the formation of

two tissue layers, one on top of the other. A ventral slit in the cup, the embryonic fissure, permits vascular contact with the inner structures of the cup; later, the fissure disappears.

The two layers of the cup eventually form all of the retina and parts of the ciliary body (including the musculature system that serves to control the shape or position of the lens) and the iris (see Fig. 2.1). The outer layer of the retinal portion of the cup (the layer closest to the optic stalk) remains a relatively simple structure consisting of a single layer of epithelial cells, the retinal pigmented epithelium. As its name suggests, this layer is pigmented: it helps to form the dark chamber needed for vision. The retinal pigmented epithelium also plays a role in the turnover of visual pigment of the specialized photoreceptor cells of the retina, rods and cones.

The inner layer of the optic cup (the layer closest to the center of the developing eye) becomes an elaborate neural structure known as the neural retina. This layer differentiates extensively before birth into a region of three main cell layers—a layer of rods and cones (the layer closest to the pigmented epithelium); a middle layer, the bipolar cell layer; and the innermost layer, the ganglion cell layer. These three neural layers form an interneuron network that is every bit as complex as the brain, the structure from which it develops directly. It is the nerve axons of the ganglion cells that form the optic nerve, the structure that carries visual information from the retina to the brain. The human retina is an inverted one. Light must travel through much of the retina before reaching the receptors, the rods and cones. At the fovea, a central retinal depression that represents the portion of the retina responsible for high-resolution vision and color vision, the ganglion and bipolar cell layers are diverted laterally and horizontally so that light hits the receptors (cones) directly.

The anterior region of the optic cup, the region adjacent to the lip of the cup, develops further to form the sphincter and dilator muscles of the iris and a deeply pigmented layer of cells on the inner surface of the iris. This

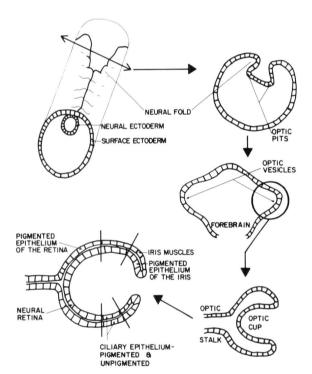

Figure 2.1 Neural ectoderm development of the eye showing the development of a dorsal hollow nerve cord and the optic cup.

layer, the pigmented epithelium of the iris, is partly responsible for the ability of the iris to control the amount of light entering the eye.

The region of the optic cup between the developing retina and the iris eventually forms the inner lining of the ciliary body. These two layers of the cup remain single layers of epithelial cells. The innermost layer remains unpigmented, whereas the layer below it (the layer that is continuous with the pigmented epithelium of the retina) also becomes pigmented.

Thus, the neural ectoderm produces all of the retina and the optic nerve and also parts of the ciliary body and iris. The rest of the ciliary body and iris develop from mesodermal tissue—the blood vessels of both structures and the actual muscle of the ciliary body, the muscle that is responsible for accommodation.

It should be noted that all ocular structures develop simultaneously. Descriptions that specify the development of one or other germinal tissues at one time do so for convenience only. Thus, while the optic cup is developing from the forebrain, a similar change is taking place in the surface ectoderm opposite the open lips of the developing optic cups (Fig. 2.2). First, the cells of the surface ectoderm thicken to form a structure known as the lens placode. Rapid growth in this region results in the invagination of the surface cells to form a lens vesicle, which ultimately separates from the surface to form a hollow spherical vesicle. The walls of this vesicle consist of a single layer of epithelial cells. Because of the inward invagination, the basement membrane of these cells is found around the outside of the vesicle. The lumen of the lens vesicle is slowly filled by elongation of the cells that form the posterior hemisphere of the original vesicle. These are known as the primary lens fibers, the embryonic nucleus of the lens (see Fig. 2.2). The lens continues to grow before and after birth. Subsequent growth (after the laying down of the primary lens fibers) takes place around the equator of the embryonic lens. New cells grow over the old fibers to form the secondary lens fibers (Fig. 2.2). A single layer of

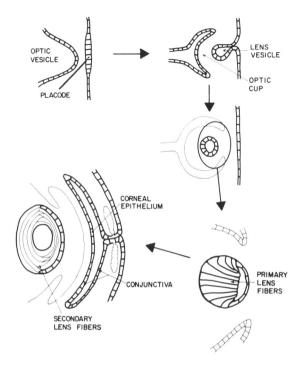

Figure 2.2 Surface ectoderm development of the eye emphasizing the formation of the lens.

cells, the lens epithelium, is left on the front surface. The basement membrane thickens and becomes the lens capsule. This capsule is, until later years, an elastic and acellular structure that plays a role in determining the shape of the lens during accommodation. Thus, the origin of the entire lens is surface ectoderm.

The mesodermal structures of the eye are formed mainly around the developing optic cup. First, a vascular and pigmented layer of mesodermal tissue is laid down to form a continuous vascular region known as the uvea (Table 2.1). The uveal tract consists of the choroid (which supplies the metabolic needs of the retinal rods and cones), the vascular and muscular part of the ciliary body, and the anterior vascular area of the iris. A second mesodermal layer of development overlies these vascular regions to form the fibrous, tough outer tunic of the eye, the sclera and the cornea. Eventually, mesodermal devel-

Table 2.1 ANATOMIC RELATIONSHIPS BETWEEN COMPONENTS OF THE OPTIC CUP AND THE UVEA

Tissue (Source)	Retina and Choroid	Ciliary Body	Iris
Optic cup (neural ectoderm)	Neural retina	Unpigmented epithelium	Pigmented epithelium
	Retinal pigmented epithelium	Pigmented epithelium	Muscles
Uvea (mesoderm)	Stroma of the choroid Epichoroid	Stroma of the ciliary body Ciliary muscle	Iris stroma

opment forms other orbital structures, such as the extraocular muscles, orbital bones, and the bulk of the eyelids.

A temporary embryonic vascular network, the hyaloid circulation, enters the optic cup from the mesodermal tissues around it through the embryonic fissure. This circulation supplies the early developing lens. Eventually, the hyaloid circulation disintegrates, often leaving behind debris. With new growth it becomes the true retinal circulation. As the embryonic fissure closes, the hyaloid vessels move to the region of the optic stalk. The growth of ganglion cell axons during the formation of the optic nerve traps the major artery and vein of the hyaloid. These vessels become the central retinal artery and central retinal vein.

The last major ocular development involves further rapid growth and invagination of the surface ectoderm. This results in the formation of the epithelium of the cornea (which joins the mesodermal part of the cornea), the conjunctiva (an epithelial cell layer, which lines the eyelids and is reflected back onto the surface of the eyeball to join with the corneal epithelium), and the glands of the eyelids.

Cornea and Crystalline Lens

The cornea and the crystalline lens are the two optical elements responsible for focusing an image on the retina. Both the cornea and the lens have the same basic problem—maintaining adequate conditions for living tissue while being part of a sophisticated optical in-

strument. Thus, both structures have evolved metabolic processes which are adequate for nonvascular conditions. Anatomically, both structures exhibit adaptations designed to minimize light scatter, but despite these and other obvious similarities, fundamental differences in embryonic development, location, and function have far-reaching consequences for ocular health.

Corneal Anatomy and Development

The cornea can be described as a collagen sandwich with epithelial tissue on both sides (8, 14). The external layer, the epithelium, consists of stratified squamous epithelial cells approximately five cell layers thick.

A mitotic basal layer of columnar cells rests on a basement membrane, whereas the superficial squamous layer is subject to a process of erosion, or sloughing. The full regenerative cycle takes about 7 days. The fact that corneal epithelial cells adhere tightly to one another by means of desmosomes and other junctional devices minimizes intercellular space and potential light scatter. Unlike the epidermis, the external and internal epithelial surfaces are relatively smooth and parallel to one another.

The innermost layer of the cornea, the endothelium, consists of a single layer of epithelial cells. In the adult eye, the endothelial cells do not exhibit a measurable regenerative cycle (14). The rest of the cornea—Bowman's membrane, stroma, and Descemet's membrane—is made up of collagen fibers. The few cells, mainly fibroblasts, are far apart. In the stroma, the collagen fibers are uniformly thick and are arranged parallel to the corneal surface. The characteristic regularity of interfiber spacing is commonly believed to produce destructive light interference, a prerequisite for corneal transparency. The corneal stroma has a very slow rate of turnover, if any (34).

The cornea starts out as a single layer of surface ectoderm cells, which reforms over the developing eye when the surface attachment of the lens vesicle has disappeared (14). These cells are joined by an internal layer of mesodermal material, which develops in concert with the condensation of mesodermal tissue around the optic cup. These cells, Descemet's mesothelium, ultimately produce the corneal endothelium and Descemet's membrane. Meanwhile, the surface layer becomes two cells thick. A second mesodermal formation develops between the cells of the surface ectoderm and the mesothelium. This tissue will form the stroma. The final multilayered structure of the surface ectoderm, the epithelium, will develop at the same time.

Lens Anatomy and Development

Lens anatomy is also characterized by regularity of structure (14), but the lens is completely cellular. A single layer of epithelial cells covers its anterior surface, and extremely elongated cells (fibers) fill the interior, extending to its posterior surface. The lens fibers are arranged in concentric shells of increasing diameter (46).

The lens fibers contain relatively few organelles, and those in the central core lack nuclei. This adaptation is undoubtedly related to the need for transparency. The fibers are intricately interconnected by means of numerous ball-and-socket articulations, which produce a highly ordered geometric pattern (46). The tight articulation between fibers reduces interfiber space and minimizes light scatter (14).

The early stages of lens development coincide with optic cup development (27, 42, 46); whereas the cup develops as an outpouching of the neural ectoderm, forming the early forebrain, the lens forms as an invagination of the surface ectoderm. The surface invagination is pinched off from the surface to form a hollow spherical vesicle in the optic cup. The posterior cells of the vesicle elongate to fill the vesicle, forming the primary lens fibers. The epithelial cells at the lens equator continue to undergo cell division before birth and throughout life (14). The new equatorial cells elongate toward the anterior and posterior lens poles, the anterior extension traveling underneath the original epithelial surface. These cells are the secondary lens fibers. Their size, shape, and interconnections determine the ultimate size and shape of the lens (38).

Location and Optical Function

Cornea

The cornea is an external ocular structure and represents the optical interface between the eye and the external environment (Fig. 2.3). The external and internal corneal surfaces are roughly parallel, so the *refractive* function of the cornea is determined by the difference between the refractive index of the medium in front of the cornea and the medium behind it (37). The latter, aqueous humor, has a refractive index (1.335) very close to that of water (1.333), so when the eye is in water, corneal refractive power is virtually nil. This is true despite the fact that the overall refractive index of the cornea (1.376) is somewhat greater than that of water.

In view of the aquatic habitat of early vertebrates, it is clear that the original function

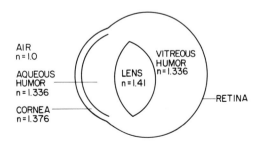

Figure 2.3 Schematic representation of the eye indicating the refractive index of the lens and cornea.

of the cornea was to provide a transparent window (37). This is reflected in the optical anatomy of modern fishes and aquatic mammals, whose lenses, the only refractive element of the eye, are spherical and have a very high refractive index (37). When the eye is in air, the refractive contribution of the cornea is considerable because of the disparity in refractive indices (air and aqueous humor). In fact, the refractive power of the human cornea is much greater than that of the lens (6).

The external location of the cornea is important for another reason. The epithelium of the cornea is the only corneal component that undergoes a significant regenerative cycle. Basal columnar cells reach the surface as squamous cells in approximately 7 days and are sloughed off to the external environment in a manner identical to the regenerative process of the epidermis. Thus, older cells are not retained.

Lens

The fact that the lens is located within the eye and that it is composed of cells of surface origin that continue to multiply throughout life has created a unique set of problems. First, because the lens is surrounded by a liquid or nearly liquid medium (see Fig. 2.3), its refractive function depends on the existence of a refractive index (the equivalent refractive index of the human lens is given as 1.41) considerably greater than that of water or corneal tissue (6). The cells of the lens have the highest concentration of protein of any body cells, presumably an adaptation to the need for a high refractive index.

Second, the internal location of the lens, coupled with the peripheral development and growth of new fibers around the equator, means that old lens tissue must be retained. In fact, the pattern of lens growth compresses older tissue toward the center. The result is a lens with a refractive index gradient, which is maximal at the center and minimal at the periphery. This gradient has the important optical consequence of helping to minimize lens spherical aberration (37).

A final point to be mentioned here is that the lens has the important function of providing the eye with a variable focal mechanism, accommodation. In humans, accommodative change in lens shape takes place in response to neural directives given to the ciliary muscle-zonule apparatus. The shape of the lens of a person in a modern urban setting may change hundreds of times each day.

The embryologic descriptions provided here make it possible to understand why the crystalline lens is the most fragile and sensitive of the two optical components of the eye, despite the fact that the external location of the cornea makes it very susceptible to mechanical damage. The high protein content of the lens creates potential molecular instability, which leads to cataract (opacification) when the lens is exposed to certain chemical agents or forms of electromagnetic radiation. The loss of accommodation with age, presbyopia, is an important consequence related to lens development and aging. In addition, age-related changes associated with continued lens growth and development lead to a variety of age-related cataract conditions. Finally, it is possible to understand why current estimates indicate that 95 percent of lenses of persons over age 65 years show cataractous change (46).

OPTICAL DEVELOPMENT DURING THE FIRST 6 YEARS

The embryonic development of the eye follows a genetically determined program which continues after birth. At this point, visual experiences appear to exert a significant influence on development.

The Gullstrand Eye

The optical components of the adult eye have been defined in several schematic, or model, eyes. Owing to the importance of such models in the study of vision, schematic eyes have been constructed by such eminent vision scientists as Helmholtz, Listing, Tscherning, and Gullstrand. A widely accepted model of the optical components consists of modifications made by Emsley to an earlier model of Gullstrand's. The parameters of this schematic have been accepted as being representative of the adult eye (Table 2.2).

Originally, the measurements were taken in vitro from enucleated eyes. Such measurements can differ from those in vivo because of blood flow reduction and artifacts arising from the preparation. Recently, ultrasonography has allowed axial distances and component thickness to be measured in vivo. The radii of curvature of the cornea and lens have also been determined in the living eye using the Purkinje-Sanson images. Only the refractive indices of the ocular media must today be determined from preparations in vitro.

A Schematic Eye of the Newborn

The optical components of the eye of a newborn differ from those of an adult. Our present difficulty is in accurately detailing the differences for each component and in charting the changes with growth. For some of the required measurements there is simply no data. Ultrasonography has provided measurements in vivo of axial length and of thickness and separation of the optical components during development. These measurements, such as those taken by Larsen (20–23), are shown in Figure 2.4 and are discussed in greater detail below.

Lotmar (24) developed a schematic eye for the newborn from photographic measurements of seven neonate eyes in vitro taken by Pflugk in 1909. The axial distances were verified with three sets of recent ultrasonographic measurements of neonates. The anterior corneal curvature measurements were replaced with more recent ones made on intact eyes of five newborns by Mandell (23). In order to complete the Gullstrand model, a refractive error of +2.4 D was selected from consideration of three reports of retinoscopic measurements of newborns (9, 15, 32). The refractive indices were given values similar to those of the adult Gullstrand model, except that the lens was given a value of 1.43 D so that the resulting overall refractive error would be +2.4 D. Lotmar's values appear in Table 2.2 beside those for the (adult) Gullstrand-Emsley eye.

It must be recognized that the neonatal values can only be approximate. They were

Table 2.2   A COMPARISON OF THE ADULT AND INFANT GULLSTRAND SCHEMATIC EYE

	Symbol	Adult	Infant
Quantity			
Anterior corneal surface	r_1	7.80 mm	6.8 mm
Crystalline lens (anterior)	r_2	10.00 mm	5.0 mm
Crystalline lens (posterior)	r_3	−6.00 mm	−3.7 mm
Spacing			
Anterior chamber depth	d_1	3.60 mm	2.6 mm
Crystalline lens	d_2	3.60 mm	3.7 mm
Depth of vitreous	d_3	16.69 mm	11.0 mm
Axial length		23.89 mm	17.3 mm
Indices of refraction			
Air	n_1	1.00	1.00
Aqueous humor	n_2	1.333	1.336
Crystalline	n_3	1.4160	1.43
Vitreous	n_4	1.333	1.334
Equivalent power		60.486 D	85.3 D
Refractive error		0.00 D	+2.40 D

taken from several different studies and, so, from different subjects. No empirical measures could be provided for the indices of refraction. The value of 1.43 for the lens could seem somewhat unlikely, as it would be expected that with growth the continued compression of the lens tissue would show a greater rather than a smaller index of refraction in adulthood, but values of this magnitude and greater have been reported (44) and they may be a consequence of a smaller water content in infant lenses. Furthermore, since the lens does not in truth have a uniform refractive index, the effective value of the Gullstrand model would also reflect shape differences (see below) between adult's and newborn's lenses.

Importantly, however, Lotmar's model provides a means by which the changes in optical components between birth and adulthood can be analyzed (see Table 2.2). Clearly, axial length increases by approximately 6 mm. Even though the neonate's eye is hyperopic, its equivalent power must be greater (85 D) than that of the adult (60 D) in order to offset the shorter axial length.

It is worthwhile considering what the result would be if the cornea and lens tissues failed to reduce their refractive power with development. The increase in axial length would render the average adult 25 D myopic. Given the rarity of such errors, it would appear that a complete breakdown in the coordination between the optical components and axial length is rare.

Growth of the Eye

Changes in the eye's axial length and the separation and thickness of the optical components of the eye can be determined by ultrasonography at various stages of development. Data on the growth of the axial dimensions of the eye have been gathered in vivo and in vitro over the past 100 years. To provide a coherent discussion of the magnitudes of these changes we have selected the comprehensive study in vivo using ultrasonography by Larsen (20–23). It should be noted that exact axial lengths differ between studies, re-

flecting variances in individual subjects and techniques. (So the values presented below differ somewhat from those of Lotmar's schematic eye in Table 2.1.) The pattern of changes is, however, consistent between studies, so it seems unnecessary to provide

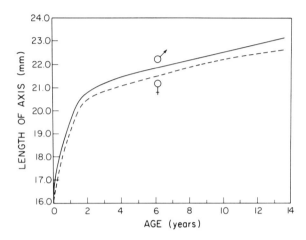

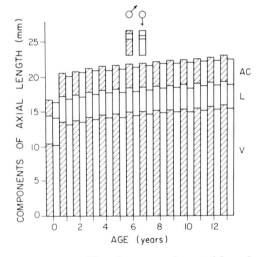

Figure 2.4(A) The change in the axial length of the eye during the first 13 or 14 years or life as measured with ultrasound. **(B)** The relative axial length of the anterior chamber (*AC*), lens (*L*), and vitreous (*V*) during 13 years of growth of the eye. (From Larsen JS: The sagittal growth of the eye. IV. Ultrasonic measurement of the axial length of the eye from birth to puberty. Acta Ophthalmol 49:882, 1971.)

an exhaustive list from all studies. An example of the overall pattern of development will illustrate the point.

Axial Length

Larsen (20) used ultrasonography to measure the axial length of the eyes of 846 infants and children aged from birth to 13 years (see Fig. 2.4A). His results show axial growth to be most rapid during the first 2 years of life when an increase of 3.8 mm is realized. Between the ages of 2 and 5 years the rate of growth is reduced (1.2 mm is added) and a slow progression up to 13 years provides another 1.4 mm. Gender differences are found where the axial lengths for boys are consistently greater than for girls at all ages. Also boys showed a greater overall change (16.78 to 23.15 mm) compared to girls (16.4 to 22.66 mm). This pattern of axial growth is consistent with other ultrasonographic studies although absolute measurements may vary within 1 to 2 mm [see (9, 12, 25)].

Vitreal Chamber

From consideration of Table 2.2, where adult and neonatal schematic eyes are compared, it would be expected that the greatest increase in axial length occurs in the vitreal chamber. This appears to be true during all stages of development: the proportion of axial length that constitutes vitreous is 62.5 percent at birth, 67 percent at 4 to 5 years, and 69.5 percent at 13 to 14 years (see Figure 2.4B). Larsen (20) found that after the age of 3 years, axial growth depends almost exclusively on an increase in the length of the vitreous. Further, he showed a high correlation between refractive state and vitreal length: myopia is associated with a long vitreal chamber and hyperopia with a short one (21).

Lens and Anterior Segment

Early anatomists (summarized in Wolff, 40) concluded that the lens of the newborn is spherical. With growth the anterior and posterior surfaces of the lens flatten (Table 2.2) to the conoid shape found in the adult eye. Larsen (22) found that the axial length of the lens decreases by 0.5 to 0.7 mm from birth to

13 years (a typical value at birth is approximately 3.9 mm). The anterior chamber increases in depth approximately 1.4 mm from birth to puberty. Three phases were identified (23). During the first 18 months, there was rapid growth (0.9 to 1.0 mm) followed by a slower phase of growth (0.3 to 0.4 mm over years one through seven) and a slow juvenile phase (0.1 mm from 8 to 13 years). The increase in depth at age 5 and thereafter is attributed to flattening of the anterior surface of the lens (20). Sivak and Dovrat (39) have recently found that this flattening is in fact initiated well before birth (between the fourth and fifth month of embryonic development). Larsen (23) found, as with the vitreous, that there was a strong correlation between anterior chamber length and refraction—the chamber was deeper in myopic than in hyperopic eyes.

Although this discussion has been limited to axial length changes with growth, it should be recognized that the eye grows in all dimensions (Fig. 2.5).

Changes in Refractive State

The changes in refractive state that occur from birth through the first 4 to 6 years of life normally follow a pattern, which has been

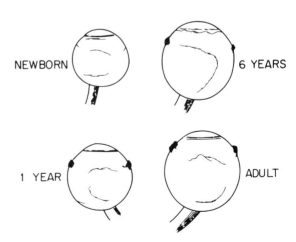

Figure 2.5 The growth of the eye after birth. (From Wolff E: Anatomy of the Eye and Orbit, 7th ed. London, HK Lewis, 1976.)

termed emmetropization. The magnitude and variance of refractive errors decline with age. Therefore, the optical components of the eye not only correct for growth but also adjust error to null, or at least reduce it (see Chap. 6).

Spherical Error

A considerable number of studies have measured the refractive state of the newborn. Banks (5) reviewed this literature. Most of these studies were, understandably, conducted with retinoscopy following the administration of a cycloplegic, although measures using ophthalmoscopy and noncycloplegic retinoscopy were also reported. Banks concluded that the refractive state of newborns shows a normal distribution with a mean of +2 D of hyperopia and a standard deviation of 2 D. Banks (5) reports that there is general agreement that hyperopia diminishes during infancy and childhood. Hirsch (13) presented data indicating that between birth and 6 to 8 years of age there is a reduction of 1 D of hyperopia and a reduction in the standard deviation from 2.73 D to 1.62 D. These results are shown graphically in Figure 2.6. It can be seen that with age the form of the distribution becomes increasingly leptokurtic at lower degrees of hyperopia. The range of refractions is reduced with age, giving rise to a smaller standard deviation. This leptokurtic distribution persists in adulthood, when the mode approaches emmetropia (40).

The Small-Eye Error   There is strong evidence that some of the hyperopia found in infants and children is a measurement artifact arising from the likelihood that in infancy (and throughout most of adulthood) the primary source of the retinoscopic reflex lies not at the plane of the receptors but at the vitreoretinal border (10, 16, 28, 29). This discrepancy will show a larger dioptric error as the axial length of the eye decreases. Specifically, the error is proportional to the inverse of the square of the focal length (10). By assuming that the focal length of the eye is a constant proportion of its axial length the extent of this error at birth has been estimated

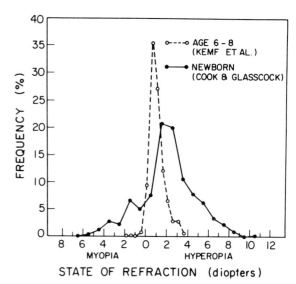

Figure 2.6 Emmetropization. With age the magnitude and variance of refractive errors decline. This process is illustrated in data from newborns and from a population of 6- to 8-year-olds. (From Hirsch MJ: The refraction of children. In Hirsch MJ, Wick RE (eds): Vision of Children. Philadelphia, Chilton Books, 1963.)

to range from 0.50 to 0.80 D (5, 16) when data from ultrasonographic measurements are considered. The error would reduce to nearly the adult level (approximately 0.37 D) by 9 months of age (16). So this error may overestimate the hyperopia, but it does not appear to explain completely the early appearance of hyperopia.

Astigmatism

Over the past decade the pattern of change in astigmatism during the first 5 years of life has been studied on infant populations in the United States and Great Britain. A consistent finding is that astigmatism is greatest during the first year of life and declines with age (2, 7, 11, 16, 18, 31). The results of a longitudinal study of 20 infants (2) conducted in the United Kingdom by Atkinson and coworkers are shown in Figure 2.7. Astigmatism was measured over the first 2 years of life. The dotted line indicates an average value

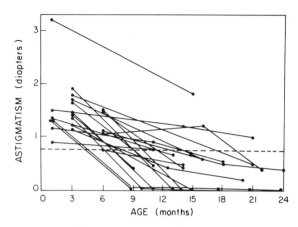

Figure 2.7 The changes in astigmatism in 20 British infants measured over the first 2 years of life. The astigmatism for each eye was determined and the mean value was plotted. The dotted line represents average adult astigmatism. (From Atkinson J, Braddick O, French J: Infant astigmatism: Its disappearance with age. Vision Res 20:891, 1980.)

(0.75 D) from a sample of adults. It is apparent that astigmatism in the first 6 months is greater than in the adult population, but there is a dramatic decline in the magnitude of the error by 18 months, when the vast majority of children have astigmatic errors no greater than those of the adult population.

The rapid decline in astigmatism during the first year of life was also observed by Mohindra and coworkers (31) in an infant population in the United States. In this group astigmatism declined more rapidly than in Atkinson's group: it appeared to peak at 11 to 20 weeks and then showed a steep decline by 5 to 6 months. Howland (16) reported that the rate of reduction of astigmatism for a population of infants in New York State was slower than that found by Atkinson and associates (2). These studies consistently show that astigmatism is reduced, but the rate of reduction presumably differs among individuals.

Is there any pattern to the major astigmatism meridians? That is, does infant astigmatism predominate in one particular form, say with-the-rule as opposed to against-the-rule.

Atkinson and Braddick (1) compared measures from refractive screenings of infants at 6 to 12 months taken in three separate locations in Britain. No single type of astigmatism predominated. One population showed more with-the-rule, whereas another showed more against-the-rule astigmatism; however, the major axes were more frequently along the vertical and horizontal meridians than the oblique meridians.

Atkinson and Braddick (1) identified infants in their 6- to 12-month-old population who were compound hyperopic astigmats where at least one meridian was +3.50 D or greater. When these infants were followed up (3) the rate of reduction of the astigmatism did vary between the differing forms. With-the-rule hyperopic astigmatism reduced significantly faster than oblique or against-the-rule types. The slowest rate of reduction was found for against-the-rule astigmatism; a preponderance of this form was found in the 1½- to 3-year-old subjects.

Three groups in the United States have studied changes in infant astigmatism over the first 5 years of life (7, 11, 18). Their results were summarized by Howland and Sayles (18) and are shown below in Table 2.3. In the main, these findings agree with the British groups: There is a steady decline in astigmatism with age and a greater frequency of against-the-rule astigmatism during the first 3 to 4 years.

Howland and Sayles (19) found that total astigmatism correlated strongly with corneal astigmatism (measured with photokeratoscopy) up to age 3 years. Astigmatism measured from 3 to 5 years showed little relationship with corneal measurements. For this population, at least, it was concluded that the astigmatism found in the first 2 years of life was primarily corneal.

Emmetropization and Its Clinical Implications

It would appear from this discussion that the growth of the eye is coordinated so that the optical components not only adjust to the increased axial length but refine their relationships during the early years of life, so that

Table 2.3 CHANGE IN ASTIGMATISM DURING THE FIRST 5 YEARS OF LIFE IN THREE POPULATIONS IN THE UNITED STATES

| | | | | Number of Subjects | | | |
| | | Cylinder | | For cylinder > 1 D | | | |
Study	Age Group (yr)	<1 D	>1 D	With-the-Rule	Against-the-Rule	Oblique	Total
Howland and Sayles	0–0.5	29	38	1	20	17	67
(18)	0.5–1.5	55	46	1	33	12	101
Noncycloplegic	1.5–2.5	14	7	0	5	2	21
Photorefraction	2.5–3.5	45	2	0	2	0	47
	3.5–4.5	59	8	0	6	2	67
	4.5–5.5	36	6	1	5	0	42
Dobson (7)	0–0.5		8	0	8	0	8
Cycloplegic	0.5–1.5		34	8	25	1	34
Retinoscopy	1.5–2.5		11	3	4	4	11
	2.5–3.5		26	9	13	4	26
	3.5–4.5		39	18	11	10	39
	4.5–5.5		44	20	15	9	44
Gwiazda (11)	0–0.5	205	235	89	111	35	440
Noncycloplegic	0.5–1.5	64	46	16	22	8	110
Retinoscopy	1.5–2.5	42	26	7	15	4	68
	2.5–3.5	88	32	10	20	2	120
	3.5–4.5	122	27	6	18	3	149
	4.5–5.5	77	20	11	9	1	97

Reprinted with permission from Howland HC, Sayles N: Photorefractive measurements of astigmatism. Invest Ophthalmol Vis Sci 25:99, 1984.

existing refractive errors are reduced. The mechanism by which this is achieved is not fully understood, so a cautious approach is needed in prescribing refractive corrections for children in this age group.

The coordination of the optical components of the eye with growth must fall into one of two general classifications. The process could be completely under genetic control and hence fully preprogrammed, or it may be self-correcting where genetic information may be influenced in part by the system's ability to recognize and correct imperfections. In the former case, the application of spectacles would not affect the reduction of ametropia. In the latter case, ophthalmic correction would reduce the "error" in the system and could, in principle, stop the emmetropization process.

Is there any evidence to guide our clinical approach here? There is some primarily from animal studies. The mechanism of emmetropization is undergoing considerable experimentation using such animals as chickens, tree shrews, cats, and monkeys (47). These studies show that emmetropization is influenced by visual experience. When the retinal image of experimental animals is degraded, emmetropization can break down. Studies show that an increase in axial myopia due to excessive vitreal chamber growth (36, 42) follows from image degradation or selective damage to retinal tissue (44). There is recent evidence that, at least in the chicken, the emmetropization process is sensitive to whether the retinal imagery is focused in front of or behind the retina and that there is an adjustment of the optical components in the appropriate direction (35).

No human study has been able to provide such a direct link between visual experience and emmetropization. However, there is evidence (33) that significant degrees of myopia can accompany various ocular anomalies which disrupt retinal imagery. Accepting that visual experience influences emmetropization does not necessarily imply that correcting infant refractive states will block their potential for emmetropization. It must be realized that the image degradations used in animal studies are extreme in comparison to most infants' blurred vision. Furthermore, uncertainty about emmetropization should not override the very important fact that prescribing spectacles for infants and children affords them clearly focused retinal images during a critical period in their development (see Chaps. 3 and 6). When, for example, astigmatism is not corrected during the first 6 years of life meridional amblyopia can arise (30). Recently Atkinson associates (3) showed that, in the first year of life, partial spectacle correction of hyperopia and hyperopic astigmatism (where one meridian was greater than +3.50 D) reduced acuity deficits during the preschool years. What is needed now are clinical models that define when and by how much a specific refractive state should be corrected.

SUMMARY

The major embryonic growth of the optical components of the eye is characterized by cell growth and differentiation of two embryonic tissues, ectoderm and mesoderm. The mechanism is programmed genetically and has been tested and refined by millions of years of evolution.

At birth the genetic program continues. The size of the eye increases most rapidly within the first 2 years of life. Axial lengthening does not result in an increase in myopia. The respective optical components adjust their refractive power. Ocular development is coordinated. Examination of the change in refractive state over the first 6 years of life shows they tend to stay within a narrow range and in fact both hyperopia and astigmatism decrease, a phenomenon referred to as emmetropization. Although postnatal developments are dictated genetically, evidence has been presented that the emmetropization process is also affected to some degree by visual experience.

It now remains for the science of pediatric optometry to develop clinical models to determine which types of refractive state need correction and which simply reflect the normal pattern of visual development.

ACKNOWLEDGMENTS

This chapter was written while WRB received support from the Natural Science and Engineering Research Council of Canada; JS was supported by the same and also by the Medical Research Council of Canada. We thank Dr. M.C. Campbell for helpful comments and Pat Anderson and Alison Zorian for preparation of the manuscript.

REFERENCES

1. Atkinson J, Braddick O: Vision screening and photorefraction. The relation of refractive errors to strabismus and amblyopia. Behav Brain Res 10:71, 1983.

2. Atkinson J, Braddick O, French J: Infant astigmatism: Its disappearance with age. Vision Res 20:891, 893, 1980.

3. Atkinson J, Braddick OJ, Wattam-Bell J, Durden K, Bobier W, Pointer J: Photorefractive screening of infants and effects of refractive correction. Invest Ophthalmol Vis Sci (Suppl) 28:399, 1987.

4. Atkinson J, Braddick OJ: Infant precursors of later visual disorders: correlation or causality. In: *20th Minnesota Symposium on Child Psychology.* A Yonas (ed) Hillsdale, NJ: Lawrence Erlbaum, 1988.

5. Banks M: Infant refraction and accommodation. Int Ophthalmol Clin 20:205, 1980.

6. Bennett AG, Francis JL: The eye as an optical system. In Davson H (ed). The Eye, vol. 4. Academic Press, New York, 101, 1962.

7. Dobson V, Fulton A, Lawson Sebiris S: Cycloplegic refractions of infants and young children: The axis of astigmatism. Invest Ophthalmol Vis Sci 25:83, 1984.

8. Duke-Elder S: System of ophthalmology. In

The Anatomy of the Visual System, vol II. London, Henry Kimpton, 901, 1958.

9. Gernet H: Achsenlange and Refraktion lebender Augen von Neugeborenen. Graefes Arch Ophthalmol 166:530, 1964.

10. Glickstein M, Millodot M: Retinoscopy and eye size. Science 168:605, 1970.

11. Gwiazda J, Scheiman M, Mohindia I, et al: Astigmatism in children: Changes in axis and amount from birth to six years. Invest Ophthalmol Vis Sci 25:88, 1984.

12. Hirano S, Yamamoto Y, Takayama H, et al: Ultrasonic observation of eyes in premature babies. Part 6. Growth curves of ocular axial length and its components. Acta Soc Ophthalmol Japon 83:1679, 1979.

13. Hirsch MJ: The refraction of children. In Hirsch MJ, Wick RE (eds): Vision of Children. Philadelphia, Chilton, 1963.

14. Hogan WJ, Alvarado JA, Weddel JE (eds): Histology of the Human Eye. Philadelphia, WB Saunders, 68, 1971.

15. Hosaka A: The significance of myopia in new born infants. In Solames, P (ed): XXI Conciliam Ophthalmologican Mexico 1970, Acta Pais I. Amsterdam, Excerpta Medica, 991, 1971.

16. Howland HC: Infant eyes: Optics and accommodation. Curr Eye Res 2:217, 1983.

17. Howland HC, Atkinson J, Braddick O, et al: Infant astigmatism measured by photorefraction. Science 202:331, 1978.

18. Howland HC, Sayles N: Photorefractive measurements of astigmatism in infants and young children. Invest Ophthalmol Vis Sci 25:93, 1984.

19. Howland HC, Sayles N: Photokeratometric and photorefractive measurements of astigmatism in infants and young children. Vision Res 25:73, 1985.

20. Larson JS: The sagittal growth of the eye. IV. Ultrasonic measurement of the axial length of the eye from birth to puberty. Acta Ophthalmol 49:872, 1971.

21. Larson JS: The sagittal growth of the eye. III. Ultrasonic measurement of the posterior segment (axial length of the vitreous) from birth to puberty. Acta Ophthalmol 49:441, 1971.

22. Larson JS: The sagittal growth of the eye. II.

Ultrasonic measurement of the axial diameter of the lens and anterior segment from birth to puberty. Acta Ophthalmol 49:427, 1971.

23. Larson JS: The sagittal growth of the eye I. Ultrasonic measurement of the depth of the anterior chamber from birth to puberty. Acta Ophthalmol 49:239, 1971.

24. Lotmar W: A theoretical model for the eye of new born infants. Graefes Arch Klin Exp Ophthalmol 198:179, 1976.

25. Luyckx J: Mesure des composantes optiques de l'oeil du nouveau-né par échographie ultrasonique. Arch Opthal (Paris) 26:159, 1966.

26. Mandell RB: Corneal contour of the human infant. Arch Opthalmol 77:345, 1967.

27. Mann I (ed): The Development of the Human Eye, 3rd ed. New York, Grune and Stratton, 316, 1969.

28. Millodot M: Reflection from the fundus of the eye and its relevance to retinoscopy. Atti Fond G Ronchi 28:31, 1972.

29. Millodot M, O'Leary D: The discrepancy between retinoscopic and subjective measurements: Effect of age. Am J Optom Physiol Opt 55:304, 1980.

30. Mitchell DE, Freeman RD, Millodot M, Haegerstrom G: Meridional amblyopia: evidence for modification of the human visual system by early experience. Vision Res 13:535, 1973.

31. Mohindra I, Held R, Gwiazda J: Astigmatism in infants. Science 202:329, 1978.

32. Molnar L: Refraktion sanderung des Auges im Laufe des Lebens. Klin Monatsbl Augenheilkd 156:326, 1970.

33. Rabin J, Van Slayters RC, Malach R: Emmetropization: a vision-dependent phenomena. Invest Ophthalmol Vis Sci 20:561, 1981.

34. Rodrigues MM, Waring III GO, Hackett J, et al: Cornea. In Jakobiec FA (ed.): Ocular Anatomy, Embryology and Teratology. Philadelphia, Harper and Row, 153, 1982.

35. Schaeffel F, Glasser A, Howland MC: Accommodation, refractive error and eye growth in chickens. Vision Res 28:639, 1988.

36. Seltner RL, Sivak JG: A role for the vitreous humor in experimentally-induced myopia. Am J Optom Physiol Opt 64:953, 1987.

37. Sivak JG: Optics of the crystalline lens. Am J Optom Physiol Opt 62:299, 1985.

38. Sivak JG: Optics of the amphibious eye in vertebrates. In Atema J, Fay RR, Popper AN (eds): Sensory Biology of Aquatic Animals. New York, Springer-Verlag, 468, 1988.

39. Sivak JG, Dovrat A: Embryonic lens of the human eye as an optical structure. Am J Optom Physiol Opt 64:599, 1987.

40. Sorsby A, Sheridan M, Leary GA: Vision visual acuity and ocular refraction of young men. Br Med J 1:1394, 1960.

41. Tripathi RC, Tripathi BJ: Morphology of the normal, aging and cataractous human lens. I. Development and morphology of the adult and aging lens. Lens Res 1:1, 1983.

42. Wallman J, Adams JI: Developmental aspects of experimental myopia in chicks: Susceptibility, recovery and relation to emmetropization. Vision Res 27:1139, 1987.

43. Weale RA: A Biography of the Eye. London, HK Lewis, 1982.

44. Wildsoet CF, Pettigrew JD: Kainic acid induced eye enlargement in chickens: Differential effects on anterior and posterior segments. Invest Ophthalmol 29:311, 1988.

45. Wolff E: Anatomy of the Eye and Orbit, 7th Ed. London, HK Lewis, 1976.

46. Worgul BV: Lens. In Jakobiec FA (ed): Ocular Anatomy, Embryology and Teratology. Philadelphia, Harper and Row, 355, 1982.

47. Yinon U: Myopia induction in animals following alteration of visual input during development: A review. Curr Eye Res 3:677, 1984.

Chapter 3

Normal Development of the Neural Pathways

Ross Beauchamp

Most important characteristics of the adult visual system are established before birth and several years thereafter, during which time the neurons of the retina and visual pathways differentiate and make their permanent synaptic connections. Among clinicians, interest in this formative period has been heightened by the knowledge that in the first 5 years of life, a child's developing nervous system may be influenced by the visual environment. The scope of this plasticity and the mechanisms underlying it are receiving widespread research attention today. New radioactive and metabolic labels for neurons have been especially useful in characterizing patterns of neural growth associated with normal vision and impaired vision.

In this chapter, normal development of the retina and visual pathways in humans is outlined. The reader should understand throughout that gaps in knowledge about the human nervous system must often be filled by extrapolating from animal research data. Readers who require more details than this brief account provides are encouraged to consult the many fine papers and reviews cited here, among them those of Movshon and Van Sluyters (87), Sherman and Spear (114), Mitchell and Timney (84), Boothe (20), Hickey and Peduzzi (54) and Lund (76). The approach of this chapter is to intersperse a brief review of the anatomy and physiology necessary to comprehend the themes under consideration with a fuller account of more current developments, especially those related to amblyopia, strabismus, myopia, and other visual dysfunctions that have a developmental component.

THE RETINA

Recent descriptions of infant human retinas (1, 134) have demonstrated a more extended period of immaturity after birth than was previously recognized (78). As we will document here, the entire retina, and particularly the fovea, continues to develop until age 4 or 5 years. The initial immaturity during the first year probably accounts for the reduced acuity and absence of central fixation often observed in infants. We first describe processes of prenatal retinal development and then changes that occur after birth.

Embryonic Period

Retinoblast Proliferation

During the first few months of gestation, the cells destined to become the neural elements of the retina are undifferentiated neuroblasts, or retinoblasts. Also out of the same population of cells will arise the glial elements of the retina, the Müller cells. At this stage, the undifferentiated neuroblasts divide rapidly, each division following a set sequence (G1 interphase, S phase, and G2 interphase) (58, 115). The mitotic cycle of a neuroblast has a rhythmic beauty as the cell's nucleus migrates back and forth within the elongated cell profile that spans the width of the incipient retina (Fig. 3.1).

For reasons not at all well understood at present, neuroblast cells at some point withdraw from the S phase and cease dividing. The precipitating conditions are likely biochemical, although the physical impediment to nucleus migration may sometimes be a factor, as when layers like the outer nuclear layer begin to form (103). In general, cytogenesis terminates first in the central retina, then a little later in the periphery, but in humans, cell division right across the retina is almost certainly over by birth (71, 77). That the undeveloped retina has its full complement of neural elements at birth is a fact of some significance. Postnatal growth of the retina must consist of redistribution of a stable cell population rather than a continuing increase in numbers of cells.

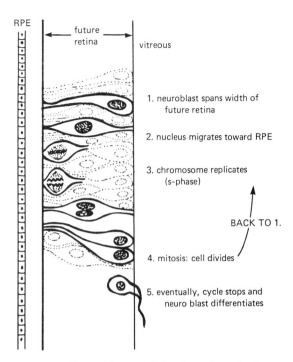

1. neuroblast spans width of future retina

2. nucleus migrates toward RPE

3. chromosome replicates (s-phase)

BACK TO 1.

4. mitosis: cell divides

5. eventually, cycle stops and neuro blast differentiates

Figure 3.1 Neuroblast proliferation: the mitotic cycle in embryonic retina. (After Farber D, Adler R: Issues and questions in cell biology of the retina. In: The Retina: A Model for Cell Biology Studies. Toronto, Academic Press, 1, 1986.)

Differentiation of Retinal Cells

Shortly after a neuroblast stops dividing, it migrates to a specific location in one of the developing layers and begins expressing characteristic differentiated properties. These include formation of dendrites and axons and acquisition of enzymes for neurotransmitter synthesis (79). By the time of birth, all retinal cells have established their identity (Fig. 3.2) as Müller cells or as one of the five neural cell types (rod or cone photoreceptors, horizontal, bipolar, amacrine, and ganglion cells). Also, the layers of the retina (photoreceptor, outer nuclear, outer plexiform, inner nuclear, inner plexiform, ganglion cell) have their adult form, at least in the periphery (see Fig. 3. 2). For details of retinal anatomy and physiology the reader may consult Rodieck (106) or Dowling (34).

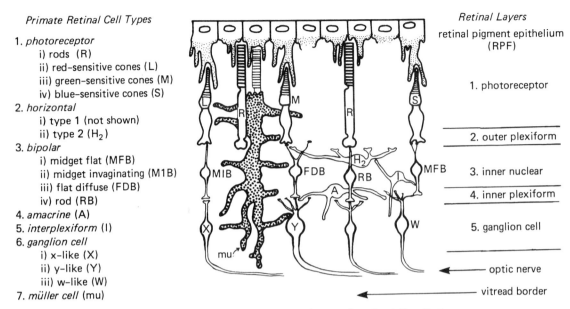

Primate Retinal Cell Types

1. *photoreceptor*
    i) rods (R)
    ii) red–sensitive cones (L)
    iii) green–sensitive cones (M)
    iv) blue–sensitive cones (S)
2. *horizontal*
    i) type 1 (not shown)
    ii) type 2 (H$_2$)
3. *bipolar*
    i) midget flat (MFB)
    ii) midget invaginating (M1B)
    iii) flat diffuse (FDB)
    iv) rod (RB)
4. *amacrine* (A)
5. *interplexiform* (I)
6. *ganglion cell*
    i) x–like (X)
    ii) y–like (Y)
    iii) w–like (W)
7. *müller cell* (mu)

Retinal Layers

retinal pigment epithelium (RPF)

1. photoreceptor

2. outer plexiform

3. inner nuclear

4. inner plexiform

5. ganglion cell

optic nerve

vitread border

Figure 3.2 Cell types and layers in postnatal retina (After Farber D, Adler R: Issues and questions in cell biology of the retina. In: The Retina: A Model for Cell Biology Studies. Toronto, Academic Press, 1, 1986.)

The process of differentiation from a neuroblast to a more specialized form begins at about 2 months' gestation and is complete by about the seventh month (35, 78). The Müller cells, about which too little is known (38), appear early as distinguishable elements, in keeping with the general rule that supportive tissues develop first to provide a sort of scaffold for later-arriving specialized tissues (78).

The ganglion cells are the first neural component to become visible under the light microscope (17-mm stage) and are the first completed layer (130-mm stage, at about 5 months) (35). Ganglion cells are generated first in the central retina and later in the periphery (113). Recent calculations indicate that there are about two ganglion cells for each cone in the central fovea out to about 2.5 degrees (110).

The photoreceptors are the last to differentiate completely, beginning at about the 48 to 65-mm stage, ending at the 170-mm stage or about 5½ months' gestation; cones come before rods. "Precursors" of photoreceptors seemingly may be identified earlier with appropriate stains, perhaps as early as ganglion cells (35). The nature and exact timing of the intracellular events underlying a "commitment" to a particular differentiated form are still not understood (38). In the interval between ganglion cell and photoreceptor differentiation, other cell types such as bipolars and amacrines arise in a species-specific sequence (89, 90, 121).

Subtypes of Retinal Cells

Of current research concern are the differentiation details of the many subtypes of cells found in the adult retina (see Fig. 3.2). In primate retina, there are three types of cone photoreceptors, red-, green-, and blue-absorbing (L, M, and S types, respectively) (4, 30), two types of horizontal cells (68, 74), three or more bipolars (67, 95), many amacrine cell types (69, 95), and three or more ganglion cell types (32, 33, 42, 93, 120). Should one or more of these retinal cell subtypes specialize only after birth, cell development would be subject to influence from the postnatal photic environment, a possibility that arouses great clinical interest.

A recent report suggests that in cats ganglion cell subtypes are present before birth (102). Alpha, beta, and gamma ganglion cell types (corresponding to Y, X, and W in the physiologic classification) could be distinguished from embryonic day 52 on (cat gestation is approximately 65 days), but the ganglion cell dendritic tree and axons often were not in the adult form, tending to be morphologically "exuberant." It remains to be seen whether the analogous ganglion cell types in primate retina are also discernible before birth.

Cell Death

In addition to proliferation and differentiation, a third process, cell death, has a strong influence on retinal topography during the embryonic period (73, 97). Most of the attrition seems to occur at the time of synaptogenesis, when cells are making contact with other cells (see reviews by Cunningham and Cowan et al) (24, 27). The scene is set for cell death during the proliferative phase, before differentiation begins, when dividing neuroblasts provide at least two to three times the number of cells required at birth. The final adult number of cells is reached only by wholesale cell death. The currently accepted theory of the mechanism of cell death holds that only those cells survive that make synaptic contact with appropriate target cells; the rest perish. For example, only ganglion cells whose axons reach the lateral geniculate nucleus (LGN), superior colliculus, or other postsynaptic center and make connections there survive.

Cells in the retina probably make many inappropriate contacts in the process of prolific sprouting, but these do not sustain the cell. A cell that possesses too large a proportion of such futile contacts is probably destined to die (79).

The mechanism of cell survival is largely speculative at present. Developing neurons seem to require a "survival supporting factor" from target neurons; and, reciprocally,

the target neurons require appropriate presynaptic input. Apparently, some sort of biochemical matching is required between the presynaptic neuron and its target, probably on the basis of neurotransmitter specificity. In addition to interneuronal contacts, other, more general, survival-promoting regulatory macromolecules are probably needed in the microenvironment. What these substances are remains a mystery (121).

Summary of Embryonic Features

By birth the numbers and types of retinal cells are, for the most part, fixed. Consequently, the postnatal form and distribution of the retina result from rearrangement of this fixed population of cells. Although cell death is a major influence in shaping the retinal mosaic, most of it seems to occur prenatally.

Postnatal Period

At birth the human retina is immature in a number of ways, and the developments discussed below must occur before the adult form is fully realized.

Expansion of the Retina

Postnatal expansion of the retina is a very important factor contributing to the adult topography of retinal cells. The area of the retina at birth is only about half that of the fully mature retina—590 mm^2 and 1250 mm^2, respectively (108, 133). The expansion of the retina must be accompanied by a redistribution and overall thinning of the photoreceptor mosaic and the cells with which they make contact (since few new cells are produced as the retina expands). The geometry of the expansion is a major factor in determining cell distribution in the adult retina.

Expansion Asymmetry Alters Cell Distributions

Postnatal expansion of the retina is non-uniform, at least in cats (73, 80); consequently some parts of the retina thin more than others (Fig. 3.3). The periphery, for example, expands faster than the central retina,

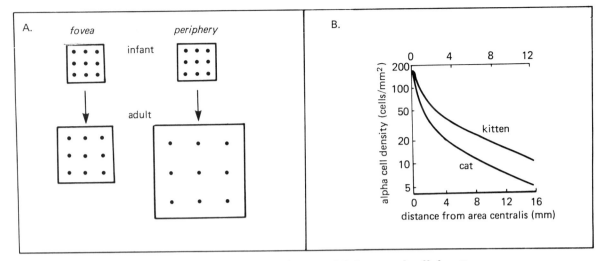

Figure 3.3 (*A*) Nonuniform expansion of postnatal retina. (*B*) Increased cell density gradient across retina. Note different abscissa scales for cat and kitten. (After Mastronarde DN, Thibeault MA, Dubin MW: Non-uniform postnatal growth of the cat retina. J Comp Neurol 228:598, 1984.)

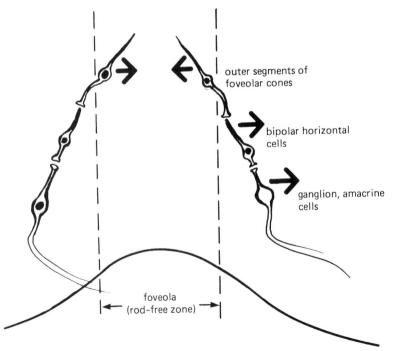

Figure 3.4 Migration of retinal cells after birth.

thus contributing to the decreased density of
ganglion cells and other cell types in the periphery (although retinal expansion is not the
whole story). Also, the temporal retina expands more than the nasal retina. This difference contributes to the higher density of photoreceptors and ganglion cells in the nasal
retina (14).

Migration of Cells

Reduction in Diameter of Foveola At the
same time the retina is expanding after birth,
the cells in the retina are migrating (Fig. 3.4),
some away from the foveola and others toward it. (The foveola is defined as the rod-
free zone in the very center of the retinal depression, the fovea). At birth, there are still
ganglion cells and inner nuclear cells such as
bipolar cells overlying the foveola. After
birth, these cells migrate away from the foveola. One result of this migration is a deepening of the foveolar depression (Fig. 3.5),
which continues until 15 months after birth
(134). The foveolar cones, on the other hand,
migrate toward the midpoint of the foveola.
As a consequence, the diameter of the rod-
free zone is reduced (see Fig. 3.5) from 1000
μm before birth to 650 to 700 μm 45 months
after birth (134). In terms of visual angle, the
area of a newborn's foveola is roughly 2.21
times that of an adult's.

Foveolar Cone Density Since a fixed number of cones (about 31,827) are condensed
into about one-fourth the foveolar area (2
mm² down to 0.4 mm²), it follows that the
density of cones must increase about fourfold
(see Fig. 3.5). According to Yuodelis and
Hendrickson's limited sample, cone density
at the midpoint of the foveola increased until
age 37 years. In the oldest eye examined, 72
years, there was a decrease in density.

Calculation of total cones in the foveola
clarified the dynamics of cone density increase. Initially, the increase in density
seems to arise solely from compacting of
cones within the foveolar border (defined by
the innermost rods). Between 22 weeks' gestation and 45 months postpartum, the number

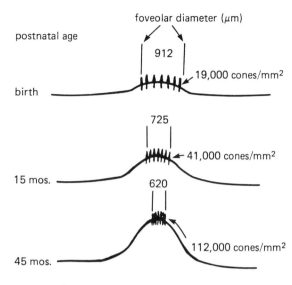

1. foveal depression deepens
2. foveola diameter (rod–free zone) decreases
3. foveolar cone density increases

Figure 3.5 Three results of postnatal cell migration. (After Yuodelis C, Hendrickson A: A qualitative and quantitative analysis of the human
fovea during development. Vision Res 26:847,
1986.)

of cones in the foveola remains constant (31,
827). It follows that no cones previously outside the foveola have migrated across the rod
border into the foveola.

Between 45 months and 37 years this
may not be true: the number of cones in the
foveola doubles to 76,282, whereas foveolar
diameter stays the same. The increase in absolute numbers of cones suggests that some
cones have migrated across the rod-cone border into the foveola. By 72 years, the number
of cones in the foveola has decreased to
48,804.

These data have interesting clinical implications, but before too much is made of
them, a larger sample of eyes must be studied. (Yuodelis and Hendrickson had only five
postnatal eyes.) The variability to be expected among individual retinas, quite apart
from age, has recently been demonstrated by
cone counts on four adult retinas: maximum

cone density varied by as much as 2.9 times among them (28).

Change in Cone Structure

Lengthening of Axon The migration of cones is accompanied by lengthening of the axon (fiber of Henle) that connects the cone inner segment to its synaptic pedicle (Fig. 3.6). This lengthening is necessary because the outer segment is moving centrad while the cone pedicle in contact with bipolar and horizontal cells is moving peripherad. The 300-μm length of the fiber of Henle indicates a considerable migration path.

Lengthening of Outer Segment At 5 days, the outer segment length of the most central foveolar cones is only 3 μm, less than one tenth its mature length (see Fig. 3.6). Interestingly, both foveolar cones and foveal cones outside the rod-free zone seem to increase in length throughout life: the longest cones, 57 μm, were those of a 72-year-old eye.

Reduction in Diameter Another change concurrent with cone migration is narrowing of cone diameters. This complements increased packing of foveolar cones between birth and 4 years. At birth the inner segment

is 6 μm wide, whereas at 45 months it is only 2 μm wide. Thereafter, there isn't much change.

Clinical Consequences

The central 5 degrees of retina is immature at birth, though peripheral regions appear well-developed and mature. Thus, over the first years—and especially the first months—of life, retinal expansion and cone migration continuously change foveolar cone density and, consequently, visual acuity.

The poorly developed outer segments of foveolar cones in the first year or so of life, and their relatively low density, probably account for the relatively poor visual acuity of many infants (see Chap. 2) (20). Also, the poorly developed foveola may account for the clinical observation that central fixation often does not seem to be present at birth (78). Vision in newborns would seem to depend mostly on extrafoveal vision (1).

During this early period of immaturity, the visual system may be susceptible to influences from the visual environment. For example, image quality might influence growth of the eye and retina through local feedback mechanisms (11). Alternatively, delays or abnormalities in foveolar maturation may influence normal development of cortical binocu-

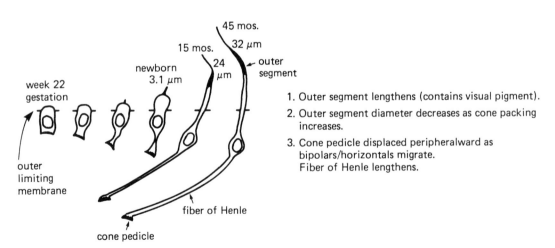

1. Outer segment lengthens (contains visual pigment).
2. Outer segment diameter decreases as cone packing increases.
3. Cone pedicle displaced peripheralward as bipolars/horizontals migrate. Fiber of Henle lengthens.

Figure 3.6 Maturation of foveolar cones. (After Hendrickson A, Yuodelis C: The morphological development of the human fovea. Ophthalmology 91:603, 1984.)

lar mechanisms (12). In short, one can hope that there may be some opportunity, largely unexplored at present, for enhancing visual capacity (acuity, peripheral motion detection) by manipulating image quality on the retina early in life.

OPTIC NERVE AND TRACT

In keeping with what we have discussed about ganglion cell numbers (cell death, above), there is an initial fourfold or so overabundance of optic fibers about midway through gestation, then a gradual attrition due to ganglion cell death, until adult levels are reached by the time of birth (113). Some nerve fibers are myelinated at birth, but myelination proceeds rapidly up to 2 years of age and less rapidly thereafter, according to Magoon and Robb (77). Another view is that myelination is complete by the beginning of the sixth month of life (52).

The optic fibers that project from the contralateral eye arrive first (101) and those from the ipsilateral eye, a little later. At first there is intermixing of the input from the two eyes, then segregation as the LGN layers begin to develop at about 22 weeks (101).

As we mentioned previously, the primate retinas, like those of cats, seem to have at least two types of morphologically distinct ganglion cells. The P beta (X-like) cells are smaller and color opponent in receptive field organization; P alpha cells are larger and have broad band spectral sensitivity. Recently, two distinct populations of fibers, one fine, one coarse, have been noted in monkey optic tract, and the reasonable suggestion has been made that these are the axons of X-like and Y-like ganglion cells, respectively (104). There is some segregation of the finer optic fibers in the middle of the optic nerve and this has been attributed to the advanced arrival of axons from the earlier-maturing P beta ganglion cells in central retina (131). The same line of thought can account for the fact that the first P beta axons to arrive terminate in the deeper (parvocellular) LGN layers, 3 to 6, and the later, thicker, P alpha fibers make connection in more ventral positions (magnocellular layers 1 and 2).

The developmental mechanisms by which optic fibers properly map out the visual field on the LGN and segregate in layers according to fiber size and function remain a mystery. The issue will continue to interest clinicians, because many visual dysfunctions are familial and probably result from faulty "neural wiring." For example, congenital strabismus in cats has been associated with aberrant projection of optic fibers onto the LGN (43, 60).

LATERAL GENICULATE NUCLEUS

LGN neurogenesis is complete by about $9\frac{1}{4}$ weeks' gestation; then there is approximately a 12-week delay before lamination begins (100). The laminae of the LGN (Fig. 3.7) begin to form about the 22nd week of gestation and are in their adult form by the 25th week (31, 55). The lamination is closely associated in time with the segregation of retinogeniculate axon terminals according to eye of origin (99).

At the time lamination is occurring, and even later at birth, most LGN cells remain immature in terms of size and dendritic arborization (52, 53). After birth rapid development of LGN cells continues. Cells in the parvocellular layers (3 to 6) reach adult size by the end of the sixth month and those in the magnocellular layers (1 and 2) near the end of the first year (54). The number of spines on LGN cell dendrites reaches a maximum about 4 months after birth and declines until 9 months, at which time dendrite morphology resembles that in adults (30a, 40a).

Little information is available on development of the small cells in the intercalated layers of the LGN which project to cytochrome oxidase patches, or "blobs," in primary visual cortex (76). These patches are thought to play a special role in color vision (75).

According to Blakemore and Vital-Durand (16, 17), the spatial resolution of monkey LGN cells representing central vision increases from 5 to 35 cycles per second

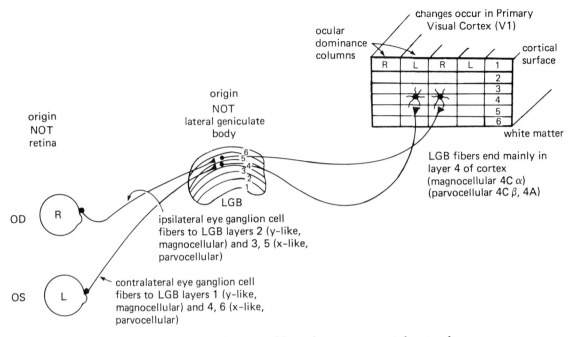

Figure 3.7 Neural origin of amblyopia. (Comparable pathway serving right visual field is not shown.)

between birth and 30 weeks of age. Similar improvements were noted in contrast sensitivity functions. Outside the central 10 degrees, there was no change after birth. Some, but not all, of the improvement in central vision could be attributed to retinal maturation.

Deprivation Conditions

At the time of birth, the optic fibers from the two eyes are segregated into alternate layers in the lateral geniculate body, in the adult layered pattern (55). So it seems unlikely that binocular interactions leading to amblyopia occur in the LGN.

A consistent finding has been that cells in LGN layers representing an occluded eye are smaller than normal (48). The pattern was confirmed in the one human eye examined to date (129). The reduction in LGN soma size is thought to be a secondary effect. The precipitating event is the failure of the LGN axon terminals to make the usual number of

synaptic connections with cortical cells. As the terminal arborization shrinks, it requires a smaller cell body in the LGN to support it (44). Although the deprived eye's LGN cells are smaller, they maintain essentially normal functional properties, such as receptive fields (19, 84). Ikeda and Tremain (63) have presented some evidence to the contrary.

PRIMARY VISUAL CORTEX

The discovery in the early 1960s by Wiesel and Hubel (132) (now Nobel laureates) that monocular lid suture of kittens led to permanent amblyopia in the occluded eye has focused attention on the events underlying development of binocular vision. In the process, a good deal has been learned about maturation of the primary cortex, for it is here that amblyopia-producing anomalies arise (84).

In this section, the appearance of binocular organization in the primary cortex will serve as a model of brain maturation in general. Other cortical networks subserving orientation selectivity, motion detection, and other perceptual abilities probably develop in much the same manner.

Arrival of Geniculocortical Fibers

Initially the geniculocortical fibers from the LGN arriving in layers 4A, 4C (Fig. 3.6), and elsewhere in the primary visual cortex (also known as visual area V1, or Brodmann's area 17) have widespread overlapping axonal branches. Inputs from left- and right-eye LGN fibers overlap (Fig. 3.8A).

Segregation of Eye-Specific Endings

Before birth, the endings representing each eye start to segregate into vertical slabs made up of cortical cells, which are contacted more often by one eye's fibers than the other's (Fig. 3.8B). The slabs are the beginnings of ocular dominance slabs or columns (12, 61). The segregation results from a retraction, or "pruning" process, during which the most widespread axonal processes withdraw toward their root axon. Probably the event that triggers retraction in a given axonal process is

failure to make viable synaptic contact with a cortical cell (see "mechanism of segregation," below).

In humans, the segregation leading to ocular dominance columns starts about day 144 of embryonic growth (98). Other specialized regions of the cortex, such as cytochrome-rich blobs, also appear about the same time (59). A similar pruning of excess axonal processes is seen elsewhere in the brain during the early postnatal period. For example, Innocenti (64) reports that more than 70 percent of the 79 million axons in the newborn kitten's corpus callosum are lost by adulthood.

The Plastic or Sensitive Period

After birth, segregation continues. Of course, now the visual system is exposed to light, and there is a period during which segregation can be influenced by visual experience. This is the so-called plastic period (also known as the critical period, sensitive period, or period of susceptibility).

How important visual experience is during normal development is still under investigation. In the cat, binocular suture after birth or rearing in total darkness abolishes the columnar periodicity usually present in layer IV (123). Between 48 and 128 hrs of

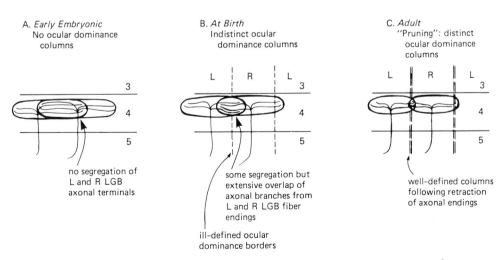

Figure 3.8 Normal development of ocular dominance columns in primary visual cortex (V1).

visual experience before 8 weeks of age seems to be necessary to drive segregation forward.

Cats also require light for onset of the plastic period. Dark rearing delays plastic period onset (29, 88). Species differences are to be expected; dark rearing does not seem to obstruct segregation in monkey, at least at the layer IV level (72).

Cell Numbers and Morphology

In monkeys the total number of neurons shows a postnatal decrease of 16 percent (92). The number of spines on cortical cells also decreases dramatically after a peak at 8 weeks of life (19a, 76a). Glial cells show a 10-fold increase from birth to adulthood (91).

Completion of segregation and synapse formation occurs sometime after birth—in monkeys and cats at about 6 weeks (84). The timing for humans is not yet known. At this point, ocular dominance columns have their adult appearance and cell properties (Fig. 3.8C).

In humans, the number of synapses increases until 8 months then slowly decreases to 60 percent of its peak value at age 11 years (62).

Plastic Period Ends

At a time not necessarily coincident with completion of segregation (72), the plastic period comes to an end. Thereafter, visual experience has little or no influence on the structure of ocular dominance columns. Estimates of the duration of the plastic period are constantly being modified as new testing procedures are employed, so current values should be taken only as indications of the most vulnerable period. The age of susceptibility in cats, for example, has recently been revised upward from 6 weeks to 4 to 7 months (82). For monkeys, the period starts near birth and extends to at least 6 to 10 weeks (72). Existing statistics suggest that the human plastic period begins at about 4 months and lasts up to age 7 to 10 years (6, 125), but there is really very little firm evidence. Susceptibility probably peaks sometime in the first few years of life (132).

The developmental events responsible for terminating the sensitive period are still not understood, but three suggestions have been put forward: (1) completion of myelination of geniculocortical fibers; (2) completion of synaptogenesis along cortical cell spines; and (3) reduction in some plasticity-enhancing neural substance such as norepinephrine (6, 39, 66, 94) (see Chaps. 4 and 6).

Mechanism of Segregation

The sorting out of the intermixed embryonic LGN terminals from the two eyes is thought to involve some form of competition for synaptic sites on cortical cells (132). Each set of fibers seeks to make contact with the same cortical cells, which at this point have no eye preference.

Apparently, cortical cells are equally open to connection with either eye's LGN fibers (removal of one eye at birth results in absence of ocular dominance columns; the remaining eye takes over all the visual cortex). Hence, the eye preference of a cortical cell depends on the proportion of its cell membrane surface occupied by the two eyes' competing LGN terminals. A similar competition probably occurs for synaptic sites on higher-order cortical cells receiving input not from LGN terminals but from other cortical cells.

Little is known about the biophysical events that drive the competition, although one recent hypothesis suggests synchronized activation of cortical cells from a number of LGN afferents may be necessary for synapse formation (10). The rather remarkable finding that implantation of a third eye can result in formation of binocular dominance columns in the normally monocular frog tectum (23) may provide an opportunity to study competition mechanisms in the brains of lower vertebrates.

Dependence on Normal Visual Environment

Normal development of the neural pathways is dependent on a normal visual environment during the plastic period. Defining the characteristics of a normal visual environment may seem intuitively easy, but in fact it requires a detailed knowledge of how the nervous system develops. In practice, the problem is approached backward, by distorting some aspect of vision in infancy then observing the consequences on neural development. Later chapters in this book will deal in more detail with deprivation conditions and their clinical implications. Here, I will limit the discussion to the more dramatic deprivation conditions that have revealed principles of normal development.

The most instructive deprivation experiments have been those in which one input to the brain is removed during development and others are left intact. For example, monocular occlusion, strabismus, or anisometropia results in one eye sending weaker signals to the brain; the other eye's signals are not affected. These experiments have clarified the distortions that may be introduced by competitive imbalance between rival fiber populations.

Monocular Occlusion and Anisometropia

After monocular occlusion or anisometropia during infancy, the deprived eye is amblyopic in adulthood, and fewer cortical cells respond strongly to it. The columns representing that eye become narrower (Fig. 3.9). In

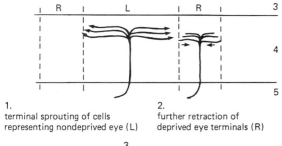

1.
terminal sprouting of cells
representing nondeprived eye (L)

2.
further retraction of
deprived eye terminals (R)

3.
consequent narrowing of deprived
eye columns; widening in nondeprived
eye columns

Figure 3.9 Monocular deprivation causes changes in column widths.

these situations the expanding column width and number of cells serving the dominant eye probably result from two processes (13). (1) The axon terminals of the nondeprived eye do not retract to the usual degree, and the terminals of the deprived eye retract farther than usual. (2) Not only do fibers representing the dominant eye retract less, they undergo renewed sprouting as well (see Fig. 3.9). Brain cells at this point in development still retain the ability to sprout and extend their axonal arborization. Why visual stimulation should increase the sprouting vigor of an LGN or cortical cell remains very much a mystery. A neurotransmitter arriving from activating cells, in addition to immediately initiating a neural signal, may trigger long-term increases in protein production and growth. Or, the neural responses themselves (membrane potentials, action potentials) may stimulate and sustain sprouting (122). Finally, there may be release of a growth-promoting substance originating from postsynaptic cortical cells once axonal processes have made synaptic contact. Current research results are inconclusive.

Strabismus

The deficits following experimentally induced strabismus in infancy are slightly different than those for occlusion or anisometropia. Both humans and monkeys with plastic period eso- or exostrabismus later exhibit stereoblindness. Whether amblyopia develops in the deviated eye depends on circumstances.

With esodeviation, the deviated eye usually does become amblyopic (25, 26, 128, 130). Both spatial and temporal resolution decrease. With exodeviation, the amblyopia is less severe or absent (see Chaps. 12, 13, and 14).

Ocular dominance slabs in the primary cortex of animals subjected to plastic period strabismus are the same width as in a normal brain, but most of the cells in each slab are monocular, responding to only one eye or the other but not both. In contrast, in a normally developing brain most cortical cells are binocular; they give a bigger action potential response to one eye but respond more weakly to stimulation of the other eye as well.

Why amblyopia should occur more often in esotropias than in exotropias in both humans and experimental animals is currently a debated issue. One proposed explanation is that exotropia is less likely than esotropia to be constant over time, as, in the former instance, voluntary or fusional convergence can pull the deviating eye inward intermittently. Hence, in the case of exotropia, the developing brain gets binocular input at least some of the time.

This constancy explanation makes intuitive sense but needs further documentation. Moreover, it is difficult to explain differential susceptibilities noted in cat and monkey experimental strabismus in these terms. When myectomy is used to create exotropia, the cut muscle would seem to preclude intermittent fusion.

An alternative explanation recently advanced is that nasal and temporal retina are asymmetric in their binocular suppression potential (37). Connections from the nasal retina are thought to have a greater cortical inhibitory influence than those from temporal retina. Hence, the foveal signal from an esodeviated eye will be competing with fibers from the nasal retina of the nondeviated eye. Suppression of the deviating foveal image is likely to result. An exodeviating eye will not be affected as much, because the competing signals will arise from the weaker temporal field of the nondeviating eye. Whatever the answer, it is still true that about 80 percent of childhood strabismus is esotropic and places the child at risk for developing amblyopia in the deviating eye (109). A percentage of those with exotropia will be affected as well.

Reverse Occlusion

In human infants, provided action is taken early enough, the deleterious effects of monocular occlusion can be reversed to some degree simply by removing the occlusion (65,

86). In the monkey, simple removal of the occluder is not sufficient.

In humans, the amblyopia recovery process is enhanced when the deprived eye is uncovered and the normal eye is occluded in addition. In the cortex, the proportion of cortical cells served by the previously amblyopic eye increases, and its binocular column width increases to normal. Unfortunately, if the reversed occlusion is sustained long enough, the previously good eye becomes amblyopic. To be effective, all of these maneuvers must take place while the brain is still in its plastic phase.

Function-Specific Plastic Periods

A new conceptual twist has been added to plastic period theorizing by the discovery that subsets of visual system pathways have their own distinct plastic periods. The Y-like, or magnocellular, system matures first. In monkey, Y-like connections are set at 3 weeks of age (72, 132). The X-like parvocellular system remains plastic until about 6 weeks. The influence of competition between the earlier arriving X-like and later arriving Y-like terminals on the timing of their respective plastic periods is not yet clear (124).

There is as yet no clear link between the identified subsets of visual pathways and specific perceptual tasks such as foveation or form perception, although most neurophysiologists are likely to accept such a link as a working hypothesis. It follows that various aspects of vision might be expected to exhibit distinct plastic periods. Initial reports to that effect are beginning to come in (45).

For example, the sensitive period for deviation of an eye leading to strabismic amblyopia is said to begin at 4 months of age (86) and continue to 7 years (9, 56). The time of onset coincides roughly with the appearance of stereopsis in infants (7, 47). Refractive (meridional) amblyopia, on the other hand, is said to begin at 6 months and continue to 6 years (8, 46, 83). Clearly, the details of timing are not known precisely enough to support theories of pathway-specific critical periods, but a conceptual framework now exists that suggests that distinct neural pathways subserve specific visual functions, each pathway having its own characteristic developmental timetable.

Clinical Significance

The animal results, together with a lot of supporting human case studies, suggest that many amblyopic conditions arise during childhood and then cannot be altered later in life because the plastic period is over. The brain has lost its capacity for adjustment, and therapies are not likely to alter the underlying neural deficiencies. Contrary to this view is the persistent clinical observation that in some cases therapy after the plastic period leads to measurable and lasting improvement in vision (5, 11, 15, 22, 41, 51, 65, 85, 96, 107, 112).

The apparent contradiction between what is known about the plastic period limitation on amblyopia reversal and the many exceptions observed clinically has yet to be resolved. A number of explanations have been advanced:

1. Some persons may retain some degree of plasticity for life.
2. Amblyopia may not arise only from a deficiency of cortical connections for the amblyopic eye. It may in fact be a two-step process. The first step may be partial reduction (but only partial) in the number of connections for a deprived eye. The second step may be active suppression by the dominant eye of the now weakened synaptic structure of the deprived eye.

The evidence supporting this point of view is twofold. First, vision in an amblyopic eye, even one resistant to reverse occlusion therapy, improves when the dominant eye is surgically removed (70, 81). Second, reduction of gamma aminobutyric acid (GABA), the neurotransmitter thought to be responsible for binocular suppression in the cortex, increases the representation from an amblyopic

eye (21, 116, 117). Further, the number of GABA-stained neurons is less in the ocular dominance columns representing a deprived eye (50).

To summarize, the best current explanation for post-plastic period improvement of human amblyopia rests on three assumptions: (1) During the plastic period, deprivation of vision in one eye may lead to a reduction (but not complete loss) in synaptic representation in the cortex for that eye. (2) The reduced synaptic representation may then be exaggerated, with suppression by the dominant eye. (3) Post-plastic period success in amblyopic therapy may depend on release of the dominant eye's suppression, which in turn allows access to the heretofore dormant cortical representation of the amblyopic eye. No doubt this preliminary model of events surrounding amblyopia treatment will improve as more information appears about development of cortical synapses and their subsequent suppression interactions.

3. A behavioral adjustment. Finally, a nondevelopmental explanation of successful adult amblyopia treatment may be performance enhancement due to the patient's increased concentration and motivation inspired by the therapist (a sort of placebo effect), or the development of new coping or seeing strategies, such as more effective fixation. There is nothing wrong with this sort of improvement, of course, but from a neurodevelopmental point of view, the underlying deficits remain (see Chap. 14).

OTHER VISUAL AND VISUOMOTOR AREAS

Very little is known about the developmental details of the many extrastriate visual areas in the cerebral cortex (at least a dozen at last count, 126) or of the complex neural circuitry responsible for eye movements and eye-body coordination (40). What little is known suggests that visuomotor structures like the superior colliculus undergo similar processes of cell death, differentiation, and plastic period modification (119).

SUMMARY

Many visual dysfunctions such as amblyopia and strabismus, of which the genetic and neurologic origin were not long ago a complete mystery, are now better understood, thanks to our increasing knowledge of developmental processes, both normal and abnormal. This chapter has outlined the normal development of the retina, optic nerve and tract, LGN, and primary cortex (with emphasis on development of binocular vision mechanisms). The developmental principles revealed by some of the more extreme deprivation conditions, such as monocular occlusion, have been described. In the next decade optometrists can look forward to further insights from research.

REFERENCES

1. Abramov I, Gordon J, Hendrickson A, et al: The retina of the newborn infant. Science 217:265, 1982.

2. Adler R: Trophic interactions in retinal development and in retinal degenerations. In vivo and in vitro studies. In Adler R, Farber D (eds): The Retina: A Model For Cell Biology Studies. New York, Academic Press, 1986.

3. Adler R: The differentiation of retinal photoreceptors and neurons in vitro. In Osborne N, Chader G: (eds): Progress in Retinal Research, 6. New York, Pergamon Press, 1987.

4. Ahnelt PK, Kolb H, Pflug R: Identification of a subtype of cone photoreceptor, likely to be blue-sensitive, in the human retina. J Comp Neurol 255:18, 1987.

5. Amos J: Refractive amblyopia. In Amos J (ed): Diagnosis and Management in Vision Care. Boston, Butterworths, 372, 1987.

6. Aoki C, Siekevitz P: The role of hormone-stimulated cAMP metabolism in visual cortical plasticity. In Hilfer SR, Sheffield JB (eds): Development of Order in the Nervous System. New York, Springer-Verlag, 143, 1986.

7. Atkinson J, Braddick O: Stereoscopic discrimination in children. Perception 5:29, 1976.

8. Banks RV: A clinical assessment of new methods of treatment for amblyopia. Aust Orthopt J 17:6, 1980.

9. Banks MS, Aslin RN, Letson RD: Sensitive period for the development of human binocular vision. Science 190:675, 1975.

10. Bear MF, Cooper LN, Ebner FF: A physiological basis for a theory of synapse modification. Science 237:42, 1987.

11. Beauchamp R: Causes of myopia. Iss Vis Physiol 1:3, 1987a.

12. Beauchamp R: Imaging ocular dominance columns in visual cortex. Iss Vis Physiol 1:3, 1987b.

13. Beauchamp R: Lazy eye. Iss Vis Physiol 1:9, 1987d.

14. Beauchamp R: Photoreceptor density and acuity. Iss Vis Physiol 1:20, 1987c.

15. Birnbaum MH, Koslowe K, Sanet R: Success in amblyopia treatment as a function of age. Am J Optom Physiol Opt 54:269, 1977.

16. Blakemore C, Vital-Durand F: Development of spatial resolution and contrast sensitivity in monkey visual cortex. Neurosci Abstr 7:140, 1981b.

17. Blakemore C, Vital-Durand F: Postnatal development of the monkey's visual system. The fetus and independent life. Ciba Found Symp 86:152, 1981a.

18. Blakemore C, Vital-Durand F: Development of contrast sensitivity by neurones in monkey striate cortex. J Physiol 334:18, 1982.

19. Blakemore C, Vital-Durand F: Development of the monkey's geniculo-cortical systems. In Stone J, Dreher B, Rapaport DH (eds): Development of Visual Pathways in Mammals. New York, Alan Liss, 463, 1984.

19a. Boothe RG, Greenough WT, Lund JS, Wrege K: A quantitative investigation of spine and dendrite development of neurons in visual cortex (area 17) of *macaca nemestrina* monkeys. J Comp Neurol 18:473, 1979.

20. Boothe RG, Dobson V, Teller DY: Postnatal development of vision in human and nonhuman primates. Ann Rev Neurosci 8:495, 1985.

21. Burchfiel JL, Duffy FH: Role of intracortical inhibition in deprivation amblyopia: Re-

versal by microionotophoretic biuculline. Brain Res 206:479, 1981.

22. Ciuffreda KJ: Visual system plasticity in human amblyopia. In Hilfer SR, Sheffield JB (eds): Development of Order in the Nervous System. New York, Springer-Verlag, 211, 1986.

23. Constatin-Patin M, Ferrari-Eastman P: Pre- and post synaptic interocular competition and segregation in the frog. J Comp Neurol 255:178, 1987.

24. Cowan WM: Neuronal death as a regulative mechanism in the control of cell number in the nervous system. In Rockstein M (ed): Development and Ageing of the Nervous System. New York, Academic Press, 1973.

25. Crawford MLJ: Abnormal early visual experience and visual function in monkeys. In Hilfer SR, Sheffield JB (eds): Development of Order in the Nervous System. New York, Springer-Verlag, 193, 1986.

26. Crawford MLJ, Von Noorden GK: The effects of short-term experimental strabismus on the visual system in *Macaca mulatta.* Invest Ophthalmol Vis Res 18:496, 1979.

27. Cunningham TJ: Naturally occurring neuron death and its regulation by developing neural pathways. Int Rev Cytol 74:163, 1982.

28. Curcio CA, Sloan KR, Packer O, et al: Distribution of cones in human and monkey retina: Individual variability and radial asymmetry. Science 236:579, 1987.

29. Cynader M, Mitchell DE: Period of susceptibility of kitten visual cortex to the effects of monocular deprivation extends beyond six months of age. Brain Res 191:5515, 1980.

30. Dartnall HJA, Bowmaker JK, Mollon JD: Microspectrophotometry of human photoreceptors. In Mollon JD, Sharpe LT (eds): Color Vision: Physiology and Psychophysics. London, Academic Press, 1983.

30a. de Courten C, Garey LJ: Morphology of the neurons in the human lateral geniculate nucleus and their normal development: A Golgi study. Exp Brain Res 147:159, 1982.

31. Dekaban A: Human thalamus: An anatomical, developmental and pathological study. II. Development of the human thalamic nuclei. J Comp Neurol 100:63, 1954.

32. de Monasterio FM: Properties of concentrically organized X and Y ganglion cells of macaque retina. J Neurophysiol 41:1394, 1978.

33. de Monasterio FM, Schein SJ: Protan-like spectral sensitivity of foveal Y ganglion cells of macaque monkeys. J Physiol (Lond) 299:385, 1980.

34. Dowling J: The Retina. Cambridge, MA, Harvard University Press, 1987.

35. Duke-Elder S, Cook C: Embryology. In: Systems of Ophthalmology, vol. 3, Normal and Abnormal Development, Pt. 1. St. Louis, CV Mosby, 1963.

36. Duke-Elder S, Wybar K: Ocular motility and strabismus. In: Systems of Ophthalmology, vol. 6. St. Louis, CV Mosby, 1973.

37. Fahle M: Naso-temporal asymmetry of binocular inhibition. Invest Ophthalmol Vis Sci 28:1016, 1987.

38. Farber D, Adler R: Issues and questions in cell biology of the retina. In: The Retina: A Model for Cell Biology Studies. Toronto, Academic Press, 1986.

39. Foote SL, Morrison JH: Development of the noradrenergic, serotonergic and dopaminergic innervation of neocortex. Curr Topics Dev Biol 21:391, 1987.

40. Fuchs AF, Kaneko CRS, Scudder CA: Brainstem control of saccadic eye-movements. Ann Rev Neurosci 8:307, 1985.

40a. Garey LJ, de Courten C: Structural development of the lateral geniculate nucleus and visual cortex in monkey and man. Behav Brain Res 10:3, 1983.

41. Garzia RP: Efficacy of vision therapy in amblyopia: A literature review. Am J Optom Physiol Opt 64:393, 1987.

42. Gouras P, Evers HU: The neurocircuitry of primate retina. In Gallego A, Gouras P (eds): Neurocircuity of the Retina. New York, Elsevier, 1985.

43. Guillery RW: An abnormal retinogeniculate projection in Siamese cats. Brain Res 14:739, 1969.

44. Guillery RW, Stelzner DJ: The differential effects of unilateral lid closure upon the monocular and binocular segments of the dorsal lateral geniculate nucleus in the cat. J Comp Neurol 139:413, 1970.

45. Harwerth RS, Smith EL, Duncan GC, et al: Multiple sensitive periods in the development of the primate visual system. Science 232:235, 1986.

46. Held R: Development of visual acuity in normal and astigmatic infants. In Cool SJ (ed): Frontiers in Visual Science. New York, Springer-Verlag, 1978.

47. Held R, Birch E, Gwiazda J: Stereoacuity of human infants. Proc Natl Acad Sci USA 77:5572, 1980.

48. Hendrickson AE, Movshon JA, Eggers HM, et al: Effects of early unilateral blur on the macaques visual system. 2. Anatomical observations. J Neurosci 7:1327, 1987.

49. Hendrickson A, Yuodelis C: The morphological development of the human fovea. Ophthalmology 91:603, 1984.

50. Hendry SHC, Jones EG: Reduction in number of immunostained GABA-ergic neurons in deprived-eye dominance columns of monkey area 17. Nature 320:750, 1986.

51. Hess RF, France TD, Tulunay-Keesey U: Residual vision in humans who have been monocularly deprived of pattern stimulation early in life. Exp Brain Res 44:295, 1981.

52. Hickey TL: Postnatal development of the human lateral geniculate nucleus: Relationship to a critical period for the visual system. Science 198:836, 1977.

53. Hickey TL, Guillery RW: Variability of laminar patterns in the human lateral geniculate nucleus. J Comp Neurol 183:221, 1979.

54. Hickey TL, Peduzzi JD: Structure and development of the visual system. In Salapatek P, Cohen L (eds): Handbook of Infant Perception, vol. 1, 1, 1987.

55. Hitchcock PF, Hickey TL: Prenatal development of the human lateral geniculate nucleus. J Comp Neurol 194:395, 1980.

56. Hohmann A, Creutzfeldt OD: Squint and the development of binocularity in humans. Science 254:613, 1975.

57. Hollenberg MJ, Spira AW: Early development of the human retina. Can J Ophthalmol 7:472, 1972.

58. Hollenberg MJ, Spira AW: Human retinal development: Ultrastructure of the outer retina. Am J Anat 137:357, 1973.

59. Horton JC: Cytochrome oxidase patches: A new cytoarchitectonic feature of monkey visual cortex. Philos Trans R Soc Lond [Biol] 304:199, 1984.

60. Hubel DH, Wiesel TN: Aberrant visual projections in the Siamese cat. J Physiol 218:33, 1971.

61. Hubel DH, Wiesel TN: Functional architecture of macaque monkey visual cortex. Proc R Soc Lond 206:419, 1977.

62. Huttenlocher PR, de Courten C, Garey LJ, et al: Synaptogenesis in human visual cortex—Evidence for synapse elimination during normal development. Neurosci Lett 33:247, 1982.

63. Ikeda H, Tremain K: The development of spatial resolving power of lateral geniculate neurons in kittens. Exp Brain Res 31:193, 1978.

64. Innocenti GM: Role of axon elimination in the development of visual cortex. In Stone J, Dreher B, Rapaport D (eds): Development of Visual Pathways in Mammals. New York, Alan Liss, 243, 1984.

65. Jacobson SG, Mohindra I, Held R: Visual acuity in infants with ocular diseases. Am J Ophthalmol 93:198, 1982.

66. Kasamatsu T: Norepinephrine hypothesis for visual cortical plasticity: Thesis, antithesis, and recent development. Curr Top Dev Biol 21:367, 1987.

67. Kolb H: Cone pathways in the mammalian retina. In Hilfer SR, Sheffield JB (eds): Molecular and Cellular Basis of Visual Acuity. New York, Springer-Verlag, 1984.

68. Kolb H, Mariani A, Gallego A: A second type of horizontal cell in the monkey retina. J Comp Neurol 189:31, 1980.

69. Kolb H, Nelson R, Mariani A: Amacrine cells, bipolar cells and ganglion cells of the cat retina: a Golgi study. Vision Res 21:1081, 1981.

70. Kratz KE, Spear PD, Smith DC: Post-critical period reversals of effects of monocular deprivation on striate cortex cells in the cat. J Neurophysiol 39:501, 1976.

71. Le Vail MM, Yasumara D, Rakic P: Cell genesis in the rhesus monkey retina. Invest Ophthalmol Vis Sci (Suppl) 24:7, 1983.

72. LeVay S, Wiesel TN, Hubel DH: The development of ocular dominance columns in normal and visually deprived monkeys. J Comp Neurol 191:1, 1980.

73. Lia B, Williams RW, Chalupa LM: Formation of retinal ganglion cell topography during prenatal development. Science 236:848, 1987.

74. Linberg KA, Fisher SK: Ultrastructural evidence that horizontal cell axon terminals are presynaptic in the human retina. J Comp Neurol 268:281, 1988.

75. Livingston MS, Hubel DH: Anatomy and physiology of a color system in the primate visual cortex. J Neurosci 4:309, 1984.

76. Lund JS: Anatomical organization of macaque monkey striate visual cortex. Ann Rev Neurosci 11:253, 1988.

76a. Lund JS, Boothe RG, Lund RD: Development of neurons in the visual cortex (area 17) of the monkey *macaca nemestrina:* A Golgi study from fetal day 127 to postnatal maturity. J Comp Neurol 176:149, 1977.

77. Magoon EH, Robb RM: Development of myelin in human optic nerve and tract. Arch Ophthamol 99:655, 1981.

78. Mann IC: The Development of the Human Eye. New York, Grune and Stratton, 1964.

79. Marc RE: The development of retinal networks. In Adler R, Farber D (eds): The Retina: A Model for Cell Biology Studies. New York, Academic Press, 1986.

80. Mastronarde DN, Thibeault MA, Dubin MW: Non-uniform postnatal growth of the cat retina. J Comp Neurol 228:598, 1984.

81. Mitchell DE: Effects of early visual experience on the development of certain visual capacities in animals and man. In Walk RD, Pick HL (eds): Perception and Experience. New York, Plenum, 37, 1978.

82. Mitchell DE: The extent of visual recovery from early monocular or binocular visual deprivation in kittens. J Physiol 395:639, 1988.

83. Mitchell DG, Freeman RD, Millodot M, et al: Meridional amblyopia: Evidence for the modification of the human visual system by early visual experience. Vision Res 13:535, 1973.

84. Mitchell DE, Timney B: Postnatal development of function in the mammalian visual system. In: Handbook of Physiology: The Nervous System III, chap. 12, 507, 1984.

85. Mitchell DG, et al: The effect of minimal occlusion therapy on binocular visual functions in amblyopia. Invest Ophthalmol Vis Sci 24:778, 1983.

86. Mohindra I, Jacobson SG, Thomas J, et al: Development of amblyopia in infants. Trans Ophthalmol Soc UK, 99:344, 1979.

87. Movshon JA, Van Sluyters RC: Visual neural development. Ann Rev Psychol 32:477, 1981.

88. Mower GD, Berry D, Burchfiel JL, et al: Comparison of the effects of dark rearing and binocular suture on development and plasticity of cat visual cortex. Brain Res 220:255, 1981.

89. Nishimura Y, Rakic P: Development of the rhesus monkey retina. I. Emergence of the inner plexiform layer and its synapses. J Comp Neurol 241:420, 1987.

90. Nishimura Y, Rakic P: Development of the rhesus monkey retina: II. A three-dimensional analysis of the sequences of synaptic combinations in the inner plexiform layer. J Comp Neurol 262:290, 1987.

91. O'Kusky J, Colonnier M: Postnatal changes in the number of astrocytes, oligodendrocytes, and microglia in visual cortex (Area 17) of the macaque monkey: A stereological analysis in normal and monocularly deprived animals. J Comp Neurol 210:307, 1982a.

92. O'Kusky J, Colonnier M: Postnatal changes in number of neurons and synapses in visual cortex (Area 17) of macaque monkey: A stereological analysis in normal and monocularly deprived animals. J Comp Neurol 210:291, 1982b.

93. Perry VH, Cowey A: The morphological correlates of X- and Y-like retinal ganglion cells in the retina of monkeys. Exp Brain Res 43:226, 1981.

94. Pettigrew JD, Kasamatsu T: Local perfusion of noradrenalin maintains visual cortical plasticity. Nature 271:761, 1978.

95. Polyak S: The Retina. Chicago, University of Chicago Press, 1941.

96. Press LJ: Amblyopia. J Optom Vis Dev 19:2, 1988.

97. Provis JM: Patterns of cell death in the ganglion cell layer of the human fetal retina. J Comp Neurol 259:237, 1987.

98. Rakic P: Prenatal genesis of connections subserving ocular dominance in the rhesus monkey. Nature 261:467, 1976.

99. Rakic P: Genesis of the dLGN in the rhesus monkey: Site of origin, kinetics of proliferation, routes of migration and pattern of distribution of neurons. J Comp Neurol 176:23, 1977a.

100. Rakic P: Prenatal development of the visual system in rhesus monkey. Philos Trans R Soc Lond [Biol] 278:245, 1977b.

101. Rakic P: Prenatal development of the visual system in rhesus monkey. Philos Trans R Soc Lond [Biol] 278:245, 1977c.

102. Ramoa AS, Campbell G, Shatz CJ: Transient morphological features of identified ganglion cells in living fetal and neonatal retina. Science 237:522, 1987.

103. Rapaport DH, Robinson SR, Stone J: Cell movement and birth in the developing cat retina. In Stone J et al (eds): Development of Visual Pathways in Mammals. New York, Alan R. Liss, 23, 1984.

104. Reese BE, Guillery RW: Distribution of axons according to diameter in the monkey's optic tract. J Comp Neurol 260:453, 1987.

105. Rhodes RH: A light microscope study of the developing human neural retina. Am J Anat 154:195, 1979.

106. Rodieck RW: The Vertebrate Retina. San Francisco, Freeman, 1973.

107. Rosenthal RJ: Treatment regimen for an amblyopic adult patient. J Optom Vis Dev 14:8, 1983.

108. Scammon RE, Wilmer HA: Growth of the components of the human eyeball. II. Comparison of the calculated volumes of the eyes of the newborn and of adults, and their components. Arch Ophthalmol 43:620, 1950.

109. Schapero M: Amblyopia. Chilton, Philadelphia, 1971.

110. Schein SJ: Anatomy of macaque fovea and spatial densities of neurons in foveal representation. J Comp Neurol 269:479, 1988.

111. Scott AB: Pharmacological treatment of strabismus. In Lennerstrand G, et al (eds): Functional Basis of Ocular Motility Disorders. New York, Pergamon Press, 199, 1982.

112. Selenow A, Ciuffreda KJ: Visual function recovery during orthoptic therapy in an adult esotropic amblyope. J Am Optom Assoc 57:132, 1986.

113. Shatz CJ, Sretavan DW: Interactions between retinal ganglion cells during the development of the mammalian visual system. Ann Rev Neurosci 9:171, 1986.

114. Sherman SM, Spear PD: Organization of visual pathways in normal and visually deprived cats. Physiol Rev 62:738, 1982.

115. Sidman RL: Histogenesis of mouse retina studied with thymidine-3H. In Smelser GK (ed): Structure of the Eye. New York, Academic Press, 1961.

116. Sillito AM, Kemp JA, Blakemore C: The role of GABAergic inhibition in the cortical effects of monocular deprivation. Nature 2911:318, 1981.

117. Sillito AM, Kemp JA, Patel H: Inhibitor interactions contributing to the ocular dominance of monocularly dominated cells in the normal striate cortex. Exp Brain Res 41:1, 1980.

118. Spira AW, Hollenberg MJ: Human retinal development: Ultrastructure of the inner retinal layers. Dev Biol 31:1, 1973.

119. Stein BE: Development of the superior colliculus. Ann Rev Neurosci 7:95, 1984.

120. Stone J: Parallel Processing in the Visual System. The Classification of Retinal Ganglion Cells and Its Impact on the Neurobiology of Vision. New York, Plenum, 1983.

121. Stone J, Malim J, Rapaport D: The development of the topographical organization of the cat's retina. In Stone J, Dreher B, Rapaport DH (eds): Development of Visual Pathways in Mammals. New York, Alan R. Liss, 3, 1984.

122. Stryker MP, Harris WA: Binocular impulse blockade prevents the formation of ocular dominance columns in cat visual cortex. J Neurosci 6:2117, 1986.

123. Swindale NV: Role of visual experience in promoting segregation of eye dominance

patches in the visual cortex of the cat. J Comp Neurol 267:472, 1988.

124. Sur M, Weller RE, Sherman SM: Development of X- and Y-cell retinogeniculate terminations in kittens. Nature 310:246, 1984.

125. Vaegan DT, Taylor D: Critical period for deprivation amblyopia in children. Trans Ophthalmol Soc UK 99:432, 1979.

126. Van Essen DC: Functional organization of primate visual cortex. In Jones EG, Peters AA (eds): Cerebral Cortex, vol. 3. New York, Plenum Press, 1985.

127. Vital-Durand F, Garey LJ, Blakemore C: Monocular and binocular deprivation in the monkey: Morphological effects and their reversibility. Brain Res 158:45, 1978.

128. Von Noorden GK: Experimental amblyopia in monkeys. Further behavioral observations and clinical correlations. Invest Ophthalmol Vis Sci 12:721, 1973.

129. Von Noorden GK, Crawford MLJ, Levacy RA: The lateral geniculate nucleus in human anisometropic amblyopia. Invest Ophthalmol Vis Sci 24:788, 1983.

130. Von Noorden GK, Dowling JE: Experimental amblyopia in monkeys. II. Behavioral studies in strabismic amblyopia. Arch Ophthalmol 84:215, 1970.

131. Walsh C, Polley EH: The topography of ganglion cell production in the cat's retina. J Neurosci 5:741, 1985.

132. Wiesel TN: Postnatal development of the visual cortex and the influence of environment. Nature 299:583, 1982.

133. Wilmer HA, Scammon RE: Growth of the components of the human eyeball. I. Diagrams, calculations, computations and reference tables. Arch Ophthalmol 43:599, 1950.

134. Yuodelis C, Hendrickson A: A qualitative and quantitative analysis of the human fovea during development. Vision Res 26:847, 1986.

Chapter 4

Visuomotor Development

Clifton Schor

Virtually no aspect of oculomotor control is fully developed at birth. Many of the characteristically immature oculomotor functions observed in infants resemble the abnormal oculomotor behavior that characterizes developmental disorders, such as strabismus and amblyopia (119) and disorders of the central nervous system, such as Parkinson's disease (34). During development, varying degrees of deficit are found in the different oculomotor subsystems. Under these circumstances, one oculomotor system (e.g., the saccadic) may substitute its function for that of a less mature system (e.g., smooth-pursuit following response). This particular example of substitution is referred to as cogwheel movements (Fig. 4.1), which can be observed in normal neonates (4) and in adults with Parkinson's disease (31) who are attempt-

ing to follow a moving object. Eventually the smooth-pursuit system develops (at 2 months), and the infant becomes capable of smooth following movements (see Fig. 4.1) (4).

In order to understand the factors underlying oculomotor development it is helpful to use heuristic descriptions of oculomotor control. Systems are defined in terms of functional behavior and afferent and efferent subcomponents. Development of oculomotor control requires maturation of sensory afferent processes that transduce the optically transformed light distribution of the retinal image into neural codes that are interpreted and that evoke efferent commands that guide oculomotor mechanisms (i.e., the intra- and extraocular muscles).

The precision of these motor responses

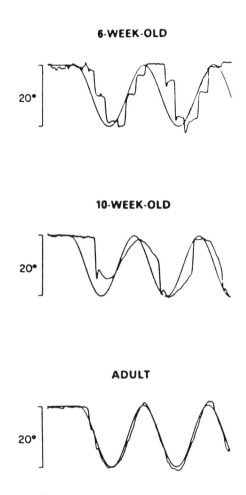

6-WEEK-OLD

20°

10-WEEK-OLD

20°

ADULT

20°

HORIZONTAL EYE POSITION

TIME

Figure 4.1 Sample eye movement tracings illustrating the developmental emergence of smooth pursuit from cog-wheel response (*top*) to horizontal target excursions (*smooth sinusoidal line*). (From Aslin RN: Development of smooth pursuit in human infants. In Fisher DF, Monty RA, Senders JW (eds): Hillsdale NJ, Earlbaum, 1981.)

develops substantially during the first 6 months of life. The foveal depression is immature in newborns (91). Prior to migration of foveal ganglion cells away from the pit (1) photoreceptors in this region are morphologically different from those in adult retinas. In neonates outer segments of foveal cones are stubby, and possibly nonexistent (1, 64, 148), whereas their extrafoveal cone morphology appears mature. In addition, the density of cones that make up the retinal mosaic is 2.5 times lower in neonates than in adults. The increased density of foveal cones is believed to result from postnatal centripetal migration of photoreceptors, because the total number of cones is believed to remain constant after birth. A major question that remains, however, is to what extent, if any, does the immature fovea limit oculomotor performance except under conditions of reduced visibility, where contrast sensitivity and visual acuity can limit target visibility. As will be discussed subsequently, these visibility limits will influence finely guided control of accommodation, pursuit tracking movements, and the precision of monocular and binocular eye alignment. In addition to retinal factors, the visual cortex is another neural locus that accounts for some of the neonate's sensory deficits. Comparative developmental studies illustrate reduced disparity tuning and contrast sensitivity of cortical neurons in kittens (98). These cortical factors influence mainly binocular vergence control, but also the motor responses discussed earlier under conditions of reduced visibility.

Other factors that limit oculomotor performance in neonates are higher-level cognitive factors such as attention, motivation, state level of alertness, distraction, fatigue, and sleepiness. These higher-level factors influence even the simplest motor reflexes. For example, the pupil tends to decrease in size during periods of inattention and just before sleep (88); this could be mistaken for a developmental difference between pupil size in infants and adults at high luminance levels. Similarly, we have observed in our laboratory that inattentive infants, who effectively sleep with their eyes open, do not exhibit an opto-

can be limited by a deficit in any of the subcomponents, but much of the limitation in infancy appears at the sensory or afferent side of the motor reflex arc. For example, the human neonate's fovea is immature in comparison to the peripheral retina (1). The fovea kinetic following reflex even when they are surrounded by a rotating textured optokinetic drum. In contrast, during an alert state, the optokinetic reflex is reliably triggered by the same stimulus; accordingly, an infant's average oculomotor behavior is not typical of its best performance or potential capability. Infants' general inability to cooperate justifies drawing attention to isolated records of unusually good performance as a measure of the potential level of oculomotor development.

METHODS AND EVALUATION

Direct Observation

The most common clinical method for evaluating eye movements is to observe directly the change in limbal position and corneal light reflex. Assuming the eye's center of rotation is 10 mm from the neonate's cornea, a 1-mm translation of the limbus corresponds to approximately 10 degrees of eye rotation. During a saccade, a 0.1-mm displacement, which corresponds to 1 degree of rotation, can be detected by an experienced observer. Detection of vertical eye rotation is enhanced by a factor of two as a result of the rocking motion of the eyelashes as the cornea pushes out the upper lid during vertical saccades.

Corneal Reflex

Changes in the position of the eye can also be judged from the location of the corneal reflex in the pupil boundary. The translation of the corneal reflex during eye rotation is the result of the corneal bulge. If the eye were spherical and the center of curvature of the cornea were at the same location as the eye's center of rotation the corneal reflex would remain motionless during eye rotation. But the center of curvature is anterior to the center of rotation, so the cornea translates in the direction of rotation during eye rotation. Paradoxically, the corneal reflex moves in the same direction as the rotating eye but more slowly than the translation of the pupil and limbus. This produces a relative motion between the corneal reflex and pupil margin that causes

the reflex to appear to move in the direction opposite that of eye rotation. Approximately 1 mm of relative displacement corresponds to 10 degrees of eye rotation (76). Although the method is less sensitive to changes in eye position than is observed by tracking of the limbus, it is more sensitive for estimating absolute static direction of gaze, because as observers we find it easier to judge the separation between two targets (a form of hyperacuity) than the absolute position of a single target.

One of the most frequent uses of corneal reflection is to estimate errors of monocular and binocular fixation. Eye position is judged from the displacement of the optical axis from the line of sight (angle Alpha) which is referred to clinically as angle Kappa. Normally the optical axis diverges 5 degrees from the visual axis, which during accurate foveal fixation of a penlight causes the corneal reflex to appear 0.5 mm nasalward in the pupil. Deviations from this normal offset are interpreted clinically as indicating foveal fixation errors, and if the angle Kappa differs in the two eyes during attempted binocular fixation, strabismus, or eye turn, is present. Early studies of binocular fixation in infants reported that the pupil centers of young infants were symmetrically divergent and that this divergence decreased during the first 2 to 3 months of life (93, 145). Although the results could indicate a lack of bifoveal fixation and exotropia, they also could indicate changes in the angle Kappa with growth of the eye. Indeed, Slater and Findlay (135) observed that optic axis discrepancy or divergence is 2 times greater in neonates than in adults and that as the axial length increases the optical and visual axes approach one another. These growth factors should not be confused with errors of monocular and binocular fixation during the first 2 to 3 months of life. Measurement error with this method has been described in detail (26, 135).

Infrared Reflection

These corneal observation techniques have been automated by electronic transducers that sense the intensity of infrared light reflected from the anterior surface of the eye. These transducers are referred to as infrared limbal trackers and are used mostly in adults because the infrared sensor must be attached near the eyes with spectacle frames and the device does not work well with small palpebral fissures. In the last decade, several commercial remote video-based infrared-sensing systems have been developed that analyze eye position and rotation from the sensed position of the corneal reflex within the boundaries of the pupil. Because infants move their heads about during recordings, a head-mounted reference is also recorded to allow the computation of eye-orbit position, regardless of head motion. These objective recording systems require data analysis by a computer to compensate for inherent nonlinearities and for the presence of head motion.

Electrooculography

The problem of head movement artifacts is eliminated by electrooculography (EOG) that uses miniature silver chloride skin electrodes attached with double-sided tape to the outer canthi and a reference electrode on the forehead. (The infant's tiny nasal canthi are too small to support electrodes.) These electrodes sense proximity of the corneal apex, which has the same electrical charge as the retina. Because the retina is insulated from the back of the eye by the pigmented epithelium, the eye acts as a dipole. This would be an excellent voltage source were it not for other sources of extraneous noise such as action potentials for the orbicularis oculis. Sucking, facial grimace, blepharospasm, and crying all generate massive amounts of noise, which obscures the EOG recording. Under the best circumstances the EOG technique has a resolving power of 0.5 to 1 degree of eye rotation up to ±30 degrees.

Retinoscopy and Photorefraction

Objective measures of infants' static accommodative state and refractive state can be obtained by observing the motion of the retinal reflex with a retinoscope (93) and from photographs of the spread of light reflected from the retina (68). In photorefraction, photographs are taken of the infant's pupil from some distance. If the infant is emmetropic the retina will be conjugate to the camera aperture and spread of light will be minimal. Myopic and hyperopic refractive states will spread reflected light onto a large area, and the pupil will appear expanded on the film plane. If the camera is slightly off axis, the reflex will also appear off center in the pupil, as it does in retinoscopy when there is a refractive error (77). Thus reflex displacement provides information about the type of refractive state (hyperopic versus myopic). Elliptical distortion of the pupil image is an indicator of astigmatism (see Chap. 7).

FIXATIONAL EYE MOVEMENTS

Monocular Fixation

The postnatal changes in morphology of the fovea described above indicate that approximately the central 5 degrees of the retina is at best partially functional at birth, whereas the structure of the parafovea resembles that in an adult's eye. Currently, it is not known whether this foveal scotoma influences the stability and accuracy of monocular fixation; indeed, infants may utilize extrafoveal sites for monocular and binocular fixation while the fovea develops during the first 3 months of life (25, 86). Given the uncertainty of the angle Kappa and the known immaturity of the fovea, it is impossible at this time to establish whether fixation is foveal or has any preferred site during the first 3 months of life. Presumably, fixation will align objects of interest with the highest-resolution retinal loci. Given the reduced visual acuity of the newborn, there is no specific site, as there is in the adult, where a fixation preference would be advantageous.

In adults, fixational movements are composed of irregular slow drifts, fixation saccades (1 to 5 per second), and a 60-Hz microtremor. The drifts and saccades are both error producing and error correcting (35, 139).

These movements tend to follow the outline of contour in the visual field (108), and they have idiosyncratic biases. These can be responses to imbalances in the vestibuloocular reflex (131).

Although it is not known what retinal site, if any, infants prefer in monocular fixation, they do stare steadily at objects (56, 86) and infrequently shift their gaze to fix on a new target (104). The tendency to refixate on new objects increases in frequency during the first 3 months of life (12, 140). This may be due to an increase in the visual field, to the development of a preference for central retinal fixation (as opposed to no preference), or to the ability to relinquish fixation and attention of one target in order to capture another one. Studies of the dynamics of fixational eye movements in infants ranging in age from 2 weeks to 1 year revealed that they tend to fixate an object to within 1 degree of some unspecified retinal locus (60); age trends were not identified within that year. Inspection of these fixation records taken by remote infrared video reveals both fixation saccades and drifts by 2 months of age (62). Preschool children and 10-year-olds are reported to have less precise fixation control than adults (80). Where the increased range of eye position is caused by large saccades, much of this difference may be attributed to attentional factors (8).

Binocular Fixation

Binocular fixation can be maintained in adults to within a range of 6 to 10 arc minutes. Static subjective measures of fixation vergence error are referred to as fixation disparity. These binocular errors rarely exceed 6 arc minutes when heterophoria is corrected with prisms (100, 120). Dynamic objective measures of binocular alignment demonstrate a similar range of variability (110, 112). The components of binocular fixation serve different roles. Yoked saccades appear to correct fixation errors of individual eyes, whereas drifts tend to be disjunctive and to correct overall vergence errors between the two eyes (112). These errors of binocular

alignment do not elicit diplopia, as the retinal image disparities that they produce fall within the range of Panum's fusional limits (130).

Rudimentary binocular alignment without a cosmetically noticeable strabismus is often present at birth; however, it is unlikely that true bifoveal fixation occurs much before 2 to 3 months of age. Using corneal photography, Slater and Findlay (134) report that newborns changed binocular convergence in response to 10- and 20-inch viewing distances but not to a 5-inch distance. Aslin (5) used corrected measures of corneal photography and found that 1-month-old infants' eyes converged and diverged in response to 12- to 22-cm/sec target movements along the midline from 57 to 15 cm (see Fig. 4.2). Two- and 3-month-olds had more accurate vergence responses, and the speed of their movements

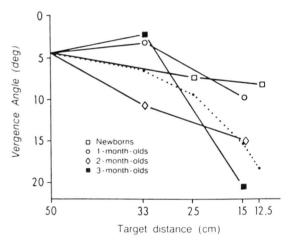

Figure 4.2 Vergence angle as a function of target viewing distance in newborns (From Slater AM, Findlay JM: Binocular fixation in the newborn baby. J Exp Child Psychol 20:248, 1975) and in older infants (From Aslin RN: Development of binocular fixation in human infants. J Exp Child Psychol 23:133, 1977.) Dotted line indicates expected value. (From Aslin RN: Normative oculomotor development in human infants. In Lennerstrand G, Von Noorden G, Campos E (eds): Strabismus and Amblyopia—Experimental Basis for Advances in Clinical Management. New York, Pergamon Press, 1988.)

increased during the first 3 months of life. These results elaborate earlier qualitative results by Ling (87). It is possible that while the fovea is immature infants use an extrafoveal retinal region during binocular fixation. The stimulus to apparent convergence is also unknown. Stimuli could evoke accommodative vergence, disparity vergence, and monocularly driven proximal vergence, and none of them requires bifoveal vergence and alignment. Clearly, binocular fixation is less accurate than in adults. Much of the time the two ocular images are not aligned on corresponding points, but since Panum's areas may be much larger in neonates than adults owing to the reduced visual acuity and possible extrafoveal fixation preference of infants fusion may result. Panum's areas in adulthood vary according to the spatial frequency or coarseness of the fusion stimulus from several arc minutes with fine detail to over 6 degrees with coarse detail (132). Reduced acuity in infancy may restrict binocular integration to coarse features, which results in an extended fusion range. (See Fig. 4.2.)

VERSIONAL (CONJUGATE) EYE MOVEMENTS

Hering's Law of Yoked Eye Movements

In addition to convergence, which allows the eyes to fuse objects binocularly at various viewing distances, binocular vision also relies on yoked conjugate eye movements to maintain a fixed vergence angle during versional saccadic and pursuit eye movements. Hering's law describes this conjugacy relationship as equal movement of the two eyes. Recent studies by Horner, Gleason, and Schor (69) demonstrate that conjugacy can be recalibrated in response to anisometropic spectacle corrections and to partial weakening of one or more muscle groups.

Ling (87) observed binocular following (conjugate) eye movements of all types and in all directions in 75 infants during the first 48 hours of life. She reported that the onset of convergence is delayed nearly 2 months in

the same infants. There are sparse reports of an apparent lack of conjugacy or independence of eye rotation in newborns (51), but these may result from an occasional combination of versional and accommodative vergence movements, both of which are present in neonates.

Saccades

Rapid shifts of attention from one portion of the visual field to another often evoke a fast, saccadic eye movement that places the image of the new target of regard on the fovea. These movements have short latencies of 180 to 200 msec and high velocities approaching 1000 deg/sec. Saccade velocity increases with saccade amplitude according to a function referred to as the main sequence plot (Fig. 4.3), which provides a means of identifying saccadic eye movements on the basis of their velocity (14).

Saccadic movements are easily observed in newborn infants during wakefulness and sleep. Initially infants are likely to hold one fixation position as opposed to shifting gaze into the periphery; however, the likelihood that a saccade will respond to a peripheral target increases with age and decreases with retinal eccentricity (12). When a novel stimulus is introduced into the periphery, 1- to 2-month-old infants approach the target with a series of small saccadic steps of equal amplitude that rarely exceed 50 percent of the target eccentricity rather than with a single large saccade (3, 12). By the second week of life the hypometric saccadic sequence reliably directs the line of sight toward a peripheral target. After the second month of life, large single saccades are used to redirect gaze to novel targets. Peripheral targets may be fixated as eccentrically as 30 degrees horizontally and 10 degrees vertically. Latencies for initiating the saccadic sequence are highly variable: median values for 1-month-olds are 800, 1320, and 1480 msec in response to step displacements of 10, 20, and 30 degrees. Median latency is reduced in 2-month-olds to 480, 429, and 1280 msec for the same step amplitudes. Intersaccadic intervals

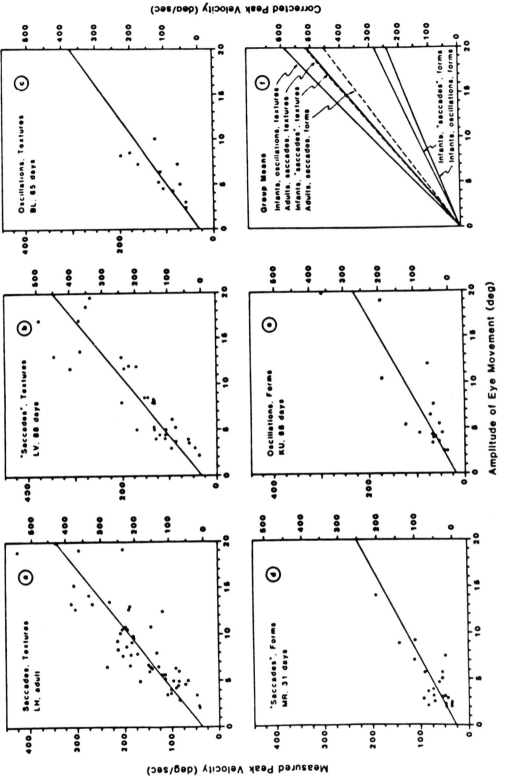

Figure 4.3 Examples of typical main sequences for peak velocity and amplitude of eye movement. The left ordinate shows measured uncorrected values for peak velocity. The right ordinate shows corrected peak velocities for each subject's main sequence (see text). The solid lines chart a linear regression fit to the data. (a) Adult subject, texture stimuli; corrected slope is 21.6, $r = 0.85$. (b) Eighty-eight-day-old infant, texture stimuli, saccades (nonoscillatory fast movements); corrected slope is 22.3, $r = 0.88$. (c) Sixty-five-day-old infant, texture stimuli, oscil-

lations; corrected slope is 18.8, $r = 0.71$. (d) Thirty-one-day-old infant, form stimuli, saccades; corrected slope is 12.3, $r = 0.81$. (e) Sixty-eight-day-old infant, form stimuli, oscillations; corrected slope is 12.8, $r = 0.85$. (f) Average main sequence for infant and adult subjects, plotted separately for form and textures. Infant curves are also shown separately for saccades and oscillations. (From Hainline L, Turkel J, Abramov I, et al: Characteristics of saccades in human infants. Vision Res 24:1771, 1984.)

of all amplitude saccades are of similar duration. Interestingly, the highly variable latencies observed in infants can be as short as 240 msec, similar to the briefest normal adult saccade latency to unpredictable target motion. The long latencies and hypometric saccadic responses may reflect spatial uncertainty, which in turn could result from the initial stage of calibrating the integration of retinotopic and eye position (motor outflow) information in the computation of visual direction. Interestingly, longer saccadic latencies have also been observed in preschool children (80) and in older children (105).

Scanning Eye Movements

Eye movement patterns that explore a static visual display are composed principally of saccadic eye movements. In his classic text, Yarbus (147) demonstrates how the saccadic pattern of eye movements reflects the points of greatest interest in the visual scene. Fantz (44) and many others have used saccades as an objective indicator to investigate the development of pattern vision in infants. Interestingly, the characteristics of saccadic movements are different under these conditions of free scan than when specific novel stimuli are presented in the periphery. When infants ranging in age from 2 weeks to 5 months are presented with a complex scene, and no attempt is made to elicit eye movements to a particular location, multiple saccades no longer occur; rather, single large saccades control fixation (57). The range of amplitudes (2 to 20 degrees) is similar to the adult range of scanning saccade amplitudes. Saccade velocity is also adultlike. Figure 4.3 illustrates the main sequence plot of saccade velocity as a function of saccade amplitude for infants viewing textured stimuli and simple geometric forms. Saccades reach adult velocities when they view textured stimuli and slow down when they view geometric forms (59). Regression analysis of developmental trends reveals that saccadic eye velocity does not increase over the 2-week to 5-month period (59). Apparently, during free scanning eye movements infants from 2 to 20 weeks make

mature saccades, whereas when targets are flashed in an otherwise empty field saccadic responses are hypometric during the first 2 months of life (12). Saccades are relatively mature compared to most other types of eye movements made by infants. This precocity forms the basis of the preferential looking (PL) techniques, in which two images, a test and control, are presented alternately to an infant. Based on the work of Fantz (44) and others, the infant is assumed to direct saccadic head and eye movements toward the most interesting or highly visible target (57, 58, 78, 84, 94, 113, 118). Because neonates exhibit saccades the PL method can be applied in very young infants.

Pursuits

Pursuit tracking eye movements are one of the oculomotor functions most susceptible to postnatal development of the fovea and to the corresponding development of contrast sensitivity. Whereas it is possible for adults to pursue extrafoveal targets (33, 141, 146), these responses have lower velocities or velocity gain (eye velocity/target velocity) than do foveal pursuit responses. In addition, the upper velocity limit for adult pursuit responses is reduced by lowering target contrast (52, 141). Normally smooth following pursuit velocity can approach 100 deg/sec for brief constant velocity targets and 30 to 40 deg/sec for continuously varying sinusoidal motion (28, 30). Latencies are shorter for pursuits to unpredictable ramp targets (130 msec) than for saccades (180 to 200 msec) (108). Pursuit accuracy is much improved by predictability (81); eye velocity can vary sinusoidally in phase with pendular target motion over a range of temporal frequencies (up to 1 Hz).

Immature foveal function in neonates is believed to be responsible for their poor smooth-pursuit performance (82). Pursuit responses by newborns have been reported for simple ramp or constant-velocity targets of short duration (56, 82, 111) but not in response to sinusoidal varying (pendular) motion (4, 136). Pursuit responses in the newborn are brief and intermittent, lasting 300 to 400 msec per episode (Fig. 4.4). These responses are interrupted by what appear to be catch-up saccades. These early pursuits are evoked by large (12-degree) targets that stimulate parafoveal regions, but early responses can also be obtained with small (1.5-degree) targets if they are made attractive with synchronized music and flashing lights (56) or by imaging cartoon characters (111). Early responses are further enhanced by reducing target velocity to under 10 deg/sec, whereas responses to higher velocities (over 15 deg/sec) can be obtained at 10 to 12 weeks of age (56, 111) (Fig. 4.5). These upper velocity limitations may result in part from increased latencies for pursuits in neonates. At high velocities, targets become eccentric or even invisible prior to the onset of the pursuit. Perceived contrast is another factor that can limit the upper velocity for immature pursuits. Contrast sensitivity improves dramatically

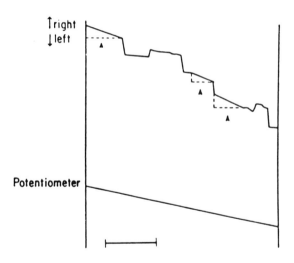

▲,--- added to highlight smooth pursuit segments

Figure 4.4 Typical segment of single-target tracking. Note periods of smooth pursuit interspersed with corrective saccades. Time calibration: 1 second. (From Krementizer JP, Vaughan HG, Kurtzberg D, et al: Smooth-pursuit eye movements in the newborn infant. Child Dev 50:442, 1979.)

during the first 6 months of life (115), and the upper velocity limit for pursuits is clearly restricted by reduced target contrast (52, 141).

Horizontal pursuit develops before vertical pursuit, and responses to constant-velocity targets appear before those to targets with variable (sinusoidal) motion in both orientations (57). Sinusoidal responses to pendular motion require prediction or anticipation of future target velocity in order to maintain a phase-locked velocity response profile. At birth, infants attempt to track pendular target motion with saccades and do not demonstrate smooth following components in their tracking response until 8 to 12 weeks of life (Fig. 4.1) (4). Even then, the pursuit component of the predictive tracking has less gain (0.5) and greater phase lags than the adult response at similar tracking frequencies (0.33 to 0.5 Hz) (4). Even a small sample ($N = 2$) of preschool children aged 4 and 5 have pursuits with increased phase lag in response to periodic target motion (80). Ten-year-old children show some pursuit phase improvement but are still worse than adults (77). These differences may be due to attentional factors. Clearly, the development of the pursuit response varies a great deal between individuals. From a clinical standpoint, failure of infants older than 4 months to pursue a hand-held moving target observed directly is likely to indicate a sensory or motor abnormality. Smooth eye movement disorders can be diagnosed by observing for the optokinetic reflex, which is normally responsive to high-velocity stimuli (>25 deg/sec) at birth.

REFLEX CONJUGATE EYE MOVEMENTS

Optokinetic Nystagmus

Reflex optokinetic following responses to large, moving, patterned fields are more easily evoked in neonates than are pursuit responses to small isolated targets (13, 38). This is due, in part, to the interaction of target size and the immature fovea. Optokinetic nystagmus (OKN) targets that exceed 5 degrees in diameter will stimulate the more devel-

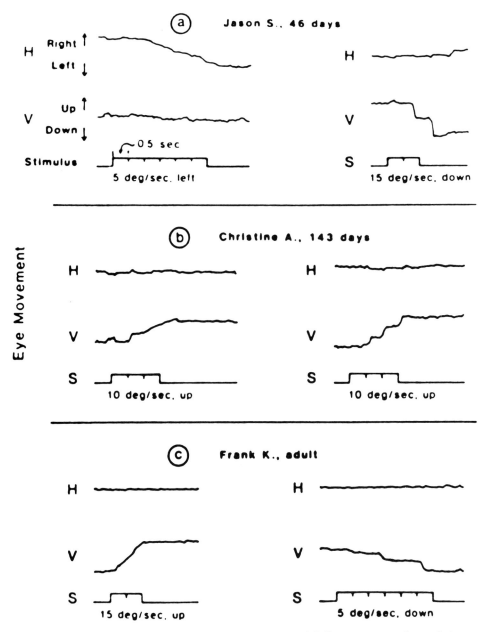

Figure 4.5 Examples of smooth pursuit from infants of different ages and an adult. The target was a 1.5-degree spot. The top trace for each example represents horizontal and the bottom trace vertical eye position, each plotted against time. Note that the younger infant (**a**) shows smooth pursuit at lower velocities but not higher velocities. The older infant (**b**) is able to show smooth pursuit to higher velocities but does not do so all the time. A naive adult subject (**c**), capable of smooth pursuit at higher velocities, also shows saccadic pursuit to lower velocities on some trials. (From Hainline L: Oculomotor control in human infants. In (Groner R, McKonkie GE, Menz L (eds): Eye Movements and Human Information Processing. Amsterdam, Elsevier, 1985.)

oped parafovea, whereas small pursuit targets can easily be restricted to the immature central retina.

The mature optokinetic reflex responds to target motion in any direction or orientation with slow following movements interrupted 2 or 3 times each second by saccadic refixation in the opposite direction. The amplitude or gain of the slow phase response to a broad range of stimulus velocities varies from 70 to 90 percent, approaching 90 deg/sec for large field stimuli. Responses to smaller fields (20 degree) are limited to lower velocities by the duration of the stimulus as it crosses the field and by the 3-Hz saccadic (fast-phase) frequency limit (128). The fast-phase frequency of OKN has two states that depend on viewing instructions. Fast-phase frequency is 1 Hz when the subject is instructed to follow individual features (look OKN), and it increases to 3 Hz when the subject is instructed not to attend to any particular feature but to maintain target visibility (stare OKN) (129). This fast-phase frequency is an indicator of the fixation mode used by infants during tests of OKN.

Traditionally, OKN has been used to evaluate visual acuity in infants (37, 44, 47). More recently it has been used to evaluate the development of binocularity. Patients with binocular anomalies of childhood strabismus, monocular cataract, or amblyopia exhibit an asymmetry of the optokinetic response. When stimulated monocularly, the slow-phase component has a higher velocity in response to nasalward and to downward than to temporalward and upward field motion (127). This asymmetry occurs for monocular stimulation of either the preferred or nonpreferred eye and is believed to result from a deficit of cortical binocularity (67). Afferent fibers from the two eyes converge on the pretectum via binocular cells in the visual cortex. In the absence of binocularity, temporal asynchrony between the two eyes' inputs is believed to result in subcortical suppression of motion signals in the temporalward, and presumably the upward, direction (67). Latent nystagmus, which is a nasalward slow-phase jerk nystagmus during monocular fixation, is another symptom of this subcortical binocular anomaly (131). Prior to the development of cortical binocularity infants exhibit a similar horizontal asymmetry of monocular OKN (13, 58, 99, 129). After 5 months of age, the infant's OKN becomes symmetric in the horizontal meridian at about the same time that stereopsis emerges (99). OKN remains asymmetric in adults who had deprived binocularity as a result of cataract (93, 127) or strabismus (127) prior to 6 years of age. Since symmetric OKN appears at 3 months of age, the loss of this symmetry later represents deterioration or loss of binocularity rather than arrest of development. The loss may persist even though normal visual acuity is restored in monocular cataract (85) amblyopia and when binocular eye alignment is regained in strabismus (127). The continued OKN asymmetry suggests that subcortical binocularity may remain disrupted after some binocular cortical functions are recovered (124).

OKN is present at birth in full-term and premature infants (82, 90). Fast-phase frequency is approximately 1 Hz (131), which suggests that infants are in the look fixation mode of OKN. Occasionally a young infant shows brief bursts of 3-Hz OKN (stare OKN) and then reverts back to the lower-frequency response. These low-frequency responses are not voluntary pursuits, because aftereffects of OKN (OKAN) continue in darkness (see Fig. 4.6) (131). Clearly, attentional factors have a strong influence on the fast-phase frequency of OKN.

The slow phase of the optokinetic response increases proportionally with stimulus velocity up to a limit. The upper limit in newborns is approximately 25 deg/sec (82). Improvement in slow-phase response occurs through the first year of life, eventually reaching adult velocity limits over 40 deg/sec. The gradual improvement in slow-following phase parallels the development of contrast sensitivity during the first 5 months of life (18). Reduced target contrast normally reduces the upper velocity limit for smooth following movements in adults (52, 141). Clearly, reduced contrast sensitivity will reduce the gain of slow-phase responses to high-velocity stimuli.

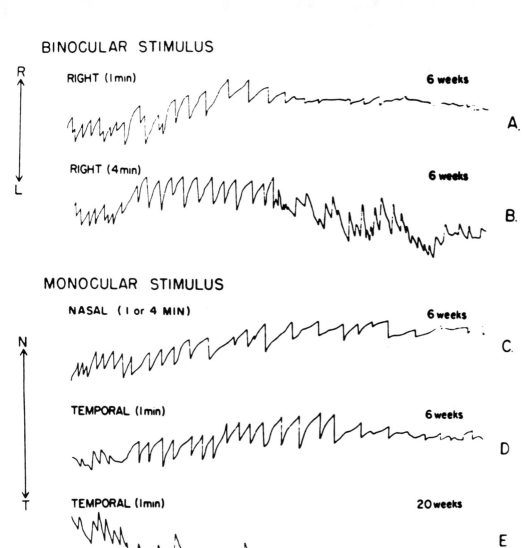

BINOCULAR STIMULUS

RIGHT (1 min)   **6 weeks**   A.

RIGHT (4 min)   **6 weeks**   B.

MONOCULAR STIMULUS

NASAL (1 or 4 MIN)   6 weeks   C.

TEMPORAL (1 min)   6 weeks   D

TEMPORAL (1 min)   20 weeks   E

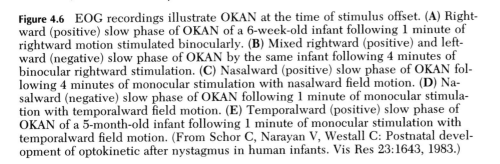

LIGHT   DARKNESS

10 SECONDS

Figure 4.6 EOG recordings illustrate OKAN at the time of stimulus offset. (**A**) Right-ward (positive) slow phase of OKAN of a 6-week-old infant following 1 minute of rightward motion stimulated binocularly. (**B**) Mixed rightward (positive) and left-ward (negative) slow phase of OKAN by the same infant following 4 minutes of binocular rightward stimulation. (**C**) Nasalward (positive) slow phase of OKAN following 4 minutes of monocular stimulation with nasalward field motion. (**D**) Na-salward (negative) slow phase of OKAN following 1 minute of monocular stimulation with temporalward field motion. (**E**) Temporalward (positive) slow phase of OKAN of a 5-month-old infant following 1 minute of monocular stimulation with temporalward field motion. (From Schor C, Narayan V, Westall C: Postnatal development of optokinetic after nystagmus in human infants. Vis Res 23:1643, 1983.)

Vestibuloocular Reflex

Direction of gaze is sustained during body movement by OKN at relatively low stimulus velocities and by vestibuloocular reflex (VOR) during acceleration. The VOR responds to even the smallest head acceleration after a 12-msec latency (31). Like OKN, the VOR to unidirectional acceleration is characterized by slow-phase compensatory eye movements interrupted by rapid flicks in the opposite direction. In addition to these dynamic posture responses, there are static gravitational reflexes in which the eyes counter roll in response to head tilt.

The vestibular system is anatomically complete and functional at birth. The endolymphatic and bony labyrinths are mature at birth (36a) and the full complements of myelinated vestibular fibers (18a), and vestibular hair cells (110a) are also present.

Both the static and kinetic ophthalmic vestibular responses are present at birth (104). The VOR is present in full-term infants but not in premature infants, and it is more robust in infants with higher birth weight (42). From 1 month of age the VOR evoked by unidirectional acceleration is of a higher amplitude and velocity than it will be later in life. Slow-phase amplitude slowly decreases in the first 7 years of life (101). These changes have been quantified by modeling the VOR as a first-order open-loop control system with a gain defined as the ratio of maximum eye velocity to acceleration, and a time constant describing the decay of slow-component velocity following termination of head acceleration (102). Time constants increase, but gains decrease as a function of the logarithm of age. The most dramatic changes occur in the first 30 months, when gain is reduced from 10 to 7.5 and time constant increases from 8 to 10 seconds. The time constant of decay reflects the viscoelastic properties of the cupula and the effect of a central neural integrator (102). Presumably, higher gains are advantageous to young infants, who constantly experience unpredictable passive body motion.

The VOR operates in an open-loop mode; that is, it has no direct feedback for its accuracy. Visual experience is required to maintain an adequate vestibular response to body motion, as is evidenced by reduced gain of the VOR in adults who were blinded at an early age (136). Visual feedback, in the form of retinal slip, alters the gain of the VOR (131). For example, optical distortions produced by a left-right–reversing prism (49) or an optical image magnifier (95) result in respective phase reversal or gain alterations of the VOR. During the first few months of life, when there is rapid visual development, including growth of the eyeball and its contents, there is a need for continued accurate calibration of the VOR in order to maintain clear vision during body movement.

The VOR shows evidence of plasticity and adaptability at birth. Adaptability is normally indicated by a reversal of the slow-phase component of VOR after nystagmus when an acceleration stimulus has ceased. During the first year of life the amplitude of this secondary nystagmus (vestibulo afternystagmus) is disproportionately greater than the primary nystagmus (101). Plasticity of the VOR, as evidenced by changes in gain produced by unidirectional optokinetic stimulation, has been demonstrated in children as young as 2 months of age (143). Development of the optokinetic response was reflected in the plasticity of the VOR. During the first 2 months of life, both nasalward and temporalward optokinetic stimulation produced an increased slow-phase gain of the nasalward VOR. After 2 months, slow-phase gain of the VOR increased in the same direction as the optokinetic stimulus. These results indicate development of direction selectivity during the first 2 months of life (129).

NEAR-TRIAD AND DISJUNCTIVE EYE MOVEMENTS

Pupillary Reflex

The near triad describes the simultaneous accommodation and vergence response of the pupil to either accommodative or vergence stimuli. Presumably the associated pupillary constriction with near-point activity is to increase the eye's depth of focus and reduce the demand on the accommodative system and to reduce chromatic and spherical aberration of the optics of the eye during critical near-point inspection tasks. The third and most obvious function is to regulate the amount of light entering the eye, particularly during the initial stages of light- and dark adaptation.

In adults, pupil diameters range from 2 to 8 mm, with variations of light level that result in a 16-fold or 1.2–log unit change in retinal illumination. The pupillary response has an initial transient or phasic component, which is followed by a sustained tonic component. The phasic component has a latency of 300 to 500 msec and a duration of 1 second (88). The tonic, or resting, state is achieved within several minutes, depending on the time course of light and dark adaptation.

Pupillary responses to light are present at birth in both full-term and premature infants (78, 104). The pupillary response is also consensual at birth. The phasic component of the pupillary response of a 2-month-old infant to increments in light (0.1 to 0.5 log ftL) has prolonged latency (567 to 467 msec) and smaller amplitude and is more sluggish than in adulthood (Fig. 4.7) (6). The tonic diameter of the infant's pupil increases during the first 2 months of life (115). Figure 4.8 illustrates mean pupil diameter in adults and in 1- and 2-month-old infants as a function of increasing background luminance following dark adaptation. The seven panels present responses to seven luminance levels (0.06 to 60.74 ftL in 0.5–log unit steps). Each luminance level was presented for 30 seconds following 10 minutes of dark adaptation. The left plot is of mean pupil diameter averaged second by second. The right plot is the mean pupil diameter averaged across the final 10 seconds of each luminance level (116). The figure illustrates that mean pupil diameter decreased by nearly 2 mm as luminance increased from very dim to very bright levels (3 log units). Pupil diameter is smaller by 1 to 2

mm at all light levels in 1-month-olds than in 2-month-olds, and absolute pupil diameter in 2-month-old infants is very similar to that of adults. The pupil diameter of young infants is highly variable, presumably owing to large variations in level of attention and state of alertness (15).

Depth of Focus

The reduced pupil size in infancy is one of several factors that contribute to greater depth of focus (DOF) in neonates. Other factors that increase DOF include reduced visual acuity, reduced receptor density at the fovea, and short (18 mm) axis (48). These factors predict that a newborn's DOF should be approximately 1.5 D compared to the 0.43 D of adults (29). A neonate's DOF approximates the average refractive state of 1.5 D of hyperopia (15, 48) (Fig. 4.9). Not until 6 to 12 months of age does the DOF fall below this level (106). Accordingly, the preferential looking procedure, which evaluates visual acuity, will not be contaminated by the average error of refraction until 6 to 12 months of age.

Accommodation

As would be expected, the magnitude and accuracy of accommodation improve as the DOF is reduced in the developing infant (15, 63). At birth, the amplitude of accommodation, extrapolated from Hofstetter's equation (68), is 18.5 D. This amplitude is reduced by 1 D every 3 years, owing to progressive sclerosis of the lens that becomes complete at approximately 53 years of age (61). In spite of their potential capacity, newborn infants do not fully utilize accommodation because their DOF is so large that large changes in target distance do not produce increases in perceived blur and, consequently, an accommodative response is unnecessary. The accuracy of accommodation agrees closely with the DOF, which, as it is reduced with age, is largely responsible for the improvement in accommodative responses (15).

Accuracy of accommodation is measured by the accommodative response curve, which

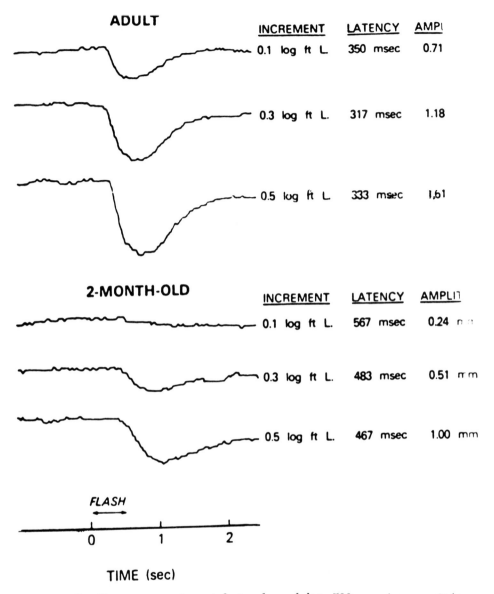

Figure 4.7 Pupillary response in an infant and an adult to 500-msec increments in luminance at intervals of 1 sec. (From Aslin RN: Motor aspects of visual development in infancy. In Salapatek P, Cohen L (eds): Handbook of Infant Perception, vol 1, chap 2. New York, Academic Press, 1987.)

plots accommodative response as a function of its stimulus. The response function slopes increase from 0.5 in 1-month-old children to 0.75 in 2-month-olds, and to about 0.8 in 3-month-olds (15), whereas the adult's slope is 0.95 (Fig. 4.10). Clearly, there is a notable

improvement in accommodative accuracy by 2 to 3 months of age.

One consequence of the inaccurate accommodation in infants is that they can accommodate incorrectly without experiencing noticeable blur. Errors of this sort are re-

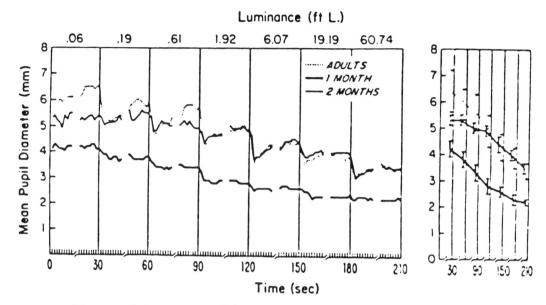

Figure 4.8 Mean pupil diameters in adults, 1-month-olds, and 2-month-olds as a function of increasing background luminance following dark adaptation. (From Salapatek P, Banks MS: Infant sensory assessment. Vision. In Minifie FD, Lloyd LL (eds): Communicative and Cognitive Abilities: Early Behavioral Assessment. Baltimore MD, University Park Press, 1978.)

ferred to as pseudomyopias; examples are space myopia and instrument myopia (65). One-month-old infants exhibit a pseudo-myopia in which they accommodate to a distance of 20 cm while viewing distant targets (63). This pseudomyopia provides an estimate of the resting focus of accommodation in infancy. Given that infants are normally 1.5 to 2 D hyperopic under cycloplegic refraction (15), at least 5 to 7 D of accommodation is needed to reach the resting focus. The average resting focus of accommodation in adults is only 1.5 D (103, 124). It is likely that proximal stimuli and large prolonged after effects of sustained near accommodation (126) contribute to the high values for the resting focus of accommodation in young infants. The pseudomyopia disappears by the third month of life, when infants begin to accommodate more accurately (16). The appearance of accommodative responses may be delayed, however, until a later age by large amounts of hyperopia and myopia which are not easily

overcome by low-level efforts of accommodation (27). Consequently, infants with large refractive states may be at risk for amblyopia and reduced contrast sensitivity as a result of deprivation from inaccurate accommodation (6). Indeed, Ingram et al. (73) report that refractive errors at 12 months are followed by development of strabismus and amblyopia.

Naturally occurring astigmatism may play an important role in the development of accommodation. Owing in part to the large angle Kappa associated with the infant's short axial length, against-the-rule astigmatism is produced by the mismatch of the visual and optical axes of the eye. This form of astigmatism is corneal and is highly prevalent (57%) during the first 6 months of life (39, 70, 96). Astigmatism effectively reduces the DOF if the DOFs for the most ametropic meridians do not overlap (70). A reasonable strategy for accommodation is to focus the retinal image in the center of the interval of Sturm. Additional information about the direction to ac-

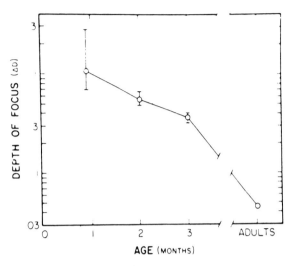

Figure 4.9 DOF values estimated from equation $(D = 7.03/P \cdot V)$ for 1-, 2- and 3-month-olds and adults. (*V*, visual acuity; *P*, pupil diameter.) The points represent the average DOFs calculated with acuity values from Allen (2), Atkinson et al., and Banks and Salapatek (18). The brackets represent the total range of DOFs calculated using those acuity values. [Reprinted with permission from Vision Res 20:827, 1980, Green DG, Powers MK, Banks MS: Depth of focus, eye size, and visual acuity. Copyright (1980), Pergamon Press plc.]

commodate can also be gained from astigmatism (29). With the development of acuity and reduction of DOF, the astigmatic information is no longer necessary. Interestingly, there is a sharp decline in the incidence of astigmatism during the second 6 months of life that coincides with the rapid improvement of visual acuity, and there is a reduction in angle Kappa due in part to an increase of axial length from 17 to 20 mm (83).

Vergence

A variety of sensory functions including relative depth perception, camouflaged form perception (as in random dot stereogram), and motion in depth perception are enhanced by binocular disparity cues. Our ability to sense

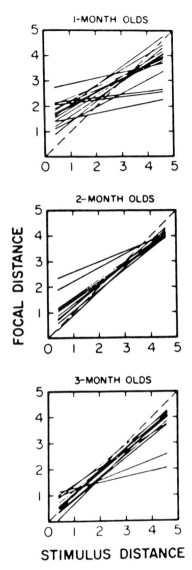

Figure 4.10 Best-fitting lines were found for each infant's accommodation functions. Those lines are plotted here. The graphs display the lines for 1-month-olds (3 to 5 weeks), 2-months-olds (7 to 9 weeks), and 3-month-olds (11 to 13 weeks), respectively. Individual infants may be represented more than once in a particular age group. Data obtained at 6 and 10 weeks are not shown. The function that would be observed if accommodation were perfectly accurate is indicated by the broken lines. (From Banks MS: The development of visual accommodation during early infancy. Child Dev, 51:646, 1980.)

or encode these disparities relies heavily on binocular alignment of the eyes to within a fraction of a degree of the object of regard. If this binocular motor alignment is not achieved during early infancy, the binocular sensory functions may not develop adequately to support binocular alignment in the future. In such cases constant strabismus may develop. Subsequent suppression of the deviating eye may deprive it of necessary stimulation during the critical period of development (98), and partial loss of sight (amblyopia) could result.

Vergence eye movements normally respond in both open-loop and closed-loop modes. The open-loop responses do not utilize feedback and are stimulated by intrinsic innervation (tonic vergence), blur (accommodative vergence), and perceived distance (proximal vergence). These responses are refined by a closed-loop response (disparity vergence) that utilizes retinal image disparity as a source of sensory feedback. Currently it is believed that the open-loop vergence responses are present at birth but that the closed-loop disparity vergence develops postnatally.

Tonic Vergence

Innervation that converges the eyes from the divergent anatomic position of rest to the physiologic position of rest is referred to as tonic. The physiologic position of rest is usually quantified with the distances phoria test and is normally found to be 1 to 2 PD exophoric (97). Dark vergence, or convergence in darkness, is another measure that some use to locate the physiological position of rest (103). In darkness the eyes frequently converge to 1.2 m (8 PD esophoria). The 10-PD difference in these two measures is not due to accommodative vergence, since accommodation and vergence are weakly correlated in darkness (79). Dark vergence appears to have a strong proximal component, because it correlates strongly with errors of perceived distance (103).

Errors of binocular fixation, described for infants earlier in this chapter, are usually di-

vergent (5, 92, 135, 145). This error would represent the physiologic position of rest if there were no fusional vergence responses operating prior to 3 to 4 months of age.

Another approach to measuring tonic vergence has been to measure binocular eye position during deep sleep (109). Approximately half of the infants examined by Rethy had 15 to 35 degrees of divergence during the first few days of life. Some of this measure may have been biased by the large angle Kappa of newborns; however the disappearance of this divergence at the third week of life suggests that angle Kappa was not the sole factor involved because the eye does not change axial length sufficiently in 3 weeks to account for the observed change. It is possible that an innervation other than tonic, such as accommodative vergence, may also have contributed to the change noted in binocular alignment during sleep.

Unlike the large divergent errors noted for neonates in sleep and while fixating distance objects, measures of dark vergence in infants aged 5 to 22 weeks reveal that the eyes converge to a distance of 33 cm (9, 11). The difference between light heterophoria and dark vergence (74) is nearly twice that observed in adults who converge to 1.2 m in darkness. Possibly the dark vergence represents a proximal vergence response to sensed distance in darkness.

Observations made by Rethy (109) suggest that there are marked changes in the tonic vergence during the first few weeks of life. These changes are long lasting, as is demonstrated by the stability of the distance heterophoria throughout life (66). The process of reducing the distance phoria is referred to as orthophorization (36) and demonstrates the plasticity of tonic vergence innervation. This plasticity is manifest in maturity as prism adaptation or adjustment of heterophoria in response to lenses and prisms worn before the eyes for a period of 15 seconds (122). Clearly, vergence adaptation would be of benefit to infants during the first 5 years of life, when there is rapid growth of the cranium and increase in interpupillary distance.

Accommodative Vergence

Accommodative vergence is another open-loop response that is believed to be present in neonates (6). During the second week of life, monocularly stimulated accommodation results in a reliable convergence of the covered eye (10). The magnitude of the accommodative convergence-accommodation (AC-A) ratio in neonates has not been determined, principally because of calibration difficulty (10). It is possible that the gain of accommodative vergence is modified during development to compensate for changes in interpupillary distance of 40 mm at birth to 64 mm in adulthood. One possible mechanism for this change would be the development of adaptable tonic accommodation. Accommodative vergence becomes reduced as the resting focus of accommodation adapts to minimize accommodative effort (125). Developmental change in DOF is still another factor that influences the effective range and amplitude of accommodative vergence. Clinically, the AC-A ratio is computed with the stimulus rather than accommodative responses in the denominator. Because accommodation lags behind its stimulus, the stimulus ratio will underestimate the actual response gain of accommodation vergence by about 10 percent. This error in measurement will be much larger in infants, because the lag of accommodation is nearly 100 percent in neonates owing to their DOF. Thus changes noted in the stimulus AC-A ratio may simply reflect changes in the DOF and accuracy of the accommodative response (134). As the DOF becomes smaller, the infant will accommodate more to near objects, and accommodative vergence will begin to emerge as a major component of the composite vergence response.

Fusional Vergence

The refinement of binocular alignment is achieved by utilizing feedback from retinal image disparity (108). Both the disparity vergence response and binocular sensory functions such as fusion and stereopsis rely on the same stimulus (retinal image disparity). Until the mechanisms that encode and process retinal image disparity develop, there can be no disparity vergence or stereoscopic depth. Studies utilizing visual evoked potentials that examine correlates of fusion and stereopsis indicate that the visual cortex first becomes functionally binocular between 3 and 5 months of age (22). Behavioral tests of stereopsis using preferential looking confirm that stereoscopic depth perception matures during the period from 4 to 6 months of age (19, 45). This postnatal development is not delayed by convergence inaccuracy because the age of onset of stereopsis is no earlier when infants are tested with periodic depth gratings that yield a stereopercept for a large range (30 degrees) of vergence angles (20). Preferential looking tests also indicate that sensory fusion and rivalry emerge at 4 months (21, 138).

The age of onset for disparity vergence has been determined by Aslin (4) using the loose prism test (75, 142). In this test, a base-out (BO) prism of 4 to 10 PD is placed before the preferred eye during binocular fixation of a distant target. The normal response to this asymmetric vergence stimulus is a yoked saccade away from the side of the prism eye, followed by a convergence of the two eyes. If both phases of this response occur, the nonpreferred eye abducts and then adducts. If fusion does not occur, there is only the abduction or no movement if the patient chooses to fixate with the nonpreferred eye. Aslin observed that 3-month-old infants demonstrated the biphasic response only once in 120 trials. Four-month-olds demonstrated the biphasic response on 2 percent of the trials with a 5-BO prism and 13 percent with a 10-BO prism. Six-month-olds demonstrated the biphasic response 45 percent of the time with the 5-BO prism and 72 percent with the 10-BO prism (Fig. 4.11). Thus motor fusional responses are emerging at the age of onset of stereopsis. It is possible that some gross fusional movements occur prior to this age and that they produce the apparent binocular alignment during the first 4 months of life. These may be peripheral fusion responses that are too sluggish or that have too long a latency to be detected on the loose prism test.

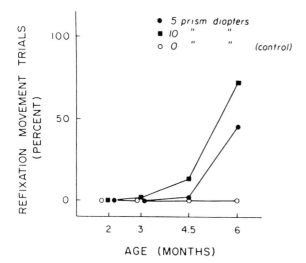

Figure 4.11 The probability of a refixation response to prism-induced binocular misalignment. (From Aslin RN: Development of binocular fixation in human infants. J Exp Child Psychol 23:133, 1977.)

Diplopia would not necessarily appear in the central visual field, owing to the immature acuity and the large Panum's limits that occur with perception of low spatial frequency detail (132). It is also possible that accommodative and proximal vergence maintain gross alignment, or perhaps that the eyes could converge on a near target by means of separate control of each eye's fixation (22). Subtle aspects of this latter possibility are seen in conjugate saccadic vergence eye movements made by normal adults during asymmetric vergence (41).

It is clear that the binocular disparity vergence system is the last of the oculomotor functions to develop. Little is known about the dynamics of these responses in immature infants (i.e., latency, velocity, adaptability) or the age at which the response is adultlike. It is remarkable that gross binocular alignment is possible in infants prior to the emergence of disparity vergence, as this is the only vergence component that utilizes sensory feedback to ensure an accurate response (closed-loop). Curiously, patients who lose their

ability to utilize disparity cues have both stereoblindness and strabismus. Apparently they no longer have access to the mechanisms utilized by neonates to maintain gross binocular alignment in the absence of the disparity vergence feedback control system. It is also possible that they have extensive suppression that blocks central and peripheral sensory fusion. It is likely that infants utilize peripheral fusion before it has developed centrally to support stereoscopic depth perception and that peripheral fusion is too sluggish to be revealed by the loose prism test of asymmetric vergence.

REFERENCES

1. Abrimov I, Gordon J, Hendrickson A, et al: The retina in the newborn infant. Science 217:265, 1982.

2. Allen S: Visual acuity development in human infants up to 6-months of age. Unpublished doctoral dissertation. University of Washington, 1979.

3. Ashmead D: Parameters of infant saccadic eye movements. Infant Behav Dev 7:16, 1984.

4. Aslin RN: Development of smooth pursuit in human infants. In Fisher DF, Monty RA, Senders JW (eds): Eye Movements: Cognitive and Visual Perception. Hillsdale NJ, Erlbaum, 1981.

5. Aslin RN: Development of binocular fixation in human infants. J Exp Child Psychol 23:133, 1977.

6. Aslin RN: Motor aspects of visual development in infancy. In Salapatek P, Cohen L (eds): Handbook of Infant Perception, vol 1, chap 2. New York, Academic Press, 1987.

7. Aslin RN: Normative oculomotor development in human infants. In: Strabismus and Amblyopia—Experimental Basis for Advances in Clinical Management. New York, Pergamon Press, 1988.

8. Aslin RN, Ciuffreda K: Eye movements of preschool children. Science 222:74, 1983.

9. Aslin RN, Dobson V: Dark vergence and dark accommodation in human infants. Vision Res 23:1671, 1983.

10. Aslin RN, Jackson RW: Accommodative-convergence in young infants: Development of a synergistic sensory-motor system. Can J Psychol 33:222, 1979.

11. Aslin RN, Jackson RW: Dark vergence in human infants. Invest Ophthalmol Vis Sci (Suppl) 20:47, 1981.

12. Aslin RN, Salapatek P: Saccadic localization of visual targets by the very young human infant. Percept Psychophysics 17:293, 1975.

13. Atkinson J, Braddick O: Development of optokinetic nystagmus in infants: An indicator of cortical binocularity? In Fisher DF, Monty RA, Sander JW (eds): Eye Movements: Cognition and Visual Perception. Hillsdale NJ, Erlbaum, 1981.

14. Bahill AT, Clark MR, Stark L: The main sequence, a tool for studying human eye movements. Math Bio Sci 24:191, 1975.

15. Banks MS: The development of visual accommodation during early infancy. Child Dev 51:646, 1980.

16. Banks MS: Infant refraction and accommodation. Int Ophthalmol Clin 20:205, 1980.

17. Banks MS: The development of spatial and temporal contrast sensitivity. Curr Eye Res 2:191, 1982.

18. Banks MS, Salapatek P: Acuity and contrast sensitivity in 1-, 2-, 3-month-old human infants. Invest Ophthalmol Vis Sci 17:361, 1978.

18a. Bergstrom B: Morphology of the vestibular nerve. II. The number of myelinated vestibular nerve fibers in man at various ages. Acta Otolaryngol (Stockh) 76:173, 1973.

19. Birch EE, Gwiazda J, Held R: Stereoacuity development for crossed and uncrossed disparities in human infants. Vision Res 22:507, 1982.

20. Birch EE, Gwiazda J, Held R: The development of vergence does not account for the onset of stereopsis. Perception 12:331, 1983.

21. Birch EE, Shimojo S, Held R: Preferential-looking assessment of fusion and stereopsis in infants aged 1–6 months. Invest Ophthalmol Vis Sci 26:366, 1985.

22. Braddick O, Atkinson J: Some recent findings on the development of human binocularity: A review. Behav Brain Res 10:141, 1983.

23. Braddick O, Atkinson J, French J, et al: A photorefractive study of infant accommodation. Vision Res 19:1319, 1979.

24. Braddick O, Atkinson J, Julesz B, et al: Cortical binocularity in infants. Nature 258:363, 1980.

25. Bronson GW: The Scanning Patterns of Human Infants: Implications for Visual Learning. Norwood NJ, Ablex, 1982.

26. Bronson GW: Potential sources of error when applying a corneal reflex eye-monitoring technique to infant subjects. Behav Res Meth Instrum 15:22, 1983.

27. Brookman KE: Ocular accommodation in human infants. Am J Optom Physiol Opt 60:91, 1980.

28. Buzza A, Schmid R, Gizi MR: The range of linearity of the smooth pursuit control system. In Gale AG, Johnson F (eds): Theoretical and Applied Aspects of Eye Movement Research. Amsterdam, Elsevier, 473, 1984.

29. Campbell FW, Westheimer G: Dynamics of the accommodation response of the human eye. J Physiol (Lond) 151:285, 1960.

30. Carpenter RHS: Movements of the Eyes. London, Pion, 1977.

31. Cogan DG: Neurology of the Ocular Muscles. Springfield IL, Charles C Thomas, 1956.

32. Cohen B, Henn V, Raphen T, et al: Velocity storage, nystagmus and visual-vestibular interactions in humans. Ann NY Acad Sci 421, 1981.

33. Collewijn H, Tamminga EP: Human fixation and pursuit in normal and open-loop conditions: Effects of central and peripheral retinal targets. J Physiol 379:109, 1986.

34. Corin MS, Teresita ES, Bender MB: Oculomotor function in patients with Parkinson's disease. J Neurol Sci 15:251,1972.

35. Cornsweet TM: Determination of the stimulus for involuntary drifts and saccadic eye movements. J Opt Soc Am [A] 46:987, 1956.

36. Crone RA: Diplopia. New York, Elsevier, 1973.

36a. Dayal VS, Farkashedy J, Kokshanian A: Embryology of the ear. Can J Otolaryngol 2:136, 1973.

37. Dayton GO, Jones MH: Analysis of charac-

teristics of fixation reflexes in infants by use of direct current electrooculography. Neurology 14:1152, 1964.

38. Dayton GO, Jones MH, Rawson RA, et al: Developmental study of coordinated eye movements in the human infant. II. An electroculographic study of the fixation reflex in the newborn. Arch Ophthalmol 71:871, 1964.

39. Dobson V, Fulton A, Sebrish L: Cycloplegic refractions in infant and young children: The axis of astigmatism. Invest Ophthalmol Vis Sci 25:83, 1984.

40. Dobson V, Howland AC, Moss C, et al: Photorefraction of normal and astigmatic infants during viewing of patterned stimuli. Vision Res 23:1043, 1983.

41. Enright JT: Facilitation of vergence changes by saccades: Influences of misfocused images and of disparity stimuli in man. J Physiol (Lond) 371:69, 1986.

42. Eviatar L, Eviatar A, Narcy I: Maturation of neurovestibular responses in infants. Rev Med Child Neurol 16:435, 1974.

43. Eviatar L, Miranda S, Eviatar A, et al: Development of nystagmus in response to vestibular stimulation in infants. Ann Neurol 5:508, 1979.

44. Fantz RL, Ordy LM, Udelf MS: Maturation of pattern vision during the first six months. J Comp Physiol Psychol 55:907, 1962.

45. Fox B, Aslin RN, Shea SL: Stereopsis in human infants. Science 207:323, 1980.

46. Fulton AB, Dobson V, Salem D, et al: Cycloplegic refractions in infants and young children. Am J Ophthalmol 90:239, 1980.

47. Gorman JJ, Cogan DG, Gellis SS: An apparatus for grading the visual acuity of infants on the basis of optokinetic nystagmus. Pediatrics 19:1088, 1957.

48. Green DG, Powers MK, Banks MS: Depth of focus, eye size, and visual acuity. Vis Res 20:827, 1980.

49. Gonshor A, Melville-Jones G: Extreme vestibulo-ocular adaptation induced by prolonged optical reversal of vision. J Physiol (Lond) 256:381, 1976.

50. Crone RA: Diplopia. New York, Elsevier, 1973.

51. Guernsey M: A quantitative study of the eye reflexes in infants. Psychol Bull 26:160, 1929.

52. Haegerstrom-Portnoy G, Brown B: Contrast effects on smooth-pursuit eye movement velocity. Vision Res 19:169, 1979.

53. Hainline L: Developmental changes in visual screening of faces and nonface patterns by infants. J Exp Child Psychol 25:90, 1978.

54. Hainline L: Eye movements and form perception in human infants. In Fisher DF, Monty RA, Senders JW (eds): Eye Movements: Cognition and Visual Perception. Hillsdale NJ, Erlbaum, 1981.

55. Hainline L: Saccades in human infants. In Gale AG, Johnson F (eds): Theoretical and Applied Aspects of Eye Movement Research. North Holland, Elsevier, 1984.

56. Hainline L: Oculomotor control in human infants. In Groner R, McKonkie GE, Menz L (eds): Eye Movements and Human Information Processing. Amsterdam, Elsevier, 1985.

57. Hainline L: Normal lifespan developmental changes in saccadic and pursuit eye movements. In Johnston CW, Pirozzolo F (eds): Neuropsychology of Eye Movements. Hillsdale NJ, Erlbaum, 1987.

58. Hainline L, Lemerise E: Infant's scanning of geometric forms varying in size. J Exp Child Psychol 33:235, 1982.

59. Hainline L, Lemerise E, Abramov I, et al: Orientational asymmetrics in small-field optokinetic nystagmus in human infants. Behav Brain Res 13:217, 1984.

60. Hainline L, Turkel J, Abramov I, et al: Characteristics of saccades in human infants. Vision Res 24:1771, 1984.

61. Hamasaki D, Ong J, Marg E: The amplitude of accommodation in presbyopia. Am J Optom Arch Am Acad Optom 33:3, 1956.

62. Harris C, Hainline L, Lemerise E, et al: Infant eye movements: Quality of fixation. Invest Ophthalmol Vis Sci (ARVO Suppl) 26:252, 1985.

63. Haynes H, White BL, Held R: Visual accommodation in human infants. Science 148:528, 1965.

64. Hendrickson AE, Yuodelis C: The morphological development of the human fovea. Ophthalmology 91:603, 1984.

65. Hennessy RT: Instrument myopia. J Opt Soc Am [A] 65:1114, 1975.

66. Hirsch MJ, Alpern M, Schultz H: The variation of phoria with age. Am J Optom Arch Am Acad Optom 25:535, 1948.

67. Hoffmann PK: Neuronal basis for changes of the optokinetic reflex with strabismus and amblyopia. In Lennerstrand G, von Noorden G, Campos E, et al: Strabismus and Amblyopia—Experimental Basis for Advances in Clinical Management. Oxford, Pergamon, 1988.

68. Hofstetter HW: Useful age—Amplitude formula. Opt World 38:42, 1950.

69. Horner D, Gleason G, Schor C: The recalibration of Hering's law for versional eye movements in response to aniseikonia. Invest Ophthalmol Vis Sci (Suppl) 28:1988.

70. Howland HC: Infant eyes: Optics and accommodation. Curr Eye Res 2:217, 1952.

71. Howland HC, Howland B: Photorefraction: A technique for study of refractive state at a distance. J Opt Soc Am [A] 64:240, 1974.

72. Howland HC, Sayles N: Photokeratometric and photorefractive measures of astigmatism in infants and young children. Vis Res 25:73, 1985.

73. Ingram RM, Traymar MJ, Walker C, et al: Screening for refractive error at age 1 year: A pilot study. Br J Ophthalmol 63:243, 1979.

74. Ivanoff A, Bourdy C: Le comportement de la convergence en nocturne. Ann Opt Ocul 3:70, 1954.

75. Jampolsky A: The prism test for strabismus screening. J Pediatr Ophthalmol 1:30, 1964.

76. Jones R, Eskridge B: The Hirschberg test—A re-evaluation. Am J Optom Arch Am Acad Optom 47:105, 1970.

77. Kaakinen K: A simple method for screening of children with strabismus, anisometropia or ametropia by simultaneous photography of the corneal and fundus reflexes. Acta Ophthalmol (Copenh) 57:161, 1979.

78. Kessen W, Salapatek P, Haith MM: The visual response of the human newborn to linear contour. J Exp Child Psychol 13:9, 1972.

79. Kotulak J, Schor CM: The dissociability of accommodative from vergence in the dark. Invest Ophthalmol Vis Sci 27:544, 1986.

80. Kowler E, Facciano DM: Kid's poor tracking means habits are lacking. Invest Ophthalmol Vis Sci (ARVO Suppl) 22:103, 1982.

81. Kowler E, McKee S: Sensitivity of smooth eye movement to small differences in target velocity. Vision Res 27:993, 1987.

82. Krementizer JP, Vaughan HG, Kurtzberg D, et al: Smooth-pursuit eye movements in the newborn infant. Child Dev 50:442, 1979.

83. Larsen JS: Sagittal growth of the eye. II. Ultrasonic measurement of the axial length of the eye birth to puberty. Acta Ophthalmol (Copenh) 49:873, 1971.

84. Leahy RL: Development of preferences and processes of visual scanning in human infant during the first 3 months of life. Dev Psychol 12:250, 1976.

85. Lewis TL, Maurer D, Brent A: Effects on perceptual development of visual deprivation during infancy. Br J Ophthalmol 70:214, 1986.

86. Lewis TL, Maurer D, Kay D: Newborn's central vision: Whole or hole? J Exp Child Psychol 26:193, 1978.

87. Ling BC: A genetic study of sustained fixation and associated behavior in the human infant from birth to six months. J Genet Psychol 61:227, 1942.

88. Lowenstein O, Lowenfeld IE: The pupil. In Davson H (ed): The Eye, vol 3. New York, Academic Press, 1969.

89. Mcfarlane A, Harris P, Barnes I: Central and peripheral vision in early infancy. J Exp Child Psychol 21:532, 1976.

90. McGinnis JM: Eye movements and optic nystagmus in early infancy. Genet Psychol Monogr 8:321, 1930.

91. Mann I: The development of the human eye. London, British Medical Association, 1964.

92. Maurer D: The development of binocular convergence in infants. Doctoral dissertation. University of Minnesota, 1975.

93. Maurer D, Lewis TL, Brent H: Peripheral vision and optokinetic nystagmus in children with unilateral congenital cataract. Behav Brain Res 10:151, 1983.

94. Maurer D, Salapatek P: Developmental changes in the scanning of faces by young infants. Child Dev 47:523, 1976.

95. Miles FA, Eighmy BB: Longterm adaptive changes in primate vestibulo-ocular reflex 1. Behavioural observation. J Neurophysiol 43:1406, 1980.

96. Mohindra I, Held R, Gwiazda J, Brill S: Astigmatism in infants. Science 202:329, 1978.

97. Morgan MW: The analysis of clinical data. Optom Weekly 65:27, 1964.

98. Movshon JA, Van Sluyters RC: Visual neural development. In Rosenzweig MR, Porter LW (eds): Annual Review of Psychology, vol 32. Palo Alto, Annual Reviews, 1981.

99. Naegele JR, Held R: The postnatal development of monocular optokinetic nystagmus in infants. Vision Res 22:341, 1982.

100. Ogle KN: Researchers in Binocular Vision. New York, Hofner, 1964.

101. Ornitz EM, Atwell CW, Water DO, et al: The maturation of vestibular nystagmus in infancy and childhood. Acta Otolaryngol (Stockh) 88:244, 1979.

102. Ornitz EM, Kaplan AR, Westlake JR: Development of the vestibulo-ocular reflex from infancy to adulthood. Acta Otolaryngol (Stockh) 100:180, 1985.

103. Owens DA, Leibowitz HW: Accommodation, convergence and distance perception in low illumination. Am J Optom Physiol Opt 57:540, 1980.

104. Peiper A: Cerebral Function in Infancy and Childhood. New York, Consultants Bureau, 1963.

105. Pirrozolo FJ: The Neurophysiology of Developmental Reading Disorders. New York, Praeger, 1979.

106. Powers MK, Dobson V: Effect of focus on visual acuity of human infants. Vision Res 22:521, 1979.

107. Rashbass C: The relationship between saccadic and smooth tracking eye movements. J Physiol (Lond) 159:326, 1961.

108. Rashbass C, Westheimer G: Disjunctive eye movement. J Physiol (Lond) 159:339, 1961.

109. Rethy I: Development of simultaneous fixation from the divergent anatomical eye position in the neonate. J Pediatr Ophthalmol 6:92, 1969.

110. Riggs LA, Neihl: Eye movements recorded during convergence and divergence. J Opt Soc Am 50:913, 1960.

110a. Rosenhall U: Vestibular macular mapping in man. Ann Otolrhinol Laryngol 81:339, 1972.

111. Roucoux A, Culee C, Roucoux M: Development of fixation and pursuit eye movements in human infants. Behav Brain Res 10:133, 1983.

112. St Cyr GS, Fender D: The interplay of drifts and flicks in binocular vision. Vision Res 9:245, 1969.

113. Salapatek P: Visual scanning of geometric figures by the human newborn. J Comp Physiol Psychol 66:247, 1968.

114. Salapatek P, Aslin RN, Simonson J, et al: Infant saccadic eye movements to visible and previously visible targets. Child Dev 51:1090, 1980.

115. Salapatek P, Banks MS: Infant sensory assessment. Vision. In Minifie FD, Lloyd LL (eds): Communicative and Cognitive Abilities: Early Behavioral Assessment. Baltimore MD, University Park Press, 1978.

116. Salapatek P, Beditold AG, Bergamon J: Pupillary response in 1- and 2-month-old infants. Paper presented at the annual meeting of the Psychonomic Society, Washington DC, 1977.

117. Salapatek P, Haith M, Maurer D, et al: Error in the corneal-reflection technique: A note on Slater and Findlay. J Exp Child Psychol 14:493, 1972.

118. Salapatek P, Kessen W: Visual scanning of triangles by the human newborn. J Exp Child Psychol 3:155, 1966.

119. Schor CM: A directional impairment of eye movement control in strabismus amblyopia. Invest Ophthalmol Vis Sci 14:692, 1975.

120. Schor CM: The relationship between fusional vergence eye movements and fixation disparity. Vision Res 19:1359, 1979.

121. Schor CM: Subcortical binocular suppression affects the development of latent and optokinetic nystagmus. Am J Optom Physiol Opt 60:481,1982.

122. Schor CM: Fixation disparity and vergence adaptation. In Schor CM, Ciuffreda K (eds): Vergence Eye Movements: Basic and Clinical Aspects. Boston, Butterworths, 1983.

123. Schor CM, Gleason G, Horner D: The variability and adaptability of Hering's law for yoked reflexive eye movements. Invest Ophthalmol Vis Sci (ARVO Suppl) 29:1988.

124. Schor CM, Johnson C, Post R: Adaptation of tonic accommodation. Ophthalmol Physiol Optics 4:133, 1984.

125. Schor CM, Kotulak J: Dynamic interactions between accommodation and convergence are velocity sensitive. Vision Res 26:927, 1986.

126. Schor CM, Kotulak J, Tsuetaki T: Adaptation of tonic accommodation reduces accommodative lag and is masked in darkness. Invest Ophthalmol Vis Sci 27:820, 1986.

127. Schor CM, Levi DL: Disturbances of small-field horizontal and vertical nystagmus in amblyopia. Invest Ophthalmol Vis Sci 19:683, 1980.

128. Schor C, Narayan V: The influence of field size upon the spatial frequency response of optokinetic nystagmus. Vision Res 21:985, 1981.

129. Schor C, Narayan V, Westall C: Postnatal development of optokinetic afternystagmus in human infants. Vis Res 23:1643, 1983.

130. Schor C, Tyler C: Spatio-temporal properties of Panum's fusional area. Vision Res 21:683, 1981.

131. Schor CM, Westall CW: Rapid adaptation of the vestibulo-ocular reflex and induced self motion perception. Perception Psychophysics 40:1, 1986.

132. Schor CM, Wood IC, Ogawa J: Binocular sensory fusion is limited by spatial resolution. Vision Res 24:661, 1984.

133. Slater AM, Findlay JM: The measurement of fixation position in the newborn baby. J Exp Child Psychol 14:349, 1972.

134. Slater AM, Findlay JM: The corneal-reflection techniques and the visual preference method: Sources of error. J Exp Child Psychol 20:240, 1975.

135. Slater AM, Findlay JM: Binocular fixation in the newborn baby. J Exp Child Psychol 20:248, 1975.

136. Shea S, Aslin RN: Development of horizontal and vertical pursuits in human infants. Invest Ophthalmol Vis Sci (ARVO Suppl) 25:263, 1984.

137. Sherman KR, Keller BL: Vestibulo-ocular reflexes in blind subjects. Invest Ophthalmol Vis Sci (ARVO Suppl) 22:271, 1983.

138. Shimojo S, Bauer J, O'Connell K, et al: Prestereoptic binocular vision in infants. Vis Res 26:501, 1986.

139. Steinman RM, Haddard GM, Skavenski AA, et al: Miniature eye movements. Science 181:810, 1973.

140. Tronick E: Stimulus control and the growth of the infant's effective visual field. Perception Psychophysics 11:373, 1972.

141. Tychsen L, Lisberger S: Visual motion processing for the initiation of smooth-pursuit eye movements. J Neurophysiol 51:952, 1986.

142. von Noorden GK, Maunamee AE: Atlas of Strabismus. St Louis, CV Mosby, 1967.

143. Westall CW: Interactions between optokinetic and vestibular systems in strabismic amblyopia and their development in infancy. Doctoral dissertation. University of California Berkeley, 1984.

144. Westheimer G, Campbell FW: Light distribution in the image found by the living human eye. J Opt Soc Am [A] 52:1040, 1962.

145. Wichelgren C: Convergence in the human newborn. J Exp Child Psychol 5:74, 1967.

146. Winterson BJ, Steinman RM: The effect of luminance on human smooth pursuit of perifoveal and foveal targets. Vis Res 18:1165, 1978.

147. Yarbus AL: Eye Movements and Vision. New York, Plenum Press, 1967.

148. Yuodelis C, Hendrickson A: A qualitative and quantitative analysis of the human fovea during development. Vis Res 26:847, 1986.

Chapter 5

Genetics and Congenital Ocular Disorders

John R. Griffin

"Parents should be blamed less for kids who have problems and take less credit for kids who turn out well." This observation of psychologist and twins researcher David Rowe of the University of Oklahoma was reported by Leo, who also summarized reports of twin studies showing that approximately half of a person's personality is shaped by heredity and that there is a trend away from the concept that environment fully shapes a person's character (15).

That personality may be profoundly influenced by heredity may shock some believing in the power of nurture, yet there is no question that many physical traits are most likely purely genetic (e.g., albinism, Fabry's disease, Stargardt's disease). Genetic traits that affect children's eyes and vision will be discussed briefly in this chapter. This chapter is a summary of the genetics of ocular disorders and is not intended to elaborate on anomalies and diseases covered elsewhere in this book. The reader is referred to these chapters and to references on genetics listed in this chapter. Definitions of anomalies, diseases, and syndromes discussed in this chapter are given in the *Dictionary of Visual Science* (2).

CONGENITAL DISORDERS

A congenital condition is one existing at, and usually before, birth, regardless of its causation (4).

Genetic versus Nongenetic Disorders

A genetic condition is any one controlled by the genes (14). Some congenital anomalies may have either a genetic or an environmental cause. Because the manifestations are the same in either case, it may be difficult to know whether the cause is genetic or environmental (32).

Some common congenital diseases are listed in Table 5.1. Since only six of these are not genetic, the implication is that the majority of common congenital ocular problems are genetic.

Not only are most congenital disorders genetic, but as Newcomb pointed out, "Due to the widespread use of antibiotics and steroid preparations, infectious diseases are no longer significant as major causes of blindness in the United States today. . . . Genetic diseases now lead the list of the most frequent causes of blindness." (21).

Anophthalmos and Microphthalmos

Anophthalmos is a rare condition characterized by the complete absence of the tissues of the eye. Sometimes it is impossible to differentiate it from an extreme case of microphthalmos. There are three types of anophthalmos. Primary anophthalmos results from the optic pit failing to form an outgrowth from the forebrain. The ectodermal elements of the eye are missing but the orbit, lids, lacrimal apparatus, conjunctival sac, extraocular muscles, and nerves may be formed (3). Secondary anophthalmos is associated with abnormal development of the entire forebrain. Degenerative (or consecutive) anophthalmos results from atrophy of the optic vessel after it forms. Almost all cases are the result of a consanguineous union; that is, the parents are related (16).

Microphthalmos presents as a small globe within the soft orbital tissues (23). It is sometimes associated with an orbital cyst, usually attached to the inferior pole of the eye in association with a coloboma. The clinical features are "marked hypermetropia, macular hypoplasia, and the late occurrence of simple glaucoma" (3). Dominant and recessive forms are known (16).

Congenital Eyelid Disorders

Epicanthal folds are congenital structural anomalies. A vertical fold of tissue is continuous with the medial upper lid margin and continues downward to conceal the medial canthus. This is an autosomal dominant trait (16).

Blepharochalasis is relaxation of the upper eyelid tissue which causes an extra skin fold to form. This defect is due to abnormal insertion of muscle fibers into the skin. It is frequently, but not always, hereditary (3, 16).

Blepharophimosis is a generalized narrowing of the palpebral fissure which gives the appearance of ptosis. This condition may be associated with other syndromes and anomalies, such as dwarfism, Down's syndrome, ectropion, and microphthalmos (3).

Coloboma of the eyelid is a notch in the lid margin. The gap is usually triangular, with rolled edges. Lashes and glands are missing from this area. Exposure keratopathy may occur if the notch is large, resulting in corneal desiccation and scarring. A true coloboma is very rare. The cause is undetermined in most cases. Congenital ptosis is usually hereditary. When so, it is an autosomal dominant trait (16).

Distichiasis is a rare, and usually familial, disorder characterized by the absence of meibomian glands. An extra row of lashes grows in place of the glands. These lashes have a tendency to turn in and touch the globe (trichiasis) (16).

Duane's Syndrome

Duane's syndrome involves the extraocular muscles and is probably hereditary in most cases. It is an autosomal dominant trait (16).

Strabismus

Congenital strabismus is probably genetic. The majority of cases of congenital strabismus are esotropic. Griffin believes that about 25 percent of the cases of constant esotropia are congenital and that onset of constant stra-

Table 5.1 EXAMPLES OF CONGENITAL OCULAR DISORDERS

Disorder	Genetic	Comments
Anophthalmos	Yes	Autosomal recessive
Microphthalmos	Yes	Autosomal recessive, autosomal dominant
Epicanthal folds	Yes	Autosomal dominant
Blepharochalasis	No?	Not always, but frequently, hereditary autosomal dominant)
Blepharophimosis	Yes	Autosomal dominant
Coloboma of the eyelid	No?	Genetic cause has not been established
Ptosis	Yes	Autosomal dominant
Distichaiasis	Yes	Autosomal dominant
Duane's syndrome	Yes	Autosomal dominant
Strabismus	Yes?	Probably multifactorial
Fetal alcohol syndrome	No	
Megalocornea	Yes	X-linked recessive
Microcornea	Yes	Autosomal recessive
Congenital aniridia	Yes	Autosomal dominant
Corectopia	Yes	Autosomal dominant
Cataract	No?	One fourth of cases may be hereditary (autosomal dominant, autosomal recessive, and X-linked recessive)
Ectopia lentis	Yes	Autosomal recessive, autosomal dominant (usually occurring with other syndromes, e.g. Weill-Marchesani, Marfan's)
Optic nerve coloboma	Yes	Autosomal dominant
Toxoplasmosis	No	
Retinoblastoma	Yes?	Although the majority of cases occur sporadically both mendelian (autosomal dominant) and chromosomal (13q−) causes are frequently proven.
Retrolental fibroplasia	No	

bismus must occur before age 6 months if it is to be classified as congenital (8). Richter reported that the inheritance of strabismus is probably multifactorial (25, 26). She investigated 697 probands aged 4 to 7 years with strabismus of various types and causes and 2206 members of their families. Griffin and associates (9) supported the multifactorial model suggested by Richter by studying only pedigrees in which probands had congenital esotropia. They suggested that risk factors for congenital esotropia include a family history of strabismus, high accommodative-convergence to accommodation (AC/A) ratio, and significantly high hyperopia. Similarly, Spivey (31) summarized that esotropia is a risk when (1) a parent has esotropia, (2) there is a family history of esotropia, and (3) both parents have very low vergence ability and sig-

nificant hyperopia. Although the multifactorial model is the most widely accepted, a codominance model (like that of A, B, AB, and O blood types) was suggested by Maumenee (18).

Howard pointed out that there is an inordinately high prevalence of strabismus in more than 300 different chromosomal errors that have been identified. For example, esotropia occurs in the entire population at a frequency of 2 to 4 percent, but in 33 percent of persons with trisomy 21 (Down's syndrome) (13).

Fetal Alcohol Syndrome

Heavy alcohol consumption by a pregnant woman commonly causes some or all of the following ocular findings in her infant: nar-

row palpebral fissures, epicanthal folds, ptosis, and strabismus. Less common are myopia, microphthalmos, and blepharophimosis.
Mental retardation, low birth weight and
short stature, cardiovascular and skeletal disorders, and a thin vermilion border of the upper lip may also be present (20).

Disorders of the Cornea

Megalocornea is an enlargement of the cornea beyond 13 mm in diameter. The corneal
curvature may be increased, the anterior
chamber is enlarged, and because there is no
enlargement of the lens, iridodonesis often
results. The cornea is usually clear and visual
acuity good, although astigmatism is common. Subluxation of the lens is also common
owing to rupture of the stretched zonular fibers. Megalocornea is bilateral and is inherited as an X-linked recessive trait (3, 16).

Microcornea is a small cornea (diameter
less than 10 or 11 mm). The entire anterior
segment of the eye is small, and the corneal
curvature is steeper than normal. Vision is
good when the refractive error is corrected,
but the patient is predisposed to glaucoma. It
is inherited as an autosomal recessive trait.

Congenital glaucoma affects the cornea
and is probably due to decreased aqueous
outflow caused by improper development of
the chamber angle. This results in increased
intraocular pressure at birth. The cornea be⊥
comes hazy; the eye becomes enlarged; and
the infant has excessive tearing and photophobia. Congenital glaucoma is inherited as
an autosomal recessive trait (16).

Disorders of the Iris and Ciliary Body

Congenital aniridia is a rare disorder in
which the iris is severely underdeveloped, so
that it is hidden behind the corneoscleral
margin. Sometimes this short iris stump adheres to the posterior corneal surface and interferes with the function of the canal of Sch-
lemm, which can lead to glaucoma later in
life. It is associated with macular aplasia that
correlates with the sensory nystagmus and
decreased visual acuity of these patients. The
condition may be inherited as an autosomal

dominant trait or may result from a spontaneous mutation (which may be passed on to successive generations as an autosomal dominant trait) (16, 23).

Corectopia is a condition in which the
pupil is displaced from its normal position.
The pupil sometimes is oval, and vision is
impaired. Lens subluxation is often associated with this disorder. It is inherited as an
autosomal dominant trait (3).

Disorders of the Lens

Congenital cataracts may be caused by diseases such as rubella and by toxic agents.
About one fourth of the cases, however, are
genetic in origin (19). Congenital cataracts
are often inherited through autosomal dominant transmission, but less frequently transmission may be autosomal recessive or X-
linked recessive (5).

Ectopia lentis may result from several
conditions. Homocystinuria may result in bilateral lens dislocation, as a result of a deficiency of cystathionine synthetase. Dislocation is usually inferior, and acute glaucoma
may result if the lens dislocates into the anterior chamber. It is an autosomal recessive
trait (16, 23). Marfan's syndrome is usually
associated with lens dislocation, which is
usually superior and rarely into the anterior
chamber (although acute secondary glaucoma may result if this happens). The patients are tall and thin and may have scoliosis, arachnodactyly, and hyperextensible
joints. It is an autosomal dominant trait (16,
23). Weill-Marchesani syndrome is characterized by small, spherical lenses that frequently dislocate anteriorly to precipitate
acute glaucoma (23). Affected persons are
short and have broad fingers and hands. Inheritance is autosomal recessive (16).

Disorders of the Retina and Optic Nerve

Optic nerve coloboma is an autosomal dominant trait that results in the failure of the most
anterior portion of the optic stalk to close.
The optic disc becomes enlarged and exca-
vated and is often vertically oval. The major-

ity of the defects are found at the 6 o'clock position (16, 32).

Congenital ocular toxoplasmosis results when the toxoplasma organism is passed from an affected pregnant mother, through the placenta, to the nerve tissue of the fetus. Acute chorioretinitis begins with severe retinal inflammation and exudation into the vitreous with secondary involvement of the choroid (1). Pigmented, circumscribed scars remain after the infection subsides. The encysted parasite may remain quiescent for many years or may reactivate at any time. The infection can also cause intracranial calcification, hydrocephalus, mental retardation, and epilepsy in newborns (29).

Retinoblastoma is a congenital malignant tumor, although not usually observed at birth but almost always before age 5 years. It is usually diagnosed initially by a whitish reflex of light observed at the pupil, and the lesion may appear in the vitreous as a pinkish-white mass with blood vessels extending over its surface (2). The majority of cases are sporadic and often may not be genetic in origin; but when it is shown to be hereditary, it follows an autosomal dominant mode of transmission. Less frequently, retinoblastoma patients have been found to have a deletion of band 4 in region 1 of the long arm of chromosome 13 (13q14) (30). Sporadic bilateral cases are always hereditary; approximately 85 percent of sporadic unilateral cases are not hereditary (7).

Retrolental fibroplasia is an acquired condition involving premature infants, usually of low birth weight. The condition develops following prolonged periods of incubator ventilation (6). The first abnormality that can be seen is dilated, tortuous retinal blood vessels. Later, the periphery of the retina becomes elevated. The retinal tissue detaches, forming a gray membrane, and comes forward, producing an opaque cast behind the lens (28).

MODES OF GENETIC TRANSMISSION

A brief discussion of chromosomal, mendelian, and multifactorial modes of transmission

follows. More complete explanations and information on this subject are presented by Fatt and Griffin (5).

Chromosomal Aberrations

The normal human has 46 chromosomes (23 pairs). There are 22 autosomal pairs and one pair of sex chromosomes. A normal male has one X and one Y sex chromosome (46 XY karyotype) and a normal female has two X sex chromosomes (46 XX karyotype). A genetic defect will occur if there are too many chromosomes (e.g., Down's syndrome, 47 XX if female or 47 XY if male) or too few chromosomes (e.g., 46 XO Turner's syndrome female—only one sex chromosome).

Occasionally there may be partial loss of a chromosome, called deletion. The most significant deletion disease for the primary eye care practitioner is retinoblastoma. As stated previously deletion of a portion of the long arm of chromosome 13 is associated with retinoblastoma. Another deletion disease of possible importance to the practitioner is the 5p⁻ (cat-cry) syndrome. A portion of the short arm of chromosome 5 is missing. An infant with this syndrome mews as a kitten does and has hypertelorism, microcephaly, optic atrophy, and other ocular problems; there is also mental retardation, usually severe (5).

Most chromosomal aberrations result in spontaneous abortion, death in early infancy, or severe physical disabilities, so, the primary eye care practitioner rarely sees many of them. The exceptions are mainly those who have Down's syndrome and, more rarely, Turner's syndrome, retinoblastoma, and cat-cry syndrome.

Mendelian Transmission

Three mendelian modes of genetic transmission are discussed here: autosomal dominant, autosomal recessive, and X-linked recessive. The X-linked dominant mode is not discussed because of the rarity of ocular traits associated with this mode.

Autosomal Dominant
An autosomal dominant trait is transmitted and expressed even if only one of an in-

herited gene pair is mutant. (A single dose will do it.) Each offspring of an affected parent has a 50-percent chance of inheriting the trait (Fig. 5.1). Because the defective gene is on an autosomal chromosome (not a sex chromosome) both males and females are generally affected equally. There are exceptions, however, when gender influences the penetrance and expressivity of certain traits. Penetrance refers to whether or not the defective gene is able to make the trait manifest at all. If not, this is referred to as a lack of penetrance, also referred to as reduced penetrance. Expressivity refers to the severity of the trait (i.e., mild, moderate, marked). For example, baldness in males (16) and Fuchs' epithelial and endothelial dystrophy of the cornea (16) are autosomal dominant traits, but women tend to have corneal dystrophy and men tend to be bald. Most reports on Fuchs' dystrophy indicate a higher penetrance in females than in males. Rosenblum and associates (27) suggest that the expression is more severe in females but that penetrance may be

the same in males and females. Nevertheless, gender influences expressivity of this autosomal dominant trait.

Lack of penetrance may result in a pedigree in which the trait "skips" a generation as seen in Figure 5.2. (Refer to the proband's mother, II-4.) This is important to keep in mind when doing genetic counseling (5). Expressivity cannot be predicted, either. A parent may have a mild form of Marfan's syndrome and the offspring a marked form, or vice versa.

Examples of traits that follow the autosomal dominant mode of transmission are listed in Table 5.2. Notice that most of these traits are structural defects (e.g., aniridia, epicanthus). This is in contrast to autosomal recessive traits, which generally are metabolic errors (e.g., Tay-Sachs disease).

Autosomal Recessive

Unlike an autosomal dominant trait, an autosomal recessive trait needs a double dose to be manifested. Usually an autosomal recessive trait appears sporadically in a family and preceding or successive generations are not affected. In such a case the father and mother of the affected child each carry one gene for the trait. This is illustrated in Figure

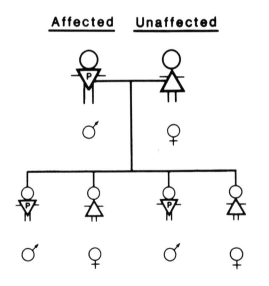

Figure 5.1 Autosomal dominant transmission showing 50-percent theoretical risk to offspring if one parent has the autosomal dominant trait. (P, phenotype.)

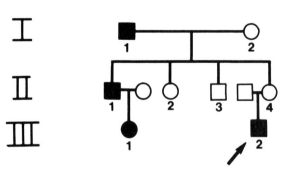

Figure 5.2 Pedigree showing autosomal dominant transmission. The trait is manifested in the proband (index case) who is designated III2 (generation III, number 2). Note that his mother (II4) has lack of penetrance. The grandfather (I1), however, shows the trait. Vertical transmission with no skipping is shown in I1 to III to III1, which is more typical in autosomal dominant transmission.

Table 5.2 EXAMPLES OF PHENOTYPES OF AUTOSOMAL DOMINANT GENETIC TRANSMISSION

Aniridia
Best's disease
Corneal dystrophy (e.g., deep, Fuchs', granular,
  lattice, Meesmann's, Reis-Bückler, fleck)
Doyne's honeycomb degeneration
Drusen
Duane's syndrome
Ehlers-Danlos syndrome
Epicanthus
Horner's syndrome
Hypertelorism
Lacrimal duct defect
Marcus Gunn jaw-winking phenomenon
Marfan's syndrome
Neurofibromatosis
Persistent pupillary membrane
Pterygium
Ptosis
Waardenberg's syndrome

(From Fatt HV, Griffin JR: Genetics for Primary Eye Care Practitioners. Chicago, Professional Press, 1983.)

5.3. Each offspring has a 25-percent chance of being affected and a 50-percent chance of being a carrier. Their chance of being genotypically and phenotypically normal is also 25 percent. In geographically isolated groups there is likelihood of consanguinity (mating with a blood relative). In Figure 5.4 consanguinity between the parents (I-1 and I-2) of the proband (II-1) is a possibility that should be investigated in genetic counseling.

General albinism, for example, is an autosomal recessive trait requiring accurate genetic counseling. If both parents are known to be carriers of the same type of general albinism, the theoretical risk to offspring is 25 percent. The exact diagnosis, however, is vitally important for genetic counseling, because there are several different types of albinism. The two basic types are tyrosinase negative and tyrosinase positive albinism. These are not allelic with each other (33); they are two entirely different genetic diseases whose phenotypes may be similar. If the father and mother, as in Figure 5.3, are carriers of different types of albinism, theoretically there is no risk to offspring. Similarly suppose two affected albinos mate (both homozygous) and have a nonalbino child. How can this happen when a double dose from each parent gives a theoretical risk of 100 percent to offspring? The answer is that if one parent has tyrosinase-negative and the other parent has tyrosinase-positive albinism, then the theoretical risk is zero. Therefore, the exact diagnosis must be determined by the hair bulb tyrosine test before any genetic advice is given to patients.

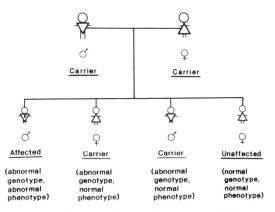

Figure 5.3 Autosomal recessive transmission showing 25-percent theoretical risk to offspring of two parents who are carriers of the trait.

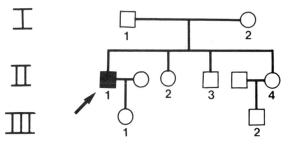

Figure 5.4 Pedigree showing autosomal recessive transmission. The trait is manifest in the proband (III1) and nowhere else. The parents (I1 and I2) are presumed carriers. Carrier status of the other unaffected members of the family cannot be determined from this pedigree. Carrier status, however, can be determined in some autosomal recessive traits by biochemical analysis.

The primary eye care practitioner, working with other health care professionals, is usually able to make diagnoses with certainty. A sample of autosomal recessive diseases is listed in Table 5.3. Pedigree analysis for carrier status is usually difficult in autosomal recessive diseases, but fortunately, blood testing can detect carriers for some of the inborn errors of metabolism. Knowing the carrier status of members in a family improves certainty in genetic counseling.

X-Linked Recessive

Some X-linked recessive diseases likely to be seen by primary eye care practitioners are listed in Table 5.4. Each almost always affect only males, because males have only one X chromosome (they are hemizygous for the X chromosome) so that, even though the condition is recessive, it takes only one dose for the phenotype to be expressed.

In the usual situation an affected male proband has unaffected parents. In order for a

Table 5.3   EXAMPLES OF PHENOTYPES OF AUTOSOMAL RECESSIVE GENETIC TRANSMISSION

Alkaptonuria
Anophthalmos
Coats' disease
Congenital optic atrophy
Corneal dystrophy (e.g., band-shaped, congenital hereditary, macular)
Cranial nerve paralysis
Friedreich's ataxia
Fundus flavimaculatus
Galactosemia
Gyrate atrophy
Marchesani's syndrome
Niemann-Pick disease
Night blindness with high myopia
Refsum's syndrome
Riley-Day syndrome
Sandhoff's disease
Sjögren's syndrome
Stargardt's disease
Tay-Sachs disease
Usher's syndrome

(From Fatt HV, Griffin JR: Genetics for Primary Care Practitioners. Chicago, Professional Press, 1983.)

Table 5.4   EXAMPLES OF PHENOTYPES OF X-LINKED RECESSIVE GENETIC TRANSMISSION

Choroideremia
Color vision deficiencies
Fabry's disease
Hunter's syndrome
Leber's optic atrophy (may be of cytoplasmic inheritance instead of X-linked recessive)
Lowe's syndrome
Norrie's disease
Ocular albinism
X-linked retinitis pigmentosa
X-linked retinoschisis

(From Fatt HV, Griffin JR: Genetics for Primary Eye Care Practitioners. Chicago, Professional Press, 1983.)

son to have the trait, his mother must be a carrier (Fig. 5.5). A typical X-linked recessive pedigree is shown in Figure 5.6. The proband (II-1) inherited the trait from his mother (the carrier status of the mother is indicated by the dot in the circle). Theoretically, sons have a 50-percent chance of having the trait and daughters have a 50-percent chance of being a carrier. Notice that the daughter (III-1) of the proband is a carrier. She is called an obligate carrier, as the only way her father

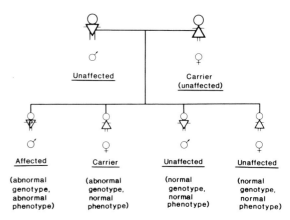

Figure 5.5   X-linked recessive transmission showing 50-percent theoretical risk to sons of a carrier mother.

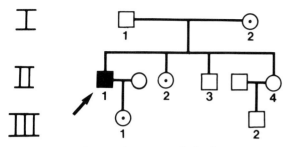

Figure 5.6 Pedigree showing X-linked recessive transmission and 50-percent theoretical risk to sons of a carrier mother. Daughters of a carrier mother have a 50-percent chance of also being carriers.

could have a girl is to donate his X chromosome, the one with the deleterious gene.

Carrier status often, but not always, can be determined by pedigree analysis. Can carrier status be determined with certainty in II-2 and II-4 by pedigree analysis alone? The answer is no. Two methods for doing so, however, include biochemical analysis and ophthalmoscopy. Three X-linked recessive ocular diseases are often detectable in a carrier female by means of ophthalmoscopy. Female carriers of ocular albinism of the Nettleship type often show a mosaic pigmented pattern in the fundus (33). This is because of the random inactivation of each X chromosome in the female (the normal gene is randomly inactivated to cause a patchy fundus). Choroideremia and X-linked retinitis pigmentosa can also be detected in carrier females in many cases.

The exact diagnosis and certainty of carrier status are important in genetic counseling in X-linked recessive diseases. A pregnant mother who is a carrier has a 50-percent chance of passing the disease on to a son, but there is no risk (other than carrier status) to daughters. In seriously debilitating diseases such as ocular albinism, a genetic counselor may advise amniocentesis for sex determination of the fetus before counseling continues. If the fetus is male, medical abortion may be discussed, with compassion and in a nondirective manner.

Multifactorial Inheritance

Multifactorial means that many genes as well as environmental factors are influencing the expression of a trait. Examples of multifactorial inheritance are height, intelligence, diabetes, and blood pressure. Good nutrition is an environmental factor in height, and good education promotes intelligence. A stressful environment may increase blood pressure, and an improper diet may exacerbate a diabetic condition, leading to diabetic retinopathy.

Other examples of multifactorial traits are refractive errors, and strabismus. The nature-versus-nurture controversy can be settled when a multifactorial explanation is given. Myopia, for example, probably has both genetic and environmental elements (5).

Empiric risks in multifactorial transmission are generally less than in theoretical risks in mendelian traits. The severity of a defect in a proband, however, increases the risk to offspring; the severity of a mendelian trait does not affect the risk to offspring (5).

OTHER GENETIC PROBLEMS

Dyslexia

Griffin found that one of the several types of dyslexia is genetic and of the autosomal dominant mode (5). This is the dyseidetic pattern of dyslexia, as found on the Dyslexia Determination Test (DDT) (10). For the other six patterns determined by the DDT no clear mendelian pattern could be found. Multifactorial inheritance is possible in these other types of dyslexia, which may account for their pedigree analyses being nebulous.

Genetic counseling is important if there is dyseidetic dyslexia in a family. Although the trait is autosomal dominant, a male-to-female ratio of 82% to 18% was reported. Some aspect of female gender reduces penetrance in females (5). Genetic counselors should keep in mind the possibility that this autosomal dominant trait can skip a generation of females who carry the gene for dyseidetic dyslexia.

Eye care practitioners should be aware of procedures in vision therapy or educational therapy that may be efficacious for different types of dyslexia. These are discussed in detail in *Therapy in Dyslexia* (11). There are three basic types of dyslexia:

Dysnemkinesa

A "motor" type of dyslexia manifested in problems of number and letter reversals in writing. Consequently, handwriting looks abnormal (e.g., *b*s and *d*s written backward).

The general therapeutic approach for dysnemkinesia is to improve laterality and directional skills (e.g., left-right problems). Later, these skills are transferred to writing and identifying numbers and letters (e.g., *b*s and *d*s). Most elementary school children who have dysnemkinesia probably can be cured.

Dysphonesia

An "auditory" type of dyslexia manifested in poor phonetic analysis, syllabication, and structural analysis in decoding during reading and poor phonetic encoding during writing and spelling. There is poor decoding of unfamiliar words that are not known by sight. Spelling often does not make sense phonetically (e.g., *solw* for *slow*).

The general therapeutic approach for dysphonesia is to emphasize the eidetic, look-say, approach initially and minimize phonics. Tachistoscopic drills of grade-appropriate words are used to increase the dysphonetic person's reading and spelling vocabulary. Later, a phonics program can be instituted to help word attack skills by building up phonetic decoding ability. Most of the children who have this type of dyslexia can improve reading skills through appropriate educational therapy; a small percentage are cured. If a multifactorial mode of transmission of dysphonesia is assumed, it is logical to assume that intervening environmental factors (e.g., educational therapy) may have an ameliorative effect on this type of dyslexia.

Dyseidesia

A "visual" type of dyslexia manifested in poor sight recognition of whole words during decoding and poor spelling and writing of words from visual memory. Reading is slow and labored because of the necessity to decode many words phonetically. Spelling is poor because of the reliance on phonetics (e.g., *laf* for *laugh*).

The general therapeutic approach for dyseidesia is to emphasize the phonetic approach (analysis of letter and syllable sounds, syllabication, structural analysis, blends, etc.) initially and minimize whole-word, look-say, eidetic decoding. Many excellent phonics programs, including computerized regimens, are in resource specialists' classrooms. Because dyseidesia is probably an autosomal dominant genetic trait, intervening environmental factors, such as educational therapy, generally have little or no effect on the dyseidetic pattern per se; the dyseidesia is not cured or changed significantly. Nevertheless, the dyseidetic person may be helped tremendously by working around the problem. Also, vision problems such as uncorrected hyperopic astigmatism, convergence insufficiency, and visual perceptual and oculomotor dysfunctions have an adverse effect on most readers, whether they are dyslexic or not. It is desirable to eliminate such obstacles, as often can be done with lenses and vision training.

Besides vision problems, other factors such as low intelligence, neurologic problems, cultural deprivation, and educational opportunity must be addressed in educational therapy for any dyslexic person.

In summary, dysnemkinetic dyslexia can be treated directly, usually with great success. Dysphonetic dyslexia must be treated both indirectly (working around the problem) and directly (for somewhat limited success in curing the condition). Even if the condition is not "cured," educational therapy can be used to work around the problem and help the individual perform in school and at work. Thus, reading can be improved in spite of dyslexia. Dyseidetic dyslexia is usually untreatable; an indirect approach is necessary. Nevertheless, a dyseidetic person can be taught to be a better reader, speller, and writer via nemkinetic and phonetic approaches in educational therapy. Dyslexia does not mean there is no hope. Most dyslexic persons can become successful in school, work, and play and lead happy and rewarding lives. Early detection is the key to prevention of school dropout, juvenile delinquency, and drug dependency. The Dyslexia Screener (TDS) (12) provides a quick assessment of dysphonesia and dyseidesia on a pass-fail basis. If a dyslexic coding pattern is suspected, full testing with the DDT is then recommended. If a dyslexia pattern is confirmed, appropriate educational therapy can address the problem.

Glaucoma

Whether transmission of glaucoma is genetic is controversial, although it is generally accepted that glaucoma runs in families. Nixon and Phelps (22) summarized reports indicating autosomal recessive transmission of congenital glaucoma. On the other hand, congenital glaucoma may be associated with other congenital diseases (e.g., aniridia) that are autosomal dominant.

Macular Dystrophies

Fatt and Griffin showed the diversity of modes of transmission of various macular dystrophies. For example, Best's disease has an autosomal dominant mode; Stargardt's disease is autosomal recessive, and juvenile retinoschisis is X linked (5).

Nystagmus

According to Martyn, "Knowledge of the complex mechanisms underlying various types of nystagmus is incomplete. . . . Nystagmus may arise from defects in the fixation mechanism, from defects in the conjugate gaze mechanisms, or from defects in the vestibular system" (17). This explains why information on modes of transmission of nystagmus is incomplete.

Nystagmus may occur in various genetic syndromes and diseases (e.g., albinism), or it may occur in isolation. Whether in association with other diseases or in isolation, nystagmus is usually genetic. McKusick reported four modes of mendelian inheritance—auto-

somal dominant, autosomal recessive, X-linked recessive, and X-linked dominant (16). Needless to say, genetic counseling is difficult in most cases of nystagmus.

Optic Atrophy

Optic atrophy may be associated with many diseases (e.g., glaucoma). Monocular optic atrophy tends not to be genetic, whereas bilateral optic atrophy tends to be genetic. Toxic optic atrophy also tends to be bilateral. Five significant types of genetic optic atrophy were summarized by Fatt and Griffin (Table 5.5). The type of optic atrophy must be established before genetic counseling is offered.

Refractive Errors

Mild refractive errors are probably multifactorial in origin (5). Severe pathologic myopia, however, has been reported to be autosomal recessive (16).

Retinitis Pigmentosa

An example of genetic heterogeneity is shown in retinitis pigmentosa. The phenotype results from autosomal dominant, autosomal recessive, or X-linked recessive transmission. Hence, the exact mode of transmission must be known before genetic coun-

Table 5.5 EXAMPLES OF TYPES OF GENETIC OPTIC ATROPHY

Type	Mode of Transmission
Leber's optic atrophy	X-linked recessive (may be cytoplasmic inheritance)
Optic atrophy with diabetes	Autosomal recessive
Behr's syndrome	Autosomal recessive
Simple recessive optic atrophy	Autosomal recessive
Dominant optic atrophy	Autosomal dominant

(From Fatt HV, Griffin JR: Genetics for Primary Eye Care Practitioners. Chicago, Professional Press, 1983.)

seling is given. Retinitis pigmentosa is also associated with other genetic diseases (e.g., Usher's syndrome) (5).

Noncongenital and Late-Onset Diseases

Many ocular diseases often appear after infancy, perhaps in middle age or later, yet, they may be genetic, at least in part. Examples include cataracts, corneal and macular dystrophies, glaucoma, optic atrophies, refractive errors, retinitis pigmentosa, and strabismus. Genetic counseling is difficult when it is not known whether the trait will appear later in a patient's life.

Table 5.6   GENETIC COUNSELING RULES

The exact diagnosis must be made.

Single-gene (mendelian) traits are unlikely to be affected by environmental factors.

Polygenic (multifactorial) traits are likely to be affected by environmental factors.

Karyotyping is important in chromosomal aberrations and for sex determination in X-linked recessive traits (male fetus is at risk if mother is a carrier).

Pedigree analysis is relatively easy for autosomal dominant and X-linked recessive but more difficult for autosomal recessive and multifactorial modes.

Theoretical risks can be calculated for purely genetic traits; empiric risks can be estimated for multifactorial traits.

Severity is variable in autosomal dominant and in multifactorial traits but much less so in autosomal recessive and X-linked recessive traits.

Biochemical analysis after blood testing of parents and amniotic fluid of the fetus may detect an abnormal genotype in many autosomal recessive and X-linked recessive traits (inborn errors of metabolism).

Genetic counselors should not force their views on patients; rather, the patients should make the decisions.

The goal of genetic counseling is to alleviate individual suffering.

(From Fatt HV, Griffin JR: Genetics for Primary Eye Care Practitioners. Chicago, Professional Press, 1983.)

GENETIC COUNSELING

Important rules in genetic counseling are listed in Table 5.6. These apply to all counselors, whether the primary eye care practitioner or the medical specialist in genetics. Referral sources for genetic counseling include most major hospitals in the United States, particularly those affiliated with university medical schools.

Genetic counselors are medical specialists who are trained to be knowledgeable and sensitive to patients' needs and wishes. Nevertheless, the primary eye care practitioner can begin informal genetic counseling. Patients should be referred for continued and formal genetic counseling in the case of serious conditions such as Down's syndrome, ocular albinism, Marfan's syndrome, Tay-Sachs disease, and Fabry's disease. On the other hand, relatively mild traits such as color vision deficiencies, epicanthus, strabismus, and refractive errors do not ordinarily require referral for formal genetic counseling. A primary eye care practitioner who is knowledgeable about genetics and sensitive to the patient's wants and needs can provide this informal counseling.

REFERENCES

1. Brown GC, Tasman WS: Congenital Anomalies of the Optic Disc. New York, Grune & Stratton, 1983.
2. Cline D, Hofstetter HW, Griffin JR: Dictionary of Visual Science, ed 3. Radnor, PA, Chilton, 1980.
3. Donaldson DD: Atlas of External Diseases of the Eye, vol. 1. Congenital Anomalies and Systemic Diseases. St. Louis, CV Mosby, 1966.
4. Dorland's Illustrated Medical Dictionary, 26th ed. Philadelphia, WB Saunders, 298, 1981.
5. Fatt HV, Griffin JR: Genetics for Primary Eye Care Practitioners. Chicago, Professional Press, 1983.
6. Flynn JT: Acute proliferative retrolental fibroplasia: Multivariate risk analysis. Trans Am Ophthalmol Soc 81:549, 1983.

7. Fung YT, Murphree AL, T'Ang A, et al: Structural evidence for the authenticity of the human retinoblastoma gene. Science 236:1657, 1987.

8. Griffin JR: Binocular Anomalies: Procedures for Vision Therapy, 2nd ed. Chicago, Professional Press, 133, 1982.

9. Griffin JR, Asano GW, Somers RJ, Anderson CE: Heredity in congenital esotropia. J Am Optom Assoc 50:1237, 1979.

10. Griffin JR, Walton HN: Dyslexia Determination Test (DDT). Los Angeles, Instructional Materials and Equipment Distributors (IMED), 1981. (Revised edition, 1987).

11. Griffin JR, Walton HN: Therapy in Dyslexia and Reading Problems Including Vision, Perception and Motor Skills. Los Angeles, IMED, 1985.

12. Griffin JR, Walton HN, Christenson GN: The Dyslexic Screener (TDS). Culver City, CA. Reading and Perception Therapy Center, 1988.

13. Howard R: Chromosomal disease and strabismus. Am Orthoptic J 27:138, 1977.

14. International Dictionary of Medicine and Biology, vol. 2. New York, Wiley and Sons, 1191, 1986.

15. Leo J: Exploring the traits of twins. Time 129:63, 1987.

16. McKusick VA: Mendelian Inheritance in Man, 8th ed. Baltimore, Johns Hopkins University Press, 1988.

17. Martyn LJ: Pediatric neuro-ophthalmology. In Harley RD (ed): Pediatric Ophthalmology, 2nd ed., vol. 2. Philadelphia, WB Saunders, 803, 1983.

18. Maumenee IH, Alston A, Mets MB, et al: Inheritance of congenital esotropia. Trans Am Ophthalmol Soc 64:85, 1986.

19. Merin S, Crawford JS: The etiology of congenital cataracts. Can J Ophthalmol 6:178, 1971.

20. Miller MT, Epstein RJ, Sugar J, et al: Anterior segment anomalies associated with the fetal alcohol syndrome. J Pediatr Ophthalmol Strabismus, 21:8, 1984.

21. Newcomb RD: Optometry and genetic counseling: The first lines of defense against blindness. J Am Optom Assoc 47:458, 1976.

22. Nixon RB, Phelps CD: Glaucoma. In Renie WA (ed): Goldberg's Genetic and Metabolic Eye Disease, 2nd ed. Boston, Little, Brown, 290, 1986.

23. Pavan-Langston D (ed): Manual of Ocular Diagnosis and Therapy, 2nd ed. Boston, Little, Brown, 1985.

24. Punnett HH, Harley RD: Genetics in pediatric ophthalmology. In Harley RD (ed): Pediatric Ophthalmology, 2nd ed., vol. 1. Philadelphia, WB Saunders, 76, 1983.

25. Richter S: Untersuchungen über die Heredität des Strabismus Concomitans. Abhandlungen aus dem Gebiet der Augenheilkunde, vol. 35. 1967.

26. Richter S: Zur Heredität des Strabismus Concomitans. Humangenetik 3:235, 1967.

27. Rosenblum P, Stark WJ, Maumenee IH, et al: Hereditary Fuchs' dystrophy. Am J Ophthalmol 90:455, 1980.

28. Silverman WA: Retrolental Fibroplasia: A Modern Parable. New York, Grune & Stratton, 7, 1980.

29. Spalton DJ, Hitchings RA, Hunter PA (eds): Atlas of Clinical Ophthalmology. Philadelphia, JB Lippincott, 10, 1984.

30. Sparkes RS, Murphree AL, Lingua RW, et al: Gene for hereditary retinoblastoma assigned to human chromosome 13 by linkage to esterase D. Science 219:971, 1983.

31. Spivey BE: Strabismus: factors in anticipating its occurrence. Aust J Ophthalmol 8:5, 1980.

32. Van Dalen JTW: Congenital Anomalies of the Eye. Amersfoort, The Netherlands, Holland Ophthalmic Publishing Center, 1, 1983.

33. Worobec-Victor SM, Bair MAB: Oculocutaneous Genetic Diseases. In Renie WA (ed): Goldberg's Genetic and Metabolic Eye Disease. Boston, Little, Brown, 492, 1986.

Chapter 6

Refractive Status of Infants and Children

William R. Baldwin

The eye may be considered as an optical system made up of two thick lenses separated by some distance (anterior chamber depth), placed in two media (aqueous and vitreous), each of which has an index of refraction. Total refractive power of this system averages about 60 D, but wide variations are common. Eyes of greater optical power tend to have shorter axial lengths. The reverse is also true. Axial length is not, however, a factor in determining total refractive power. Whatever the optical power of a given eye, if it is without an astigmatic component, it is emmetropic when the fovea lies at the posterior principal focus of the system. The posterior principal focus is the point at which a distant point source is imaged as a point. This definition excludes the effects of diffraction and aberrations of the optical system. Although axial

length is independent of the eye's optical power, refractive status is not. It is the resultant of the optical power of a given eye, its anterior chamber depth, and its axial length.

All departures from emmetropia commonly have been characterized as refractive errors. Steiger (197) introduced the concept of biologic variants to the study of refraction. He suggested that, as with such characteristics as stature and interpupillary width, there is a range of variations from emmetropia that are within normal limits for human populations. This implies that the terms *refractive anomaly* and *refractive error* are misleading. The terms *refractive status* and *refractive state* are sometimes preferred because they do not connote abnormality.

Steiger believed that refractive status resulted from a free association of the ocular optical and axial components, but it has been demonstrated subsequently that development and change of these components is correlated in such a way as to produce emmetropization of most eyes from birth to adulthood. Donders (45) presaged this conclusion much earlier when he stated, "A priori it might be supposed, and it has been not only supposed, but also asserted, that less convexity of the cornea and of the crystalline lens is peculiar to the hypermetropic eye. So far as the cornea is concerned, I am justified by the results of numerous accurate determinations, in denying the assertion. . . . In the highest degrees of hypermetropia, I have found the radius even less than normal."

To the extent that we can measure the ocular and axial components and changes in them we can determine refractive state with precision by knowing the contributions of each. If one or more of these components lies near the limit of the range of distribution, giving rise to a significant and predictable ametropia, the term refractive anomaly may be used. It is appropriate to speak of refractive abnormalities when those refractive conditions—usually of severe degree—are associated with disease or with ocular malformations. Often we cannot clearly distinguish between what may be a normal variation or a refractive condition caused by abnormal processes.

In practice we measure refractive status as an entity. The validity of all methods of measuring refractive conditions is dependent on the status of accommodation at the time of measurement. Attempts are made to control accommodative posture by eliminating all near stimuli, by inhibiting action of the ciliary muscle while the patient actively fixates a visual target placed at a real or simulated distance of 6 m or more, or by applying a cycloplegic agent. Although stimuli to accommodation can be eliminated and dosages controlled, accommodative response is almost never established during measurement of refractive status. Recent evidence suggests that tonic accommodation may have a different baseline value for hyperopia and myopia, being highest in hyperopia, lower in juvenile

myopia, and lowest in young adult-onset myopia (142, 143). Persons with late-onset myopia have the greatest amplitude of accommodation and those with hyperopia the least when matched for age (144). Indeed we are not certain whether making an ideal measurement of refractive state requires complete relaxation of the ciliary muscle or some residual tonus that produces an accommodative posture that can be further inhibited but is "at rest." This is an even more complicating factor in refractive measurements of infants and of children who are unable to comply with the test requirement of active fixation on a distant target. Practically, we assume that refractive state of a given eye is established when, without stimulus to accommodation or after prescribed instillation of a cycloplegic agent the retinal image is as well-defined as it can be by application of spherical and cylindrical lenses. The subjective correlate is maximization of visual acuity.

In demographic studies of refractive status reported to date accommodation has not been fully controlled, nor its status known. Differences between cycloplegic and noncycloplegic refraction vary as much as 4.0 D among infant populations. Children 5 years of age and older demonstrate much less variation. In studies in which hyperopic and myopic subjects are evaluated separately, hyperopic children and young adults exhibit a mean of 0.50 to 1.0 D greater hyperopia under cycloplegia. Mean differences of myopic populations range from 0.0 to 0.50 D less myopia. Except for age groups under 5 years, and particularly when data for myopes and hyperopes are segregated, cycloplegic and noncycloplegic results may be compared directly by taking into account these mean differences.

While mean spherical equivalent refraction (SER) provides adequate information concerning spherical ametropia, it tells us nothing about how astigmatism and anisometropia are distributed and how they change from birth to adulthood. Most of what we know of astigmatism comes from a modest number of studies reported in the last quarter

century. Little demographic information
about anisometropia is available. High ametropias are defined here as refractive anomalies or refractive abnormalities, depending
on whether they are related to other congenital defects.

This chapter is divided into three major
topical units. The first is concerned with ametropia expressed as the spherical equivalent
of the two major refractive meridians. Emphasis is on prevalences and changes in SER
from infancy to young adulthood. Astigmatism, anisometropia, and refractive variants
other than those characterized by SERs
within the range of normal biologic variation
are discussed next. Refractive status of the
eye is the result of its combined optical and
axial properties. The third section of this
chapter describes how these components
change from birth through adolescence and
how changes in the components relate to refractive changes.

SPHERICAL EQUIVALENT REFRACTION

Premature Infants Without Ocular Complications

About one in 20 white infants and one in
eight nonwhite neonates born in the United
States weigh less than 2500 g at birth (108).
These are identified as low–birth weight
(LBW) infants. Birth weights between 1500 g
(3.3 lb) and 2500 g (5.5 lb) may occur in full-
term infants. When the gestation period is 37
weeks or less, the birth is classified as premature. About half of infants that weigh more
than 1500 g and almost all that weigh less are
estimated to be premature, although in individual births gestational age often cannot be
determined. Intrauterine growth retardation
(IUGR) signifies LBW, and probable prematurity, and is usually associated with inadequate nutrition or maternal disease.

Retrolental fibroplasia (now labeled retinopathy of prematurity, ROP) with congenital high myopia is a complication of administration of pure oxygen to premature infants.
Premature infants without ROP have a higher

prevalence of myopia then those born at full
term (73, 81, 85, 109, 160, 176). Fletcher and
Brandon (58) reported that many premature
infants who did not develop ROP were myopic at birth (up to −6.0 D) but when compared to ROP cohorts, paired for similar birth
weights, myopia was less prevalent and
milder. Mukherji et al. (160) found that 44
percent of newborn infants weighing less
than 2500 g were myopic in at least one principal meridian, whereas less than 5 percent
of those weighing more had this condition.
Banks (15) presented five studies of premature neonates and 10 studies of full-term
newborns in which cycloplegic refraction
was determined shortly after birth. Table 6.1
provides the mean SERs and ranges of premature and full-term newborns from all studies in which these data were available. Table
6.2 compares prevalence of myopia and birth
weight reported by three investigators.

Mean cycloplegic SER of newborn premature infants without ROP is similar to or
slightly less than SER of normal term infants
at 3 years of age and older. Table 6.3 presents
longitudinal studies (77, 89, 176, 177) of
those born prematurely that demonstrate emmetropization and hyperopic change. Forty-
six percent of those with congenital myopia
in one sample (176) became emmetropic or
hyperopic. Most eyes in these studies that
were hyperopic or emmetropic at birth remained stable throughout the 7-year period.

Some investigators (82, 172, 182) report
no distinguishable differences in SER between infants born prematurely and those
born after term, when both groups are compared at ages from 2 to 10 years. Others (26,

Table 6.1 COMPARISON OF DATA FROM REFRACTIVE STUDIES OF PREMATURE AND FULL-TERM NEONATES

	Mean of Mean SERs (D)	Range of Mean SERs (D)
Full-term neonates	+1.8	+0.6–+2.6
Premature neonates	+0.24	−1.3–+1.1

Table 6.2 RELATION OF PREVALENCE AND DEGREE OF MYOPIA AT BIRTH TO BIRTH WEIGHT

Investigator	Number of Subjects	Gestational Age or Birth Weight	Myopia (%)
Graham (85)	82	1815–2500 g	21
	52	1360–1785 g	42
Kalina (121)	1126	1300–2400 g	6
	273	<1300 g	78
Mukherji (160)	500	40–42 wk	6
	328	38–40 wk	21
	172	36–38 wk	24

(From Graham MV, Gray OP: Refraction of premature babies' eyes. Br Med J 1:145, 1963; Kalina RE: Ophthalmic examination of children with low birth weight. Am J Ophthalmol 67:134, 1969; and Mukherji R, Roy A, Chatterjee SK: Myopia. Indian J Ophthalmol 31:705, 1983.)

55, 176) have found mean SER of children born prematurely to be about 0.50 D less than those born at term when the two groups are compared at ages 7 to 18 years.

Normal Full-Term Neonates

When premature infants and those with birth defects are excluded from refractive studies of neonates, refractive distribution data yield a binomial curve. The apex is at +2.0 D mean SER or higher when refraction is performed under atropine cycloplegia (59, 110, 149, 166, 227). Goldschmidt (79) reported the results of 20 prior studies of infant refraction. Myopia was extremely rare when measures were performed with cycloplegia. Mean SER was from +2.3 to +4.8 D. Means near the lower end of this range were reported in retinoscopic studies; means were higher when

Table 6.3 LONGITUDINAL STUDIES (SER) OF INFANTS AND CHILDREN BORN PREMATURELY

Investigator	At Birth (D) Mean	SD	Elapsed Time	At End (D) Mean	SD
Gleiss (77)	+0.50		3 mo	+1.2	
Grignola (89)	−1.2		6 mo	−0.1	
Scharf (177)	−1.3	3.2	6 mo	−0.1	1.9
Scharf (176)	−1.3	3.2	7 yr	−0.2	1.4

(From Gleiss J, Pau H: Die Entwicklung der Refraction vor der Beburt. Klin Monatsbl Augenheilkd 121:440, 1952; Grignola A, Rivara A: Biometry of the human eye from the sixth month of pregnancy to the tenth year of life (measurements of the axial length, retinoscopy refraction, total refraction, corneal and lens refraction). In Vanysek J (ed): Diagnostica Ultrasonic in Ophthalmologica. Brno Czechoslovakia, University J.E. Purkyne, 251, 1968; Scharf J, Zonis S, Zelter M: Refraction in Israeli premature babies. J Pediatr Ophthalmol 12:193, 1975; and Scharf J: Refraction in premature babies: A prospective study. J Pediatr Ophthalmol 15:48, 1977.)

ophthalmoscopic assessments were made. Goldschmidt's own study involved 356 infants from 2 to 10 days old and with birth weight greater than 2500 g. He found a much higher prevalence of myopia (24.2 percent) than was found in all but two of the earlier reports. Mean SER for his sample was +0.55 D (standard deviation, 2.26). Plausible explanations for these variations in results include differences in method and technique, variations in sample, and difficulty in achieving full cycloplegia. Goldschmidt emphasized

that there are wide variations in developmental age among newborn infants, even when birth weight is considered normal.

Figure 6.1 shows distribution of SER from three studies in which atropine was administered repeatedly to large numbers of newborn infants before refraction was measured. Wibaut's (219) sample was drawn from the files of several ophthalmologists in Germany. Goldschmidt's (79) study was conducted in a Danish hospital. The Cook and Glasscock (31) sample included 630 black in-

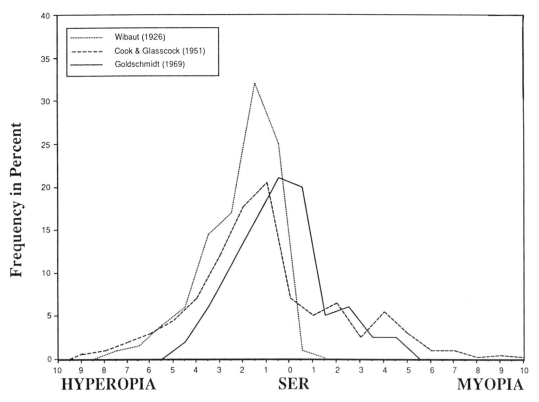

Figure 6.1 Wibaut's (219) sample was collected from several sources and numbered 2398 newborn infants. Cook and Glasscock's (31) 1000 infants were examined from 30 to 36 hours after birth. This study and Goldschmidt's (79)—whose subjects were 2 to 10 days old—involved a consecutive series. In the former only severely malformed infants were excluded; in the latter all with health problems or with birth weight below 2500 g were excluded. (From Wibaut F: Uber die Emmetropisation und den ursprung der spharischen refraktion-sanomalien. Graefes Arch Clin Exp Ophthalmol 116:596, 1926; Goldschmidt E: Refraction in the newborn. Acta Ophthalmol (Copenh) 47:570, 1969; and Cook RD, Glasscock RD: Refractive and ocular findings in the newborn. Am J Ophthalmol 34:1407, 1951.)

fants and 370 white infants born in a hospital in the southern United States. Ten infants in this sample were known to be premature. Black infants had a lower mean birth weight and accounted for 44 of the 56 instances of myopia greater than −4.0 D. Differences between the two groups are as likely to be based on socioeconomic factors as on racial differences (49). Wibaut's sample contained only three cases of myopia and no hyperopia more severe than +8.0 D. Cook and Glasscock found one infant to be 12 D hyperopic.

These are representative presentations of distribution of refraction under cycloplegia in newborn infants. The German and Danish studies underrepresent extremes and, therefore, may serve as better examples of distribution among healthy normal term infants; the 1950 study better reflects distribution among all live-born infants, excluding only neonates with severe malformations or disease. Wibaut's data includes some ophthalmoscopic assessments, which give higher means and shifts toward hyperopia. Figure 6.2 compares mean SERs from several studies of normal term and premature infants.

All but one of these studies (98) were conducted shortly after birth, involved a series of consecutive infants that met study criteria, and employed retinoscopy after repeated administration of a cycloplegic agent.

Studies of neonates without cycloplegia have been conducted employing retinoscopy and photorefraction. Both methods have been found to give reliable measures (8, 21, 111, 156, 184) but consistently result in lower mean SERs than cycloplegic studies. The first to report examination of neonates without cycloplegia was von Jaeger (212). He found that 78 of 100 eyes of infants less than 3 weeks old were myopic. Ely (52) repeated von Jaeger's investigation after instilling 0.5-percent atropine. He reported that only 17 percent of his neonate sample were myopic. In full-term neonate noncycloplegic samples, 2 to 4 D less SER is commonly found than with cycloplegic studies, shifting noncycloplegic distribution curves toward myopia (21). When a single group of newborns were examined with and without cycloplegia,

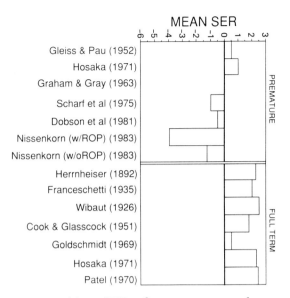

Figure 6.2 Mean SERs of term neonates and premature neonates were obtained retinoscopically except for Herrnheiser's, who used an ophthalmoscope. All were done under cycloplegia. Hosaka's premature subjects (109) were selected on the basis of birth weight less than 2500 g, so they included many term infants. Dobson's (42) were born after 36 weeks or less gestation. Sharf's (177) weighed from 1250 to 1750 g. All term infants were less than 1 week old. Most premature infants were less than 1 month old. Nissenkorn's (163) mean SERs are for infants who were myopic (50 percent of ROP infants, 16 percent of non-ROP infants). (From Hosaka A: The ocular findings in the premature infant, especially on the premature signs. Jpn J Ophthalmol 7:77, 1963; Dobson V, Fulton AB, Manning K, et al: Cycloplegic refractions of premature infants. Am J Ophthalmol 91:490, 1981; Scharf J, Zonis S, Zelter M: Refraction in Israeli premature babies. J Pediatr Ophthalmol 12:193, 1975; and Nissenkorn I, Yassus Y, Masshkowski D, et al: Myopia in premature babies with and without retinopathy of prematurity. Br J Ophthalmol 67:170, 183.)

mean SERs were +2.4 D and −2.2 D, respectively.

Millidot (151) suggested that all retinoscopic measures include a systematic error and that the actual mean SER refraction of newborn infants is near emmetropia because the retinal layer from which light is reflected during retinoscopy is in front of the receptor layer; therefore, the actual refractive power of the eye is underestimated. This effect would be significantly greater with the very short axial lengths of newborns. Cycloplegic studies might indicate that infant refraction is actually near emmetropia. If Millidot's correction factor is applied to noncycloplegic studies, mean SER would increase toward greater myopia.

Mean differences in SER between studies done with and without cycloplegia involve two factors. Accommodation is undoubtedly more active in noncycloplegic studies, although differences at later ages are small. Astigmatism is reported much more frequently in noncycloplegic techniques, resulting in lowered SER (66, 111, 155). It also appears that there was no attempt to record the degree of astigmatism in many retinoscopic studies following cycloplegia.

From Infancy to 7 Years

During the first years of life several changes take place in distribution and prevalence of SER. Mean SER under atropine changes from more than +2.0 D to about +1.0 D. This is due to the emmetropizing effect of developmental changes in ocular optical components (see Tables 6.20 and 6.22). Noncycloplegic SER means also move toward emmetropia, and myopia associated with uncomplicated prematurity regresses. At 1 year of age premature infants show much less variation from normal age peers in distribution and prevalence of ametropia. Emmetropization is a major ocular characteristic of early infancy.

This decreased dispersion in refractive distribution is accompanied by refractive stability. Most extreme spherical errors present at 1 year change little, if at all. Infants who were severely hyperopic at birth, both under cycloplegia and without it, are likely to remain hyperopic at about the same level. Hyperopia that is significantly greater under cycloplegia than without it is more likely to regress. Seldom does it progress. Only if myopia is significantly milder under cycloplegia than without is it likely to regress. Although uncomplicated congenital high myopia more often remains stable, if it changes it is toward greater myopia. Progression of high ametropia, when it occurs during the first year, is most often associated with other neonatal abnormalities that are themselves progressive.

Table 6.4 gives mean annual change in SER between the ages of 1 and 10 years found in three different studies and mean spherical equivalent at each age.

Brown's (24) and Slataper's (186) data include a number of subjects with strabismus. The Krause (129) subjects were randomly selected. This may account for the difference in direction of change at younger ages. A large group of Finnish school children from which this study was made had a prevalence of 1.9 percent myopia (>0.50 D) at ages 7 to 8 years and 21.8 percent at 14 to 15 years. Tassman (203) reported 1 percent of the eyes in a large sample from age 1 to 5 years were myopic more than −0.50 D (SER). By this criterion 8.6 percent of those aged 5 to 10 years were myopic. Kalogjera (122) compared the cycloplegic SER of rural and urban children in Yugoslavia at ages 3 to 7 years. Table 6.5 shows the prevalence at each 1-D level of spherical equivalents throughout this period. Figure 6.3 gives comparisons of distribution at 3 and 7 years. Table 6.5 and Figure 6.3 demonstrate the stability of refractive status from 3 to 7 years of age and confirm that myopia is rare in this age group.

Hirsch's (99) noncycloplegic data for 5- to 6-year-old children give a distribution similar to cycloplegic studies at that age. Only 4 percent of the group were myopic (SER −0.50 D or more). The mean SER of this group was +0.72 D. This is about 0.50 D less than the mean of cycloplegic studies.

It has been pointed out that cross-sectional age-related studies obscure the nature of changes in subgroups. Longitudinal investigations often suffer from small sample size and selection processes that make them poor predictors of general incidence, prevalence, and variation within selected populations. However, longitudinal studies of changes in

Table 6.4 CHANGES IN MEAN SER FROM 1 TO 10 YEARS

Age (yr)	Annual Mean Change			SER General Population (129) (D)
	Clinic Patients (24) (D)	Clinic Patients (186) (D)	General Population (129) (D)	
1				+1.45
2	+0.41	+0.26	−0.12	+1.33
3	+0.42	+0.34	−0.20	+1.13
4	+0.27	+0.31	−0.28	+1.41
5	+0.23	+0.23	0	+1.41
6	+0.17	+0.16	−0.31	+1.20
7	−0.02	+0.07	−0.30	+0.90
8	−0.11	−0.21	−0.26	+0.64
9	−0.19	−0.15	−0.20	+0.44
10	−0.27	−0.24	−0.36	+0.08

(From Brown EVL, Kronfeld P: Net average yearly changes in refraction of atropinized eyes from birth to beyond middle life. Arch Ophthalmol 19:719, 1938; Slataper FR: Age norms of refraction and vision. AMA Arch Ophthalmol 43:466, 1950; and Krause U, Krause K, Rantakillio P: Sex difference in refractive errors. Acta Ophthalmol (Copenh) 60:917, 1982.)

Table 6.5 FREQUENCY OF 1-DIOPTER SER INTERVALS FROM AGE 3 YEARS TO 7 YEARS

Diopter	Age (yr)				
	3 (%)	4 (%)	5 (%)	6 (%)	7 (%)
≥−3.0	0.0	0.97	0.46	0.0	0.8
−2.0	0.0	0.0	0.0	0.0	0.8
−1.0	3.1	2.9	0.0	2.9	0.8
0.0	3.0	4.8	10.65	20.6	9.1
+1.0	37.5	29.1	46.8	41.2	40.1
+2.0	37.8	43.7	24.1	25.5	34.9
+3.0	9.7	10.7	11.1	6.4	10.3
+4.0	5.6	2.9	1.8	0	1.4
+5.0	1.4	2.0	2.3	1.5	0.4
+6.0	1.0	0.5	0.9	0	0.4
+7.0	0.7	1.0	1.8	1.0	0
+8.0	0	0.5	0	1.0	0.0
+9.0	0	1.0	0	0	0
Mean D(SD)	+1.6 (1.2)	+1.5 (1.8)	+1.5 (1.3)	+1.1 (1.3)	+1.3 (1.2)

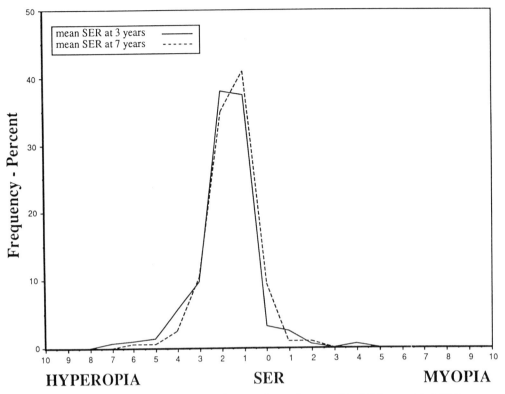

Figure 6.3 Comparison of distribution of SER of 144 3-year-old children with 126 7-year-olds in a Yugoslav urban population unselected except for age (122). Children were tested within a few days after their birth date. This cross-sectional comparison suggested stability of refractive status during this period. (From Kalogjera T: Refractive error in Yugoslav urban children aged between 3 and 7 years. Child Care Health Dev 5:439, 1979.)

refraction from birth to 6 or 7 years also indicate that this period can be characterized as one of emmetropization and refractive stabilization. Healthy infants who are either mildly hyperopic or myopic tend to change toward emmetropia. This is reflected by a much more sharply peaked refractive distribution curve at age 3 years. Even so, there remains a strong correlation between the degree of refractive spherical equivalents at birth and at 3 years.

It is very unlikely that a significant number of eyes of healthy youngsters that are near emmetropia at birth develop significant ametropia before age 6 years. Some sub-groups may show change during this age period of general stability. Some children who contract one of the febrile diseases that are common at these ages may become myopic (187). Measles specifically has been implicated (101). Near emmetropes in this age range, especially those who have against-the-rule (AR) astigmatism, are at risk to develop juvenile myopia.

Juvenile Myopia and Young-Adult Myopia

From age 3 to 6 years there is virtually no change in mean refractive status (about +1.00

D when determined after repeated administration of atropine). More than 80 percent of all 5- to 7-year-olds exhibit cycloplegic SERs between +0.50 D and +3.0 D. Less than 5 percent exhibit hyperopia greater than +5.0 D. Fewer than 3 percent are myopic in any degree. Extreme ametropias result almost exclusively from congenital refractive abnormalities and inherited myopia or severe astigmatism. Refractive anomalies following febrile illness or trauma may be sources of a few extreme ametropias in this age group (101, 187).

After age 8 years, cross-sectional means drop at a rate of 0.15 to 0.35 D per annum then become stable again in the mid- to late teens. This trend could result from very slight changes toward myopia among a large proportion of the total juvenile population or from onset and progression of significant myopia in a small subgroup.

Since the mid-19th century, when Cohn (30) reported an increasing incidence of myopia among school children as they progressed academically, a multitude of studies have shown that many children who are not myopic at age 6 years develop myopia between 7 and 12 years of age, which progresses until 15 to 17 years, then stabilizes. Harman (94) provided a striking example of this change in distribution of refractive anomalies. He cited a 1931 British Board of Education report containing the information that when almost all (1166) children in a school district between 4 and 5 years of age were examined retinoscopically following cycloplegia only five were found to be myopic. Two were at the level of −1.0 D, one at −2.0 D, one at −5.0 D, and one at −11.0 D. Harman repeated the study in another district. Of 368 children aged 4 to 7 years, only six were myopic. At about the same time an unselected sample of 1702 children in an English school district between ages 5 and 14 years were examined. Twenty-one percent were −0.50 D myopic or more.

Cycloplegic and noncycloplegic SERs become more similar from infancy, until at 5 years of age and upward, cycloplegic and noncycloplegic refractive data are usually in close agreement (16, 22). With hyperopia the mean difference is no more than 0.75 D. Myopic persons, as a group, exhibit no more than 0.25 D mean difference, although rarely—as in hyperopia—individual differences as great as 2.0 D are encountered (16, 22). For most purposes, prevalence data of populations aged 5 years and older acquired under both sets of conditions may be compared.

This most common form of myopia and most prevalent static refractive change after infancy is called juvenile myopia. The subgroup that develop juvenile myopia represent perhaps half or more of those who have an SER between +0.50 D and emmetropia at age 5 or 6 years. Depending on criteria for myopia and on population characteristics, this represents from 15 to 30 percent of the juvenile population.

If, in addition to having low hyperopia or emmetropia, a child exhibits 0.25 D or more AR astigmatism at 5 years, juvenile myopia is more likely to follow. Children who are among the approximately 4 percent of the population at age 5 or 6 years whose SER is between −0.12 D and −1.0 D will almost certainly develop significantly greater myopia than the mean for juvenile myopes. Esophoria has also been implicated as a predictor of juvenile myopia. Three other predictive associations have been reported. Children who have suffered from febrile diseases during early childhood are at greater risk to develop juvenile myopia (101). Children with tuberculosis are also predisposed to develop myopia (210). A relationship between dental malocclusion and juvenile myopia (80, 103, 139) has been suggested, but this association is less clear (125).

Onset of juvenile myopia may occur at any time between the ages of 6 and 15 years. The earlier the onset, the more severe the myopia is likely, ultimately, to be (205). Incidence figures drop to insignificance from about 15 years to about 18 years (84), after which another series of mean changes and greater variation in SER indicate that another subgroup are experiencing myopic onset and progression. This is labeled young-adult myopia.

The rate of progression of juvenile myopia varies, but it appears to be monotonic in almost all instances, averaging about −0.50 D per year for as much as 6 years. If myopia develops before 9 years of age it seldom progresses less than 2 D and has a mean SER of about −4.0 D. If it appears first after the age of 10 years it seldom progresses more than 3 D and has a mean SER of about −1.75 D. Myopia greater than about −6.0 D is quite rare among those who become myopic after age 5 years. When all juvenile myopia is considered, the mean spherical equivalent is about −3.0 D.

Children who are less than 1 D hyperopic between ages 7 and 13 years may show slight changes toward myopia without becoming myopic. Those who are at least 1 D hyperopic are much less likely to show change in this direction. On the other hand mild hyperopia and emmetropia very rarely change toward higher hyperopia during youth. Hyperopic progression is not common under any circumstance, but the greater the initial hyperopia, the greater the likelihood that it will progress and the greater the degree of progression is likely to be. Table 6.6,

constructed from Hirsch's study, demonstrates the tendency for mild hyperopia and emmetropia to become myopia, for higher hyperopia to remain stable, for mild myopia to progress, and the likelihood of patients with AR astigmatism to develop myopia. Table 6.7 gives distribution of various degrees of myopia among a population of young myopes ages 12 to 17 years who were selected only for age and presence of myopia.

A distinctive new form, young-adult myopia, appears at about 18 to 20 years (90). It affects primarily college students and those working extensively at near-point tasks. About 20 percent of those with very mild hyperopia or emmetropia develop a low degree of myopia (−1.0 D or less) under these conditions. More than half of all juvenile myopes show renewed progression as college students. Likelihood of progression and rate of progression among those who were initially myopic are greater for persons whose initial degree of myopia is greater. Total myopic progression may be as great as 2 or 3 D (90). Young-adult myopia usually involves axial elongation, although a few incidents of cor-

Table 6.6   ASTIGMATISM AND SER CHARACTERISTICS AT AGE 5 YEARS OF CHILDREN WHO ARE MYOPIC AT AGE 14 YEARS

At Age 5 Years			At Age 14 Years		
			SER		
	Astigmatism		Myopia −0.01 to −0.49 (%)	Emmetropia −0.50 to −0.99 (%)	Hyperopia ≥+1.00 (%)
	(No.)	(%)			
None or W/R	218	84	33	43	24
Against-the-Rule	43	16	58	26	16
SER (D)	261	100			
>+1.25	41	16	0	1	99
+1.00−+1.24	31	12	6	48	46
+0.75−+0.99	66	25	23	62	15
+0.50−+0.74	59	22	36	56	8
+0.25−+0.49	41	16	90	10	0
0.00−+0.24	13	5	54	46	0
<−0.01	10	4	100	0	0

Table 6.7 DISTRIBUTION OF VARIOUS DEGREES OF MYOPIA AMONG A POPULATION OF MYOPIC CHILDREN AGED 12 TO 17 YEARS

Degree of SER (D)	Myopic Subjects (No.)	(%)
−0.10−−1.9	1900	48
−2.0−−3.9	1068	27
−4.0−−5.9	633	16
−6.0−−8.6	356	9
Total	3957	100

neal power increase, leading to very mild myopia, have also been reported.

Young adults who do not continue their education beyond the secondary level later demonstrate a much lower prevalence of myopia. It has not been determined that high school graduates who are college bound have a higher prevalence of juvenile myopia than their age peers, but prevalence figures among college freshmen suggest that this is so. Young-adult myopia may represent reinitiation of the same fundamental factor that led to juvenile myopia.

Whatever the causes, the prevalence of myopia (SER >−0.50 D) among the adult population from 21 to 40 years is the sum of congenital (1 to 2 percent), juvenile (15 to 30 percent), and newly initiated young-adult myopia (20 percent of those entering college who are not myopic—about 8 to 10 percent of all young adults), or a total prevalence of myopia of about 25 to 40 percent. This total is in close agreement with studies of adult prevalence that employ the criterion of −0.50 D or greater SER to define myopia.

Gender Differences in Retractive Status

Distribution of refractive status by gender is similar for premature and normal term neonates, except that premature female infants show a slightly higher prevalence of high myopia (>−6.0 D) and high astigmatism (>3.0 D) (28).

Gender comparisons of mean SER annually from 1 year to 16 years are presented in Figure 6.4. No clear SER differences exist between girls and boys until age 10 or 11 years, when girls exhibit a greater mean decrease in SER (100). Increased incidence and progression of myopia from about 8 years to the middle teens results from very low hyperopia and emmetropia becoming myopia, then progressing (juvenile myopia). McIlroy and Hamilton (145) studied gender differences in the incidence of myopia for subjects from age 4 to 18 years (Fig. 6.5). Changes in mean refraction (see Fig. 6.4) confirm the tendency of girls to become myopic at a slightly earlier age. This disparity has been attributed to difference in physiologic age of boys and girls and to hormonal changes associated with puberty. McIlroy found earlier onset of menarche among myopic girls than among those who were hyperopic.

Most extreme ametropias probably are congenital. Congenital high myopia is two to three times more prevalent than congenital high hyperopia. Prevalence of myopia greater than −6.0 D in general populations ranges from about 2 percent in the United States to as high as 10 percent in certain countries and among some ethnic groups (116). When gender differences in prevalence of high myopia have been determined in adult populations, females usually show a prevalence more than twice as great as males.

Studies of prevalence among clinic and nonclinic adult populations in which high myopia was excluded show 5 to 15 percent greater prevalence among males. As the prevalence of severe myopia in females is about twice that in males, it is likely that juvenile myopia, and perhaps young adult myopia as well, affects males slightly more often than females. Occidental studies of college students report virtually equal proportions for both sexes. Males predominated among college populations during the late nineteenth and early twentieth centuries, when most prevalence studies were made. College pop-

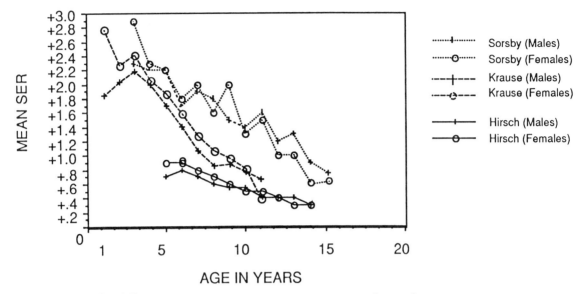

Figure 6.4 Gender differences in mean retinoscopic SER at annual ages from 1 to 16 years. Sorsby's (192) (England) and Krause's (129) (Finland) studies followed administration of cycloplegia. Hirsch (99) (United States) did not use cycloplegics. (From Sorsby A, Leary G: A longitudinal study of refraction and its components during growth. Medical Research Council, Special Report Series No. 309:1. London, Her Majesty's Stationery Office, 1969; Krause U, Krause K, Rantakillio P: Sex difference in refractive errors. Acta Ophthalmol (Copenh) 60:917, 1982; and Hirsch MJ: The changes in refraction between the ages of 5 and 14, theoretical and practical considerations. Am J Optom Arch Am Acad Optom 29:444, 1952.)

ulations consistently show a higher prevalence of myopia; this may account for the apparently greater prevalence among adult males.

Almost all prevalence studies indicate no significant gender difference in mild and moderate hyperopia at any age.

Ethnic Differences

Valid evidence of ethnic differences in distribution of SER can be drawn only from studies that make comparisons in which common criteria are applied and common protocols are followed. White and black children have been compared from birth through secondary school years. Black infants have a higher prevalence of severe myopia than white infants, but blacks are much less likely to

develop juvenile myopia or young-adult myopia.

Cook and Glasscock (31) found that in white newborns the prevalence of hyperopia +4.0 D and above is greater (23 versus 16 percent). Blacks had greater prevalence of myopia more than −3.0 D (15 versus 4 percent). While 10 infants were identified as premature (seven white and three black), none had ROP. The difference in prevalence of more extreme myopia may be related to ethnic or socio-economic differences in incidence of ocular abnormalities associated with inherited congenital defects or maternal disease. Figure 6.6 provides prevalence comparisons between black and white infants for SER at 1-D intervals. Callan (25) studied prevalence of myopia among more than 900 black children in the first six grades of pri-

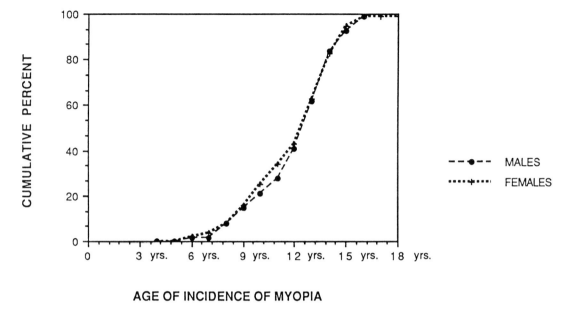

Figure 6.5 Gender differences in incidence of myopia between 3 years and 16 years constructed of data from McIlroy and Hamilton's (145) study of an English school district population. At 10 to 12 years, incidence is slightly greater among girls. No other gender differences in onset of myopia are apparent. (From McIlroy J, Hamilton R: Investigation into increase and progress of myopia in children. London County Council Report 4, 3:690, 1932.)

Figure 6.6 Comparison of distribution of SER of black and white newborn infants from data of Cook and Glasscock (31). White neonates show less dispersion, higher prevalence of moderate hyperopia, and less high myopia. (From Cook RC, Glasscock RE: Refractive and ocular findings in the newborn. Am J Ophthalmol 34:1407, 1951.)

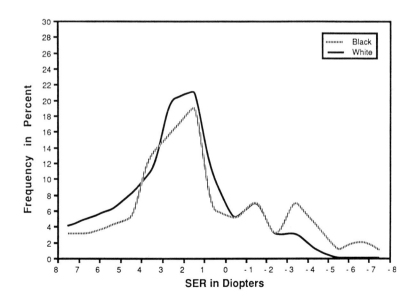

Table 6.8 PREVALENCE OF MYOPIA AMONG BLACKS AND WHITES IN VARIOUS AGE GROUPS

	All (%)	12–17 yr (%)	18–24 yr (%)	25–34 yr (%)	35–44 yr (%)	45–54 yr (%)
Blacks	13.0	11.7	9.5	12.8	13.7	17.0
Whites	26.5	25.7	29.7	25.0	24.4	24.9

mary schools in the United States: 2.3 percent were myopic. He did not provide prevalence figures for their white age peers but indicated that they were somewhat greater. About the same time Agnew (1) reported prevalence of myopia among white students in primary grades one through four to be 10 percent and among grades five through eight to be 14 percent.

Sperduto et al. (196) compared myopia prevalence of blacks and whites in several age groups. A significant difference was found in all. Standard deviations were considerably greater for blacks at all ages except 18 to 24 years. These data support the conclusion that blacks have a significantly greater prevalence of congenital severe myopia but less mild to moderate myopia. Table 6.8 is extracted from Sperduto's study.

Angle and Wissmann (6), like Sperduto et al. (196), obtained data from an unselected population. They, too, found a significant difference in prevalence of myopia between blacks and whites (25 versus 33 percent at ages 12 to 17 years).

Jewish children have been compared to others in the same locale in many countries (67, 176, 188, 195). All such studies report greater prevalence of myopia and a significantly greater mean degree of myopia among Jews (123). The only studies in which severe myopia was found to be as prevalent in males as in females involve Jewish children and adults. Table 6.9 provides comparisons of myopic prevalence between Jewish and non-Jewish children in a study reported by Sorsby (188). The difference in prevalence in this sample results from a much higher incidence of juvenile myopia among Jewish boys. Some believe this reflects greater near-work demands.

Chinese and Japanese youth appear to have a higher prevalence of myopia than whites—especially of high myopia (164, 169, 173, 202). Japanese draftees had a greater prevalence of myopia than U.S. draftees by a ratio of 3:2 (162). Figure 6.7 shows the prevalence of ametropia in several ethnic groups of children in one school district in Hawaii (33). Children of Chinese, Japanese, and Ko-

Table 6.9 PREVALENCE OF MYOPIA AMONG JEWISH AND NON-JEWISH SCHOOL CHILDREN OF ENGLAND

	Age		5–14 yr	
	5–9 yr (%)	10–14 yr (%)	Males (%)	Females (%)
Jews	9.1	33.5	43.2	26.0
Non-Jews	10.2	25.5	21.7	27.2

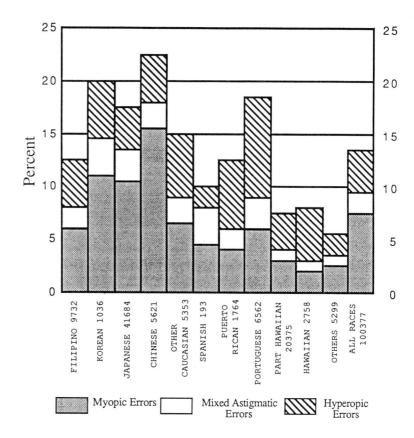

Figure 6.7 Prevalence of various ametropias (≥1.0 D) among racial groups in a Hawaiian school district (33). Children's ages are 6 to 11 years. (From Crawford HE, Hammond GG: Racial analysis of ocular defects in the schools of Hawaii. Hawaii Med J, 9:90, 1949.)

rean descent had the highest prevalences of myopia. Japanese school children have been found to have a lower prevalence of myopia than Chinese age peers in at least one other comparative study (13 vs 22 percent) (207).

Dzen (48) compared prevalence of hyperopic and myopic SER of more than 500 clinic patients not selected for age in each of two groups—Caucasian and native Chinese. Table 6.10 gives these comparisons. Similar results have been reported in other studies.

School children of Asian Indian origin have been examined in different locales within and outside India (147, 167, 183). Refractive data are characteristic whether the children reside in India or abroad. No significant differences exist between them and U.S. age peers, but Indian children have a higher prevalence of myopia than African age peers living in the same communities (147).

Comparisons of Caucasian ethnic groups have not yielded clear distinctions. Tenner (204) compared groups of children of different nationalities in a New York City school (Table 6.11). If there is a distinction among Caucasian ethnic groups it is most likely that Germans have the highest prevalence of myopia of all degrees.

In most underdeveloped countries the prevalence of juvenile myopia is low but severe myopia is more frequent than in highly industrialized nations. Those comparisons in which differences in prevalence of myopia seem to be clearly established indicate low prevalence among black children in all countries and high prevalence among Chinese and Jewish children. The prevalence among Eskimo (4, 159, 224) and Japanese (165, 173) children appears to be high at the present time and has increased during the past sev-

Table 6.10   COMPARISON OF PREVALENCES IN REFRACTIVE STATUS OF CHINESE AND CAUCASIAN CLINIC PATIENTS

Diopter Range	Hyperopia		Myopia	
	Chinese (%)	Caucasian (%)	Chinese (%)	Caucasian (%)
0–+1	23.0	27.0	13	6
1–2	16.0	33.0	9	7
2–3	3.5	10.0	6	3
3–4	0.7	3.5	5	2
4–6	0.9	2.4	8	3
6–10	1.4	0.2	6	1
10–14	0.5	0.4	5	0
	46.0	76.5	52	22

eral decades. Eskimos (20, 185) of earlier generations were rarely myopic. In Japan (164, 207) prevalence of myopia was high early in this century then fell during the World War II era. Prevalence has increased steadily among Japanese children residing in Japan during the last four decades (165, 173).

It is very likely that ethnic differences in prevalence of mild to moderate myopia are due in large part to differences in prevalence of juvenile myopia and young adult-onset myopia.

Table 6.11   COMPARISON OF PREVALENCE OF MYOPIA AMONG SCHOOL CHILDREN OF EUROPEAN BACKGROUND

Ethnic Background	Prevalence of Myopia (%)
German	35.0
Russian (mostly Jews)	24.5
American	31.0
Austrian	30.0
Irish	27.0
Italian	23.8

OTHER REFRACTIVE VARIANTS

Astigmatism

Astigmatism greater than 2 D is common among premature infants at birth but less common after 1 year, and it rarely persists in this magnitude into childhood. At birth the horizontal meridian is more often the meridian of maximum refractive power (astigmatism against the rule). The cornea (and perhaps the lens) is implicated in the high prevalence of moderate to high AR astigmatism among premature newborns. Dobson et al. (42) made refractive measurements of the eyes of 146 infants between 32 and 37 weeks' gestational age. Those with detectable ROP or other ocular disease were excluded. Prevalence and degree of myopia and astigmatism increased as gestational age decreased. Sixty-eight percent of the total group had at least 1 D of astigmatism in one or both eyes. More than 80 percent of this astigmatism was AR. Myopia and astigmatism associated with uncomplicated prematurity tend to occur together; both typically regress. By the age of 1 year, infants born prematurely but without ROP show distribution and mean of astigmatism similar to their normal term cohorts.

Santonastaso (172) was the first to assess astigmatism of full-term infants during the first week of life. He found that seven of 15 showed astigmatism between 1.0 and 2.0 D under cycloplegia and that 13 had 1.0 D or more of astigmatism when retinoscoped without cycloplegia. Franceschetti (59) reported meridional mean refractions of 200 infant eyes examined retinoscopically under cycloplegia 3 to 16 days after birth. He reported mean values of +1.4 D in the horizontal meridian and +2.5 D in the vertical. Cook and Glasscock (31) did not report the degree but estimated that 25 percent of their newborn subjects had astigmatism.

From 1935 to 1975 virtually no effort was made to distinguish the astigmatic component of ametropia. This led to the general assumption that astigmatism was not prevalent among infants. Recent studies—both cycloplegic and noncycloplegic—clearly indicate that AR astigmatism is not unique to prematurity. Figure 6.8 gives prevalence data for premature and full-term newborns.

It is likely that the severity and prevalence of astigmatism are greater among premature neonates. Dobson et al. (42) found that degree and prevalence increase as gestational age decreases. Hosakas' infants were below 2500 g birth weight (109). No more than half of infants that weigh less than 2500 g are expected to be premature.

One notable exception to the high prevalence of AR astigmatism among infants was reported by Thorn et al. (206), who compared prevalence of astigmatism greater than 0.50 D among Chinese and white cohorts. About 50 percent of the Chinese infants had astigmatism with-the-rule (WR) and about 15 percent had AR. These prevalence figures were reversed for the white subjects (206).

Prevalence and mean degree of AR astigmatism increase during the first year of life then decrease. Table 6.12 presents prevalence data at various age levels from birth to 5 years.

Figure 6.9 compares prevalence of AR and WR astigmatism. There is no clear difference between premature and full-term newborns; however, the proportion of AR declines significantly with age.

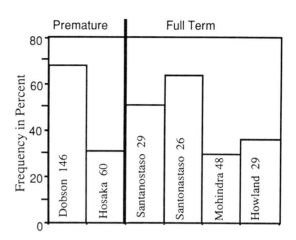

Figure 6.8 Comparison of prevalence of astigmatism of 1.0 D or more among premature and normal term neonates less than 1 month after birth. Number of subjects is indicated in each bar. Santonastaso (172) found the prevalence to be higher when 26 of 29 infants examined retinoscopically under atropine were later tested without cycloplegia. Mohindra (155) performed retinoscopy without cycloplegia; Howland (111), performed photorefraction without cycloplegia. (From Santonastaso A: La refraziene oculare nei primi anni di vita. Ann di Ottal e Clin Ocul (Italy) 848:1930; Mohindra I, Held R, Swiazda J, et al: Astigmatism in infants. Science 202:329, 1978; and Howland HC, Atkinson J, Braddick O, et al: Infant astigmatism measured by photorefraction. Science 202:331, 1978; Hosaka A: The ocular findings in the premature infant, especially on the premature signs. Jpn J Ophthalmol 7:77, 1963; Dobson V, Fulton AB, Manning K et al: Cycloplegic refractions of premature infants. Am J Ophthalmol 91:490, 1981.

Longitudinal studies of children who were healthy infants show that this high prevalence of AR astigmatism during infancy reduces sharply (9, 43, 66). Mild WR astigmatism becomes the norm. Those few who have WR astigmatism as infants do not show shifts in axis, although their astigmatism infrequently may progress (84).

Sometime during the first year of life as many as half of all infants exhibit AR astigmatism of 0.50 D or more. Less than 12 percent

Table 6.12 PREVALENCE OF ASTIGMATISM OF VARIOUS DEGREES AT 1-YEAR INTERVALS IN SEVERAL PUBLISHED STUDIES

Investigator	Age Range	Astigmatism (D)	No. Subjects	Prevalence (%)	Eyes Chosen	Method
Santonastaso (1930)	0–1 yr	1–2	108	56	——	Atropine retinoscopy
	0–1 yr	>2	100	49	——	Noncycloplegic retinoscopy
Friedman (1976)	1–2.5 yr	1–2.5	84	22	More ametropic eye	1% cyclopentolate retinoscopy
	1–2.5 yr	3–6	84	7		
Howland (1978)	0–1 yr	≥1	117	64	Most astigmatic eye	Photorefraction
	1–2 yr	≥1	61	42		
	2–3 yr	≥1	29	20		
	3–4 yr	≥1	60	11		
	4–5 yr	≥1	70	12		
Mohindra (1978)	0–4 wk	≥1	48	29	Right	Noncycloplegic retinoscopy
	5–8 wk	≥1	27	48		
	9–16 wk	≥1	78	55		
	17–32 wk	≥1	70	63		
	33–64 wk	≥1	50	42		
	65–128 wk	≥1	39	37		
	129–256 wk	≥1	81	33		
Ingram (1979)	1 yr	≥1.5	1648	13	More hyperopic eye	1% cyclopentolate retinoscopy
	3.5 yr	≥1.5	1648	5		
Fulton (1980)	0–1 yr	≥1	133	20	Right or nonamblyopic eye	1% cyclopentolate retinoscopy
	2–3 yr	≥1	94	12		
	0–1 yr	≥1	22	26	Amblyopic eye	
	1–2 yr	≥1	18	12		
	2–3 yr	≥1	21	46		

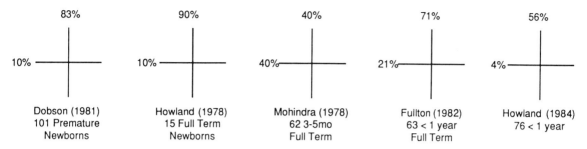

Figure 6.9 Percentage figures above vertical lines indicate prevalence of AR astigmatism; at left of horizontal lines, prevalence of WR astigmatism. Difference between sums of the two and 100 percent gives prevalence of oblique astigmatism among all astigmatic infants. Number of subjects is indicated before age designations.

of 4-year-olds have AR astigmatism in any significant degree (221). By age 6 years (102) approximately 80 percent have 0.25 D or less of astigmatism; about 12 percent are WR astigmatic between 0.25 and 0.75 D; and about 5 percent have WR astigmatism greater than 0.75 D. Only about 3 percent demonstrate AR astigmatism of any degree, none more than 1.25 D. The extreme of WR astigmatism for eyes without ocular malformations is about 6 D. Much of the change from AR astigmatism takes place during the first 2 years of life, but the trend continues. Greater corneal flattening in the horizontal meridian over this period probably is almost exclusively responsible for the refractive change.

From 8 years to adolescence, and beyond, there is virtually no change in mean refractive astigmatism (7, 102), nor in mean corneal curvature (135). Cross-sectional and longitudinal studies show that, with few exceptions, refractive astigmatism changes 0.25 D or less during this period; and very few persons who have no refractive astigmatism at 5 or 6 years develop astigmatism greater than 0.25 D. Two minor trends are observed. Slight increases in WR astigmatism occur in perhaps as many as 20 percent of those who had WR astigmatism at 5 or 6 years and the incidence of AR astigmatism increases slightly. The former trend is probably the result of continued corneal flattening in the horizontal meridian among a few. The latter

trend is associated with the increased incidence of AR refractive astigmatism with onset and progression of juvenile myopia. This is probably due to corneal flattening in the vertical meridian. As many as 40 percent of myopic juveniles exhibit AR astigmatism, rarely greater than 1.0 D. The only other children above 6 years of age who have been found to have a high prevalence of AR astigmatism are those affected by the fetal alcohol syndrome (FAS) (150). These children typically exhibit very steep corneas (as much as 56 D) and severe, permanent AR astigmatism (68).

A longitudinal study has shown that in advanced age eyes again tend to develop AR refractive astigmatism, at least in part because the horizontal corneal meridian tends to become steeper as the vertical meridian tends to remain the same (13). Both the neonatal and late adult changes in corneal astigmatism may be due to changes in tension of the eyelids (87, 136) combined with decreased scleral rigidity among neonates and in advanced age (27). Severe noncorneal astigmatism is extremely rare. Virtually all of the astigmatism that is not corneal (presumably lenticular) is AR and normally is distributed within a very narrow range (one standard deviation is about 0.25 D) about a mean of 0.5 D (106). When present, high noncorneal astigmatism is associated with congenital defects of the crystalline lens that are in turn associated with other ocular malformations.

The prevalence of WR astigmatism is significantly greater in native American children than in other ethnic groups (137, 148, 157, 220, 222). Although it is greater in degree their astigmatism is like that of the general population in other respects (Fig. 6.10).

These cross-sectional data give evidence that prevalence of corneal and refractive astigmatism changes very little from 5 to 13 years of age (102, 112).

Figure 6.11 shows that mean corneal astigmatism of all native American groups is higher than that of Caucasians. Comparison of A1 with A2 and B1 with B2 and comparisons in Figure 6.10 indicate that most refractive astigmatism is corneal astigmatism. Severe astigmatism is not characteristic of other aboriginal groups (71, 224).

It is not known whether astigmatism of native American children is congenital or acquired. Twin studies and pedigrees suggest that congenital astigmatism is chiefly hereditary (11, 191, 194, 214); however, it is also clear from FAS studies that severe corneal astigmatism can be produced by nonhereditary causes (199). There are many FAS children among native American populations. Most have very steep corneas and severe AR astigmatism. In contrast, general populations of native American children have a high prevalence of moderate to high WR astigmatism and tend to have flat corneas. Zuni Indians are reported to have a high rate of consanguinity and a high prevalence of albinism, which is one of few hereditary abnormalities highly correlated with corneal astigmatism (95). The more severe the astigmatism of native American children, the greater the hyperopia component is apt to be. When astigmatism is greater in one eye, that eye almost invariably is more hyperopic than its fellow eye. Native American children show a higher prevalence of mild to moderate hyperopia and less high spherical ametropia. Anisometropia appears to be more common, especially among those who are astigmatic (93).

Anisometropia

Anisometropia is believed by Duke-Elder (47) to be genetically determined, except for that caused by monocular disease or injury, but he also reported that the hereditary control mechanisms are obscure. Most studies of refractive states of neonates fail to report incidence of anisometropia because they present SER of one eye only or, less often, the mean of both eyes.

Among children and adults, if one eye is at or near emmetropia, significant anisome-

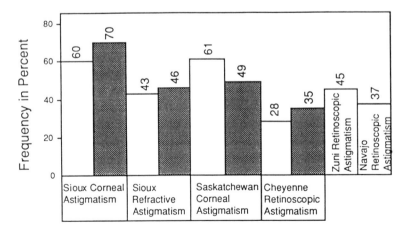

Figure 6.10 Prevalence of astigmatism of at least 1.0 D among native American children of 5 or 6 years compared to prevalence at 11 to 13 years, taken from several cross-sectional studies. Open bars represent prevalence at younger ages; closed bars at older ages. Retinoscopic means compared to keratometric means of Sioux children indicate that corneal astigmatism is partially compensated by noncorneal astigmatism of opposite power. Number of subjects is given above each bar.

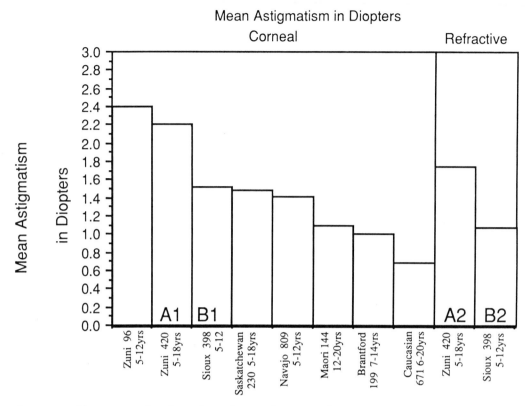

Figure 6.11 Mean corneal astigmatism of several groups of native American children and white children. A1-A2 and B1-B2 are 0.5 and 0.4 D, approximating the mean of noncorneal astigmatism. Number of subjects is indicated before age range below each bar.

tropia is seldom found. A difference greater than 3.0 D is very rare. In large errors (more than +5.0 D or −6.0 D), the difference between the two eyes is more likely to be significant (more than 1.0 D). Myopic children are anisometropic much more often than those who are hyperopic.

Anisometropia is more common among all premature infants than among normal term neonates; however, significant differences between the two eyes are much less prevalent among children who were born prematurely but who did not develop ROP than among those who did.

Neonate studies of anisometropia were reported in an ophthalmic screening program in Israel of 38,000 children between 1.5 and 2.5 years of age (64). Anisometropia of 2 D or more was found in 9.4 percent of the 360 cases of esotropia identified. Of the children discovered to have some "significant" degree of ametropia, 9 percent exhibited 2 D or more of anisometropia. The authors reported that anisometropia was particularly frequent in persons with constant unilateral esotropia.

Atkinson et al. (10) found only 1.3 percent of a sample of infants between the ages of 6 and 9 months had more than 1.0 D anisometropia. Goldschmidt (79) found that 2.5 percent of boys and 2.9 percent of girls who were myopic had anisometropia of 3.0 D or more.

Monocular amblyopia is the most common feature of high anisometropia, affecting the eye with the greater refractive error. If that eye is not congenitally malformed, the amblyopia may be subject to orthoptic treatment following correction of the refractive anomaly.

Refractive Anomalies

The term refractive anomalies is reserved for moderate to severe ametropias that result from significant variation from population means of one or more ocular optical components but that are not associated with congenital ocular malformations. Distinctions are seldom made between those mild to moderate ametropias that are produced by variations of the ocular optical components within the limits of normal biologic variation and those identified here as refractive anomalies. As measures of ocular optical components become more refined and more often employed, these distinctions will become clearer.

Uncomplicated severe congenital hyperopia probably results from a shortened axial length. The corneal power of neonates who are highly hyperopic, as Donders (45) noted over a century ago, typically is greater than normal. The role of the crystalline lens is less clear. Based on pedigrees and twin studies, most high hyperopia is very likely inherited, although the mode of inheritance is not clear (60). The condition has also been linked to underdevelopment of the fetal eye; however, uncomplicated prematurity is characterized by curvature myopia. Hyperopia greater than +8.0 D is extremely rare in nonaphakic eyes. Among 2398 newborns Wibaut (219) found 5 percent to be greater than +5.0 D and none greater than +8.0 D.

Cook and Glasscock (31), whose sample included only a few premature infants, found hyperopia above +5.0 D in 10.5 percent of their 1000 neonates. Three percent had myopia over −5.0 D. Wibaut found less than 7 percent to be myopic in any degree; none more than −4.0 D (see Fig. 6.1). Other investigators report that 1.0 percent or less of all newborns show congenital severe myopia.

In general U.S. population samples from which those affected by significant congenital malformations are excluded, myopia greater than −6.0 D is found in about 20 percent of all myopic subjects. This represents a prevalence of about 4 percent. Prevalence of high myopia is considerably greater among young and mature adults than among young children. This indicates that some of this myopia is acquired or developmental, although myopia that appears after infancy may be influenced by heredity (i.e., abiotrophic). Another possibility is that acquired severe myopia may be associated with hereditary predisposition but may be expressed only if certain environmental factors intervene. When both parents are severely myopic, their offspring are severely myopic much more often than offspring of only one very myopic parent. Monozygotic twins show extremely high concordance for high ametropia, high anisometropia. Heterozygotic twins show much lower concordance (41).

Significant choroidal and retinal degeneration are almost always present with high myopia, whereas it is found very rarely with emmetropia and almost never with hyperopia (37, 39, 210). These processes occur in the form of posterior scleral ectasia with temporal crescent, or tesselation (179, 213), and, less often, rupture of Bruch's membrane (36). A decrease in index of refraction of the vitreous may also be present, increasing the degree of myopia. The term pathologic myopia traditionally has been used to describe this form. Curtin (38) presents a thorough discussion of ocular characteristics in pathologic myopia. Most conditions of the posterior globe associated with myopia are probably consequences of axial elongation. More severe forms, especially in high myopia, may reflect primary connective tissue abnormalities or mesodermal dysplasia that initiate axial elongation.

When high myopia (at least −6.0 D) does not progress after early childhood and when the eyes are free of degenerative retinal and choroidal anomalies, the child is perhaps most likely to have large globes accompanied by refractive surfaces that are less curved than normal (37, 133).

Pedigrees indicate that extreme corneal

astigmatism, although rare, commonly affects family cohorts. Waardenburg (213) reported that differences in corneal refraction between corresponding eyes of monozygotic twins never exceeded 2.0 D, whereas those of dizygotic twins and in general populations varied as much as 8 D. It is not known whether this refractive abnormality is congenital or, like keratoconus, is abiotrophic. When keratoconus is unilateral, the cornea of the fellow eye is often highly astigmatic. It is possible that severe congenital astigmatism is present in at least some individuals at risk for keratoconus and that early treatment with contact lenses would prevent some of the consequences.

Severe oblique astigmatism is most commonly associated with high myopia. In myopic anisometropia the more myopic eye is likely to be more astigmatic as well. Both severe astigmatism and severe myopia, commonly found together, are sometimes progressive. It has been speculated that uncorrected astigmatism in infants, which does not decrease significantly at an early age, causes progression of myopia by producing meridional blur. It is known that uncorrected astigmatism produces meridional amblyopia in young children. It is evident that—except for rare malformations of the crystalline lens—differences in principal meridians of the cornea are responsible for significant degrees of astigmatism. Changes in astigmatism probably involve nonhereditary influences, perhaps imposed on hereditary predisposition.

High spherical ametropias at ages 2 to 6 years frequently are associated with strabismus and amblyopia (115, 120). Some investigators have found 50 percent or more of persons with severe ametropia to have strabismus, at least intermittently (114); however, many children with strabismus have no significant ametropia.

After the age of 5 years, the prevalence of high myopia (more than 6.0 D) is at least twice as great for females as for males. It is not known whether a disparity of this magnitude is present at birth or during infancy. High hyperopia (more than +5.0 D) is equally prevalent in both sexes after age 5

years, and probably throughout life (115). Gender differences in prevalence and degree of astigmatism and anisometropia have not been studied thoroughly. As indicated earlier, premature female neonates more frequently exhibit severe astigmatism than do males. Girls and women also have a greater prevalence of astigmatism greater than 3.0 D.

Refractive Abnormalities

Severe ametropia associated with patent ocular malformation or disease is defined here as a refractive abnormality. Severe myopia occurring with ROP is the most common example of a postpartum disease that results in refractive abnormalities. Fletcher and Brandon (58) were the first to distinguish between refractive states of premature infants with ROP and those without retinal complications. They reported, "It is striking that almost all of the high myopia seen in our clinic during the past 4 years has been in infants who previously had acute retrolental fibroplasia." Several others have reported myopia with a range of −4.0 to −24.0 D among infants with ROP during the first year of life when retinoscopic results were attainable. Kushner (130) found a much greater prevalence of all forms of significant ametropia as well as strabismus and amblyopia among premature infants with ROP than among premature neonates without ROP.

ROP can regress and result in a normal-looking fundus, even though vascularization of the retina is not normal (124). A 5-year follow-up study of 84 percent of all infants born at one hospital who weighed 1815 g (4 lb) or less found that most eyes in which ROP was diagnosed at birth had good visual acuity and many appeared normal (226). Table 6.13 presents refractive data for various subgroups of this cohort classified by presence and degree of ROP at birth. These data support the conclusion that, at 5 years, premature infants who do not develop ROP at birth show a prevalence of myopia only slightly higher than that among term infants, and no severe myopia. Children who have ROP on the other hand show a much greater prevalence at 5 years, much of it moderate to severe.

Table 6.13   VISUAL DATA AT 5 YEARS FOR SUBJECTS WHO WEIGHED LESS THAN 1815 GRAMS AT BIRTH

	No ROP	Mild ROP (Dilation & Tortuosity)	Moderate (New Capillary Growth)	Severe A (Incomplete Retrolental Membrane)	Severe B (Complete Retrolental Membrane)
Study population	299	68	51	27	21
Affected subjects (%)	72	10	11	4	3
Best corrected VA ≥20/30 (%)	88	91	75	56	18
Myopia (SER ≥0.25 D) (%)	5	12	21	54	35
Myopic astigmatism (%)	3	2	14	27	10
SER <3.0 D) (%)	3	10	16	15	0
SER 3.0 to 6.0 D (%)	1	2	2	19	5
SER ≥6.0 D (%)	0	3	4	19	24

These results have been confirmed by other studies.

Congenital myopia associated with ROP is often severe at birth but usually remains stable during the first 5 to 8 years of life. Longitudinal data from Fledelius' (54–57) studies (see Tables 6.14 and 6.15) show that severe myopia of ROP children also tends to remain relatively stable from 10 to 18 years.

Genetic syndromes that include ocular malformations are rare (108), but when they occur severe ametropia is a common consequence. Table 6.16 lists the refractive anomalies that are most often associated with congenital ocular malformations.

Refractive abnormalities are also associated with three other ocular conditions. Severe myopia occurs with myelinated optic nerve fibers (51, 107). Hittner and Antoszyk (104) reported on a series of 12 such subjects; seven had a mean myopia of −13 D. They also had macular defects and poor visual acuity. The remaining five patients with a mean myopia of −3.75 D obtained good visual acuity after conventional amblyopia therapy. The myopia associated with myelinated nerve fibers is axial.

Retinitis pigmentosa (RP) is an inherited ocular disease that typically is not present at birth but appears between age 2 years and early adulthood. Multiple syndromes, including pigmentary degeneration (Laurence-Moon-Biedl and Usher's syndrome are examples) often include middle ear deafness. Myopia is more prevalent among RP patients generally, but Heckenlively (96) reported hyperopia ranging from +3.0 to +6.0 D in five persons (mean, +3.77 D) in a sample with onset of RP between ages 3 and 6 years. All five exhibited a unique pattern of retinal pigmented epithelium under retinal arterioles. This pattern occurs in less than 1 percent of RP patients.

Hoyt (113) reported monocular axial myopia of −4.25 to −7.0 D following neonatal eyelid closure that occluded the visual axis. Causes included third nerve palsy, blepharoptosis, or edema of eyelids from obstetric trauma. The corneas were not affected. Axial length difference between the two eyes varied from 1.6 to 2.8 mm. The typical refractive anomaly associated with blepharoptosis was hyperopia. The subjects' ages were 7 weeks to 19 months; the data were drawn from a series of 64 infants who exhibited eyelid closure.

Refractive abnormalities associated with congenital ocular malformations are present at birth. They are also found in the presence of certain hereditary craniofacial malforma-

Table 6.14 COMPARISON OF OCULAR OPTICAL AND AXIAL COMPONENTS IN VARIOUS DEGREES OF MYOPIA

Degree of Myopia	No. Eyes	Axial Length (mm)			Vitreous Depth (mm)			Lens Thickness (mm)		Anterior Chamber Depth (mm)		Radius of Corneal Curvature (mm)			Corneal Power (D)		Lens Power (D)		
		Mean	SD	Range	Mean	SD	Range	Mean	SD	Mean	SD	Mean	SD	Range	Mean	SD	Mean	SD	Range
Grade I <6 D	30	25.6	0.77	24–27	17.7	0.80	15–19	3.56	0.18	3.37	0.15	7.65	0.29	7.2–8.1	44.1	2.10	15.3	2.6	11.3–21.2
Grade II 6–15 D	63	27.5	1.49	24.5–30.0	19.1	1.38	17–22	3.69	0.26	3.64	0.89	7.57	0.37	6.9–8.3	44.8	2.76	14.3	1.7	8.1–25.1
Grade III >15 D	28	32.6	1.98	30.0–38.5	24.1	1.85	22–29	3.47	0.26	3.67		7.66	0.26	7.2–8.2	44.1	1.92	12.6	3.1	9.2–16.5

Table 6.15   COMPARISON OF REFRACTIVE DATA AT 10 YEARS AND 18 YEARS OF PREMATURE AND TERM COHORTS

| | Premature Infants | | | | Normal Term Infants | |
| | Group I, 20 Eyes | | Group II, 26 Eyes | | Group III, 26 Eyes | |
	Mean	SD	Mean	SD	Mean	SD
	(LBW with ROP)		(LBW, no ROP who develop juvenile myopia)		(who develop juvenile myopia)	
At 10 yr	−5.15		−0.33		−1.16	
At 18 yr	−6.76	4.77	−2.43	2.03	−3.50	2.00
Mean change from 10 to 18 yr	1.61	1.77	−2.10	1.49	−2.34	1.32

tions. Extreme ametropia may be congenital, in which case it is more likely to remain stable, or it may develop sometime during childhood and progress. Table 6.17 lists genetic syndromes that commonly include refractive abnormalities.

Inborn errors of metabolism produce biochemical defects of enzyme systems from reduction or absence, overproduction, or substitution of specific enzymes, or of enzyme systems. These defects affect body functions and often produce tissue damage. The abnormalities often become apparent sometime after birth, but metabolic dysfunction is present at birth. Renal dysfunction is a common component of congenital syndromes; several can be diagnosed by urinalysis. More than 3000 enzymes have been identified; abnormal production of any may result from a genetic metabolic error. Table 6.18 lists diseases resulting from inborn errors of metabolism that are associated with refractive abnormalities.

Passage of toxic agents through the placenta or deficiency of oxygen or other essential substances can cause spontaneous abortion, premature birth, or fetal deformation. Congenital myopia and cataract are the two most common ocular complications of mater-

nal disease. Table 6.19 presents diseases of pregnancy that are associated with refractive abnormalities.

We cannot clearly distinguish between toxemias and deficiencies of pregnancy and prematurity in considering prevalence based on cause; nor do reports of prevalence always permit us to distinguish between congenital severe ametropias that are static, those that progress or regress, and those that develop sometime after birth. When severe ametropia is related to inborn errors of metabolism or to maternal disease, often it is not known whether it is congenital or develops during early childhood.

OCULAR OPTICAL AND AXIAL COMPONENTS

At Birth

There is a greater prevalence of myopia even among premature infants without ROP than among normal term infants (121, 163, 215). Prevalence increases as birth weight or gestational age decreases. Mean axial length is less as birth weight and gestational age decrease, but corneal power and lens power are substantially greater. This is shown in Gor-

Table 6.16 REFRACTIVE ABNORMALITIES ASSOCIATED WITH CONGENITAL OCULAR MALFORMATIONS

Congenital Ocular Malformation	Associated Refractive Abnormality			
	Myopia	Hyperopia	Astigmatism	Anisometropia
Anterior polar cataracts (72)		Axial		Lenticular
Blue sclera (128)	High, only when associated with other ocular defects			
Buphthalmos (61)	High axial			
Coloboma with microcornea (14, 117)	High, with posterior staphyloma			
Cornea plana (62, 128)		6–10 D		
Cortical cataracts (18, 128)		If without dehydration		Lenticular
Idiopathic nystagmus (72)			Very common	
Keratoglobus (61)				
Megalocornea (61)		Low to moderate corneal	High, WR corneal	
Microcornea with microphthalmos (17)	Very high			
Microphthalmos (72, 117)	With lenticonus or glaucoma	Without other involvement, often very high axial		
Microspherophakia (34)	High without ectopia	High, with ectopia		
Neonatal lid closure (17, 75)	Moderate axial			
Nyctalopia (105, 146)	Medium to high			
Pigmentary glaucoma (131, 208, 217)	High			Axial

Table 6.17 REFRACTIVE ABNORMALITIES ASSOCIATED WITH CONGENITAL CRANIOFACIAL AND OTHER NONOCULAR SYNDROMES

| Syndrome | Associated Refractive Abnormality | | | |
	Myopia	Hyperopia	Astigmatism	Anisometropia
De Grouchy (2)	Medium			
Down (180)	Medium to high not progressive 10 to 20% prevalence			
Hydrocephalus (138)	>5.0 D in about 20% of children			
Knies (40)	High at birth, stable, retinal detachment			
Marchesini (75, 141)	Lenticular, with microphakia	High, without microphakia		
Marfan (40, 44, 141)	High with low corneal power		With ectopia	High
Spondyloephyseal dysplasia (2, 119)	Moderate to high			
Sturge-Weber (2,118)	Appears after age 3; progressive retinal detachment			
Syndromes that include congenital hearing loss (40, 141)	Moderate to high			
Turner (40)	Low to medium	With microcornea		
Van der Hoeve (72)	Appears after 2 or 3 yrs			
Wagner-Stickler (3, 134, 171)	Appears after age 3; is progressive			

don's (82) and Grignold's (89) data for premature infants in Table 6.20. Therefore, it appears that myopia of uncomplicated prematurity, unlike juvenile myopia, is caused primarily by greater than average refractive power of the cornea and lens, the lens contributing more when severe myopia is present. Table 6.21 shows mean differences in ocular diameters taken from different samples of those premature and full-term infants who survived less than 1 week after birth. Table 6.21 indicates that premature eyes are smaller in all dimensions than the eyes of full-term infants. Table 6.20 gives mean axial length, corneal power, and crystalline lens power at various intervals after conception for full-term infants as well.

Data of normal term infants at birth (39 to 41 weeks' gestational age) are similar in both studies (Table 6.20). At 3 months (12 months' gestational age, Gringolo) mean axial length has increased but corneal and lens power have decreased. Cycloplegic SER (+2.53) is similar to that reported in other studies (182)

Table 6.18 REFRACTIVE ABNORMALITIES ASSOCIATED WITH INBORN ERRORS OF METABOLISM

Disease	Time of Onset of Clinical Signs	Enzyme or Deficiency	Associated Refractive Abnormality			
			Myopia	Hyperopia	Astigmatism	Other Defects
Albinism (62)	From birth	Tyrosinase deficiency	Moderate to severe	Least common	Severe, most common	(See text)
Ehlers-Danlos syndrome (132)	3 wk–2 yr	Lysyl hydroxylase deficiency	Moderate to severe, stable			Ectopia lentis, blue sclera, tissue fragility
Homocystinuria (132)	1–2 yr	Cystathionine deficiency		Usually after 2 yr, with ectopia		Mental retardation, osteoporosis, scoliosis, ectopia lentis
Kenny's syndrome (140)	3 wk (convulsions)	Mucopolysaccharidosis	Moderate to severe with partial syndrome, stable	Severe with greater microphthalmos		Dwarfism, microphthalmia, anemia
Krabbes' disease (29)	12 wk–8 yr	Lipidosis		Moderate to severe		Mental retardation, slow reaction time, corneal dystrophy
Niemann-Pick (40, 132)	1–6 yr	Lipidosis		Moderate to severe		Progressive hypotonia
Tay-Sachs (40, 132)	3–6 mo	Lipidosis		Moderate to severe		Cherry red macula, motor weakness, mental deterioration

Table 6.19   REFRACTIVE ABNORMALITIES ASSOCIATED WITH MATERNAL DISEASE

Disease	Associated Refractive Abnormality		
	Myopia	Hyperopia	Astigmatism
Alcohol abuse syndrome (5, 69, 150, 200)	High		Very common, with steep corneas
Diabetes mellitus (23, 35, 209)	Four times more prevalent than in normals at 8 years		
Rubella (50)	Probably abiotrophic		
Toxemia of pregnancy (70)	At birth with prematurity		
Toxoplasmosis (126)	Moderate		

(see Fig. 6.2). Gordon's data for infants from birth to 9 months illustrate continuing increase in mean axial length and decrease in power of the optical components.

Biologic Variation from Infancy to Maturity

Normal eyes of cadavers of various ages gave us norms of globe mass and diameter as early as 1925 (175). X-ray measures of axial diameters were introduced in the 1930s (170). More recently, ultrasound and phakophotometry have led to refinement and extension of axial measures and refracting surfaces of the eye (63, 76, 78, 88, 168, 223). From birth to maturity the globe increases in mass and volume about threefold (133). This corresponds approximately to growth of the brain, whereas body mass increases from 20 to 30 times from birth to adulthood. Figure 6.12 compares cross-sections of eyes at 8 months' gestational age, at full term, and at maturity.

In normal eyes mean axial length increases about 6 mm during the first 3 years of life and only about 1 mm thereafter. The normal cornea flattens about 5 to 6 D, and the lens about 10 or 12 D during this period. The resultant refractive change is seldom more than 1 or 2 D (toward emmetropia) by age 3 years. Relatively few eyes change as much as 0.50 D in refractive status between age 3 and 7 years. A significant proportion do from age 7 to 12 years. Almost all of them become less

hyperopic or become myopic. These changes are shown in Table 6.22, which is a compendium of ocular optical component and axial data from many studies. Rates of change are quite different for the various components (190). Spherical equivalent corneal power typically changes from about 50 D at birth to about 44 D between age 2 and 3 years then remains relatively stable. The unaccommodated crystalline lens contributes about 32 D to total refractive power of the eye at birth, and about 24 D between age 2 and 3 years. Lens radii of curvature increase into early adulthood. The lens continues to add sub-

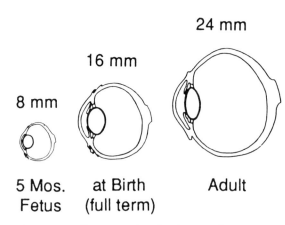

Figure 6.12   Cross-sectional schema of eyes at three stages of development. Dimensions approximate actual average dimensions at 5 months fetal age, at birth, and after full growth.

Table 6.20 REFRACTIVE DATA OF PREMATURE INFANTS AND TERM INFANTS

	Premature Infants					Term Infants			
	(89)			(82)		(89)		(82)	
Gestational Age	25 wk	30	35	30–35 wk	35–39 wk	39–41 wk	12 mo	39–41 wk	Birth–1 yr
No. Eyes	22	40	34	11	14	36	68	10	11
Mean SER (D)	−6.5	−3.8	−1.0	−1.0	+0.3	+0.52	+2.53	+0.40	+0.90
Mean axial length (mm)	12.1	14.4	16.8	15.1	16.1	17.0	19.4	16.8	19.2
Mean corneal power (D)	62.0	59.2	53.2	53.6	52.6	54.3	50.5	51.2	45.2
Mean lens power (D)	96.0	62.3	43.5	43.5	36.9	37.8	25.3	34.4	28.7

(From Grignola A, Rivara A: Biometry of the human eye from the sixth month of pregnancy to the tenth year of life (measurements of the axial length, retinoscopy refraction, total refraction, corneal and lens refraction). In Vanysek J (ed): Diagnostica Ultrasonic in Ophthalmologica. Brno, Czechoslovakia, University J.E. Purkyne, 251, 1968 and Gordon RA, Donzis PB: Refractive development of the human eye. Arch Ophthalmol 103:785, 1985.)

Table 6.21 OCULAR DIAMETERS OF PREMATURE AND TERM NEWBORNS

| | No. Eyes | Mean Diameter | | | | |
| | | Globe | | | Cornea | |
		Sagittal (mm)	Transverse (mm)	Vertical (mm)	Transverse (mm)	Vertical (mm)
Premature	27	14.8	14.7	14.0	7.9	8.5
Term	50	17.8	18.2	17.3	9.8	10.5

stance throughout life; it is unique in this respect (32).

Changes in anterior chamber depth contribute much less to total refractive power, but the effect of the approximately 1-mm change (from 2.8 to 3.8 mm), like that of the cornea and lens, is to create less refractive power of the system from birth to the time when the globe is fully formed. Total decrease in power from these combined sources (cornea, anterior chamber depth, crystalline lens) is 15 to 18 D.

At birth the mean axial length is about 17 mm. At 2 to 3 years, the mean is about 22 mm. This change would produce an increase of about 18 D in total refractive status, assuming an effective 3.0 D change for each 1-mm change in axial length (each unit of axial length change has greater refractive influence at birth when axial length is least). These comparisons also assume no changes in refractive indices.

Mean cycloplegic SERs change from about +2.0 D at birth to about +1.5 D at age 2 to 3 years. Longitudinal studies indicate that mean SER moves toward greater hyperopia during the first few months after birth. Mean cycloplegic SER may be as much as +3.0 D at 6 months. Noncycloplegic SER roughly approximates +0.75 D at 3 years, from a mean of −1.0 D to −2.0 D of myopia at birth. This would indicate that the emmetropizing process influences eyes when accommodation is functioning normally as well as when it is partially or fully deactivated.

If eyes that become myopic after age 7 years are excluded, mean spherical equivalent refraction does not change significantly from 3 years of age until adulthood. It appears that most but not all hyperopic eyes are stable during this period; a few show some increase in hyperopia, and others decrease slightly in hyperopia.

This is not a precise analysis, but it demonstrates the remarkable relationship between these variables. Each ocular optical component is normally distributed during the first 3 years, and each changes significantly. Refractive stability during this period undoubtedly results from optical compensation of axial elongation by increases in radii of curvature of the cornea and lens and, to a lesser extent, deepening of the anterior chamber.

Changes in ocular optical components between ages 6 and 18 years and adult studies of subjects who became myopic as juveniles show that axial elongation (without fully compensating changes in the anterior segment) accounts for juvenile myopia. When axial lengths of myopic juveniles are related to degree of ametropia, they show high correlation. When mean axial lengths of adults who developed myopia as juveniles were compared to general adult populations they were greater by 1.2 mm. The mean difference in SERs was 3.2 D (12). In myopic adults axial length difference accounts for most of their anisometropia (12, 193).

Table 6.23 compares ocular optical components of myopic young adults, myopic juveniles, and a general adult population not selected for refractive status. When compared to random samples of adults, the most

Table 6.22 MEANS OF REFRACTIVE COMPONENTS FROM BIRTH TO ADULTHOOD

Age (yr)	Birth	0.5	1	2	3	4	5	6	7	10	15	18	Adults 18+
Mean SER (D)	+2.2	+2.0	+1.5	+1.3	+1.3	+1.3	+1.2	+1.0	+0.90	+0.50	+0.40	+0.40	+0.50
Axial length (mm)	17.2	18.0	19	20.5	21.4	21.8	22.0	22.1	22.2	23.4	23.7	23.8	23.8
Anterior chamber depth (mm)	2.8				3.3				3.4				
Corneal power (D)	50		45	44.5	44	43.5				43			43
Lens power (D)	32		27	25.5	24	22	21	19.5	19	18.5	18	17.5	17

Table 6.23   COMPARISON OF MEAN OCULAR OPTICAL COMPONENTS OF YOUNG ADULTS

	Emmetropia (Range of Means)	Myopia (−1.5 to −6.0 D)	Juvenile Myopia	Young Adult General Population
Axial length (mm)	22.6–23.8	25.63	25.14	24.0
Vitreous depth (mm)	15.6–17.2	17.66		16.5
Anterior chamber depth (mm)	3.04–3.6	3.42		3.5
Lens thickness (mm)	3.60–4.01	3.60		4.0
Corneal power (D)	42.1–44.3	43.8	43.7	43.6
Lens power (D)	17.8–22.2	15.3	16.2	20.0

significant single component corresponding to mean SER change is axial length; of those compensating mechanisms of the anterior segment, lens power provides the most compensation.

We do not know what processes initiate interaction between the ocular optical components that result in emmetropization and refractive stabilization, as each of the components undergoes significant change. Whatever the initiating process, it is likely that stabilization of refractive status of most children that is maintained from 4 or 5 years onward and juvenile myopia both result mainly from interaction between changes in axial length and crystalline lens power (46, 189).

Premature and Normal Term Cohorts from Infancy to Adulthood

Because much of the myopia of premature infants who are not afflicted with ROP disappears during the first year, it may be assumed that most non-ROP premature infants suffer little or no retardation of ocular development. Some premature infants without ROP retain greater than average hyperopia, myopia, or astigmatism, indicating that the ocular development of some is arrested. In infants without congenital ocular defects whose normal development is arrested, axial length may remain shortened while the cornea and crystalline lens develop normally (axial hyperopia);

or axial length may develop normally as development of cornea or lens remains arrested (curvature myopia). The greatest hyperopia retention reported among children born prematurely is +3.0 D; though it is rare, myopia as severe as −15.0 D has been found. In exceptionally severe myopia it is probable that cornea and lens development sometimes are retarded and the axis elongates extraordinarily as well.

Table 6.24 compares SER and optical and axial component means of nearly emmetropic children between 5 and 9 years of age who were born prematurely with those of children born at term. Mean differences are small but

Table 6.24   COMPARISON AT 5 TO 9 YEARS OF AGE OF NEARLY EMMETROPIC CHILDREN BORN PREMATURELY AND AT FULL TERM

	Premature	Term
Mean SER (D)	+0.54	+0.60
Mean axial length (mm)	23.1	23.5
Anterior chamber depth (mm)	3.8	3.9
Mean lens thickness (mm)	3.6	3.5
Mean corneal power (D)	43.8	43.0

Table 6.25   GENDER COMPARISONS OF AXIAL LENGTH AND CORNEAL POWER OF PREMATURE AND TERM INFANTS AT VARIOUS AGES

	At Birth (189)		At 5–9 Years (216)		At 10 Years (55)		At 18 Years (55)	
	Male	Female	Male	Female	Male	Female	Male	Female
				Axial Length (mm)				
Premature	14.8	14.9	23.4	22.7	23.3	22.7	24.2	23.4
Term	17.9	17.7	23.6	23.4	23.5	23.3	24.2	23.7
				Corneal Power (D)				
Premature			43.5	44.2	44.0	44.6	44.0	44.5
Term			42.7	43.2	42.5	43.0	42.5	43.0

(From Weale RS: Ocular anatomy and refraction. Doc Ophthalmol 55:361, 1983.)

suggest slight retardation of ocular development among many premature infants or significant retardation among a small subgroup (216). Differences that indicate retardation of ocular development are also suggested by the data in Table 6.25 (55,192, 216), which also demonstrates gender differences in components. At all age levels, among those born

prematurely and at term, males show greater mean axial length and less corneal power.

Fledelius (54–57) made longitudinal comparisons of refractive and component data of children born prematurely and at term. Table 6.26 provides comparisons suggesting that in severe myopia 2 types of change may be occurring in different sub-

Table 6.26   COMPARISON OF REFRACTIVE COMPONENTS OF PREMATURE AND TERM COHORTS AT 10 YEARS AND 18 YEARS (SEE TABLE 6.15)

	Group I, 20 Eyes		Group II, 26 Eyes		Group III, 26 Eyes	
At Age 18 Yr	Mean (LBW, no ROP)	SD	Mean (Normal term)	SD	Mean (LBW with ROP)	SD
Axial length (mm)	25.65	1.98	24.26	1.37	25.27	0.98
Lens thickness (mm)	3.77	0.19	3.60	0.18	3.58	0.21
Corneal power (D)	44.5	1.8	44.5	1.7	42.9	1.4
Anterior chamber depth (mm)	3.84	0.21	4.02	0.27	4.14	0.19
Mean Change from 10–18 yr						
SER	1.61	1.77	2.10	1.49	2.34	1.32
Axial length	1.01	0.65	1.00	0.73	1.24	0.67

groups. Neither group is likely to include myopic juveniles. Those with severe myopia (Groups II and III) show considerably more dispersion than does Group I. The variation in dispersion of lens power between Group II and Group III could be accounted for by subgroups that developed severe myopia in various ways. One subgroup may have become severely myopic in spite of normal functioning of the optical components of the emmetropization process because of excessive axial elongation; others may have become severely myopic because the emmetropization process functioned at less than a normal or usual capacity as axial length progressed at a less excessive rate.

Table 6.26 gives refractive data for three groups of children studied by Fledelius (55) over a 10-year period. Group I was made up of those born prematurely with ROP. Group II were LBW infants without ROP. Group III were normal term infants. All in Groups II and III were presumed to have developed myopia as juveniles. Mean SER of those born prematurely who developed ROP (Group I) was at the level of high myopia, with widely dispersed distribution, but myopic change between 10 and 18 years was less than that of premature or term infants who did not become myopic until they became juveniles. Table 6.26 also provides refractive and axial data at age 18 years for these groups as well as mean change between 10 and 18 years for axial length and SER (54, 55). Axial length was greater for those in Group I than the mean for adults and greater than the mean for Group II or III, uncompensated by means of any of the other ocular components, but mean SER changed somewhat less toward increased myopia from 10 to 18 years among these children, who probably had congenital severe myopia, than among the myopic juveniles, even though axial length change was similar for all three groups. This provides evidence that refractive abnormalities associated with ROP are relatively stable because compensating change occurs as axial length increases during this period.

Virtually all significant myopic progression appears to be the result of axial elongation in the absence of fully compensating optical changes in the anterior segment. Corneal power did not change significantly between 10 and 18 years. The lowest means for corneal power were found when full-term subjects who become myopic juveniles were grouped together. Mean anterior chamber depth increased slightly for all groups. The greatest mean increase (0.17 mm) was for myopic juveniles who had been normal term infants, whose mean anterior chamber depth at age 10 was already deeper (3.89 mm) than that of any other group. Lens thickness was least at 10 years and 18 years for this group. Children who were born prematurely tended to have smaller eyes and shorter corneal and lens radii of curvature than those born after normal term, but both are equally prone to develop juvenile myopia, and the condition progresses in similar fashion in both.

The Fledelius studies are reported in detail because they are the only longitudinal investigations to date that provide both refractive and ocular optical component data of several subgroups over an extended period.

Astigmatism and Other Variables

It has been established that virtually all astigmatism that is not corneal (presumably lenticular) is normally distributed within a very narrow range (SD about 0.25 D) about a mean of about 0.50 D (106). The limited infant studies of refractive astigmatism indicate that most astigmatism is caused by differences in corneal radii of curvature. AR astigmatism is common at birth but regresses as corneal astigmatism changes by age 5 or 6 years to WR. Pedigrees and twin studies involving older children and adults demonstrate that severe astigmatism is inherited (194).

When there is significant difference in degree of myopia between two eyes at birth the more myopic eye usually develops more marked signs of posterior staphyloma and is more likely to suffer retinal detachment later.

Most significant myopic anisometropia is axial. The more myopic eye is likely to be more astigmatic as well (12, 193). Hyperopic anisometropia is usually of lesser degree and more often due to curvature differences between the two corneas. In hyperopic anisometropia greater than 3 D, axial length differences probably become the dominant factor. It is very likely that, when corneal curvatures of the two eyes are similar, anisometropia is almost always the result of axial differences. One extremely rare exception involves monocular congenital lenticonus. Another less rare exception occurs in the development of age-related cataract in which nuclear sclerosis is more advanced in one eye.

Anthropometric studies indicate no correlation between myopia or ocular optical components and cranial or general growth (12, 154).

Correlation of Ocular Optical and Axial Components

Many investigators have found that axial elongation is negatively correlated with corneal power, crystalline lens power, and the optical effect of anterior chamber depth (12, 169, 170, 198, 216).

The first investigator to provide extensive factor analysis of ocular optical components was van Alphen (211). Calculation of partial correlations and multiple correlations led him to propose three basic factors for determining refractive outcomes. One factor, with loading in axial length and corneal power, points to hereditary differences in globe size. Loadings in axial length, lens power, and anterior chamber depth suggest a stretch factor differentiated from the size factor. The stretch factor may result from hereditary predisposition or from environmental influence. The third factor, which results from loading in all five variables, can be due to excessive stretching of the globe relative to total refractive power of the eye. According to van Alphen, evidence for these stretch factors is also found in the higher incidence of retinal detachment, glaucoma, and other structural anomalies in myopic eyes. The theory of van Alphen is based on the assumption that the eye is a self-focusing mechanism (i.e. that the accommodative mechanism acts autonomically) causing the facultative hyperopic eye of the infant to expand until the total refractive power is compensated by adjusted axial length increase, and perhaps initiating offsetting changes in other ocular optical components as well. Changing tension produced by ciliary muscle, which counteracts intraocular pressure, is assumed to be the mechanism that generates emmetropization, or, in the presence of influences initiating stretching of the globe, juvenile and young-adult myopia.

In Table 6.27 van Alphen's third-order partial correlation coefficients and selective multiple correlation coefficients are pre-

Table 6.27 CORRELATION COEFFICIENTS OF OCULAR OPTICAL COMPONENTS

	Refraction	Axial Length	Anterior Chamber Depth	Mean Corneal Power	Mean Lens Power
Third-Order Partial Correlation Coefficients					
Refraction	x	−0.97	+0.40	−0.93	−0.89
Axial length		x	+0.48	−0.94	−0.90
Anterior chamber depth			x	+0.46	+0.33
Mean corneal power				x	−0.87
Multiple Correlation Coefficients					
Five variables	0.98	0.98	0.61	0.95	0.91

sented. The values of third-order correlation coefficients are high in all instances in which influence of anterior chamber depth is excluded. This probably occurs because the regression between refraction and anterior chamber depth is not linear. This may also be explained by the fact that anterior chamber depth is partially age dependent, tending to decrease with age, according to van Alphen, as the lens continues to grow in thickness and diameter. The fact that the remaining third-order correlations are near unity tells us that the regression equations are linear and that all significant variables are included. If the regression is indeed linear and all variance is accounted for, the five-variable multiple correlation coefficient should equal 1.0. Therefore, the multiple coefficient correlations reinforce conclusions drawn from the partial ones. More recently other investigations have confirmed the linearity of refractive change.

Van Alphen's work extends Steiger's (197) proposition that normal biologic variables combine independently by making it clear that there is a harmony to these combinations (we have labeled this emmetropization) and that an aberrating factor acts to produce myopia by stretching the globe. Van Alphen theorized that this stretching is due to loss of elasticity or thinning of scleral tissue near the posterior pole. Greene (86) has demonstrated that short-duration pulses of high intraocular pressure cause irreversible stretching of the posterior globe in experimental animals. Traction of extraocular muscles on the sclera during convergence has also been suggested as a cause.

SUMMARY AND CONCLUSIONS

Present Status

Between birth and adulthood, emmetropization and stability characterize the refractive status of most children. Compensating changes in the optical and axial components of refraction are responsible for both phenomena. Refractive powers of the cornea and lens decrease and anterior chamber depth increases, whereas axial elongation occurs in the posterior segment. The refractive status of most children changes little after age 2 years, with three significant exceptions. Young children who suffer from febrile disease—and perhaps those with certain other constitutional dysfunctions—may develop myopia. Some who have very mild hyperopia or emmetropia at ages 5 or 6 years develop mild to moderate myopia between ages 7 and 13 years. Others may develop mild myopia or myopia may again progress between ages 18 and 21 years. More than half of those who develop myopia as juveniles show significant myopic progression later if they become college students. A child who does not have congenital hyperopia and anisometropia is unlikely to develop either to a significant degree. Most congenital astigmatism is AR and transient. Moderate WR astigmatism then may develop from environmental influences. Extreme ametropias are most often congenital and relatively stable. It is not known what initiates or controls any of these processes, but they usually operate binocularly. Significant anisometropia is not common.

As far as juvenile myopia is concerned it may be that at age 8 to 10 years anterior segment optical components have lost the capacity to compensate fully for further changes in axial length. Few studies measure ocular optical components during the period when juvenile myopia develops and progresses. Data from those that do suggest that only power of the lens continues to decrease with axial elongation. If the proximal cause of juvenile myopia is initiation of axial elongation in an eye that no longer responds or compensates with optical changes of the anterior segment, the question that remains is, what causes juvenile axial elongation? Almost every conceivable explanation has been advanced. Proponents of the use abuse theory propose that sustained accommodation may produce axial lengthening, either by increasing pressure in the vitreous chamber or by creating choroidal traction from ciliary muscle contraction. Others believe that an hereditary predisposition to juvenile myopia exists that either is expressed in all cases as an abiotrophic phenomenon or may be triggered by near work or by some other environmental condition. Growth rate, hormonal changes, nutrition, and metabolic processes all have been considered factors in the development of juvenile myopia. A great variety of theories of cause and a great number of studies have appeared in ophthalmic literature over the past 150 years. Early investigators argued either that myopia was caused by sustained near work (and was, therefore, lenticular) or by hereditary fiat (therefore axial). We now know that the mechanism for juvenile myopia is axial elongation, but we know little about the initiating cause or causes.

Recent investigations of the relation between accommodative characteristics and refractive states cannot be extrapolated to explain the process whereby emmetropization occurs; however, they do suggest that changes in tonic state of accommodation and in accommodative amplitude may take place in infancy and early childhood as part of the developing interaction between sympathetic and parasympathetic systems.

Relationships have been found between physiologic activity of the autonomic nervous system and personality traits. Physiologic indices of autonomic balance were developed by Wenger in 1939 and were later validated (218). Eysenck (53) and others (161, 181) have proposed that parasympathetic dominance is reflected in introverted personality and that extroverted behavior is dominated by the sympathetic nervous system. These associations have led some to conclude that parasympathetically dominant persons became myopic through some process initiated by overactive accommodation leading to axial elongation. It may be relevant that near-accommodative amplitude of myopic children is greater than that of hyperopic or emmetropic age peers. There is increased parasympathetic activity in ciliary muscle during accommodation. Activation of accommodation also produces some increase in vitreous pressure. These have been proposed as mechanisms that produce juvenile and young adult myopia. The technology to test this theory is available.

Myopic children tend to be more successful students at all educational levels than nonmyopic ones (19, 158, 225); however, no consistent significant correlation has been found between refractive status and intelligence when subjects are matched for age and other dependent variables (225). What is clear is that myopic children spend more time reading and perform better on reading tests. The relationship is virtually unchanged if axial length is substituted for refractive status. Myopic students also spend considerably more time reading at all ages. This correlation increases with age or education level. Myopic students are significantly overrepresented in college honors programs and in graduate schools.

A number of studies indicate that some relationship exists between prevalence of refractive anomalies and social class. Prevalence of myopia is greater as family income increases, according to studies in the United States (196). Prevalence of myopia is also greater among children of college professors and of clerical workers than among children of farmers and of laborers not engaged in close work. No one yet has disentangled cause from effect in the relationships among ametropia and ethnicity, scholastic success, and personality traits.

Treatment

Stable ametropias of significant degree should be corrected as soon as they are discovered. Consequences of uncorrected refractive anomalies and refractive abnormalities include strabismus, amblyopia, anomalous correspondence, and performance deficits (91, 97, 152, 153). Monocular amblyopia is a common feature of anisometropia greater than 3.0 D, and prevalence increases with degree. Uncorrected astigmatism results in meridional amblyopia. If the amblyopic eye is not congenitally malformed visual acuity may be improved by vision training after optical correction. Anisometropic prescriptions can produce induced aniseikonia. Therefore, it is important to distinguish between axial and curvature ametropias of significant degree. Spectacles may be the treatment of choice if anisometropia is axial, or if anisometropia is present when corneal curvatures are equal. Contact lenses should be considered to limit induced size effects if corneal or lens curvatures account for high anisometropia.

Vision training—biofeedback training, contact lenses, and bifocals—have all been advocated as methods for preventing or controlling myopia. The only treatment that consistently has proven successful in preventing the development of ametropia is the use of atropine in the eyes of children at risk for juvenile myopia, but this is an arduous and lengthy procedure. It also produces side effects that make this method impractical. Evidence concerning the effectiveness of contact lenses or bifocals in preventing or retarding progression of myopia is mixed (14). Clinical trials now in progress suggest that contact lenses may have some effect, but bifocal lenses have none, except perhaps when near esophoria is present.

Surgical procedures that produce corneal flattening represent another form of optical correction for myopia. These have not been recommended for children. The long-term effects of surgical procedures are not known. In any event they do not affect the increased risk that myopes have of retinal detachment, open-angle glaucoma, and perhaps cataract.

The only treatment mandate that is clear, based on the present state of knowledge, is this: Every stable ametropia of significant degree should be corrected in full and as soon after birth as possible.

REFERENCES

1. Agnew CR: Near sightedness in the public schools. NY Med Record, 12:34, 1877.

2. Aita JA: Congenital facial anomalies with neurologic defects. Springfield, Charles C Thomas, 1969.

3. Alexander RL, Shea M: Wagner's disease. Arch Ophthalmol 74:310, 1965.

4. Alsbirk PH: Anterior chamber of the eye. A genetic and anthropological study in Greenland Eskimos. Hum Hered 25:418, 1975.

5. Altman B: Fetal alcohol syndrome. J Pediatr Ophthalmol 13:255, 1976.

6. Angle J, Wissmann DA: The epidemiology of myopia. Am J Epidemiol 3:220, 1980.

7. Anstice J: Astigmatism—its components and their changes with age. Am J Optom Arch Am Acad Optom 48:1001, 1971.

8. Atkinson J, Braddick OJ: The use of isotropic photorefraction for vision screening in infants. Acta Ophthalmol (Copenh) 157:36, 1982.

9. Atkinson J, Braddick O, French J: Infant astigmatism: Its disappearance with age. Vision Res 20:891, 1980.

10. Atkinson J, Braddick OJ, Durden K, et al: Screening for refractive errors in 6–9 month old infants by photorefraction. Br J Ophthalmol 68:105, 1984.

11. Avetisov ES: Unterlagen zur Entste-Hungtheorie der Myopia: 2. Mitteilung der genetische Faktor in der Enstehung der Myopie. Klin Monatsbl Augenheilkd 176:394, 1980.

12. Baldwin WR: Factors in Myopia. Ph.D. Dissertation. Bloomington, Indiana, Indiana University, 1964.

13. Baldwin WR, Mills DA: A longitudinal study of corneal astigmatism and total astigmatism. Am J Optom Physiol Opt 58:206, 1982.

14. Baldwin WR, West D, Jolley J, et al: Effects of contact lenses on refractive corneal and axial length changes in young myopes. Am J Optom Physiol Opt 46:903, 1969.

15. Banks MS: Infant refraction and accommodation. Int Ophthalmol Clin 20:1980.

16. Bannon RE: Use of cycloplegics in refraction. Am J Optom Arch Am Acad Optom 24:513, 1947.

17. Bateman JB, Maumenee IH: Colobomatous microphthalmia with microcornea. Ophthal Paediatr Genet 4:59, 1984.

18. Bercovitch L, Donaldson DD: The natural history of congenital sutural cataracts: Case

report with long-term follow-up. J Pediatr Ophthalmol Strabismus 19:108, 1982.

19. Bjerrum J, Philipsen H: Beretninger fra ojen-laegerne. Bilag II til: Beretninger af den under 23. juni 1882 nedsatte kommission til at tilvejebringe oplysninger om mulige sanitaere misligheder og mangler i ordningen af skolevaesenet, og til at fremkomme med forslag til sadannes fremtidige forebyggelse. Kobenhavn, 1884.

20. Boniuk V: Refractive problems in Native peoples (the Sioux lookout project). Can J Ophthalmol 8:229, 1973.

21. Borghi RA, Rouse MW: Comparison of refraction obtained by "near retinoscopy" and retinoscopy under cycloplegia. Am J Optom Physiol Opt 62:169, 1985.

22. Bothman L: A comparative study of homatropine and atropine cycloplegia. AMA Arch Ophthalmol 7:388, 1932.

23. Breidahl HD: The growth and development of children born to mothers with diabetes. Med J Aust Feb 12:268, 1966.

24. Brown EVL, Kronfeld P: Net average yearly changes in refraction of atropinized eyes from birth to beyond middle life. Arch Ophthalmol 19:719, 1938.

25. Callan PA: Examination of colored school children's eyes. Am J Med Sci 69:331, 1875.

26. Castren J: The significance of prematurity on the eye. Acta Ophthalmol [suppl] (Copenh) 44:7, 1955.

27. Castren J, Pohjola S: Refraction and scleral rigidity. Acta Ophthalmol 39:1011, 1961.

28. Chatterjee SK, Mukherji R: Myopia in newborn. J Indian Med Assoc 73:4, 1979.

29. Christomanou H, Jaffe S, Martinius J, et al: Biochemical, genetic, psychometric, and neuropsychological studies in heterozygotes of a family with globoid cell leucodystrophy (Krabbe's disease). Hum Genet 58:179, 1981.

30. Cohn H: Untersuchen der augen von 10060 Schulkindern nebst Vorsehlangen zur Verbesserung der Augen nachteiligen Schuleinrichtungen. In: Eine atiologische Studie. Leipzig, Verlag von Friederich Fleischer, 1867.

31. Cook RC, Glasscock RE: Refractive and ocular findings in the newborn. Am J Ophthalmol 34:1407, 1951.

32. Coulombre J, Coulombre A: A lens development: IV. Size, shape, and orientation. Invest Ophthalmol 4:411, 1965.

33. Crawford HE, Hammond GE: Racial analysis of ocular defects in the schools of Hawaii. Hawaii Med J 9:90, 1949.

34. Cross HE: Differential diagnosis and treatment of dislocated lenses. Ed: Bergsma, Bron, and Cotlier. Birth Defects: Original Article Series, vol XII, 335, 1976. New York, Alan R. Liss.

35. Cummins M, Norrish M: Follow-up of children of diabetic mothers. Arch Dis Child 55:259, 1980.

36. Curtin BJ: The pathogenesis of congenital myopia. Arch Ophthalmol 69:60, 1963.

37. Curtin BJ: Physiologic vs. pathologic myopia: Genetics vs. environment. Arch Ophthalmol 86:681, 1979.

38. Curtin BJ: The Myopias: Basic Science and Clinical Management. Philadelphia, Harper & Row, 1985.

39. Curtin BJ, Teng CC: Scleral changes in pathological myopia. Am Acad Ophthalmol Nov–Dec 62:777, 1958.

40. Daentl DL (ed): Clinical, Structural, and Biochemical Advances in Hereditary Eye Disorders. New York, Alan R Liss, 1982.

41. Danning H: Twin study on myopia. Chin Med J [Engl] 94:51, 1981.

42. Dobson V, Fulton AB, Manning K, et al: Cycloplegic refractions of premature infants. Am J Ophthalmol 91:490, 1981.

43. Dobson V, Fulton A, Sebris SL: Cycloplegic refractions of infants and young children: The axis of astigmatism. Invest Ophthalmol Vis Sci 25:83, 1984.

44. Donaldson DD: Atlas of External Diseases of the Eye, vol III. Cornea and Sclera. St Louis, CV Mosby, 5, 1971.

45. Donders FC: Accommodation and refraction of the eye. Sydenham Society, 1864.

46. Duane TD, Jaeger AE (eds): Biology of the eye as an optical system. In: Clinical Ophthalmology, vol I, ch 34, Philadelphia, J.B. Lippincott, 1, 1986.

47. Duke-Elder S: System of ophthalmology, vol V. St Louis, CV Mosby, 280, 1970.

48. Dzen T: Refraction in Peking medical college. Nat Med J China 6:153, 1921.

49. Eberstadt N: Economic and material poverty in the U.S. The Public Interest 90:54, 1988.

50. Ehlers JA, Stafford WR, Brady HR: Rubella pigmentary retinopathy in triplets. J Pediatr Ophthalmol 11:193, 1974.

51. Ellis GS, Frey T, Gouterman RZ: Myelinated nerve fibers, axial myopia, and refractory amblyopia: An organic disease. J Pediatr Ophthalmol Strabismus 24:111, 1987.

52. Ely ET: Boebachtungen mit dem Augenspiegel bezuglich der Refraktion der Augen neugeborener. Arch Augenheilkd 9:431, 1880.

53. Eysenck HJ: The biological basis of personality. Springfield IL, Charles C Thomas, 1967.

54. Fledelius HC: Prematurity and the eye. Ophthalmic 10-year follow-up of children of low and normal birth weight. Acta Ophthalmol [Suppl] (Copenh) 128, 1976.

55. Fledelius HC: Ophthalmic changes from age 10 to 18 years. A longitudinal study of sequels to low birth weight. IV. Ultrasound oculometry of vitreous and axial length. Acta Ophthalmol (Copenh) 60:403, 1982.

56. Fledelius HC: Is myopia getting more frequent? A cross-sectional study of 1416 Danes aged 16 years+. Acta Ophthalmol (Copenh) 61:545, 1983.

57. Fledelius HC, Stubgaard M: Changes in refraction and corneal curvature during growth and adult life. A cross-sectional study. Acta Ophthalmol (Copenh) 64:487, 1986.

58. Fletcher MC, Brandon S: Myopia of prematurity. Am J Ophthalmol 40:474, 1955.

59. Franceschetti A: Zur Refraktionskurve des Neugeboren. Klin Monatsbl Augenheilkd, 95:98, 1935.

60. Francois J: Heredity in ophthalmology. St Louis, CV Mosby, 1961.

61. Francois J (ed): Symposium on Surgical and Medical Management of Congenital Anomalies of the Eye. Transactions of the New Orleans Academy of Ophthalmology. St Louis, CV Mosby, 1968.

62. Francois J, Deweer JP: Albinisme oculaire lie au sere et alterations caracteristiques du fond d'oeil chez les femmes heterozygoted. Ophthalmologica 126:209, 1953.

63. Francois J, Goes F: Comparative study of ultrasonic biometry of emmetropes and myopes, with special regard to the heredity of myopia. In: Ophthalmic Ultrasound: Proceedings of the fourth International Congress of Ultrasonics in Ophthalmology. Philadelphia, St. Louis, Mosby, 165, 1968.

64. Friedman Z, Neumann E, Hyams SW, et al: Ophthalmic screening of 38,000 children, age 1 to 2½ years, in child welfare clinics. J Pediatr Ophthalmol Strabismus 17:261, 1976.

65. Fulton AB, Dobson V, Salem D, et al: Cycloplegic refractions in infants and young children. Am J Ophthalmol 90:239, 1980.

66. Fulton AB, Hanson R, Peterson R: The relation of myopia and astigmatism in developing eyes. J Ophthalmol 89:298, 1982.

67. Gallus E: Refraction of Jews. Z Augenheilk 48:215, 1922.

68. Garber JM: Corneal curvature in the fetal alcohol syndrome: Preliminary report. J Am Optom Assoc 53:641, 1982.

69. Garber JM: A fetal alcohol syndrome landmark. J Am Optom Assoc 55:595, 1984.

70. Gardiner PA, James G: Association between maternal disease during pregnancy and myopia in the child. Br J Ophthalmol 44:172, 1960.

71. Garner L, Grosvenor T, McKellor M, et al: Refraction and its components in Melanesian school children in Vanutu. Am J Optom Physiol Opt 65:182, 1988.

72. Geeradets MD: Ocular syndromes. Philadelphia, Lea & Febiger, 279, 1976.

73. Gerhard JP: Myopia in premature infants. Bull Soc Ophthalmol Fr 83:221, 1983.

74. Gil-Gibernau J, Galan A, Callis L, et al: Infantile idiopathic hypercalciuria, high congenital myopia, and atypical macular coloboma: A new oculo-renal syndrome? J Pediatr Ophthalmol Strabismus 19:7, 1982.

75. Gillum WN, Anderson RL: Dominantly inherited blepharoptosis, high myopia, and ectopia lentis. Arch Ophthalmol 100:282, 1982.

76. Gitter KA, Kenney AH, Sarin LK, et al (eds): Ophthalmic Ultrasound: Proceedings of the fourth international Congress of Ultrasonography in Ophthalmology. St Louis, CV Mosby, 1969.

77. Gleiss J, Pau H: Die Entwicklung der Refraction vor der Beburt. Klin Monatsbl Augenheilkd 121:440, 1952.

78. Goldmann H, Hagen R: Zur direkten Messung der Totalbrechkraft des Lebendigen menschlichen. Auges Ophthalmologica 104:15, 1942.

79. Goldschmidt E: Refraction in the newborn. Acta Ophthalmol (Copenh) 47:570, 1969.

80. Goldstein JH, Vukcevich WM, Daplan D: Myopia and dental caries. JAMA 281:1572, 1971.

81. Gonzalez TJ: Consideraciones en torno a la refraccion del recien nacido. Arch Soc Oftal Hisp Am 25:666, 1965.

82. Gordon RA, Donzis PB: Refractive development of the human eye. Arch Ophthalmol 103:785, 1985.

83. Gorzino A: Modificazione del collagene sclerale nella miopia malignz. Rass Ital Ottal 25:241, 1956.

84. Goss DA: Characteristics of myopia progression. Researches on Refractive Anomalies: Clinical Applications, ch 5. London, Butterworth, 1990.

85. Graham MV, Gray OP: Refraction of premature babies' eyes. Br Med J 1:1452, 1963.

86. Greene PR: Mechanical Aspects of Myopia. Ph.D. Dissertation. Cambridge MA, Harvard University, 142, 1978.

87. Grey C, Yap M: Influence of lid position on astigmatism. Am J Optom Physiol Opt 63:966, 1987.

88. Grey RHB, Perkins ES, Restori M: Comparisons of ultrasonic and photographic methods of axial length measurements of the eye. Br J Ophthalmol 61:423, 1977.

89. Grignolo A, Rivara A: Biometry of the human eye from the sixth month of pregnancy to the tenth year of life (measurements of the axial length, retinoscopy refraction, total refraction, corneal and lens refraction). In Vanysek J (ed): Diagnostica Utrasonica in Ophthalmologica. Brno Czechoslavakia, Universita J. E. Purkyne, 251, 1968.

90. Grosvenor T, Flom M: Young adult onset myopia. Researches on Refractive Anomalies: Clinical Applications, ch 5. London, Butterworth, 1990.

91. Gwiazda JE, Scheiman M, Held R: Meridional amblyopia in former astigmats. ARVO abstracts. Invest Ophthalmol Vis Sci (suppl) 22:127, 1982.

92. Gwiazda JE, Scheiman M, Mohindra I, et al: Astigmatism in children: Changes in axis and amount from birth to six years. Invest Ophthalmol Vis Sci 25:88, 1984.

93. Hamilton JE: Vision anomalies of Indian school children: The Lame Deer Study. J Am Optom Assoc 47:479, 1976.

94. Harman NB: The findings of eye examinations. Br Med J (suppl) 2:214, 1936.

95. Heard T, et al: The refractive status of Zuni Indian children. Am J Optom Physiol Opt 53:120, 1976.

96. Heckenlively JR: Preserved para-arteriole retinal pigment epithelium (PPRPE) in retinitis pigmentosa. Birth Defects 18:193, 1982.

97. Held R, Mohindra I, Gwiazda J, et al: Visual acuity of astigmatic infants and its meridional variation. ARVO Abstracts. Invest Ophthalmol Vis Sci 16 (suppl):65, 1977.

98. Herrnheiser J: Die Refractionsentwicklung des menschlichen Auges. Z Heilkunde 13:342, 1892.

99. Hirsch MJ: The changes in refraction between the ages of 5 and 14, theoretical and practical considerations. Am J Optom Arch Am Acad Optom 29:445, 1952.

100. Hirsch MJ: Sex differences in the incidence of various grades of myopia. Am J Optom Arch Am Acad Optom 30:135, 1953.

101. Hirsch MJ: The relationship between measles and myopia. Am J Optom Arch Am Acad Optom 34:289, 1957.

102. Hirsch MJ: Changes in astigmatism during the first eight years of school—An interim report from the Ojai longitudinal study. Am J Optom Arch Am Acad Optom 40:127, 1963.

103. Hirsch MJ, Levin JM: Myopia and dental caries. Am J Optom Arch Am Acad Optom 50:484, 1973.

104. Hittner HM, Antoszyk JH: Unilateral peripa-

pillary myelinated nerve fibers with myopia and/or amblyopia. Arch Ophthalmol 105:943, 1987.

105. Hittner HM, Borda RP, Justice J: X-linked recessive congenital stationary night blindness, myopia, and tilted discs. J Pediatr Ophthalmol Strabismus 18:15, 1981.

106. Hofstetter HW, Baldwin WR: Bilateral correlation of residual astigmatism. Am J Optom Arch Am Acad Optom July, 388, 1957.

107. Holland PM, Anderson B: Myelinated nerve fibers and severe myopia. Am J Ophthalmol 81:597, 1976.

108. Holmes LB: Current concepts in genetics. New Engl J Med 295:204, 1976.

109. Hosaka A: The ocular findings in the premature infant, especially on the premature signs. Jpn J Ophthalmol 7:77, 1963.

110. Hosaka A: The significance of myopia in newborn infants. XXI. Concilium Ophthalmologicum Mexica, 1970. Acta Pass I:991, 1971.

111. Howland HC, Atkinson J, Braddick O, et al: Infant astigmatism measured by photorefraction. Science 202:331, 1978.

112. Howland H, Sayles N: Photorefractive measurements of astigmatism in infants and young children. Invest Ophthalmol Vis Sci 25:93, 1984.

113. Hoyt CS, Stone RD, Fromer C, et al: Monocular axial myopia associated with neonatal eyelid closure in human infants. Am J Ophthalmol 91:197, 1981.

114. Ingram RM: Refraction of 1-year old children after atropine cycloplegia. Br J Ophthalmol 63:343, 1979.

115. Ingram RM, Walker C, Wilson JM, et al: Prediction of amblyopia and squint by means of refraction at age 1 year. Br J Ophthalmol 70:12, 1986.

116. Jain IS, Jain S, Mohan K: The epidemiology of high myopia-changing trends. Indian J Ophthalmol 31:723, 1983.

117. Jakobiekc FA: Ocular Anatomy, Embryology and Teratology. Philadelphia, Harper & Row, 167, 1982.

118. Johnston MC, Sulik KK: Some abnormal patterns of development in the craniofacial region. Birth Defects XV:23, 1979.

119. Judisch GF, Martin-Casals A, Hanson JW, et al: Oculodentodigital dysplasia. Arch Ophthalmol 97:878, 1979.

120. Kaakinen K, Kaseva H, Kause E-R: Mass screening of children for strabismus or ametropia with two-flash photoskiascopy. Acta Ophthalmol (Copenh) 65:105, 1986.

121. Kalina RE: Ophthalmic examination of children with low birthweight. Am J Ophthalmol 67:134, 1969.

122. Kalogjera T: Refractive error in Yugoslav urban children aged between 3 and 7 years. Child Care Health Dev 5:439, 1979.

123. Kantor DW: Racial aspects of myopia in compositors (racial factors in degree of myopia). Br J Ophthalmol 16:45, 1932.

124. Keith CG, Kitchen WH: Ocular morbidity in infants of very low birth weight. Br J Ophthalmol 67:302, 1983.

125. Keller JR: Evaluation of the relation between myopia and dental caries. Am J Optom Physiol Opt 55:661, 1978.

126. Kimball AC: Congenital toxoplasmosis: A prospective study of 4048 patients. Am J Obstet Gynecol 111:211, 1971.

127. King M: Retrolental fibroplasia. Arch Ophthalmol 43:694, 1950.

128. Kivlin JD: Developmental abnormalities of the eye. Int Ophthalmol Clin 24:55, 1984.

129. Krause U, Krause K, Rantakillio P: Sex difference in refractive errors. Acta Ophthalmol (Copenh) 60:917, 1982.

130. Kushner BJ: Strabismus and amblyopia associated with regressed retinopathy of prematurity. Arch Ophthalmol 100:256, 1982.

131. Kwitko ML: Glaucoma in Infants and Children. New York, Appleton-Century-Crofts, 1973.

132. Kwitko ML: Congenital anomalies related to metabolic disorders of the eye. In Haddad HM (ed): Metabolic Eye Disease. Springfield IL, Charles C Thomas, 1974.

133. Larsen JS: The sagittal growth of the eye: IV. Ultrasonic measurement of the axial length of the eye from birth to puberty. Acta Ophthalmol (Copenh) 49:873, 1971.

134. Liberfarb RM, Holmes LB: The Wagner-Stickler syndrome: A study of 22 families. J Pediatr 99:394, 1981.

135. Lyle WM: Inheritance of Corneal Astigmatism. Ph.D. Dissertation. Bloomington IN, Indiana University, 1965.

136. Lyle WM: Changes in corneal astigmatism with age. Am J Optom Arch Am Acad Optom 48:467, 1971.

137. Lyle WM, Grosvenor T, Dean KC: Corneal astigmatism in Amerind children. Am J Optom Arch Am Acad Optom 49:517, 1972.

138. Mankinen-Keikkinen A, Mustonen E: Ophthalmic changes in hydrocephalus, a follow-up examination of 50 patients treated with shunts. Acta Ophthalmol (Copenh) 65:81, 1987.

139. Manna F, Mackiewicz B: Refraction of the eyes of children with congenital anomalies of bite conditioned by deformation of the alveolar arch of the maxilla (in Polish). Klin Oczna, 45:407, 1976.

140. Majewski F, Rosendahl W, Ranke M, et al: The Kenny syndrome, a rare type of growth deficiency with tubular stenosis, transient hypoparathyroidism and anomalies of refraction. Eur J Pediatr 136:21, 1981.

141. Maumenee IH: The eye in connective tissue diseases. Clinical, Structural, and Biochemical Advances in Hereditary Eye Disorders. New York, Alan R Liss, 53, 1982.

142. McBrien NA: A biometric investigation of late onset myopic eyes. Acta Ophthalmol (Copenh) 65:461, 1987.

143. McBrien NA: Differences in adaptation of tonic accommodation with refractive state. Invest Ophthalmol Vis Sci 29:460, 1988.

144. McBrien NA, Millodot M: Amplitude of accommodation and refractive error. Invest Ophthalmol Vis Sci 27:1187, 1986.

145. McIlroy J, Hamilton R: Investigation into increase and progress of myopia in children. Lond County Council Report 4, no. 3:690, 1932.

146. McLaren DS: Nutrition and eye disease in East Africa, experience in lake and central provinces, Tanganyika. J Trop Med Hyg 63:101, 1960.

147. McLaren DS: The refraction of Indian school children, a comparison from East Africa and India. Br J Ophthalmol 45:604, 1961.

148. McMullen WV: The refractive state in Hopi children. Optom Weekly Jan: 31, 1972.

149. Mehra KS, Khare BB, Vaithilingam E: Refraction in full-term babies. Br J Ophthalmol 49:276, 1965.

150. Miller M, Epstein RJ, Sugar J: Anterior segment anomalies associated with the fetal alcohol syndrome. J Pediatr Ophthalmol Strabismus 21:8, 1984.

151. Millidot M: Retinoscopy and the refraction of infants. Ophthalmol Opt 12:113, 1972.

152. Mitchell DE, Freemen RD, Millodot M, et al: Meridional amblyoia: evidence for modification of the human visual system by early visual experience. Vision Res 13:535, 1973.

153. Mitchell DE, Wilkinson F: The effect of early astigmatism on the visual resolution of gratings. J Physiol (Lond) 243:739, 1974.

154. Mohindra I: The relationship between axial length and certain anthropometric data. Masters Thesis. Bloomington IN, Indiana University, 1962.

155. Mohindra I, Held R, Swiazda J, et al: Astigmatism in infants. Science 202:329, 1978.

156. Mohindra I, Held R: Refraction in humans from birth to five years. Doc Ophthalmol 28:19, 1981.

157. Mohindra I, Nagaraj S: Astigmatism in Zuni and Navajo Indians. Am J Optom Physiol Opt 54:121, 1977.

158. Morgan MW: Relationship of refractive error to bookishness and androgyny. Am J Optom Arch Am Acad Optom 37:171, 1960.

159. Morgan RW, Munro M: Refractive problem in northern natives. Can J Ophthalmol 8:226, 1973.

160. Mukherji R, Roy A, Chatterjee SK: Myopia in newborn. Indian J Ophthalmol 31:705, 1983.

161. Mull MK: Myopia and introversion. Am J Psychol 61:575, 1948.

162. Nakamura Y: Postwar ophthalmology in Japan. Am J Ophthalmol 38:413, 1954.

163. Nissenkorn I, Yassur Y, Masshkowski D, et al: Myopia in premature babies with and without retinopathy of prematurity. Br J Ophthalmol 67:170, 1983.

164. Otsuka J: Genesis of myopia. Bull Tokyo Med Den Univ 3:1, 1956.

165. Otsuku J: Acquired myopia. First International Conference on Myopia. New York, Myopia Research Foundation, 1964.

166. Patel AR, Natarajan TS, Abreu R: Refractive errors in full-term newborn babies. J All-India Ophthalmol Soc 18:59,1970.

167. Pendse GS, Bhave LS, Dandekar VM: Refraction in relation to age and sex. Arch Ophthalmol 52:404, 1954.

168. Perkins ES, Hammond B, Milliken AB: Simple method of determining the axial length of the eye. Br J Ophthalmol 60:266, 1976.

169. Rasmussen OD: Incidence of myopia in China. Br J Ophthalmol 20:350, 1936.

170. Rushton RH: The clinical measurement of the axial length of the living eye. Trans Ophthalmol Soc UK 58:136, 1938.

171. Saksena SS, Bixler D, Yu P: Stickler syndrome: A cephalometric study of the face. J Craniofac Genet Dev Biol 3:19, 1983.

172. Santonastaso A: La refraziene oculare nei primi anni de vita. Annu Ottal Clin Ocul (Italy) 58:852, 1930.

173. Sato T: The Causes of Acquired Myopia. Tokyo, Kanahara Shuppan, 1957.

174. Saunders RA, Andrews III, CJ: Refractive changes in children under general anesthesia. J Pediatr Ophthalmol Strabismus 18:38, 1981.

175. Scammon RE, Armstrong EL: On the growth of the human eyeball and optic nerve. J Comp Neurol 38:165, 1925.

176. Scharf J: Refraction in premature babies: A prospective study. J Pediatr Ophthalmol 15:48, 1977.

177. Scharf J, Zonis S, Zeltzer M: Refraction in Israeli premature babies. J Pediatr Ophthalmol 12:193, 1975.

178. Schmerl E: Higher refractive anomolies; their frequency in different groups and countries. Am J Ophthalmol 32:561, 1949.

179. Scott JD: Congenital myopia and retinal detachment. Trans Ophthalmol Soc UK 100:69, 1980.

180. Shapero M, France TD: The ocular features of Down's syndrome. Am J Ophthalmol 99:659, 1985.

181. Shapero M, Hirsch MJ: The relationship of refractive error and Guilford-Martin temperament test scores. Am J Optom Arch Am Acad Optom 29:32, 1952.

182. Shapero M, Yanko L, Nawratzki I, et al: Refractive power of premature children at infancy and early childhood. Am J Ophthalmol 90:234, 1980.

183. Shulka KN: Myopia. Indian J Ophthalmol 6:7, 1945.

184. Sjostrand J, Abrahamsson M, Fabian G, et al: Photorefraction: A useful tool to detect refraction errors. Acta Ophthalmol (Copenh) 157(suppl):46, 1982.

185. Skeller E: Anthropological and ophthalmological studies on the Angmagssalik Eskimos. Thesis. Copenhagen. 1954.

186. Slataper FJ: Age norms of refraction and vision. AMA Arch Ophthalmol 43:466, 1950.

187. Sonder T: Influence of diseases in children on progressive myopia. Arch Ophthalmol 37:290, 1920.

188. Sorsby A: Race, sex, and environment in the development of myopia. LCC Report, vol IV, II. London, 55, 1933.

189. Sorsby A: Correlation of ametropia and component ametropia. Vision Res 2:309, 1962.

190. Sorsby A, Benjamin B, Sheridan M: Refraction and its components during the growth of the eye from the age of three. Medical Research Council, Special Report Series #301. London, Her Majesty's Stationary Office, 1961.

191. Sorsby A, Fraser GR: Statistical note on the components of ocular refraction in twins. J Med Genet 1:47, 1964.

192. Sorsby A, Leary G: A longitudinal study of refraction and its components during growth. Medical Research Council, Special Report Series No. 309:1. London, Her Majesty's Stationery Office, 1969.

193. Sorsby A, Leary GA, Richards MJ: The optical components in anisometropia. Vision Res 2:43, 1962.

194. Sorsby A, Sheridan J, Leary G: Refraction and its components in twins. Medical Research Council, Special Report Series No. 303. London, Her Majesty's Stationery Office, 1962.

195. Sourasky A: Race, sex, and environment in

the development of myopia (preliminary investigation). Br J Ophthalmol 12:197, 1928.

196. Sperduto RD, Seigel D, Roberts J, et al: Prevalence of myopia in the United States. Arch Ophthalmol 101:405, 1983.

197. Steiger A: Die Entstehung d. sparischen Refraktionen des menschlichen Auges. Berlin, Karger, 1913.

198. Stenstrom S: Untersuchungen uber die Variation und Kovariation der optischen Elemente des menschlichen Auges. Acta Ophthalmol (Copenh) 24 (suppl):1, 1946.

199. Stromland K: Ocular abnormalities in the fetal alcohol syndrome. Acta Ophthalmol (Copenh) 63 (suppl):7, 1985.

200. Stromland K: Ocular involvement in the fetal alcohol syndrome. Surv Ophthalmol 31:277, 1987.

201. Takahashi T: Study of the preventive medicine for myopia. Natl Hyg 16:66, 1939.

202. Tamura K: An experimental examination concerning the etiology of myopia. Acta Soc Ophthalmol Jpn 36:17, 1932.

203. Tassman IS: Frequence of the various kinds of refractive errors. Am J Ophthalmol 15:1044, 1932.

204. Tenner AS: Refraction in school children: 4800 refractions tabulated according to age, sex and nationality. NY Med J 102:611, 1915.

205. Thomson E: Some statistics of myopia in school children with remarks thereon. Br J Ophthalmol 3:303, 1919.

206. Thorn F, Fang L, Held R: Orthogonal astigmatic axes in Chinese and Caucasian infants. Paper given at the annual meeting of the Association for Research and Vision in Optometry. Sarasota, FL, 1984.

207. Tokoro T, Suzuki K: Significance of changes of refractive components to development of myopia during seven years. Nippon Geka Gakkai Zasshi 72:1472, 1968.

208. Traboulsi EI, Levine E, Mets MB, et al: Infantile glaucoma in Down's syndrome (trisomy 21). Am J Ophthalmol 105:389, 1988.

209. Tuncer M: A long-term study of children born to diabetic mothers. Turk J Pediatr 16:59, 1974.

210. Ulrich G: Refraktion und Papilla optica der Auge der Neugeborenen. Thesis. Konigberg, Germany, 1884.

211. Van Alphen GW: On emmetropia and ametropia. Acta Ophthalmol (Copenh) 142:1, 1961.

212. Von Jaeger E: Ueber die Einstellung des dioptrischen Apparates im. menschlichen Auge. LW Seidel U Sohn, UV Wasson Wien, 1861.

213. Waardenburg PJ: Over Myopie bei jeugdige Kinderen. Maandschr Kingergeneesk 1:451, 1932.

214. Waardenburg PJ: Genetics in Ophthalmology, vol 2. Neuro-ophthalmological Part. Springfield IL, Charles C Thomas, 1963.

215. Wagner G: Augenbefunde bei Fruhgeburten. Klin Monatsbl Augenheilkd 131:326, 1957.

216. Weale RA: Ocular anatomy and refraction. Doc Ophthalmol 55:361, 1983.

217. Weinberger D, Wissenkorn I, Snir M, et al: Combined congenital glaucoma, pigmentary glaucoma, and high myopia in an infant. J Pediatr Ophthalmol Strabismus 22:147, 1984.

218. Wenger MA, Cullen TD: Studies of autonomic balances in children and adults. In Greenfield NS, Sternback RA (eds): Handbook of Psychophysiology. New York, Holt Rinehart & Winston, 535, 1972.

219. Wibaut F: Ueber die Emmetropisation und den Ursprung der spharischen Refraktionsanomalien. Graefes Arch Clin Exp Ophthalmol 116:596, 1926.

220. Wick B, Crane S: A vision profile of American Indian children. J Optom Physiol Opt 53:34, 1976.

221. Woodruff ME: Cross-sectional studies of corneal and astigmatic characteristics of children between the twenty-fourth and seventy-second months of life. Am J Optom Physiol Opt 48:650, 1971.

222. Woodruff ME, Samek MJ: A study of the prevalence of spherical equivalent refractive states and anisometropia in American populations in Ontario. Can J Public Health 68:414, 1977.

223. Yankov L: Ocular biometry in neonates. J Fr Ophthalmol 5:237, 1982.

224. Young FA, Leary GA, Baldwin WR, et al: The transmission of refractive errors within Eskimo families. Am J Optom 53:676, 1969.

225. Young FA, Singer RM, Foster D: The psychological differentiation of male myopes and nonmyopes. Am J Optom Physiol Opt 52:679, 1975.

226. Zacharias L, Chisholm JF, Chapman RB: Visual and ocular damage in retrolental fibroplasia. Am J Ophthalmol 53:337, 1962.

227. Zonis S, Miller B: Refractions in the Israeli newborn. J Pediatr Ophthalmol 2:77, 1974.

PART TWO

General Diagnosis and Management

Chapter 7

The Optometric Examination and Management of Children

Michael W. Rouse

Julie M. Ryan

Early childhood is characterized by rapid neurologic development and physical growth of the visual system. The rationale for the early examination of children is based on evidence that normal development of vision can be disrupted by the early onset of visual anomalies. Unfortunately, the onset of many significant visual anomalies occurs in the first 6 years of life, when they can have the most profound impact. If not diagnosed and treated during this critical period, these anomalies may have serious as well as lasting consequences. Early diagnosis and treatment are essential to successfully eliminate the adverse physiologic effects on visual development, and perhaps more importantly, the possible adverse effects on the child's cognitive, emotional, and psychosocial development and performance.

As the primary care vision practitioner, the optometrist has the responsibility of ensuring the normal development of the visual system through these critical early years; however, many practitioners are intimidated and frustrated by these small patients, who are sometimes uncooperative and with whom communication is often difficult. The real challenge in meeting this responsibility is to develop age-appropriate examination and management strategies. Many of the examination techniques used with young children are procedures that the optometrist routinely uses with older children and adults. These may require only age-appropriate modifications of instructions and targets to be effective with younger children. Other techniques are specifically designed to take advantage of the cognitive and behavioral characteristics

of the young child. The expanding development of these child-oriented procedures allows the optometrist to probe the child's visual system in far more detail than was
possible in the past. The reality of examining
children is that the optometrist is forced to
rely heavily on objective information that he
may feel is not as accurate or reliable as he
would like.

At what ages should children be examined to ensure that the visual system is developing normally? Many authors, ourselves included, suggest that all children be seen
before the end of the first year of life. If there
is a family history of strabismus, amblyopia,
high refractive error, or early vision loss, the
infant should be examined by 6 months of
age. If parents observe any unusual appearance of the child's eyes or visual behavior,
they should be advised to have the child
evaluated as soon as possible. Following this
early evaluation and providing no vision
problem is present, the child should routinely be seen again between the ages of $2\frac{1}{2}$
and $3\frac{1}{2}$ years, just before kindergarten, and
then yearly through elementary school. This
examination schedule will initially ensure
early detection of major visual anomalies that
might adversely affect normal visual development, and later, the timely discovery of
more subtle visual anomalies that might affect the child's general performance.

The examination of children is both a
challenging and a rewarding aspect of optometric practice. We hope that this chapter
provides the optometric student or practitioner with the management principles and
basic examination strategy to provide primary care optometric services for the pediatric population.

PEDIATRIC PRACTICE MANAGEMENT

The practitioner who offers pediatric vision
care services should consider the child's
point of view. Most optometrists have designed a pleasing environment that satisfies
their concept of comfort and welcome for a
mostly adult population; however, children's
psychological, emotional, and developmental
characteristics need to be addressed when
designing an office that conveys a welcoming
message to children.

Children enter the optometric office under circumstances that are not usually under
their control. This can lead to fear or anxiety,
which can make the examination unpleasant
for both child and optometrist. Some advanced planning can help avoid these problems. The reception area can be prepared to
convey that children are welcome by adding
a children's corner containing a small table,
chairs, and low shelves that hold books, puzzles, and games (37). The receptionist should
schedule young children for their best time
of the day. Most parents are aware of their
child's daily rhythm and can select the appointment time at which the practitioner can
expect optimal attention and cooperation.
For most young children this time seems to
follow the nap and precede the feeding. Re-
ceptionists should suggest that parents of infants and toddlers bring appropriate snacks
(i.e., dry cereal, raisins) or the child's bottle
for use during the examination.

Small but meaningful changes can also
be made in the traditional examination setting. Children's books and puzzles can be
placed in view, while normal wall plaques
can be replaced with pictures of familiar cartoon characters. A stuffed animal placed in
the lowered exam chair also helps to reduce
the intimidating appearance of ophthalmic
equipment. The optometrist may choose to
conduct the examination in street clothing,
removing the doctor's white coat, which is
often associated with painful experiences.

Clinical Management of Infants and Toddlers

The babe in arms is truly an attentive and
cooperative patient. Infants until about 6
months of age are clearly entertained by simple targets and lights. They not only look intently but often smile and laugh. At 4 to 6
months of age, they begin to gain purposeful

motor control and actively attempt to reach out to hold the presented targets. After 6 months of age, the rapid physical and neural growth infants are experiencing is evident as they learn to sit alone (6 months), crawl (7 months), say simple syllables (7 months), and walk (12 months). During this time, they also begin to interact with the examiner. Playing simple games (i.e., peek-a-boo) in order to keep their attention becomes a necessary component of the examination. It is not necessary to baby talk to infants, but gentleness in manner and voice are recommended (89). It is equally important to work quickly, as infants fatigue and lose interest rapidly. Prolonged cooperation can be enhanced by allowing the infant to take a bottle or pacifier. This is especially useful when ophthalmoscopy and retinoscopy are being performed (83). Infants will feel secure and more cooperative if held by a parent during the examination. If an infant arrives in the car seat and appears comfortable there is no reason to disturb the baby. The exam can be conducted with the infant in the car seat placed on an office table at an appropriate height.

As infants learn to walk they pass into the toddler stage (ages 14 months to $2\frac{1}{2}$ years). Toddlers behave in many ways as infants do. They look intently at a cute target, but only once, and they attempt to grab everything. They respond well to one-word instructions (i.e., look, see) and fast-paced testing. They become fatigued very quickly and do not hide their boredom. Toddlers are usually more comfortable seated on a parent's lap; wiggling and fidgeting are normal. Occasional trips out of the exam chair for breaks are necessary. Treats are often useful rewards for a toddler who has difficulty holding still. As toddlers reach 2 years of age they have command of a great number of words and can interrupt while the practitioner is trying to talk. The examiner can keep the pace moving by nodding or smiling to acknowledge the child's conversation while giving the next instruction. As these children pass $2\frac{1}{2}$ years of age, they develop a wider command of language and improved motor control and enter the preoperational stage of cognitive development as they enter preschool.

Clinical Management of Preschoolers

If the optometrist can observe the parent-child interaction in the reception room, valuable insights about the preschool child's temperament and behavior can be gained. In the few seconds between opening the door to the reception room and calling the patient's name, the doctor can speculate on whether the child is frightened or shy, angry or upset, or hyperactive.

The shy or cautious child is generally not involved in play activity and may even be clinging to the parent. This child often hides in the parent's shoulder when his or her name is called. It is generally useful to initiate conversation with the parent and allow her or him to act as liaison between the doctor and child. The optometrist and the parent will need to draw the child out by referring to the games to be played or characters to be seen, carefully avoiding provocative terminology such as tests or drugs. This child will probably need the parent for comfort and should sit in the parent's lap during the examination. The examiner may need to communicate indirectly through hand puppets or toys. As the child becomes more comfortable, direct fixation on the optometrist rather than the puppet or toy will occur. Personal rapport and more direct communication can then be established.

Far from the ideal situation is the child who is crying or angry while waiting in the reception room. If a child is upset, it is generally due to events that precede the visit to the office. Most parents attempt to help the child recover composure. If the optometrist's judgment from afar is that the parent's efforts are succeeding, then interference at that time is not recommended until the child is soothed. If the child remains upset, no more time need be wasted; the child can be moved to the exam room, where the optometrist can attempt to distract the child and gain his or her trust and cooperation. The doctor can attempt tests in confrontation position with the use of cute and attractive targets, magic tricks, or light games (i.e., penlite on-off). Children usually relax when confronted with persistent attempts to entertain. In the event that no amount of parental comforting or entertainment will sooth the child, it may be advisable to schedule another appointment, but prior to terminating the initial visit, the optometrist should set the stage for the next visit by explaining briefly what will occur, how everyone will work together, that certain instruments (lights) will be used, and that good behavior is expected. This might be a good time to send home visual acuity practice sets to improve readiness for the next appointment. The parent should be asked to reschedule for the child's best time of day.

The hyperactive child flits from one activity to the next in the reception room. No toy or person can hold this child's attention very long. Most come eagerly when their name is called and some rush ahead of parent and doctor through the office. This might be avoided by simultaneously calling the child and offering a hand to be held while walking to the exam room. Care must be taken to store valuable instruments out of sight and reach. The exam should proceed quickly, the optometrist changing fixation toys often during testing in order to hold the child's attention. Allowing the child to hold fixation targets and exchange them back and forth during the exam helps minimize the child's desire to touch or play with the phoropter or slit lamp. Behavior modification games using intermittent rewards for appropriate behavior (e.g., sitting still, looking for a long enough period of time) can be especially useful. Change is the key to remember when examining the hyperactive child. Attention can be enhanced if the doctor changes voice tones (i.e., occasionally whispers, talks slower or faster) or movement patterns (i.e., moves in slow motion).

Examining preschool children requires flexibility, ingenuity, and creativity. Even the most cooperative child can become apprehensive during specific procedures. If the child responds adversely to simple procedures, other procedures that yield similar or the same information should be substituted. For example, if the child shies from a bright light, the light source may be dimmed or covered with a cute yellow finger puppet, or a procedure that does not use lights may be used. The original procedure may be resumed later, if necessary. By changing the methods and routine the practitioner can avoid conveying negative messages of failure or creating a struggle unnecessarily.

Children of this age respond to the facial expression, body language, and inflections of the doctor as much as they do to the actual instruction. Optometrists who deal with children must learn to talk *to* children and not *at* them. Positive and complete instructions, not questions or commands, need to be used. For example, "Look at Big Bird while I move my paddle in front of your eyes," should replace "Would you like to look at Big Bird?" or "Look at Big Bird!" The first instruction tells the child what to expect during the entire procedure, so nothing comes as a surprise (89).

Intermittent reinforcement of desired behavior during the examination is an example of behavior modification and is an effective method of shaping behavior. The examiner decides which behaviors are desirable and necessary to achieve reliable results. Generally, children are rewarded for cooperation and not for the correctness of their answers. When the child cooperates, the examiner rewards on an intermittent, irregular schedule (partial reinforcement). The reward can be tangible, such as a star or sticker placed on an index card, which is then displayed next to the examination chair in full sight and awaiting more rewards (Fig. 7.1). In some examiners' minds this is bribery. The difference is clear: a bribe is the act of bestowing a favor or reward that serves to induce the child to a given line of conduct ("If you sit in the chair, I will give you this."). This method makes it necessary to bribe continuously. On the other hand, behavior modification achieves its goals by occasionally rewarding any one or several of the previously designated behaviors. The child does not know when or for which behavior a reward will be given. After

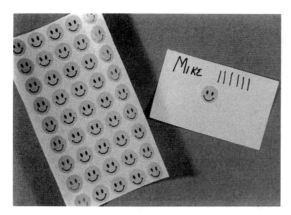

Figure 7.1 Reward system for behavior modification during the examination.

it is bestowed it is important to let the child know why the reward is given, ("That was excellent looking! You get a star for that."). A pattern of conduct is acknowledged, reinforced, and, ideally, sustained by the child.

To modify negative behavior, explicit expectations must be clearly defined for the child. The required behavior is then reinforced on an intermittent schedule and negative behavior is not rewarded. The child quickly learns that only certain behaviors are desired and rewarded. To enhance good attentive behavior, a "working position" can be established: the child is directed to sit straight, with legs crossed and hands on arms of the chair. When the child sits in working position for an individualized period of time, a reward can be given. Between procedures, the child is allowed out of working position, and the doctor provides playthings (Fig. 7.2) so that interest does not turn to the optometric instruments. All participants in the examination know what is expected and can therefore work together more effectively.

Clinical Management of School-Aged Children

Children are socially trained during the elementary school years in the rules for acceptable behavior. As a result most children of this age group are cooperative and attentive,

which allows the practitioner to follow a fairly standard examination routine. However, it is our experience that most youngsters thrive on small rewards (tangible ones or verbal praise) for good cooperation and behavior. The behavior modification techniques described earlier may be useful for managing children of this age.

School-aged children enjoy learning and are naturally curious. The practitioner can gain their trust and cooperation by spending a few minutes throughout the exam describing what each instrument or procedure is testing and how the eyes work. A truthful explanation of what is going to happen is critical, because the child's trust may be lost if there are unpleasant surprises. Saying it is not going to sting when a mydriatic or cycloplegic is instilled does not prepare the child for what is really going to happen. Rapport provides a foundation for the child's understanding of a vision problem and of the prescribed treatment.

Communication with Parents

Parents bring their child for a visual evaluation because they are concerned about the child's eyes, and they usually state their main concern directly and describe signs of possible problems. Many, however, harbor hidden fears and anxieties. Parents may wonder: whether the child will fail the vision test or fail in school because of poor vision, whether they passed on an inherited problem, whether they sought treatment too late to correct the problem, or whether the child is going blind. Therefore, it is important to recognize that any comments the optometrist makes may have unexpected consequences. In order to communicate more effectively it is essential the parents express fears and concerns. The practitioner who senses a hidden concern should simply state, "You are concerned about Sandy's condition [name the condition or consequences]." A parent who is concerned generally responds positively ("yes, I am"). If the word "concerned" is too weak or strong, the parent will naturally correct the doctor ("no, I am very worried").

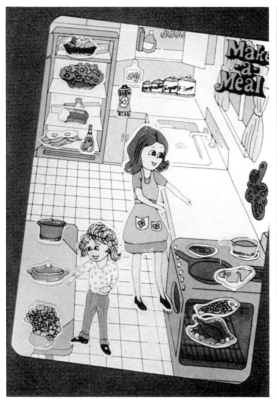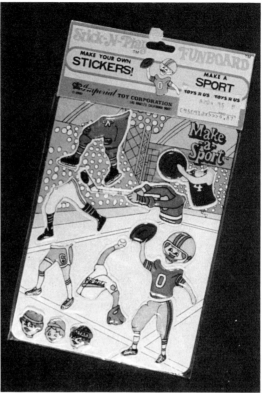

Figure 7.2 Simple games for behavior modification during the examination.

Once the intensity of feeling is expressed, the parent's concerns can be completely addressed.

During the examination many parents experience awkwardness regarding their role. To avoid this, the optometrist should clearly outline the parents' involvement. With very young children, the parent may help the doctor by holding the child and helping with testing. With most preschool-aged children this is no longer necessary. The parent needs to sit back and observe the exam with little or no comment. This is often difficult because as they observe the exam, their memories are stimulated and they think of something they feel is important to add or ask. Supplying a clipboard and paper on which to jot notes helps to control interruptions yet allows the parent to note special concerns. Parents also

enjoy reading pamphlets on vision care for children while waiting. On the whole, parents will follow the optometrist's lead and will interact with the child at the level permitted.

VISUAL EXAMINATION STRATEGY

The examination of any patient is expedited by an efficient and thorough examination strategy and recording method, and this is especially true for young children. The Problem-Oriented Record (POR) (2, 9, 42, 110) provides the structure for the logical examination, management, and follow-up of young patients.

The POR is composed of four parts: the *data base, problem list, initial plan,* and *progress note.* The data base is composed of two parts, a minimum or defined data base (information that is routinely gathered for a comprehensive exam) and a problem-specific data base (information collected in regard to specific patient concerns or symptoms). The choice of procedures that comprise the defined data base is usually based on the optometrist's experience and philosophy. The POR encourages a problem-solving approach but keeps the practitioner from reacting only to signs and symptoms by requiring collection of important screening or baseline information included in the defined data base. The defined data base requires the optometrist to think in terms of ensuring the patency of each major visual system or function rather than which specific tests should be conducted. The defined data base can be subdivided into the diagnostic areas outlined in Table 7.1.

From the results of data base evaluation the optometrist will assess the patient's problems and construct a numbered problem list. Those well-defined problems make up an index of the patient's record called the master problem list, which provides an overview of the patient's problems and eliminates the need for extensive review of the file prior to future visits. The problem list serves as the basis for the development of a numbered plan list, consisting of the numbered problem, therapeutic plan, and patient education recommendations. This sequence sets the stage for the initial management of the patient's problems. The progress note is used to follow up on the initial management plans and is outlined in SOAP notation (Table 7.2).

Table 7.2 PROGRESS NOTE FORMAT OF THE PROBLEM-ORIENTED RECORD

S *Subjective:* Information provided by patient about course of signs and symptoms, compliance with the management plan, understanding of patient education, and new concerns
O *Objective:* The practitioner's examination findings
A *Assessment:* The practitioner's interpretation of the status of the problems following initial management
P *Plan:* Any modification of the initial plan

The advantage of this style of record keeping is the completeness of the patient record and the logical progression from data collection to diagnosis and management.

CASE HISTORY

The case history is one of the optometrist's most important diagnostic tools. The information gained will affect the examination strategy, especially the problem-specific data base, the accuracy of the diagnosis, the formulation of a reasonable prognosis, and the development of a sound management plan. In addition, the case history is an excellent place to establish a compassionate and caring relationship with the parent. A general outline for a pediatric case history is presented in Table 7.3.

Table 7.1 EXAMINATION STRATEGY

Case history
Refractive status
Visual acuity status
Binocular status
   Motor
   Sensory
Accommodative status
Ocular health status
Developmental perceptual motor status

Table 7.3 PEDIATRIC CASE HISTORY

Chief complaint
Signs and symptoms
Patient eye history
Patient medical history
   Prenatal
   Perinatal
   Postnatal
Family eye and medical history

Chief Complaint

It is critical that the parent have the opportunity to explain completely the reason for the visit, including not only her or his observations but fears and concerns. Addressing all aspects of the chief complaint is an important component of a successful case presentation. In the majority of cases, infants and preschoolers react to visual disorders with relatively few signs or symptoms, and the entering complaint revolves around observations by the parent or another adult. In our experience, the major presenting complaints are the following ones:

1. The child appears to have an "eye turn" or the eyes "don't look right." The parent may associate the eye turn with a specific time (when the child is tired) or task (looking up from coloring or eating). Often parents do not notice an eye turn itself but report abnormal head positions (turns, tilts, or tips), abnormal eye positions in different directions of gaze, or covering, winking or squinting one eye.
2. The child rubs the eyes, blinks frequently or forcibly, or has red or watery eyes or asymmetric lid position. Less commonly, the child may complain of itching, burning, pain, foreign body sensation, or sensitivity to light.
3. There is a family history of high refractive state, strabismus, amblyopia, or eye disease.
4. The school-aged child may have failed a school vision screening, indicating deficient visual acuity, binocular coordination, or perceptual skills.
5. The parent may be bringing the child for a routine vision examination prior to entry into school.
6. The parent may be bringing the child for a second opinion, because she or he is confused or uneasy about a previously suggested management plan.

Patient's Eye History

The optometrist needs to inquire about previous vision care, including (1) glasses: reason prescribed, suggested wearing schedule, and compliance; (2) occlusion: reason for and schedule of patching, compliance, success; (3) eye disease: age at diagnosis, medication record, compliance, outcome of treatment; (4) eye injury: age, location of injury, severity, treatment administered (medication, patching, hospitalization); (5) eye operations: reason for operation, age at surgery, which eye, immediate postoperative and long-term results. A thorough understanding of the patient's previous care sets the stage for a successful case presentation. The optometrist can put suggested current management in perspective with past management, outlining possible differences in approach.

Patient's Medical History

The patient's medical history should be structured around the three time periods of prenatal, perinatal, and postnatal development. This history is useful for identifying factors or events that may put a child at risk for certain visual anomalies (116). This knowledge alerts the optometrist to the importance of evaluating specific visual functions and ocular structures more closely.

The prenatal history should center on whether the mother experienced a normal pregnancy. Exposure to toxic agents (tobacco, alcohol, drugs, medications), poor nutrition, or infectious diseases (rubella, syphilis, chlamydia), especially during the first trimester, should be identified. Prenatal influences are the most significant cause of vision loss in children under age 5 years (1).

The perinatal history should determine whether the pregnancy was carried to term and whether the delivery, birth weight, and Apgar score were normal (3, 4).

The postnatal history should investigate the child's medical history, development and growth, psychosocial adjustment, and school achievement. The optometrist should identify any specific events that may have affected the child's normal development, such as trauma and acute or chronic childhood disease. Parents should be questioned about the child's general development, the ages at which prominent motor and cognitive milestones were achieved (e.g., crawling, walking, and speaking first words). A review of the child's school achievement is valuable for identifying signs and symptoms of potential vision problems that may be contributing to poor classroom performance. The parent can be asked two simple questions to investigate school achievement. First, Are you [the parent] satisfied with the child's school achievement? Second, Is the teacher satisfied with the child's schoolwork and achievement? If the answer is no, the practitioner should ask what specific skill the child is having difficulty learning. Many parents have only general knowledge of the child's problems, and written or telephone contact with the teacher may be necessary to clarify the child's problems.

Family Eye and Medical History

Identification of possible hereditary anomalies, either ocular or systemic, allows the practitioner to evaluate the potential risk to the patient and to any siblings. The optometrist should be especially interested in reports of early strabismus, amblyopia, wearing of glasses, ocular disease (especially those resulting in early vision loss), and early-onset systemic diseases such as diabetes.

The history serves as a critical starting point for the formal evaluation of the pediatric patient. If it is done carefully and thoroughly the information should suggest a list of tentative diagnostic hypotheses that the optometrist can use to start the diagnostic thought process.

REFRACTION

The objective evaluation of a child's refractive status is a critical part of the visual evaluation that may help explain entering signs and symptoms, account for binocular anomalies, and help predict future visual problems. Most importantly, it is the starting point in a successful management plan. An objective evaluation is emphasized, because subjective refraction is many times beyond a child's cog-

nitive and attentional abilities before about age 5 or 6 years. Refractive status is assessed routinely in children with static and cycloplegic retinoscopy methods, and possibly keratometry, although automated refractors, photorefraction, and techniques using visual evoked potentials have been reported.

Noncycloplegic Retinoscopy

Static retinoscopy, conducted initially under noncycloplegic (dry) conditions, is in most cases the standard method for evaluating refractive status in children. Two significant problems encountered during static retinoscopy are accurate control of fixation and of accommodation. In an attempt to control these factors, a cartoon or slide is often projected to gain the patient's attention and relax accommodative effort at far point. Having the parent talk about the action in the cartoon helps maintain a younger child's attention. The examiner can ask an older child to describe what is happening in the cartoon. The use of a loose lens or lens bars is preferred to the phoropter for most children under 5 or 6 years. Lens bars are less intimidating and allow the optometrist greater patient control (Fig. 7.3). Often trial framing significant initial retinoscopy findings and scoping over those lenses helps to control accommodation and reach a stable end point, especially in

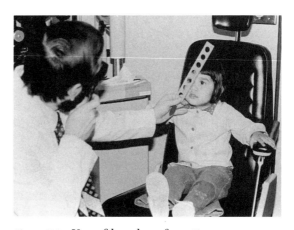

Figure 7.3 Use of lens bars for retinoscopy.

cases of simple or anisometropic hyperopia. Some children, especially infants and toddlers, are more interested in the retinoscope light than in the projected images. The examiner can take advantage of this fact by using the near retinoscopy method (NRM) (81, 82).

The NRM is conducted by having the patient fixate the retinoscope light monocularly at a distance of 50 cm in a completely dark room. One eye is occluded by an elastoplast patch or by the parent's hand. The examiner may need to make sounds (e.g., animal noise, clicking) or call the child's name to attract the child's attention to the retinoscope light. Lens bars are used to determine the neutralizing powers of the major meridians and the gross spherocylinder power (in minus cylinder form) is determined. From this, a 1.25 D adjustment factor is subtracted from the sphere power, but the cylinder power and axis remain unchanged. For example, if the gross findings were +3.25 − 0.75 × 180, the net findings would be +2.00 − 0.75 × 180. The 1.25-D adjustment factor was initially determined empirically (82) and was later confirmed in the laboratory (86). NRM has been suggested as an alternative to cycloplegic refraction (83), although Maino (74) found the two techniques were within ±0.50 D only 35.7 percent of the time and questioned this practice. Borghi and Rouse (12) conducted a similar study and found, on average, NRM revealed 0.50 to 0.75 D less plus than cycloplegic retinoscopy; 68.5 percent of the time NRM showed less plus, 18.5 percent of the time more plus, agreeing within ±0.50 only 34.8 percent of the time. Statistically, the two techniques were not found to give the same refractive amount, but the correlation between the two methods was high ($r = +0.85$).

The optometrist should view the NRM as a supplemental refractive method when cycloplegia may be contraindicated or undesirable. The practitioner can anticipate that the NRM results will be less hyperopic but will correlate reasonably well with a cycloplegic refraction. There will be a greater need for short term follow-up to reevaluate the patient for additional hyperopia if the NRM results are used to determine the refractive correction.

Cycloplegic Retinoscopy

Cycloplegic refraction is indicated when the child is found to have: strabismus, amblyopia, anisometropia, hyperopia associated with esophoria or a high lag of accommodation, unstable end point for sphere and cylinder power or axis on static retinoscopy, or when the child is uncooperative or inattentive during static retinoscopy. Given the typical presenting complaints and the general nature of children, cycloplegic refraction will be indicated in a significant number of cases. Cycloplegic refraction does not guarantee that the optometrist will determine the child's refractive status. Even the most effective cycloplegic agent does not guarantee that the examiner can successfully scope the child. A small percentage of children are too restless or just cannot be persuaded to cooperate. In addition, cycloplegia has a number of disadvantages: possible incomplete or unequal cycloplegia, improperly timed retinoscopy, increased aberrations, decreased depth of focus, altered accommodation-convergence relationships, occasional toxic or allergic effects, and added inconvenience for patient, parent, and doctor. Because of these problems, a cycloplegic drug should be administered only after a preliminary evaluation of the patient's visual acuity and refractive and binocular status.

At the present time we feel the drug of choice is cyclopentolate (see Chap. 13). The onset of action is relatively quick (25 to 45 minutes) which makes it ideal for office use. The duration of action is also reasonable; accommodation returns in 8 to 24 hours. For patients older than 1 year of age the recommended regimen is 1.0-percent solution, 1 gtt followed 5 minutes later by 1 gtt; for patients under 1 year, it is 0.5-percent solution, 1 gtt, followed 5 minutes later by 1 gtt. The reduced concentration decreases the risk of potential systemic side effects such as restlessness, aimless wandering, irrelevant talking, hallucinations, memory loss, or faulty orientation to time and place. Cyclopentolate causes considerable burning on instillation, but a prior drop of topical anesthetic (0.5-percent proparacaine) helps to alleviate this problem. In addition, there is also some information (5) that suggests the topical anesthetic may improve the absorption of cyclopentolate, thus improving its effectiveness. Even with these potential benefits, the use of the topical anesthetic (which also stings slightly) is often dispensed with, especially for children under age 5, to improve the chances of instilling the 2 drops of cyclopentolate. Some authors also suggest a drop of 2.5-percent phenylephrine or 0.5-percent tropicamide to ensure complete cycloplegia and maximum mydriasis, which are necessary for indirect ophthalmoscopy of the fundus.

To instill the drops in infant eyes, the examiner can lay the child on the parent's lap, head toward knees, having the mother hug the child's arms and legs. The examiner then quickly uses the thumb of the free hand to pin the upper lid against the superior orbital rim and with the third or fourth finger of the hand holding the bottle pulls down the lower lid and instills the drop into the lower cul de sac or directly on the globe. Toddlers and preschoolers can sit in the parent's lap while the parent cradles the child firmly, holding in the arms and legs and leaning the head back. The same instillation procedure is suggested. Children's responses to the drops vary, but the examiner can expect some crying from most children. A small number do not cry, and others who are extremely fearful kick and cry quite a bit. In some cases, a referral for examination under sedation may be necessary, although this is very rare in our experience. It is very helpful to get the child playing as soon as possible after the drops have been instilled. Toys, games, or a furry animal friend can help them recover quickly.

The refraction should be performed approximately 30 to 40 minutes after the last drop. The examiner can have the child view a distant target, such as projected cartoons. Or simply have the child fixate the light of the retinoscope, which, if done monocularly, ensures on-axis refraction in cases of strabismus. For infants, the examiner can have the mother withhold feeding until the examination is started. Most infants are unconcerned with their surroundings during feeding, which provides the examiner with an excellent opportunity to perform retinoscopy. With the lens bars the optometrist will determine the gross spherocylinder correction and subtract his working distance to arrive at the net refraction.

In certain cases atropine cycloplegia may be indicated. In the past atropine was the most popular and frequently used cycloplegic drug, even though it has a number of disadvantages that make it less than the ideal routine office cycloplegic agent. First, atropine has a delayed action (maximum cycloplegia in 3 to 6 hours), which necessitates that parents instill the drug at home prior to the office visit. Second, the duration of cycloplegia is prolonged (10 to 18 days). Third, there is an increased risk of systemic side effects such as dryness of the skin and mouth, flushing of the face, fever, tachycardia, and irritability. When atropine is indicated, the recommended dosage regimen is home instillation of 1.0-percent solution three times a day or 0.5-percent ointment at bedtime 3 days prior to refraction. Parents should be well-informed of potential side effects, so they can modify the dosage or discontinue the medication.

In our experience, comparing atropine and cyclopentolate, few patients are found to have significantly larger amounts of hyperopia with atropine. Based on the literature and the fact that cyclopentolate is a convenient, fast, and effective cycloplegic drug for office use, the suggested routine is to use cyclopentolate. The initial prescription would be based on this data, with the understanding that repeated cyclopentolate refraction (usually 4 to 6 weeks after dispensing of glasses) are important to reveal any additional hyperopia in cases of esotropia. If there are significant variations in the magnitude of the strabismus, even though cyclopentolate refraction shows no additional hyperopia, then an atropine refraction is indicated to rule out additional latent hyperopia as the cause (93).

Keratometry

If the patient is cooperative enough, keratometry serves as a helpful adjunct in confirming retinoscopic determinations of astigmatic power and axis. Keratometry can be completed routinely with children 5 years and older and with some cooperative younger children. Pretending to take the child's picture or to play a space game helps to gain the child's attention. Assistance from the parent may be necessary to stabilize the child's head in the instrument. For younger children, especially infants and toddlers, where standard keratometry is impractical, a keratoscope (Placido's disc or Klein keratoscope) can be substituted to evaluate corneal astigmatism. With some practice the optometrist can detect about 1.50 D of corneal cylinder. In addition to the information about corneal astigmatism, the keratoscope permits evaluation of the corneal surface integrity.

The real value of including some keratometric method is to provide objective problem specific data, in addition to retinoscopy findings, that will increase the optometrist's confidence in the final refractive correction.

Autorefraction

Objective and subjective autorefractors are becoming more common in the busy optometric office. Two studies have evaluated the usefulness of objective autorefraction with children (29, 50). Both studies reported comparable results for cylinder power and axis, and sphere power with cycloplegic autorefraction and cycloplegic retinoscopy. Results were unreliable under noncycloplegic conditions. Helveston reported that the majority of children 3 years and older could be successfully autorefracted under cycloplegic conditions. In addition, they found the autorefractor was especially helpful in saving time

with patients who had extreme refractive anomalies.

Our experience with autorefractors has also confirmed their usefulness for children over 3 years, but we are more likely to rely on retinoscopy results when writing the final prescription. The autorefractor is an expensive instrument that requires a reasonably cooperative patient, precisely the type who is as easily refracted by retinoscopy. So the autorefractor may be helpful as either a pre-examination refractive estimate or a secondary confirmation of retinoscopy results, but it is not viewed as a reasonable substitute for the primary refracting method of retinoscopy.

Photorefraction

Photorefraction is a photographic technique that was developed and promoted as a rapid screening method for detecting significant refractive anomalies in infancy that might later result in strabismus or amblyopia (56, 57). A number of techniques have been described in the literature: orthogonal (54), isotropic (6), and photographic skiascopy (11, 21, 46, 62, 85). These systems photograph the image of a flash source that has been refracted on entry and exit from the eye. The flash source is either coaxial with the camera (6, 7, 54) or slightly off axis (46, 62, 63). In each of the techniques the photograph must be developed and analyzed to arrive at an estimate of the refractive state. Studies (7, 21) have indicated that the techniques are valid and reliable in detecting significant refractive anomalies. The time necessary to develop the photograph and do the analysis makes this technique unsuitable for routine clinical refraction. Refinements in the technique and the analysis, combined with its speed, may make photorefraction a helpful adjunctive refractive technique for infants and uncooperative patients in the future. (See Chapter 2.)

Electrodiagnostic Refraction

The visual evoked potential (VEP) has been reported as a method to physiologically refract the visual system (27, 74, 90). The amplitude of the pattern evoked potential is extremely sensitive to optical blurring (45, 80), and by using various lens combinations the largest VEP response, representing the best optical correction, can be determined. The technique has been refined to the point where both sphere and cylinder correction can be determined quickly, and the results compare well with those of subjective refraction methods (90). But, as Sokol (105) pointed out, the VEP technique does not appear to offer much advantage over retinoscopy. The VEP technique requires a reasonably cooperative patient and takes more time, and the equipment is cumbersome, expensive, and requires a level of technical skill usually available only at large centers. The significant difference between retinoscopy, which reveals the optical state, and the VEP technique is that the VEP reflects the cortical activity and thus can be used to determine how well the visual system is processing the clearly formed images. Kuroda and Adachi-Usami (68), Lovasik and Woodruff (73) and Spafford et al. (108) have reported cases where the VEP has provided direct physiologic evidence of the value of corrective lenses. Although VEP refraction is not a practical office procedure, having access to electrodiagnostic services may be useful in evaluating the efficacy of lens therapy for nonverbal or mentally retarded children and adults.

Assessment of Visual Acuity

Recent studies have shown that visual acuity can be assessed accurately and monitored during the critical developmental years (23). Reliable assessment of infants and young children can be accomplished by selecting visual acuity methods that are appropriate for the child's cognitive or chronologic age. Such a developmental approach is used to improve both the number of children testable and the reliability of visual acuity testing.

Methods of Testing Infants' Visual Acuity

The common methods used to screen for amblyopia in infants are fixation maintenance and fixation preference, whereas optokinetic nystagmus (OKN), forced-choice preferential looking (FPL), and visually evoked response (VER) provide quantitative measures of visual acuity.

An optometrist can infer that visual acuity is adequate if fixation is central and steady. Taking advantage of the infant's fascination with lights, a light is shined directly at each eye while the other eye is occluded with the examiner's hand or thumb. The position of the corneal light reflexes (angle Kappa (Lambda)) is estimated for each eye and the two are then compared. Usually the corneal reflections of the two eyes are displaced nasally from center of the pupil by about +0.5 mm. Any deviation of the light reflex in one eye relative to the other eye suggests the presence of eccentric fixation and amblyopia.

Fixation preference can be judged when obvious strabismus is present. It is inferred that the eye that is preferred for fixation has better acuity. The infant is observed fixating an attractive toy or penlight, and the fixating eye is noted. Next, the fixating eye is occluded, to force fixation to the nonpreferred eye, and then uncovered. The fixation pattern is observed again. If fixation is sustained with the nonpreferred eye or fixation alternates between the eyes, then visual acuity is assumed to be nearly equal. If fixation is not maintained as described, amblyopia is assumed to be present (88). Fixation preference testing is ineffective for patients who present with small-angle strabismus or suspected anisometropic amblyopia, because the fixating eye cannot be determined easily by observation.

To test these patients a modified fixation preference method is recommended (119). Placing a dissociating vertical prism (10-Δ) before one eye creates diplopia if deep suppression does not exist. Fixation preference can then be judged while the infant views through the prism. Alternation of fixation between the two images indicates nearly equal visual acuity. If fixation does not alternate, the preferred eye is occluded, forcing the nonpreferred eye to fixate, and then uncovered. If the infant is able to hold fixation for at least 5 seconds or through a pursuit or freely alternates fixation between the two eyes, visual acuity is assumed to be nearly equal. If fixation reverts to the preferred eye, then amblyopia should be suspected (118).

OKN has been used over the years to investigate infant visual acuity (22, 36). By varying the angle subtended by a striped drum, visual acuity can be measured (Fig. 7.4). The angular subtense for testing is accomplished by increasing the viewing distance of the fixed stimulus drum to the maximal distance to which a response can still be observed. This requires two examiners, one to observe the eye movements and another to hold and turn the drum. In addition, it is difficult, and at times almost impossible, to obtain the infant's attention as the viewing distance increases. Clinically OKN is generally used to establish the presence or absence of vision, although it is not foolproof. Any optom-

etrist who seriously suspects there may be major vision reduction should consider referring the child for electrodiagnostic workup (72).

Adapted from research methods developed during the late 1950s (30, 31) FPL has provided a rapid and reliable method to test visual acuity clinically (23, 44). The infant is presented with two targets simultaneously, one consists of stripes (sine- or square wave gratings) and another of matched-luminance gray. If the infant can resolve the grating target, the examiner will observe the infant fixating the pattern (Fig. 7.5).

The infant is seated on the parent's lap at the appropriate fixation distance and is positioned so that the paired targets and central fixation light are at the infant's eye level. In order to control bias, the parent's view of the test targets may be occluded with blurring spectacles or a guard placed between the parent and targets. The examiner is positioned to view the infant's response to each test pair but is blind to the actual location of the grating. Between presentation of the test targets, the infant's fixation is directed to the center of the instrument with fixation lights.

When the fixation light is extinguished, the test targets are illuminated and the infant's fixational behavior is observed. The observer judges the infant's first fixation, duration of fixation, or facial expression as an

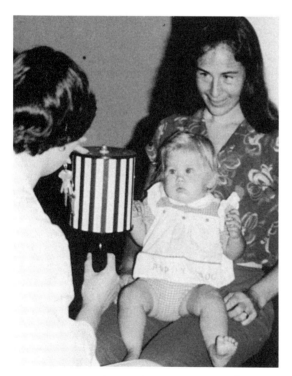

Figure 7.4 Use of OKN drum to assess infants' visual acuity.

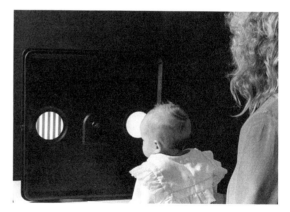

Figure 7.5 Force-Choice Preferential Looking to assess infant visual acuity.

indication of fixation direction. The test is continued until the infant shows no preference for either target or until the gray target is preferred more often than the striped target.

Overall, the data accumulated by various FPL methods have shown good agreement when acuity is estimated using sine- or square wave gratings and a similar-luminance stimulus. The reliability of the technique and the fact that high-quality grating targets and FPL instruments are now commercially available have made FPL a valuable clinical procedure.

Infant visual acuity can be estimated by the use of steady-state VER (76, 105). A checkerboard stimulus, phase altered at a rate of 6 cycles per second (cps), is presented (Fig. 7.6). The VER is the summed cortical response that results from the temporal change of characteristics and is typically recorded with electrodes placed on the scalp over the occipital lobe. The peak-to-trough amplitude of the resulting response is measured. The check size that produces the peak amplitude response generated is compared to VER data of adults with different degrees of visual acuity.

VER testing demands sophisticated equipment that the average practitioner usually does not have available. However, in certain situations other clinical acuity methods may not be successful or a particular ocular or visual condition may necessitate objective acuity testing. The only requirement is that the infant attend to the stimulus during testing; therefore VER can be performed on the very young.

A practical strategy for evaluating infant visual acuity may be, first, to observe fixation maintenance and preference compared to ocular health and refractive information, to infer whether equal acuity is present, and second, FPL, to quantify the visual acuity level of each eye. If these are unattainable and the optometrist suspects amblyopia or delayed visual development, referral for a VER is recommended.

Methods of Testing Toddlers' Visual Acuity

Many toddlers (aged 14 months to $2\frac{1}{2}$ years), even though they can speak, are unable to respond to picture card visual acuity tests, so methods that do not require verbal responses are often necessary. In order to maintain the child's attention, it is often necessary to use operant conditioning to reinforce responses and cooperation.

Operant preferential looking (OPL) uses the basic FPL method described above for infants (77). OPL includes a training phase in which the toddler is shown a pair of targets and is asked to look at the striped one. Each time the child fixates the stripes (or grating), a reward is given (e.g., a toy is activated, a treat is dispensed). Reinforcement is continued as the examiner proceeds to the testing phase. The test is continued until the child shows no preference for either target or prefers the gray target more often. FPL criteria are used to designate acuity.

The Dot Visual Acuity Test (DVAT) was designed specifically to increase the testability of older toddlers and preschool children. (65). The instrument contains a back-illuminated white field on which dots, sized from 20/20 to 20/800 equivalences, are presented. A black mask with a 3-inch hole is placed around the dot (Fig. 7.7). The mask is movable so that the dot can be made to appear in different locations within the aperture. The child is placed at a distance of 10 inches and is asked to touch the dot each time it appears.

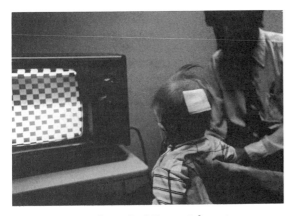

Figure 7.6 Visual Evoked Potential testing.

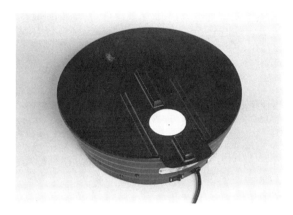

Figure 7.7 Dot Visual Acuity Test.

The dot is gradually reduced in size until it can no longer be detected by the child. Operant conditioning is used (verbal praise or a token is given) each time the child responds correctly. The DVAT is particularly valuable because so few instructions are necessary and no verbal responses are required from the child.

A practical strategy for evaluating toddler visual acuity is, first, to observe fixation maintenance and preference and then attempt to quantify by administering the DVAT or OPL.

Methods of Testing Preschoolers' Visual Acuity

At about 3 years of age most children can actively participate in visual acuity testing. They can understand a series of instructions, respond verbally, and sustain attention on the task. Some preschool children may not have enough language skills, and nonverbal matching methods may be necessary. Most are motivated to perform without the optometrist's use of operant conditioning, but reinforcing good behavior is often helpful.

A child can respond to The Lighthouse Flash Card Test (32) verbally or by matching items. It is most frequently used as a verbal response test, since the target optotypes are three simple figures: house, apple, and umbrella. The test consists of 12 flash cards on which one symbol is printed on each side in

sizes that represent a range of visual acuity from 20/10 to 20/200 (Fig. 7.8).

Administration of the Lighthouse Test begins with familiarization. Each of the 200-foot figures is presented at a close viewing distance and the child is asked to name it. After the examiner is satisfied that the child has grasped the concept the examiner can test at 10 feet. During testing it is important to randomize the sequence in which the figures are presented in order to control habituation and guessing. It is suggested that a minimum of four presentations be given at each acuity level. The visual acuity is assigned as the last Snellen equivalent for which the child correctly identified four of four presentations.

The Broken Wheel Test (BWT) uses the Landolt C optotype as the salient test item (91). The child is asked to select between two alternatives one of which is a car with broken wheels and the other a car with intact wheels (Fig. 7.9). The BWT's great advantage is that the child simply locates the broken wheels (which represent the C) and does not have to identify the direction of the opening.

The cars are presented on seven pairs of cards designed for use at 10 feet, providing Snellen equivalents from 20/20 to 20/100. A familiarization and training phase includes first pointing out the differences between the cars using the 20/100 targets at a close distance and, second, holding two cards in front of the child and asking the child to point to

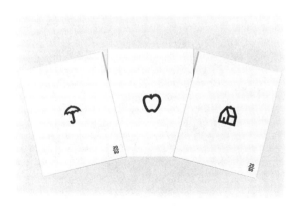

Figure 7.8 Lighthouse Flash Card Test.

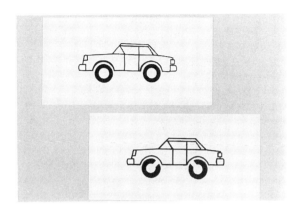

Figure 7.9 Broken Wheel Visual Acuity Test.

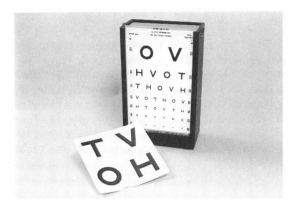

Figure 7.10 HOTV Visual Acuity Test.

the car with the broken wheels. If the child points correctly then the cards are held behind the examiner's back and changed randomly from hand to hand before being presented again. Usually the optometrist can tell whether the child has grasped the concept after two or three trials and testing can begin. The paired cards are now presented in the same manner as they were during the training phase, but at the 10-foot viewing distance. The examiner will have to remind the child to look at both cards before responding. Visual acuity is designated as the last Snellen equivalent for which the child got four of four presentations correct.

Four common letters, H, O, T, V, comprise the HOTV visual acuity test (64). The test chart, composed of Snellen equivalents from 10/10 to 10/100 is placed at a distance of 10 feet. A heavy plastic card bearing the letters is placed before the child as the "response panel" (Fig. 7.10). Four separate training flash cards are presented to familiarize the child with the letters. At this point the examiner can determine whether a verbal or nonverbal method best suits the child. If the nonverbal method is selected the child practices placing his hand on the same letter of the response panel. Verbal responses are discouraged unless the examiner is sure the child knows the letters. Testing proceeds until fewer than two of six letters per line are identified correctly.

A practical strategy for evaluating preschoolers' visual acuity would be first, to observe fixation maintenance and preference and then to attempt to quantify visual acuity, usually by selecting Lighthouse cards for the young preschooler and one of the other tests for the older preschooler.

Methods of Testing Visual Acuity of School-Aged Children

The Tumbling E Test is the classic acuity test that was used before appropriate preschool optotypes were designed. The Tumbling E Test was intended for use with illiterate persons who could name or point out the direction in which the E was presented. Many children can participate in the "E game" by pointing their hands or a model E in the same direction; however, this requires demonstration, pretraining, and practice to ensure reliability. Once the child has grasped the task, testing can be accomplished by the use of either a wall or projected chart or individual flash cards. Testing is terminated when the direction of Es is identified correctly fewer than two of six times at any acuity level on a chart or fewer than three of four times on flash cards. Clinically the use of the Tumbling E Test is slow compared to the other tests available, and often it can be particularly difficult for children because of the directionality demand.

Snellen visual acuity testing is appropriate for children who demonstrate the ability to consistently name individual letters. This skill is usually mastered around 5 years of age, but it can be learned as early as age three. Children can recite the alphabet long before they recognize, discriminate, and read letters. An examiner who is sure the child can read the ABCs can select to use Snellen letters.

Optometrists will find that selection of a visual acuity test for any child is based on the child's cognitive level and ability to communicate and on the optometrist's comfort and skill with any particular test. Recommendations made by chronologic age can be found in Table 7.4.

Evaluation of Binocular Vision

The prevalence of pediatric binocular anomalies behooves the optometrist not only to be familiar with the most prevalent conditions but also to be proficient in evaluating and diagnosing them. The breadth and depth of the optometrist's investigation should be appropriate to the child's age and cognitive development. For infants and toddlers, the examination centers around identifying gross binocular anomalies, such as strabismus, that may interfere with the normal development of visual acuity and binocular sensory processing. As children approach school age the investigation should become more sophisticated, not only identifying gross binocular anomalies but also probing for more subtle anomalies, such as convergence insufficiency, which might cause inefficient or uncomfortable vision. This progressive examination strategy ensures that the child will have the binocular visual skills necessary to meet the changing visual demands accompanying growth and maturity.

Evaluation of Binocular Alignment

The primary diagnostic question with regard to binocular alignment is whether the child has strabismus. If strabismus is present, the examiner should investigate the characteristics of the deviation outlined in Table 7.5. If it is not, the examination shifts to determining whether a heterophoria exists and identifying its direction, magnitude, and concomitancy. In addition to these motor characteristics of the deviation, the patient's sensorimotor fusion (vergence) abilities need to be evaluated to complete the patient's binocular

Table 7.4 SUGGESTED VISUAL ACUITY TESTS FOR DIFFERENT AGE GROUPS

Test	Infant (Birth–14 mo)	Toddler (14 mo–2.5 yr)	Preschooler (3 yr–5 yr)	School-Aged (>5 yr)
Fixation Maintenance	++	+	+	+
Fixation Preference	++	+	+	+
OKN	++	+	+	+
Forced-Choice Preferential Looking	++			
VER	++	+	+	+
Operant Preferential Looking		++	+	
Dot Visual Acuity		++	+	+
Lighthouse Cards		+	++	+
Broken Wheel Cards		+	++	+
HOTV			++	+
Tumbling E			+	++
Snellen			+	++

++, Preferred test
+, Optional test

Table 7.5 CHARACTERISTICS OF OCULAR DEVIATION

Direction (eso, exo, vertical, cyclo components)
Frequency (heterophoria, intermittent, or constant)
Magnitude (amount in Δ at both far and near)
Eye laterality (unilateral or alternating; if alternating, which eye is preferred for fixation?)
AC/A ratio (low, normal, high)
Cosmesis (poor, fair, good)
Concomitancy (Is magnitude equal in all fields of gaze and with either eye fixating?)

vision profile. This profile of characteristics will have a significant bearing on the optometrist's final diagnosis, subsequent prognosis, and management plan.

The binocular vision evaluation should start with a general observation of the patient's eyes and facial characteristics (Table 7.6). The optometrist should be looking for signs of obvious strabismus and for characteristics that might conceal or exacerbate the appearance of strabismus, such as the size of the patient's head, interpupillary distance, nose bridge, asymmetries in lid, pupil, or orbit position, and the presence of epicanthal folds. When the combination of wide, broad nasal bridge and epicanthal folds are present, many cases of suspected strabismus are actually diagnosed as pseudostrabismus (20). In these cases, the optometrist may need to actually pinch the bridge of the nose, pulling the epicanthal folds up and away, to convince the parent that no strabismus is present. The

Table 7.6 SEQUENCE OF TESTING FOR BINOCULAR ALIGNMENT

Observation
Hirschberg test
Krimsky Reflex Prism Test
Bruckner test
Unilateral Cover Test
Alternate Cover Test
Four–Base Out Test

examiner should look closely for any atypical head position, such as tilts, turns, or tips, that might indicate the presence of a nonconcomitant deviation. The importance of careful preliminary observation, using a mental checklist of these factors, cannot be overemphasized.

We feel it is helpful in all cases, but especially in infants and preschoolers, to begin the quantitative evaluation of binocular alignment with the Hirschberg Test (61). It allows an objective examination of the patient's undisturbed binocular alignment and requires only minimal patient cooperation and attention. The procedure involves having the patient fixate the examiner's penlight or transilluminator at a distance of ~50 cm. The examiner evaluates the relative placement of corneal reflexes in relationship to the center of the pupils. Binocular alignment is observed as a symmetric displacement of the reflexes (e.g., +0.5 mm RE, +0.5 mm LE (+ indicates nasal and −, temporal displacement). Asymmetric displacement suggests that strabismus is present; that is, +0.5 mm RE, −1.0 mm LE would suggest left esotropia of about 33 Δ using the conversion factor, 1 mm displacement = ~22 Δ (38, 61, 114). The sensitivity of the Hirschberg Test depends on the examiner's skill, but with practice it is commonly 0.5 mm displacement, or about 10 Δ. If the optometrist is unsure about estimating the displacement in millimeters, the Krimsky Reflex Prism Test (67) can be administered. This test is especially helpful for estimating the magnitude of infant strabismus in children with a blind or deeply amblyopic eye with or without eccentric fixation. The optometrist first observes the Hirschberg results (e.g., +0.5 mm RE, −1.0 mm LE) then places increasing powers of neutralizing prism in front of the fixating eye (RE) until the reflex of the deviated eye (LE) is moved to equal the fixating eye's original location (+0.5 mm). The amount of prism (~30 Δ BO in this example) is an estimate of the deviation's magnitude. To improve an infant's attention to the target for either of these techniques, the room lights should be dimmed so the penlight is the dominant stimulus in the room. For older children, the examiner can play games (e.g., "blowing out the birthday candle") that sustain attention and give the examiner enough time to evaluate the results.

The Hirschberg Test can also assist the examiner in screening for gross concomitancy. The examiner simply moves the penlight into each of the diagnostic muscle action fields (DAFs), noting any change in the relative position of the corneal reflexes. Alternately, the examiner can move the patient's head so the eyes are positioned in each DAF. A routine minimum comparison should be made between primary, up, down, right, and left gaze. If a vertical strabismus or a vertical oculomotor anomaly is found, the optometrist may wish to conduct Park's Three-Step Test (87) to isolate the affected muscle. The procedure involves simple comparisons: Which eye is hyperphoric or hypertropic in primary gaze? On which gaze (right or left) does the hyperphoria or hypertropia increase? And finally, on head tilt to which shoulder does the hyperphoria or hypertropia increase? The practitioner can refer to tables (40) or use a simple circling technique (66) to identify the affected muscle.

Some patients with dark irides are difficult to evaluate with the Hirschberg technique described above, because the border between the dark pupil and iris is difficult to distinguish. The optometrist can observe the Hirschberg reflex against a brightly illuminated pupil by administering the Bruckner Test (109). The patient fixates the ophthalmoscope light at a distance of about 1 m, while the optometrist focuses the ophthalmoscope beam, large enough to illuminate both eyes at the same time, on the patient's face. The optometrist then judges the relative position of the corneal reflexes. The optometrist can also evaluate binocular alignment by observing the relative whiteness and brightness of each pupillary reflex. If strabismus is present, the turned eye's pupil will appear brighter and whiter than the fixating eye's pupil (Fig. 7.11). Strabismus of only a few prism diopters can be detected with this method. The

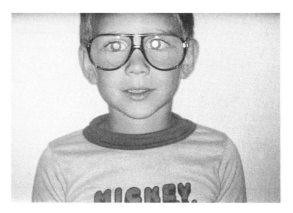

Figure 7.11 Bruckner Test. Left eye appears brighter and whiter, suggesting left-eye strabismus.

Bruckner test is very simple to administer, and the phenomenon is observed most easily in infants, less easily in older children, and with difficulty in adults. The reduced visibility with age appears to be related to changes in retinal pigmentation, because even in young Spanish or Asian children the phenomenon is difficult to observe. Keeping these limitations in mind, the Bruckner test serves as a helpful adjunct for detection of strabismus (41). In addition to the clinical method described above, a photographic application of the Bruckner Test (62, 63) has also been shown to be a reliable method for detecting strabismus.

For many infants and toddlers and some preschool children the techniques described above may be the only binocular alignment tests possible. For other children, the examiner will base binocular alignment decisions primarily on the results of the Unilateral Cover Test (UCT). Although the procedure is familiar to all optometrists (13), a few hints for working with children may be helpful. The type of targets used is very important, and the examiner should have a variety available. Infants are attracted to brightly colored toys, especially if they make a sound or light up. For older children, familiar cartoon characters or animals the child might have as a pet are extremely valuable. When the near UCT is conducted the target should include fine detail, coloring or features, that the examiner can use to focus the child's attention. The child should then be given simple verbal commands of *Ready* and *Look* for each movement of the occluder. The small details and repetitive verbal commands help maintain the child's attention and accommodative accuracy. Significant esophoria or intermittent esotropia is easily missed if accommodation is not accurately controlled. Sometimes, children are more interested in the movement of the examiner's occluder than in the target. To avoid this, the optometrist's thumb can be used as an occluder. The optometrist's hand can be positioned above or on the child's head; some children resist having the head touched, and the thumb can be casually extended down to occlude the patient's eye.

Maintaining the child's attention to assess binocular alignment is often more difficult at a distance than near. Brightly colored pictures of familiar characters or animals allow the examiner to attract the child's attention. Children respond best to action, so mechanical toys, a dancing bear, barking dog, or cymbal-clanging monkey, that make sounds or blink lights work extremely well. The optometrist needs to assess the child's level of maturity and attention to select the best target for the specific test distance.

Following the UCT, the Alternate Cover Test (ACT) with prism neutralization (loose prism or prism bar) provides an objective method for quantifying any detected deviation. For cooperative nonstrabismic children, 6 years and older, the phoropter can be used to measure the heterophoria, but we prefer to rely on out-of-instrument objective measures for younger children. In addition to neutralizing the magnitude of the deviation in primary gaze, the optometrist should routinely screen a minimum of up, down, right, and left gaze to detect any nonconcomitant component to the deviation. If the deviation has a vertical component the optometrist may wish to conduct Park's Three-Step Test, described above, to isolate a cyclovertical muscle as the possible cause. Depending on the child's

age and maturity, subjective methods, such as the red lens, Maddox rod, and Hess-Lancaster test, can also be used to confirm the diagnosis.

If the patient's attention to a static target on the ACT is poor, a moving target can be employed by administering the Kinetic Cover Test (40). As the fixation target is moved toward the patient, the ACT is conducted and the examiner estimates the magnitude at 10-cm intervals. The same procedure is used as the fixation target is moved away. By evaluating the observed change in heterophoria as the target is moved toward and then away from the patient, the optometrist can classify the patient's vergence anomaly.

In certain cases where small-angle esotropia is suspected, the optometrist may administer the Four Base Out Test (58, 59) to confirm the presence of an associated small central suppression scotoma. The test requires a fairly cooperative patient, but we have successfully conducted the test on children as young as 3 years of age. The technique involves placing a 4 BO prism over the normally fixating eye and observing the movements of the suspected strabismic eye. If the results are negative (normal) the examiner will observe a slight version (outward movement) then vergence (inward movement) of the suspected eye. If the results are positive (abnormal) the examiner will observe version and no vergence. To confirm the suspected central suppression the prism would be placed over the suspected strabismic eye and no movement of the normal eye would be observed. The Four–Base Out Test requires keen observation skills, and, unfortunately, there are a number of atypical normal responses that can complicate interpretation of the results (92).

This testing sequence requires only a few minutes and should yield sufficient information to develop a fairly complete profile of the deviation's motor characteristics. In addition to these motor characteristics, the patient's sensory and motor fusion (vergence) abilities need to be evaluated to complete the patient's binocular vision profile.

Evaluation of Sensory Fusion

The strategy for evaluating sensorimotor fusion ability varies both with the patient's age and the motor characteristics of the deviation. A significant requirement for probing sensorimotor fusion, especially sensory fusion, is the need for reliable subjective responses. Unfortunately, these responses are very individualized. A small percentage of 3-year-olds are able to give excellent almost adultlike responses, while consistently reliable responses are usually not expected until age 6 or 7 years. Even at this age, a small percentage of children give surprisingly poor responses. In addition to the issue of reliable patient responses, the motor characteristics of the deviation affect the examination strategy. If the patient has constant or high-frequency strabismus, the optometrist needs to conduct, or refer for, problem-specific testing to establish whether correspondence is normal or anomalous (40). If the patient has heterophoria or low-frequency (<50 percent) intermittent strabismus, the optometrist can usually assume that correspondence is normal (although there are exceptions) and proceed to probe sensorimotor fusion based on this premise.

The requirement for reliable subjective responses represents a major obstacle to evaluating sensory fusion before age three years. The optometrist will have to rely primarily on inferential means to judge the status of sensory fusion prior to this age. If the child is found to have binocular alignment, equal visual acuities and a low equal refractive state, the optometrist can, with a certain degree of confidence, assume that the sensory system is intact. The optometrist may be able to support this assumption by demonstrating a normal motor fusion (vergence) response to a 10- to 15-Δ BO prism placed in front of one eye. If the response is positive, the disparity vergence and sensory system are grossly intact. The clinical testing of stereopsis is typically unreliable before age three (18, 35); a large number of young children are unable to respond or refuse to wear the Polaroid glasses. A modification of the Frisby stereotest (34, Fig. 7.12) that does not require the use of

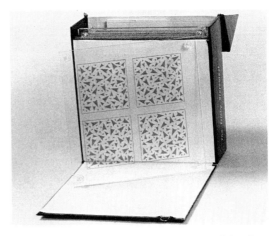

Figure 7.12 Frisby Stereo Test. One of the four squares contains the correct stereo response of a circle floating in depth.

Polaroid glasses reportedly improved the stereo testing of children as young as 30 months (43). The Lang stereotest (69), which also does not involve wearing Polaroid glasses, has shown promise for screening younger children (60, 70) (Fig. 7.13). Research using preferential looking (PL) techniques has shown adult levels of stereoacuity by 4 months of age (33, 49). Using this information, a newer method using operant condi-

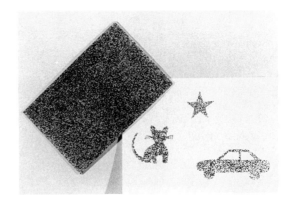

Figure 7.13 Lang Stereotest, shown with response card of figures that are seen when random dot stereopsis is present.

tioning PL has shown a significant increase in the number of children that can be tested (17).

When children reach approximately the age of three, more reliable sensorimotor fusion testing can be achieved. Children begin to respond to second-degree (flat) fusion tests, which allow sampling of sensorimotor fusion and specifically the detection of suppression. The target selected and the instructions given should be geared to the child's age. For example, the Special Three-Character Test is excellent for children between the ages of 3 and 5 years. The child wears red-green glasses and reports whether anaglyphically tagged pictures of a girl, an elephant, and a basketball are present. For the older children the Worth Four-Dot Test is effective if the child receives pretest training in the task. For example, the examiner needs to know whether the child knows how to count. He can ask, but it is best to have the child demonstrate by playing a finger-counting game in which the child responds verbally or holds up the same number of fingers as the examiner. Once the child can demonstrate the ability to count at least to five, the test can be administered. Children often give verbal responses that are impossible ("I see 8 dots"). Modifying the instructions to include a motor component, such as, "shoot out" or "point to" or "touch each of the dots," often improves reliability. We seldom use the Red Lens Test, because the subtle difference between one pink light, the fusion response, is often too difficult for the child to discriminate from one red light, a suppression response. The Pola-Mirror and Vis-à-Vis Polaroid techniques allow for the evaluation of suppression under more normal seeing conditions than the colored filter techniques above. In the pola-mirror (39) technique the child wears Polaroid glasses and looks into a mirror. The optometrist asks whether the child can see both eyes at the same time. If the patient is suppressing, that eye will appear black in the mirror. In Vis-à-Vis technique (40) optometrist and patient both wear Polaroid glasses, and the patient reports whether he or she can see both of the examiner's eyes.

The child who is suppressing will point to the examiner's eye on the same side.

Stereopsis testing is a way to confirm bifixation and to demonstrate high-level sensory processing. Stereo tests can be divided into two types, lateral contour (Stereo Fly and Stereo Reindeer) and random dot tests (Random Dot E, Randot Test, TNO, Frisby, and Lang Stereo Test). The lateral disparity designs suffer from the presence of monocular contour and displacement cues but are useful clinical tests if these limitations are kept in mind. Random dot stereograms eliminate the monocular cues and provide an excellent method for confirming bifixation (Fig. 7.14). The optometrist should have both lateral disparity and random dot tests available. A good test that incorporates both designs is the Randot Stereotest (Fig. 7.15). It is also desirable to have either the Frisby or Lang stereo test for children who refuse to wear Polaroid glasses. Children's reliability on stereo tests improves from age three, reaching adult levels by age seven (19). When administering the tests, good instructions and concrete models of the correct response help increase the number of children able to respond and the reliability of their responses. For example, with the Randot Test's random dot forms, showing the child the figures on the cover of the instruction booklet helps them know what figures may be present and the figures' approximate size and appearance on the random dot background. To increase

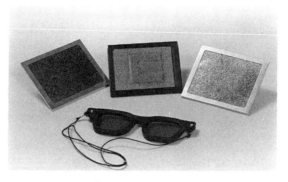

Figure 7.14   Random Dot E, example of pure random dot stereo design.

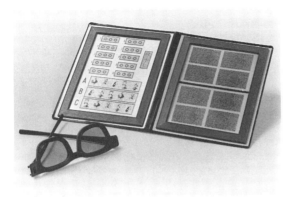

Figure 7.15 Randot Stereotest combines pure random dot stereo test with lateral disparity components.

the child's interest in the task the optometrist can make up stories. Story telling gets children excited and interested in the task. Even if the child does not respond to the quantitative portions of the stereotests, having the child attempt to pinch the stereo-reindeer's nose or stereo-fly's wings gives the optometrist information that the child has at least some gross stereopsis.

Evaluation of Motor Fusion (see Chaps. 10 to 12)

The initial step in assessing motor fusion involves examining the near point of convergence (NPC). A normal NPC is present as early as 8 weeks of age, and the optometrist should expect an NPC of at least 8 to 10 cm on all children. Testing reliability can be improved by using a detailed familiar cartoon character target and talking to the child about the figure ("Do you see him winking his eye?") as the target is moved closer and closer. The optometrist should observe for the break point and should ask the child to report when the target is doubled.

The next step in evaluating motor fusion is to examine the child's relative vergence ranges. This can be assessed best by loose prisms or a prism bar. Two different strategies can be used to assess motor fusion

ranges: (1) a smooth change in prism power until break and recovery are reported subjectively or observed objectively; (2) a jump vergence method where the prism is suddenly placed in front of the patient's eye and the recovery response is noted. A normative study (99) on smooth vergence skill of elementary school children recommended that near break and recovery findings below 15/10 BO or 7/3 BI, for 7- to 12-year-olds and 12/5 BO or 7/2 BI for 6-year-olds be considered abnormal. Actual normative information on preschool children has not been collected, but the recommendations for 6-year-olds serve as a useful guideline if there is no significant phoria and the optometrist is simply trying to establish the patency of the vergence system. The problems with using this technique for preschoolers is that their subjective responses of break and recovery are typically unreliable and objective observation of the small vergence changes is very difficult. We prefer the jump vergence method for preschoolers because it is quick, the vergence response is much easier to observe objectively, and the subjective response is more straightforward (see Fig. 7.16). Minimum recovery values of 10 BO/3 BI at near can be used as guidelines (99, 112). The optometrist's criteria should be adjusted if a significant phoria or intermittent strabis-

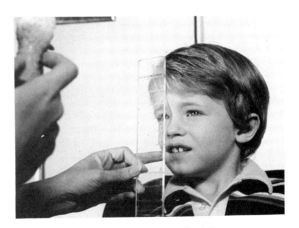

Figure 7.16 Jump vergence method (using prism bar) of assessing motor fusion ability.

mus is detected on the cover test. The optometrist should be concerned not only that the minimum expected vergence is met but also that the patient has sufficient vergence ability to comfortably compensate for the phoria. To judge whether vergence ability is adequate, Sheard's criteria (vergence = 2 × phoria) can be used if the patient is exophoric and Percival's criteria (phoria is in middle third of vergence ranges) if the patient is esophoric (103, 104). For children 7 years and older, routine phorometry can be conducted using the above criteria and established norms (52) to evaluate the results. In addition, children of these ages can respond to more sophisticated measures of vergence ability, such as vergence facility (40) and forced vergence fixation disparity methods (102).

At the conclusion of the binocular vision evaluation the optometrist should be able to generate a profile of the patient's binocular status that includes the deviation's motor characteristics and the patient's sensory and motor processing abilities.

Evaluation of Accommodation

A thorough examination of accommodative function involves the evaluation of accommodative amplitude, accuracy (lag), and facility (52, 113). Accommodative response characteristics have been reported by a number of investigators (8, 15, 48) to approximate adult abilities by 3 to 4 months of age, but routine clinical assessment of accommodative function usually is not attempted before age 4 or 5 years, and the majority of children cannot be tested reliably by traditional subjective clinical methods until age 6 or 7 years.

For children of all ages, but especially younger children, dynamic retinoscopy provides one of the few practical objective methods of assessing accommodative function. Dynamic retinoscopy is not only a valuable clinical tool; it has been used in a number of investigations into the development of accommodative function (8, 16, 47, 48). Other objective methods have been reported, for example, VEP (79) and photorefraction (14),

but these represent primarily research rather than clinical procedures. The monocular estimate method (MEM) has been shown to be a valid and reliable (95) measure of accommodative response. MEM retinoscopy is performed under normal reading conditions, including habitual refractive correction and working distance, target demand, illumination, and patient's posture. The technique is performed by having the patient read words or call out pictures that are arranged around a central hole in a card attached to the examiner's retinoscope. An estimate of the magnitude of the motion is made, and monocular lenses are then interposed until the lag of accommodation is neutralized. The lenses are interposed only briefly, so there is only minimal interference with the habitual accommodative response. The normal range of accommodative lag expected for 5- to 12-year-olds is plano to +0.75 D (97). If the lag value is greater than +0.75 D, efforts should be made to rule out (latent) hyperopia and ocular or systemic pathology, accommodative/convergence imbalances, subnormal accommodation, and medication-induced effects. If the lag values are negative, spasm of accommodation or accommodation-convergence imbalance should be ruled out as the cause. MEM retinoscopy results often provide useful objective information that influences prescribing decisions (55, 96). In addition, Bieber (10) has suggested that dynamic retinoscopy could be used to monitor accommodative response during amplitude and facility testing, thus eliminating the need for subjective responses. This would be especially helpful with nonverbal and mildly mentally retarded patients.

By age 4 or 5 years, the subjective testing of accommodative amplitude on a large percentage of children can be accomplished by either Donder's push-up method (25) or the minus lens method (101). Donder's method involves moving a finely detailed target toward the spectacle plane until the target blurs. A slight modification, which we have found helpful, involves first pushing the target to the point of first blur then pushing it up to spectacle plane and slowly withdrawing it until the child can first identify the letter or picture. This point is recorded as the accommodative amplitude. Duane (26) established normative data for children 10 years and older; later Wold (115) presented data for 6- to 10-year-olds. Based on Duane's data, Hofstetter (53) developed formulas to predict the expected range of accommodative amplitude at different ages. The minimum formula ($D = 15 - 0.25$ age in years) has been used extensively as a clinical guideline. Sheard (101) pointed out a number of problems with the push-up method, such as increased visual angle of the approaching target, and suggested that the minus lens method would provide a more accurate measure. Wold (115), and later Woodruff (117), provided normative data for children 3 to 11 years. The minus lens method values are consistently lower than those of the push-up method, which stresses the importance of referring to appropriate normative data.

The subjective evaluation of accommodative lag using the cross-cylinder method is difficult before age of six or seven. In addition, there is some concern about the procedure's validity in prepresbyopes. We prefer to use dynamic retinoscopy (MEM), regardless of the child's age, to evaluate accommodative lag. The reliable evaluation of accommodative facility starts at approximately 7 years of age. A number of studies have established normative values for different age groups (99, 120), and a strong link has been found between these normative values and the prevalence of symptoms (51, 71).

Evaluation of Ocular Health

The strategy for examining the ocular health of a child is to systematically evaluate the anterior and posterior segments to ensure normal growth, health, development, and functional status of the ocular structures (see Chap. 14). Although the examination strategy is essentially the same as for an adult patient, the actual task of evaluating a young patient's ocular health, especially of the internal structures, is often the practitioner's greatest challenge. The importance of a comprehensive evaluation of ocular health cannot be over emphasized. In certain cases the diagnosis of an ocular disease or developmental anomaly may help account for other presenting conditions (e.g., strabismus, reduced visual acuity), or it may signal a sight- or life-threatening condition that requires immediate referral. In most cases the evaluation of ocular health is left until the end of the examination, at which time the examiner has established rapport with the child, which lessens the threat from the bright lights and proximity of the examiner to the child's face.

Evaluation of Anterior Segment

The evaluation of ocular health starts the moment the patient enters the examination room and is done concurrently with other confrontation procedures. The optometrist surveys the anterior segment visually—orbital size, shape, and position; lid position, appearance, and action; lash position and appearance; scleral and conjunctival color and vascular appearance; corneal size and clarity; iris appearance and color; anterior chamber depth and clarity, and general appearance of the lens.

With infants and toddlers, who are generally too small and uncooperative to sit before a slit lamp, a penlight or transilluminator combined with a hand-held magnifier allow the optometrist to do a fairly complete evaluation of the anterior segment. The preschool child will usually cooperate in a slit-lamp examination, either sitting on the parent's lap or standing on the examination chair footrest. Often a hand-held slit lamp is useful, especially for the exceptional or handicapped child. The optometrist should be able to follow his normal slit lamp routine with school-aged children.

In addition to observation it is useful to palpate the lid and orbital area to detect any subtle orbital, lid, or lacrimal system abnormalities. Lid eversion is suggested when a child presents with red, irritated eyes or when eye rubbing or excessive blinking is reported. For children who present with unequal fissure size, exophthalmometry is recommended. Pupil function (direct, consensual, accommodative, and afferent pupil integrity) should be evaluated in each patient. Infant pupils are typically miotic and do not reach normal size and function until about 6 months of age, when the dilator muscle develops fully.

Evaluation of Posterior Segment

The posterior segment should be evaluated grossly during such procedures as retinoscopy or Hirschberg or Bruckner tests. Obvious lenticular or vitreal opacities and developmental anomalies or gross retinal disease (e.g., retinoblastoma) may be observed as a distorted red reflex. Ophthalmoscopy then allows the optometrist to inspect clarity of vitreous; optic disc color, cup-to-disc ratio, depth and vascular topography; retinal background color and appearance; retinal vascular topography, tortuosity, and arterial/venous ratio; macular color and appearance.

The problem with children is not necessarily the size of their pupils; often it is commanding sustained attention and fixation stability to allow an adequate evaluation of the retina. This is especially problematic when performing direct ophthalmoscopy, whereas the large field of view afforded with a monocular indirect (MIO) or binocular indirect ophthalmoscope (BIO) through a dilated pupil reduces the impact of poor fixation. The large retinal view during BIO allows evaluation of the optic nerve head and macula while the child fixates the light, something almost all children enjoy doing. The BIO also allows a greater distance between observer and patient, making the internal examination less threatening than with direct ophthalmoscopy. During the examination it is wise to keep the BIO light only as bright as necessary. Gentle separation of the lids is often essential; direction of gaze is controlled by targets held by an assistant or parent. The patient should be given constant encouragement and reassurance during the procedure. Often the child has undergone cycloplegia to investigate the refractive component, and the addition of MIO or BIO requires little additional time.

With all ophthalmoscopy procedures the trick is to command steady fixation, if only for brief periods. Infants less than 6 months of age are usually easy to examine lying supine on the parent's lap (Fig. 7.17). Children between 1 and 3 years of age present the greatest challenge. Children older than three can usually be persuaded to play games, which helps to promote attention and steady fixation. Fixation toys or stuffed animals can be held by parents. Older children can count the number of fingers mom is holding up, describe the action in a projected cartoon, or fixate cartoon posters in the upper corners of the room. Children enjoy performing little jobs for the doctor, for example, "Watch the cat's mouth and tell me if he sticks out his tongue" promotes accurate fixation. Telling the child that you are going to look in his eyes to see how good a job he is doing promotes prolonged attention.

If the optometrist cannot get an adequate view of the fundus and there is reason for concern, such as strabismus, monocular or bilateral reduced visual acuity, or other signs and symptoms suggestive of reduced vision, then the optometrist has two choices: consult with a general medical practitioner about the concern and the need for an examination of the fundus under sedation or refer to a pediatric ophthalmologist for a fundus evaluation under sedation or general anesthesia.

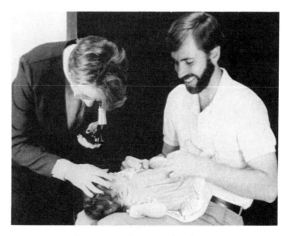

Figure 7.17 Supine position of infant for ophthalmoscopy.

Electrodiagnostic Evaluation

In certain cases, referral for electrodiagnostic testing helps the optometrist make the diagnosis. The electroretinogram (ERG) is an objective electrophysiologic test that measures the retina's functional reaction to light and is dependent on the existence of intact receptor cells. It is especially helpful when an infant or young child presents with congenital nystagmus of unknown cause. ERG responses help to identify whether Leber's congenital amaurosis, achromatopsia, or congenital stationary night blindness may be the cause. The ERG is also recommended for persons who are suspected of having tapetoretinal degeneration or who have a family history of retinitis pigmentosa.

VEP and VER have already been presented as a possible objective refraction method and a useful clinical test for estimating visual acuity. The VEP is also a useful objective diagnostic procedure for evaluating (primarily) macular function at the level of the visual cortex. For patients suspected of having cortical blindness or amblyopia or who are visually impaired, the VEP helps determine whether optic nerve pathway transmission anomalies account for the reduced visual function.

Tonometry

On children under age 5 or 6 years, tonometry is seldom accomplished reliably without sedation. Cooperation for standard clinical applanation tonometry (e.g., Goldmann Applanation Tonometry) is difficult to obtain before 8 or 10 years of age. New hand-held applanation instruments have increased the percentage of testable children, especially those with physical and mental impairments. Noncontact tonometry is often an effective alternative to applanation techniques for the school-aged population. The routine evaluation of IOP without accompanying signs and symptoms is usually not performed until the teenage years.

For an infant, toddler, or preschooler who presents with signs and symptoms suggestive of congenital or early-onset glaucoma (enlarged corneal diameter, hazy cornea, asymmetric cups, ocular or systemic anomalies that have a predilection to cause glaucoma), referral for evaluation of IOP under sedation or general anesthesia is recommended.

Visual Field Screening

Standard perimetric techniques are useful with school-aged children. They can be tested with the standard confrontation methods with a self-illuminated wand. They also respond well to tangent screen evaluations. In both of these tests, the perimetrist should work quickly, giving verbal reinforcement throughout to help the child maintain attention and fixation. The newly available visual field analyzers so closely simulate computer games that children are often eager to participate in testing. The optometrist should be prepared for more time-consuming testing, as attention wanes, resulting in more frequent loss of fixation.

Variations of confrontation field testing are generally recommended for younger children and infants. The optometrist can use a "refixational" technique for screening hemiretinal integrity in infants. Cute toys, stuffed animals, or the examiner's face can be used as the initial central fixation target. Miniature toys or pencil-toppers can be placed on the end of a black pencil or plastic knitting needle to serve as the peripherally presented target. The examiner knows when the target has been moved from a unsighted to a sighted field when one of the following behaviors is observed: a shift in fixation, head movement toward the target, pointing toward the target, or a change in facial expression of a young infant.

Preschool children who can count or play the mimicking game can have hemiretinal and quadrant integrity tested. In a modified confrontation method, the examiner holds his hand in the visual field to be tested presenting a certain number of fingers, while the child maintains fixation on the examiner's face. The child either holds up or reports the number of fingers presented.

In field testing it is important to remember that children vary tremendously in their responses. The optometrist can help confirm that a visual field defect may be present by observing the child's attempt to navigate an obstacle course, by observing the child collecting toys, blocks, or beads spread on the floor, or by obtaining observations of parents and others about the child's day-to-day behavior. The diagnosis of visual field defects of young infants and children is possible and the rewards of the examination are considerable.

Color Vision Screening (see Chap. 19)

Color vision deficiencies should be identified as early as possible in a child's life. This is particularly desirable because elementary sequencing and math concepts often employ color coding. A color deficient child could be erroneously labeled learning disabled or wrongly accused of laziness or carelessness (28). Furthermore, these color vision tests can be useful adjuncts in the differential diagnosis of ocular disease.

The Ishihara Color Test for Children is a pseudoisochromatic test that uses either a circle or a square as the test pattern. Preschool children can either name or trace over the pattern (see Fig. 7.18). If a child makes errors

on these plates, more diagnostic color vision testing may be considered.

The City University Color Vision Test consists of 10 test plates. The targets are four colored paper chips arranged in a diamond shape around a central test dot. The child is asked to select the dot in the surrounding diamond that is closest in color to the center dot. The child can point to the dot, being careful not to touch it, or can call out top, bottom, right, or left. The pattern of errors made allows for a quantitative diagnosis of the color deficiency.

The Isihara test provides the examiner with a very quick screening test which is applicable with children of a wide range of abilities. The City University Test allows quick diagnosis (except for anomalous trichromats, see Chap. 19) of the extent of the color vision defect and does not depend on the child's capacity to order items sequentially, as is necessary, for example, in the D-15 Color Test.

Developmental Visual Perceptual-Motor Screening

As a primary entry point into the health care system, optometry has expanded its scope to screen for medical conditions. Screening for developmental lags or developmental-perceptual lags is one area in which the optometrist can serve the child by detecting a significant deviation or lag that may be treated or that demands referral to other professionals (see Chap. 21). The importance of screening for these skills is evidenced in the correlation between visual processing, readiness, and reading in elementary years (98, 107). The optometrist should use screenings tests that are efficient in time, space, equipment, and personnel (94).

The Denver Developmental Screening Test (DDST) is a valid reliable instrument for use with children under the age of 5 years. It allows the examiner to survey key developmental skills that are expected for the patient's age in categories of personal-social, fine motor adaptive, gross motor, and lan-

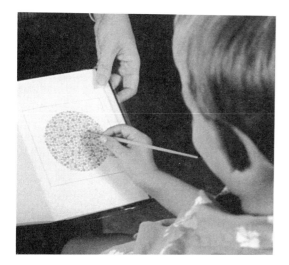

Figure 7.18   Patient tracing pattern on Ishihara Color Test for Children.

guage (see Fig. 7.19). Criteria for administering and scoring each skill within each category are clearly defined. Testing is individual for each child and depends on the child's abilities (78). Skills that a child is expected to have mastered (passed by 90 percent of children at that chronological age) but fails are considered delays. The presence of delays is the feature on which the screening is finally judged as normal, abnormal, or questionable.

The advantages of the DDST include the following: The child's age is corrected for prematurity, if necessary. It covers a wide range of skills, has an easy to use direction and recording form, and would fit the time constraints of most practices. These features make the DDST a valuable clinical tool.

With children 4 or 5 years of age, a more focused and sophisticated evaluation of visual perceptual motor skills can be accomplished. The screening battery should be broad enough to detect deficiencies that are likely to be related to the signs and symptoms of this age group. For example, four standardized tests were selected by the faculty of the Southern California College of Optometry Pediatric Service to comprise the SCCO Modified Visual Perceptual Screener (SCCO Modified). These tests were chosen for their speed, ease of administration, reliability, and repeatability in this age group. The skills tested at this age are laterality and directionality, visual perception, visual motor integration, and auditory discrimination.

The Piaget Right-Left Awareness Test provides the examiner with a consistent sequence of questions to investigate the child's capabilities in identifying his own right and left (laterality), those of another person, and the directional placement of inanimate objects (directionality; see Chap. 21). Visual perception is screened by use of the Motor Free Visual Perceptual Test (MVPT). To screen visual discrimination, visual figure-ground, visual memory, and visual closure, 36 multiple-choice test targets are presented, one at a time, to the child. Subtests include a demonstration item, and specific instructions are provided for the examiner. The number of correct items is tallied and compared to

age norms to determine an age-equivalent score. The Developmental Test of Visual Motor Integration (VMI) is used to test visual motor integrative skill. This test provides up to 24 test figures, which the child is requested to accurately duplicate. Testing is terminated when three consecutive figures are not completed correctly according to the provided guidelines. The number of correct figures is compared to norms to determine an age-equivalent score. The final test of the SCCO Modified is the Wepman Auditory Discrimination Test. The child is faced away from the optometrist, then the examiner recites 40 pairs of words. Following each pair the child reports whether the words sounded the same or different. A tally of errors is kept and used to convert to an age-equivalent score.

Once the practitioner is familiar with the administration, recording, and scoring of these tests the SCCO Modified can be completed quickly and a profile of the child's age-equivalent ability will begin to emerge.

Many tests are available to screen and quantify visuoperceptual development (106). These have been selected for their simplicity, speed, and effectiveness. The strategy is to survey significant visual processing skills to identify children who are at risk. If the optometrist does not routinely screen for perceptual motor development, these tests comprise a battery that can be used for children who present with signs or symptoms of possible perceptual motor problems.

Case Presentation

The successful conclusion of a pediatric examination rests heavily on the optometrist's ability to communicate the results and recommendations to the parent. In our experience, case presentation is the most critical part of the examination (see Chap. 23). The optometrist needs to spend adequate time outlining the child's visual problems, sequence of therapy and addressing the parent's questions and concerns. If parents leave the examination feeling unsure what the problem is, their confidence in the doctor and compliance with the prescribed treatment will suffer.

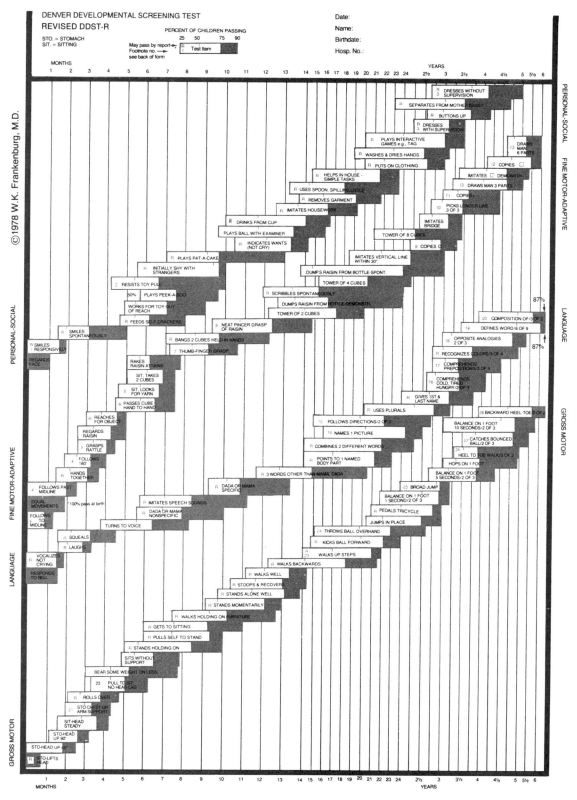

Figure 7.19 Denver Developmental Screening Test response sheet.

A successful presentation should outline the child's status in each of the major diagnostic areas listed in Table 7.1. The optometrist should explain all major conditions that represent current problems or that could cause problems in the future. If medical terms to describe the condition are used, follow-up with simplified explanations using lay terms and analogies to daily life is critical. The use of medical jargon is probably one of the major frustrations that parents have with health care providers. It is also very helpful to use line drawings, photos, and models to show parents the condition in concrete terms. It is also helpful to follow up the presentation with pamphlets on the condition that the parent can take home.

Once the parent has a reasonable understanding of the condition, it is important to specify the management options, highlighting the advantages and disadvantages of each approach. This fulfills the optometrist's responsibility of obtaining informed consent, allowing the parent to make a decision based on the complete picture of available options. Once a treatment path is selected the optometrist should outline the anticipated treatment sequence. This prepares the parent for what is coming and avoids surprises (for example the need to change a prescription). Scheduling a follow-up visit immediately emphasizes the importance of continuous care. The optometrist should encourage the parent to call if any additional questions arise. In certain cases it is advisable to follow up the presentation with a summary of the child's condition in a letter that sets forth the recommended treatment and comments on how, for example, the condition might affect development or school performance.

Finally, the optometrist should recall the chief complaint and primary concerns and fears elicited during the case history. All parents have basic fears about their child's vision (e.g., Will he have to wear glasses forever?). The optometrist needs to relate to the emotional concerns of the parent. The risk, if this is not accomplished, is that the parent may continue to search for a doctor who addresses this need. Whether vision problems are discovered or not, parents should be informed about the dynamic nature of vision during the early years and the importance of regularly scheduled subsequent examinations.

REFERENCES

1. Amos CS: Ocular disease in the pediatric patient. South J Optom 20(4):14, 1978 and 20(5):8, 1978.

2. Amos JF: The problem-solving approach to patient care. In Amos JF (ed): Diagnosis and Management in Vision Care. Boston, Butterworths, 1, 1987.

3. Apgar V: Evaluation of the newborn infant; second report. JAMA 168:1985, 1958.

4. Apgar V: A proposal for a new method of evaluation of the newborn infant. Curr Res Anesth Analg 52:260, 1953.

5. Apt L, Henrich A: Pupillary dilation with single eyedrop mydriatic combinations. Am J Ophthalmol 89:553, 1980.

6. Atkinson J, Braddick OJ, Ayling L, et al: Isotropic photorefraction: A new method for refractive testing of infants. In Maffei I (ed): Pathophysiology of the Visual System. Documenta Ophthalmologica Proceedings Series, vol. 30. Boston, The Hague, 217, 1981.

7. Atkinson J, Braddick OJ, Durden K, et al: Screening for refractive errors in 6–9 month-old infants by photorefraction. Br J Ophthalmol 68:105, 1984.

8. Banks MS: The development of visual accommodation during early infancy. Child Dev 51:646, 1980.

9. Barresi BJ: Problem orientation. In: Barresi BJ (ed): Ocular Assessment. Boston, Butterworths, 3, 1984.

10. Bieber JC: Why nearpoint retinoscopy with children? Optom Weekly 65:54, 1974 and 65:78, 1974.

11. Bobier WR: Quantitative photorefraction using an off center flash source. Am J Optom Physiol Opt 65:962, 1988.

12. Borghi RA, Rouse MW: Comparison of refraction obtained by "near retinoscopy" and retinoscopy under cycloplegia. Am J Optom Physiol Opt 62:169, 1985.

13. Borish IM: Clinical Refraction. Chicago, Professional Press, 149, 1970.

14. Braddick O, Atkinson J, French J, et al: A photorefractive study of infant accommodation. Vision Res 19:1319, 1979.

15. Brookman KE: Ocular accommodation in human infants. Am J Optom Physiol Opt 60:91, 1983.

16. Brookman KE: A retinoscopic method of assessing accommodative performance of young human infants. J Am Optom Assoc 52:865, 1981.

17. Ciner EB, Scheiman MM, Schanel-Klitsch E, et al: Stereopsis testing in 18- to 35-month-old children using operant preferential looking. Optom Vis Sci 66:782, 1989.

18. Cooper J, Feldman J: Operant conditioning and assessment of stereopsis in young children. Am J Optom Physiol Opt 55:532, 1978.

19. Cooper J, Feldman J, Medlin D: Comparing stereoscopic performance of children using the Titmus, TNO, and Randot stereo tests. J Am Optom Assoc 50:821, 1979.

20. Costenbader FD: Infantile esotropia. Trans Am Ophthalmol Soc 59:367, 1961.

21. Day SH, Norcia AM: Photographic detection of amblyogenic factors. Ophthalmology 93:25, 1986.

22. Dayton GO, Jones MH, Aiu P, et al: Developmental study of coordinated eye movements in the human infant. I. Visual acuity in the newborn human: A study based on induced optokinetic nystagmus recorded by electro-oculography. Arch Ophthalmol 71:865, 1964.

23. Dobson V, Teller DY: Visual acuity in human infants: A review and comparison of behavioral and electrophysiological studies. Vision Res 18:1469, 1978.

24. Dobson V, Teller DY, Lee CP, et al: A behavioral method for efficient screening of visual acuity in young infants. I. Preliminary laboratory development. Invest Ophthalmol Vis Sci 17:1142, 1978.

25. Duane A: An attempt to determine the normal range of accommodation at various ages. Trans Am Ophthalmol Soc 11:634, 1908.

26. Duane A: Studies in monocular and binocular accommodation with their clinical applications. Am J Ophthalmol 5:865, 1922.

27. Duffy FH, Rengstorff RH: Ametropia measurements from the visual evoked response. Am J Optom Arch Am Acad Optom 48:717, 1971.

28. Espinda SD: Color vision deficiency: A learning disability? J Learn Disab 6:163, 1973.

29. Evans E: Refraction in children using the RX1 auto-refractor. Br J Orthop 41:46, 1984.

30. Fantz RL: Pattern vision in young infants. Psychol Rev 8:43, 1958.

31. Fantz RL, Ordy JM, Udelf MS: Maturation of pattern vision in infants during the first six months. J Comp Physiol Psychol 55:907, 1962.

32. Faye EE: A new visual acuity test for partially sighted nonreaders. J Pediatr Ophthalmol 5:210, 1968.

33. Fox R: Stereopsis in human infants. Science 207:323, 1980.

34. Frisby JP, Mein J, Saye A, et al: Use of random-dot stereograms in the clinical assessment of strabismic patients. Br J Ophthalmol 59:545, 1975.

35. Gilman G, Gottfried AW: Development of stereopsis in infants and young children. J Am Optom Assoc 56:878, 1985.

36. Gorman JJ, Cogan DG, Gellis SS: An apparatus for grading the visual acuity of infants on the basis of opticokinetic nystagmus. Pediatrics 19:1088, 1957.

37. Greenspan SB, Weisz CL: Psychological factors in pediatric optometry. J Am Optom Assoc 48:79, 1977.

38. Griffin J, Boyer FM: Strabismus measurement with the Hirschberg test. Optom Weekly 65:863, 1974.

39. Griffin JR: Screening for anomalies of binocular vision by means of the Polaroid mirror method. Am J Optom Arch Am Acad Optom 48:689, 1971.

40. Griffin JR: Binocular Anomalies: Procedures for Vision Therapy. Chicago, Professional Press, 12, 54, 97, 142, 399, 1982.

41. Griffin JR, Cotter SA: The Brückner test: Evaluation of clinical usefulness. Am J Optom Physiol Opt 63:957, 1986.

42. Grosvenor TP: The patient history. In: Primary Care Optometry: A Clinical Manual. Chicago, Professional Press, 75, 1982.

43. Gruber J, Dickey P, Rosner J: Comparison of a modified (two-item) Frisby with the standard Frisby and Random-Dot E stereotests when used with preschool children. Am J Optom Physiol Opt 62:349, 1985.

44. Gwiazda J, Brill S, Mohindra I, et al: Preferential looking acuity in infants from two to fifty-eight weeks of age. Am J Optom Physiol Opt 57:428, 1980.

45. Harter MR, White CT: Effects of contour sharpness and check size on visually evoked cortical potentials. Vision Res 8:701, 1968.

46. Hay SH, Kerr JH, Jayroe Jr RR, et al: Retinal reflex photometry as a screening device for amblyopia and preamblyopic states in children. South Med J 76:309, 1983.

47. Haynes HM: Clinical observations with dynamic retinoscopy. Optom Weekly 51:2243, 1960.

48. Haynes HM, White BL, Held R: Visual accommodation in human infants. Science 148:528, 1965.

49. Held R, Birch E, Gwiazda J: Stereoacuity of human infants. Proc Natl Acad Sci USA 77:5572, 1980.

50. Helveston EM, Pachtman MA, Cadera W, et al: Clinical evaluation of the Nidek AR auto refractor. J Pediatr Ophthalmol Strabismus 21:227, 1984.

51. Hennessey D, Iosue RA, Rouse MW: Relation of symptoms to accommodative infacility in school-aged children. Am J Optom Physiol Opt 61:177, 1984.

52. Hoffman LG, Rouse MW: Referral recommendations for binocular function and/or developmental perceptual deficiencies. J Am Optom Assoc 51:119, 1980.

53. Hofstetter HW: Useful age-amplitude formula. Optom World 38(12):42, 1950.

54. Howland HC, Howland B: Photorefraction: a technique for study of refractive state at a distance. J Opt Soc Am 64:240, 1974.

55. Hutter RF, Rouse MW: Visually related headache in a preschooler. Am J Optom Physiol Opt 61:711, 1984.

56. Ingram RM: Refraction as a basis for screening children for squint and amblyopia. Br J Ophthalmol 61:8, 1977.

57. Ingram RM, Walker C: Refraction as a means of predicting squint or amblyopia in preschool siblings of children known to have these defects. Br J Ophthalmol 63:238, 1979.

58. Irvine SR: A simple test for binocular fixation: Clinical application useful in the appraisal of ocular dominance, amblyopia ex anopsia, minimal strabismus, and malingering. Am J Ophthalmol 27:740, 1944.

59. Jampolsky A: The prism test for strabismus screening. J Pediatr Ophthalmol 1:30, 1964.

60. Johnstone R, Brown S: A comparative assessment of the Lang, TNO, and Titmus stereo tests. Aust Orthop J 22:27, 1985.

61. Jones R, Eskridge JB: The Hirschberg test—A re-evaluation. Am J Optom Arch Am Acad Optom 47:105, 1970.

62. Kaakinen K: A simple method for screening of children with strabismus, anisometropia or ametropia by simultaneous photography of the corneal and the fundus reflexes. Acta Ophthalmol (Copenh) 57:161, 1979.

63. Kaakinen K, Tommila V: A clinical study on the detection of strabismus, anisometropia or ametropia of children by simultaneous photography of the corneal and the fundus reflexes. Acta Ophthalmol (Copenh) 57:600, 1979.

64. Kastenbaum SM, Caden BW, Greenspan SB: Relationship between binocularity and bilaterality. J Am Optom Assoc 45:596, 1974.

65. Kirschen DG, Rosenbaum AL, Ballard EA: The dot visual acuity test—A new acuity test for children. J Am Optom Assoc 54:1055, 1983.

66. Koch PS: An aid for the diagnosis of a vertical muscle paresis. J Pediatr Ophthalmol Strabismus 17:272, 1980.

67. Krimsky E: The binocular examination of the young child. Am J Ophthalmol 26:624, 1943.

68. Kuroda N, Adachi-Usami E: Evaluation of pattern visual evoked cortical potentials for prescribing spectacles in mentally retarded infants and children. Doc Ophthalmol 66:253, 1987.

69. Lang J: A new stereotest. J Pediatr Ophthalmol Strabismus 20:72, 1983.

70. Lang JI, Lang TJ: Eye screening with the Lang Stereotest. Am Orthop J 38:48, 1988.

71. Levine S, Ciuffreda KJ, Selenow A, et al: Clinical assessment of accommodative facility in symptomatic and asymptomatic individuals. J Am Optom Assoc 56:286, 1985.

72. London R: Optokinetic nystagmus: a review of pathways, techniques and selected diagnostic applications. J Am Optom Assoc 53:791, 1982.

73. Lovasik JV, Woodruff ME: Increasing diagnostic potential in pediatric optometry by electrophysiological methods. Can J Optom 45:69, 1983.

74. Ludlam WM, Meyers RR: The use of visual evoked responses in objective refraction. Trans NY Acad Sci 34:154, 1972.

75. Maino JH, Cibis GW, Cress P, et al: Noncycloplegic vs cycloplegic retinoscopy in preschool children. Ann Ophthalmol 16:880, 1984.

76. Marg E, Freeman DN, Peltzman P, et al: Visual acuity development in human infants: Evoked potential measurements. Invest Ophthalmol 15:150, 1976.

77. Mayer DL, Dobson V: Visual acuity development in infants and young children as assessed by operant preferential looking. Vision Res 22:1141, 1982.

78. Miller LJ, Sprong TA: Psychometric and qualitative comparison of four preschool screening instruments. J Learn Disabl 19:480, 1986.

79. Millodot M, Newton I: VEP measurement of the amplitude of accommodation. Br J Ophthalmol 65:294, 1981.

80. Millodot M, Riggs LA: Refraction determined electrophysiologically: Responses to alternation of visual contours. Arch Ophthalmol 84:272, 1970.

81. Mohindra I: A technique for infant vision examination. Am J Optom Physiol Opt 52:867, 1975.

82. Mohindra I: Near retinoscopy—An objective noncycloplegic refraction technique. Optom Monthly 71:28, 1980.

83. Mohindra I, Molinari JF: Near retinoscopy and cycloplegic retinoscopy in early primary grade schoolchildren. Am J Optom Physiol Opt 56:34, 1979.

84. Mohindra I: Comparison of "near retinoscopy" and subjective refraction in adults. Am J Optom Physiol Opt 54:319, 1977.

85. Morgan KS, Johnson WD: Clinical evaluation of a commercial photorefractor. Arch Ophthalmol 105:1528, 1987.

86. Owens DA, Mohindra I, Held R: The effectiveness of a retinoscope beam as an accommodative stimulus. Invest Ophthalmol Vis Sci 19:942, 1980.

87. Parks MM: Isolated cyclovertical muscle palsy. Arch Ophthalmol 60:1027, 1958.

88. Parks MM: Ocular motility diagnosis. In Apt L (ed): Diagnostic Procedures in Pediatric Ophthalmology. Boston, Little Brown, 115, 1963.

89. Pickwell D: Communication with children. Optom Today (Lond) 27:322, 1987.

90. Regan D: Rapid objective refraction using evoked brain potentials. Invest Ophthalmol 12:669, 1973.

91. Richman JE, Petito GT, Cron MT: Broken wheel acuity test: A new and valid test for preschool and exceptional children. J Am Optom Assoc 55:561, 1984.

92. Romano PE, von Noorden GK: Atypical responses to the four-diopter prism test. Am J Ophthalmol 67:935, 1969.

93. Rosenbaum AL, Bateman JB, Bremer DL, et al: Cycloplegic refraction in esotropic children: Cyclopentolate versus atropine. Ophthalmology 88:1031, 1981.

94. Rosner J: Question #8: Is the patient's developmental status appropriate for his age. In: Pediatric Optometry. Boston, Butterworth, 275, 1982.

95. Rouse MW, London R, Allen DC: An evaluation of the monocular estimate method of dynamic retinoscopy. Am J Optom Physiol Opt 59:234, 1982.

96. Rouse MW, Polte L: Accommodative involvement with Adie's pupil. Am J Optom Physiol Opt 61:54, 1984.

97. Rouse MW, Hutter RF, Shiftlett R: A normative study of the accommodative lag in elementary school children. Am J Optom Physiol Opt 61:693, 1984.

98. Satz P, Sparrow S: Specific developmental dyslexia: A theoretical reformulation. In

Bakker DJ, Satz P (eds): Specific Reading Disability: Advances in Theory and Method. Rotterdam, Rotterdam University Press, 17, 1970.

99. Scheiman M, Herzberg H, Frantz K, et al: Normative study of accommodative facility in elementary schoolchildren. Am J Optom Physiol Opt 65:127, 1988.

100. Scheiman M, Herzberg H, Frantz K, et al: A normative study of step vergence in elementary school children. J Am Optom Assoc 60:276, 1989.

101. Sheard C: Dynamic Ocular Tests. The Sheard Volume. Philadelphia, Chilton, 93, 1957.

102. Sheedy JE: Fixation disparity analysis of oculomotor imbalance. Am J Optom Physiol Opt 57:632, 1980.

103. Sheedy JE, Saladin JJ: Phoria, vergence, and fixation disparity in oculomotor problems. Am J Optom Physiol Opt 54:474, 1977.

104. Sheedy JE, Saladin JJ: Association of symptoms with measures of oculomotor deficiencies. Am J Optom Physiol Opt 55:670, 1978.

105. Sokol S: Visually evoked potentials: Theory, techniques and clinical applications. Surv Ophthalmol 21:18, 1976.

106. Solan HA, Groffman S: Understanding and treating developmental and perceptual motor disabilities. In Solan HA (ed): The Treatment and Management of Children with Learning Disabilities. Springfield IL, Charles C Thomas, 168, 1982.

107. Solan HA, Mozlin R: The correlations of perceptual-motor maturation to readiness and reading in kindergarten and the primary grades. J Am Optom Assoc 57:28, 1986.

108. Spafford MM, Lovasik JV, Holterman JA: Modification of cortical activity by low plus lenses. Am J Optom Physiol Opt 60:535, 1983.

109. Tongue AC, Cibis GW: Bruckner Test. Ophthalmology 88:1041, 1981.

110. Weed LL: Medical records that guide and teach. N Engl J Med 278:593, 1968.

111. Weed LL: Medical Records, Medical Education and Patient Care. Cleveland, Case Western Reserve, 1969.

112. Wesson MD: Normalization of prism bar vergences. Am J Optom Physiol Opt 59:628, 1982.

113. Wick B, Hall P: Relation among accommodative facility, lag, and amplitude in elementary school children. Am J Optom Physiol Opt 64:593, 1987.

114. Wick B, London R: The Hirschberg Test: Analysis from birth to age 5. J Am Optom Assoc 51:1009, 1980.

115. Wold RM: The spectacle amplitude of accommodation of children aged six to ten. Am J Optom Arch Am Acad Optom 44:642, 1967.

116. Woodruff ME: A preventive approach to vision care emphasizing detection and treatment in early life. J Am Optom Assoc 46:997, 1975.

117. Woodruff ME: Ocular accommodation in children aged 3 to 11 years. Can J Optom 49:141, 1987.

118. Wright KW, Edelman PM, Walonker F, et al: Reliability of fixation preference testing in diagnosing amblyopia. Arch Ophthalmol 104:549, 1986.

119. Wright KW, Walonker F, Edelman P: 10-Diopter fixation test for amblyopia. Arch Ophthalmol 99:1242, 1981.

120. Zellers JA, Alpert TL, Rouse MW: A review of the literature and a normative study of accommodative facility. J Am Optom Assoc 55:31, 1984.

SOURCE LIST

1. Broken Wheel Visual Acuity Test, City University Color Vision Test, Exophthalmometers, Frisby Stereo Test, Hand-Held Slit Lamp, Ishihara Color Test for Children, Klein Keratoscope, Lang Stereo Test.
Haag-Streit Services, Inc, 7 Industrial Park, Waldwick, NJ 07463.

2. Denver Developmental Screening Test. LADOCA Publishing Foundation, 5100 Lincoln Street, Denver, CO 80216.

3. Dot Visual Acuity Test, HOTV Visual Acuity Test.
Good-Lite Co, 1540 Hannah Ave, Forest Park, IL 60130.

4. Four-Rack Retinoscopy Lens Rack.
Bernell Corporation, 750 Lincolnway East, P.O. Box 4637, South Bend, IN 46634.

5. Luneau loose prism set. Opticokinetic drums, Prism Bar, Random Dot E Screening Test, Randot Stereo Tests, Single-rack retinoscopy lens rack.
Keeler Instruments, 456 Parkway Ave, Broomall, PA 19008.

6. LightHouse Flash Card Test.
LightHouse Low Vision Services, New York Association for the Blind, 111 E 59th Street, New York, NY 10022.

7. Motor Free Visual Perception Test, Developmental Test of Visual Motor Integration.
Academic Therapy Publications, 20 Commercial Blvd, Novato, CA 94947-6197.

8. Piaget J: Piaget Right-Left Awareness Test Judgment and Reasoning in the Child.
Rowman, Littlefield & Adams, 81 Adams Dr., Totowa, NJ 07512.

9. PL 20/20 Infant Tester.
Optical Technology Corporation, 515 E 22nd Terrace, Lawrence, KS 66046.

10. Special Three-Character Test, Stereo Fly Test, Stereo Reindeer Test, TNO Stereo Test, Tumbling E Visual Acuity Test.
Cal Coast Ophthalmic Instruments, 20675 South Western Ave, Torrance, CA 90501-1864.

11. Teller Acuity Cards.
VisTech Consultants, Inc, 1372 North Fairfield Road, Dayton, OH 45432.

Chapter 8

Spectacles for Children

Michael H. Cho

Bradford W. Wild

Children pose special optometric challenges, especially when it comes to the prescribing, fitting, and dispensing of spectacles (4). As we become increasingly sensitized to the value of early diagnosis and remediation of vision problems and the importance of regular prophylactic eye care, more and more professional attention is being directed toward children.

Since optometrists have expanded this area of vision care, they have necessarily had to delegate some of the less critical yet time-consuming details of patient care to assistants or technicians. Paraprofessionals are often given responsibility for selecting, fitting, and dispensing spectacle frames and lenses and for maintaining them with periodic adjustments.

In spite of the fact that the most common complaints about optometric services deal with poorly designed and fitted optical appliances, this delegation of care will undoubtedly continue, largely for economic reasons. It therefore behooves optometrists to understand completely the special requirements of children and to make certain that their assistants have the knowledge, skills, and motivation to work with children.

Eye care does not stop at the office door. Parents also are potentially valuable assistants, but they, too, must be adequately informed of procedures and implications. Children do not always reliably report specific problems they may have with their glasses. Instead they may wear them incorrectly or even reject them altogether. Careful observations by the parent may help identify problems. Because parents are probably the major force in ensuring compliance with optometric advice beyond the office, their assistance must be enlisted and they must be trained.

In the first section of this chapter we outline some of the implications that wearing eyeglasses may have for children, with particular attention to the psychological aspects of wearing spectacles. In the second section we discuss the choices and recommendations of optical devices available for child patients.

DIFFERENCES BETWEEN CHILDREN AND ADULTS

Physical Differences

Children's faces are not just adult faces in miniature. Children's faces are not yet fully developed, so care must be taken to select frames that do not restrict growth. For instance, it is probably better to choose frames that fit at the moment (which will be frequently adjusted and then replaced) than frames that the patient must "grow into." Children have relatively small, flat noses and relatively pronounced cheeks. Careful fitting of spectacle bridges is necessary to ensure that the frames rest securely on the nose and not on the cheeks. Without good support spectacles can rest so close to the child's face that the eyelashes touch the lenses. This can be physically bothersome, and the lashes leave oily smears on the lenses.

Children can often tolerate more irritation than adults. Their skin is more flexible and elastic and can withstand more pressure than adults' skin. They seem to adapt rapidly to glasses. It is not clear whether this is due to immature somatosensory development or to an ability for quick sensory adaptation. Even so, optometrists and parents need to check for sores stemming from poorly fitting frames.

Activity Differences

Anyone who has been around toddlers and elementary school children knows how incredibly boisterous and physical their play is. Children are much more active than adults, and their games are more likely to involve toys and physical contact that can damage spectacles. Children are less careful about their glasses, so much more attention should be given to durability, stability, and protection in children's spectacles. Again, choice of frame and lens materials and fit are essential.

Psychological Differences

It may be trite, but it is nonetheless helpful to reiterate that optometrists' patients, youngsters and adults, are persons with psychological characteristics. To ignore the psychology of the patient is to provide incomplete professional care. The basic point is that optometrists and parents should be sensitive to the possibility that eyeglasses can produce social and psychological side effects. With this knowledge, practical strategies for controlling such effects can be devised.

Glasses may have a negative affect on social appeal but may also have a positive effect on task-relevant attributes (5, 6). And wearing glasses may expose the wearer to discomfort in social interactions (1, 9). In America, girls and women are more likely than boys and men to be concerned with the social effects of glasses and may be less subject to the positive aspects of task-relevant attributions (12). This may be one of the reasons why females are much more likely than males to want contact lenses. Glasses may also affect the wearer's identity by lowering self-image (11).

It behooves the optometrist to be certain that the parents understand completely and concur with the reasons for the optical correction and that their expressed attitudes toward the necessity for spectacles are supportive and positive.

OPHTHALMIC MATERIALS

Frames

Plastic
Although the material of most plastic frames is still referred to as zyl, modern frames are made from other materials such as

proprionate, polyamide, carbon fiber graphite, and nylon. Zyl is short for zylonite, a term used for frames made from cellulose nitrate, which is no longer used because the material was flammable. Each material has advantages and disadvantages.

Most frames today are made from cellulose acetate. This plastic is durable, flexible, and heavier than the other materials. These plastic frames have the advantages of being flexible and resiliant to low impact or bumping. The material maintains adjustments and absorbs shock to protect the lenses. These frames generally have few places where the frame can break, although this is not always the case. They are safer because there are rounded edges that will not cut a child.

Plastic frames can easily be repaired or modified by adding nose pads or replacing hinges. These frames come in a wide choice of colors.

A disadvantage is that the material is sensitive to temperature. Hot weather can easily throw the frame out of adjustment, whereas cold weather can cause the frame to become brittle. Over time, most plastic frames fade and discolor and become more and more brittle. The bridge fit must be more accurate, and there are fewer adjustment options than with other materials without modifying the frame.

Proprionate can be handled much like cellulose acetate. It is lighter than cellulose acetate, so frames generally feel lighter to the patient. It has greater flexibility, allowing frames to keep their shape better.

Polyamide is a new generation of nylon material that is becoming more popular. It is strong and flexible. Frames require very little heat to insert lenses. Excessive heat causes the frame to shrink.

Optyl plastic is rigid and lightweight. It has a higher melting point, so these frames are very resistant to bubbling or pitting from salt pans. Optyl has a "memory": when heated the frame returns to its original molded shape. The advantage to this is that the frames maintain their shape even after multiple lens insertions. Common adjustment problems, such as rolled or warped eyewires, are easily reshaped. The disadvantage is that the frames do not maintain their shape after major adjustments. If the frame is reshaped slightly to fit a small lens, it will gradually return to its original size when reheated or left in a warm environment, and as a result the lens will loosen. The same thing will occur if the temples are reshaped. Optyl plastic cannot be shrunk to fit a small lens as can cellulose acetate, and it can easily break if the frame is not heated adequately before bending. This material does not withstand as much impact as other materials and should not be chosen for active children.

Frames made of carbon whisker and graphite have higher tensile strength and are lighter, so frames can be made thinner and lighter than zyl frames and still maintain their shapes. More heat is required for adjustments and lens insertion.

Nylon is usually used for sports frames. It is lighter than zyl. Since it is very flexible, it withstands greater impact. This material is not widely used for dress frames because it is very difficult to adjust. Some companies prefer to use this material for sunglasses.

Metal

Metal frames are made of various alloys electroplated to give them a gold or silver finish. There is a larger variety of colors available than a few years ago because these frames can now be painted with accent colors. Although metal frames are strong, they are inflexible and do not hold adjustments on active children. The frame can be easily bent or twisted if the glasses are bumped.

Most metal frames are available with adjustable nose pads. This is beneficial because of the flat bridges most children have. Adjustable nose pads afford the added advantage of raising or lowering the frame and changing the vertex distance. Formfit or unifit bridges do not fit many children and can lead to most of the weight being borne by a small area of the nose. In addition to adjustment problems, metal frames do not hold up well with active children because the eyewire loosens and lenses fall out as the frame becomes more abused.

Bridge Types

Three types of bridges are available with plastic frames. The first type is a keyhole bridge, so named because it is shaped like a keyhole. It is fitted so there is a clearance between the crest of the nose and the bottom of the bridge of the frame. Many keyhole bridges have fixed nose pads to support the weight of the frame on the sides of the nose.

A saddle bridge has the shape of a saddle. It is designed so that the weight is distributed over the crest of the nose. Fitting this bridge with clearance between the crest of the nose and the bottom of the bridge may put too much weight on the sides of the nose. Saddle bridges do not fit most young children properly. Until their noses develop, children need support at the sides of the bridge.

A modified saddle has the same appearance as a saddle bridge except that it has fixed nose pads. The nose pads give added support on the sides of the nose, so there can be clearance between the crest of the nose and the bridge of the frame. Modified saddle and keyhole bridges with fixed nose pads better fit children's noses because of the added support on the lower sides of the nose.

Universal or unifit bridges are plastic and similar to saddle bridges and are attached to the bridge area of metal frames. They are designed so that weight is distributed over the crest of the nose as well as to the sides. Unless the child has an adequate bridge to support the frame, there are likely to be problems, but if the frame fits correctly, the bridge gives the comfort of a plastic frame.

Adjustable nose pads can provide better support for the weight of the frame, because the nose pads can be adjusted to fit the contour of the child's nose. This is especially useful for children whose nasal bridge is flat. The height of the frame and the vertex distance can be adjusted for the most desirable cosmesis and fit of bifocal heights. Various sizes and types of nose pads are available in hard and soft plastic and silicone. The larger the surface area in contact with the nose, the more widely the weight will be distributed and the more comfortable will be the fit.

Temples

Skull temples are the most common temples available on frames today. They bend behind the ear and follow the contour of the skull. The temple bend should begin 2 to 3 mm behind the crotch of the ear. The temple end piece should extend 3 to 4 cm behind the ear to provide adequate surface contact area behind the ears and against the skull.

Riding bow temples are adjustable plastic temples that curve behind the crotch of the ear to the earlobe. These temples should be 2 to 3 cm longer than skull temples and should be adjusted to exert greatest pressure against the ear rather than the skull.

Comfort cable temples are similar in design to the riding bow temples except that the curved portion that fits around the crotch of the ear is made of flexible, coiled cable. Plastic temple covers can be put on the flexible portions of these temples. Like riding bow temples, these should be 2 to 3 cm longer than the skull temples.

Elastic-banded temples have a shortened modified shaft to which any elastic adjustable headband is attached. This design resembles that seen on adult sports frames. Some skull temples have a hole at the end of the temple where an elastic band can be attached.

Hinges

Hinges are classified by the total number of barrels when the hinges of the temples and front are interlocked. They consist of three, five, and seven barrels.

In many plastic frame fronts the hinge plate is embedded into the frame front without rivets. These are called hidden hinges because they cannot be seen from the front.

Standard hinges are characterized by a shield on the end piece of the frame front. They are stronger than hidden hinges because rivets run through the frame to secure the hinge plate.

Spring hinges are becoming increasingly popular. These temples flex wider than standard hinges and spring back to their normal positions. Upon impact to the frame, the temple hinge flexes, alleviating stress to the hinge area. This reduces the likelihood of damaging the hinge and endpiece. Spring hinges also provide constant pressure by the temples and reduce the amount of stretching of the frame front endpieces. The problem with spring hinges is that the pressure applied by the temples cannot be increased when needed. As a result, pressure in other areas may need to be increased, and this may lead to pressure points and sore areas. Spring and standard hinges are available on both plastic and metal temples.

Pin hinges are usually found on less expensive sunglass frames. Some sunglass companies use them to reduce the cost of the glasses. A pin hinge is a non-threaded pin or rivet in a three-barrel hinge.

Rimless

Rimless (or semirimless) frames are not recommended for children. Children frequently fall and without a frame to protect the lenses, this can create a safety hazard. The edge of the lenses are sharp and unprotected and can easily cut a child's face on impact. In addition, the lenses can easily chip, leaving an even sharper edge. Chips on lenses also reduce the impact resistance. Rimless frames do not hold lenses as securely as plastic or full metal frames. The lenses are more likely to pop out and injure the child if there is impact.

If a child is given a rimless frame, plastic lenses should be used. Glass lenses are not recommended for rimless or semirimless frames because they are more susceptible to chipping and cracking than plastic lenses. If a child is active, a rimless frame may be a problem because these frames tend to lose their adjustment easier than plastic or full metal frames.

Frame Warranties

Frame warranties are an important consideration in choosing children's frames. Most children are inexperienced in taking care of spectacles and tend to lose or break them. Many frames do not withstand a child's vigorous activity, so if a frame is not warranted, the replacement cost could be quite high. A lifetime warranty may sound good, but most children outgrow their spectacles within a couple of years. So a lifetime warranty becomes a low-risk offer for the manufacturer. A 1- or 2-year warranty may be just as practical in most cases. Conditions of warranties vary. A limited warranty covers any breakage due to a manufacturer's defect. An unlimited warranty covers frame breakage regardless of cause.

Frame Selection

Minimizing adjustment problems begins at the time of frame selection. Thoughtful frame selection can prevent many adjustment problems from ever occurring. All too often patients dictate the selection instead of the optometrist, and the patient may select a frame that is unsuitable. Ultimately, success or failure of the glasses reflects on the optometrist, so frame selection should be directed.

The optometrist should identify any unusual fitting problems and the solutions to these problems. In some instances, modifications may have to be made on the frame to achieve a proper fit. For example, because of children's flat noses and full cheeks, adjustable nose pads may have to be added to prevent the glasses from resting on the cheeks. It is best to know this before the glasses are ordered so adjustments can be made on the measurements.

Frames that are too large should be avoided. Many practitioners believe that children's frames should be large so that the child can grow into them instead of out of them. This should be considered only if the larger frame fits as well as the smaller size and is not optically contraindicated. If the frame is fitted too large, the child may become self-conscious and not want to wear the glasses, or the glasses may be out of adjustment frequently. Children often break or change their glasses before they grow into them anyway, so fitting large may be unnecessary.

Examine the bearing areas when a frame is tried on. The more surface area of the frame in contact with the skin, the more comfortable the fit. Sore spots are caused by excessive pressure in a localized area. If the weight of the frame is spread over a larger area, it is less likely that sore spots will occur. And, again, the frame should not rest on the cheeks.

Styling

A child should always be consulted as well as the parent about his or her preference for certain styles. The patient can be directed to frames that best meet the fitting requirements and allowed to select a frame from this group. No more than two or three frames should be presented at one time, otherwise the child may get confused.

Color should be selected by the child. To make the choice easier, the child may be guided to frame colors that also satisfy the parent. Unless the selection is clearly unsatisfactory, every effort should be made to respect the child's preference.

Children today have nearly as many options on the type of eyewear as adults. Everybody is so fashion conscious that it is not uncommon for a frame to be associated with a famous designer, celebrity, or cartoon character. Although the name has nothing to do with the quality of the frame, it does imply an important concept. Everyone wants to look good in glasses and to keep up with fashion trends. The days of having glasses only to see with are gone. Patients are educated when selecting frames. They look for function, durability, and cosmesis. Most children have one pair of dress frames and use them for everything. Selecting an inappropriate dress frame could be disastrous.

More athletic frames are becoming available for children. With increasing numbers of boys and girls participating in sports, one pair of spectacles may not be enough. Dress frames are not designed to withstand the rigors of most sports. Athletic frames, on the other hand, are not designed primarily for cosmetic appearance and comfort. Parents should be educated in the safest protection for a particular sport for their child.

Athletic frames are designed for protection. They are made of zyl, nylon, and various other plastics. The construction depends on the type of sport for which the frames will be used. Frames for high-impact sports, such as racquetball, will be heavier than those for swimming. Most frames can have prescription lenses inserted or they can be adapted to hold prescription lenses. Frames used in contact sports usually have sponge rubber pads.

Lenses

Materials

There are various lens materials available today with different refractive indices. The higher the refractive index, the flatter the curves needed to produce a given prescription. While this reduces the edge thickness of the lens, it may also, unfortunately, increase the various aberrations. Because of the way lenses can be surfaced, the effect is seen more with high minus prescriptions than with high plus prescriptions. It should be remembered that because children use smaller eyesizes, edge thickness will not be as apparent as in an adult's prescription.

CR-39, with an index of 1.498, is the most commonly used lens material. In addition to its availability in various powers and lens types, it is compatible with most tints and coatings. Since it has the lowest refractive index of all lens materials, it is also the thickest.

Among the various high-index plastics currently on the market, polycarbonate (index of refraction, 1.586) is especially well-known for its impact resistance. Its strength is attributed to the flexibility of the material, not its hardness. Although it is the most impact-resistant material used for ophthalmic lenses, the material is naturally soft and easily scratched, even when it has a scratch-resistant coating. (Both surfaces must be coated if it is to be used as an optical lens.) The scratch-resistant coating applied in laboratories is not as good as that on most factory coated CR-39 lenses. This should be a consideration when selecting lenses for children. Polycarbonate lenses are available in single-vision, flat-top 25, flat-top 28 bifocals as well as PALs, and should be the material of choice whenever protection is a consideration. Unfortunately, the optical clarity is poorer than with other materials, and it may not be as readily available from laboratories.

Various lens companies produce plastic lenses with indices of 1.56, 1.58, and 1.60. This material is not polycarbonate and it can be treated similarly to CR-39; it can also be edged, tinted, and coated. It is available in single-vision and flat-top bifocals. This material should be coated on both sides to reduce its susceptibility to scratches.

Crown glass lenses are used less frequently because of the preference for plastic lenses. With a refractive index of 1.523, these lenses are approximately 4 to 8 percent thinner than CR-39 lenses, but glass lenses weigh twice as much as CR-39 lenses and can crack or chip easily even after being hardened. One advantage of glass lenses is their natural scratch resistance; they do not need to be coated. Photochromic glass lenses are also available.

High-index glass is available in 1.60, 1.70, and 1.80 refractive indices. These lenses are considerably thinner and lighter than crown glass after about ±6.00 D. Because children wear smaller frames, these savings are not significant, so these lenses are not used by children as frequently as by adults. Reflections increase as the index increases, making the lenses look unattractive and thicker than they really are. An anti-reflective coat or a slight pink tint often helps in this regard.

Single-Vision

Most pediatric vision problems can be optimally corrected with single-vision lenses, but, as single-vision lenses correct for only one distance, precise evaluation of the child's needs is necessary. If multiple distances require optimal correction, a single-vision lens may be inappropriate.

It may be necessary for the child to have different spectacle prescriptions to correct for different distances. In this event, the instructions to the patient may not be too complicated. An adult can be told to use one pair of glasses for distance and another pair for near viewing, but active children may find it too difficult to remember which eyeglasses are for which use. It is important to make the use of spectacles as easy as possible.

Proper measurements should be taken for the distance at which the prescription will be used. For high prescription, the distance PD and optical centers should be centered near the pupils during primary gaze if the glasses are to be used for distance. If they are to be used for near viewing, a near PD is used and the optical centers are set slightly below the primary gaze.

Multifocals

The most common type of multifocal lens used by children is a bifocal. These lenses are usually fitted when the child has a general binocular dysfunction or strabismus. The segment is fitted so that the top of the segment bisects the pupil to make it more likely that the child will use the near add for near tasks (Fig. 8.1.)

Executive-type bifocals are the most common multifocals prescribed for young children. A wide segment provides a wide range for the child and helps minimize head turning. As a child gets older, the segment size is usually reduced for cosmetic purposes. Segment heights can be lowered as the child learns to use the add.

The disadvantages of using an executive-type bifocal are the weight, thickness, and appearance of the lenses. A flat-top 35 bifocal

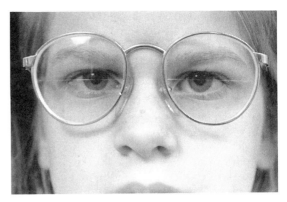

Figure 8.1 Executive bifocals should be fitted to bisect the child's pupils.

is a viable alternative. The lens provides an adequate reading area for the child with the benefits of reduced weight and thickness and the less noticeable segment line. Trifocals are not commonly used on children. They have too many segment lines for children to adapt to.

Progressive addition lenses (PAL) are being used more commonly on children. Studies have shown that these lenses have been successful for children with binocular dysfunction and strabismus (7, 8, 14).

It is recommended that children's PAL lenses be fitted with the optical center at the center of the pupil. Normally PALs are fitted with the fitting cross at the pupil, but with children the fitting cross is located 2 to 4 mm above the optical center, depending on the PAL, to allow the child to progress into the reading add sooner (Fig. 8.2). There is very little change in the prescription between the fitting cross and the optical center, so acuity is minimally compromised.

Do not attempt to "overplus" the add, as this will cause the child to use the intermediate area for reading and thus reduce the reading field. A PAL has no segment line to avoid, so the child is more likely to use the add.

Also, because of the absence of a segment line, the lenses are often better accepted by

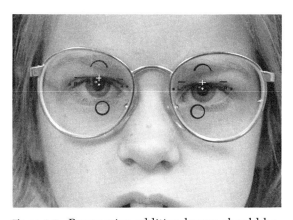

Figure 8.2 Progressive addition lenses should be fitted with the fitting cross fit 2 to 4 mm above center pupil. The fitting cross and optical center have been highlighted.

parent and child. Most parents do not like an unattractive line in the middle of their child's lenses, and a child who becomes self-conscious of the line may be reluctant to wear conventional bifocal glasses. As a result, compliance may be better with PALs.

Safety Standards

Polycarbonate should be the lens of choice whenever protection is a consideration, and for infants and children this is always. As infants and children are active and prone to eye injuries, eye protection should be a high priority. A great majority of sports-related eye injuries affect children and are preventable (2, 3), but eye injuries are not restricted to sports; most eye injuries occur around the home (3).

There are varying opinions as to the lens of choice for each situation, but it is the legal obligation of the optometrist to inform parents that CR-39 and glass provide only limited impact resistance (2).

Scratch-Resistant Coatings

The various scratch-resistant coatings have different degrees of hardness. Some offer adequate protection; others are no more than an added film on the lens. Some lenses are coated only on the front surface, and others are coated on both surfaces. One should not assume that just because a scratch-resistant coating was ordered both sides were coated. Quite often laboratories do not coat the back surface of the lens if the lens was generated from semifinished blanks. This is often the case for multifocals and special lenses. Finished stock lenses are customarily coated on both surfaces.

Factory-supplied coatings usually offer better protection than those supplied by laboratories. Most inexpensive coating units are inadequate. Solutions or creams that can be rubbed onto the lens offer almost no protection.

Scratch-resistant coatings are beneficial on most children's lenses. Infants often scratch their lenses by throwing their glasses down or while playing with their toys. Children are often impulsive and careless and do not always use care when handling their glasses.

Antireflection Coatings

Antireflection coatings (ARC) increase the transmission of light and reduce the amount of bothersome reflections. There are two general types of ARCs. Single-layer coatings reduce reflections by 50 percent. Multilayered coatings reduce reflections and increase transmission by 8 to 9 percent.

These coatings improve the appearance of the lenses by reducing annoying reflections from the lenses. Reflections interfere with eye contact and maintaining optimal intimacy during social interactions. On the other hand, the coating tends to show oil and fingerprints and is more difficult to clean, and because the coating scratches easily, it requires care of its own.

An ARC is always the last coating on a lens. It can be applied to glass or plastic lenses, although the type of coating may differ for each material.

ADJUSTMENTS AND MODIFICATIONS

The same considerations made for adults can be applied to children and infants. Depending on the age of the child, certain adjustments may be more important than others.

It is important to maintain as much surface contact area with the frame as possible. Distributing the weight affords a more comfortable fit. Once contact is made, only a small amount of pressure is necessary. Too much pressure will create a sore spot or may reduce contact somewhere else.

The temples must not be adjusted too tightly behind the ears. This creates excessive pressure on the bridge of the nose and may deform it.

Infants

Infants are prone to impact. They have not yet learned to protect themselves from falls and bumps. Plastic frames should be used, because they are less likely to have sharp edges that could cut into the infant's face. Plastic frames also absorb more shock than metal frames and stay in better adjustment.

Infants have special needs when it comes to frame and lens selection. Because of the small size and structure of their faces, a desirable fit is more difficult to obtain than with older children or adults. Eyesizes as small as 30 mm are available. Since infants have flat nose bridges, the contour of the frame bridge should also be flat to allow maximal surface contact and minimize the chance of sore spots developing. More importantly, poorly fitted frames could alter the growth of developing bone.

Skull, riding bow, cable temples and special harnesses are available that allow the frames to stay on the infant's head. Some special infant's frames have an elastic band secured to the temples that can be adjusted to vary the pressure of the frame. The elastic band should not be too tight, as it could eventually restrict growth of the infant's head. Spring hinges are also available.

Polycarbonate lenses should be considered for all infants. They ensure maximal protection if the infant falls.

Adjustments

Glasses should be aligned before dispensing or before any major adjustments are made. This will provide a starting point and help identify the precise adjustments needed. If the necessary adjustment is not identified, other incorrect adjustments may inadvertently be made to compensate for the problem which only compounds the problems.

The fit is evaluated using the normal way the patient wears the glasses as a basis. Some patients prefer to wear their glasses higher up on the nose than others. The frame width should approximate the patient's head width, allowing temples to be straight and parallel to the sides of the head, making contact only slightly anterior to the ears. This provides adequate pressure on the sides of the head.

The top of the eyewire should approximate the height of the eyebrows but should not totally obscure them. The eyebrows should be visible, so facial expressions can be seen. The top of the eyewire should follow the contour of the eyebrows for a better cosmetic appearance.

The bottom of the eyewire should not touch the cheek. The lenses will fog and become greasy if there is not some distance between the frame and the cheeks. In addition, constant contact may irritate a child's cheeks. A slight touch of the frame on the cheeks when the child smiles is acceptable as long as the glasses do not move. If the glasses lift up when the child smiles, this will reposition the frame on the nose, resulting in a loose fit. The bridge must provide adequate surface area contact; if not, sore spots will develop regardless of what type of nose pads are used.

From the side, the temples should appear straight and rest on the crotch of the ear. A space between the temple and the crotch of the ear may indicate that the earpiece bend or the earpiece is ill-fitted.

The earpiece bend should begin approximately 2 to 3 mm behind the crotch of the ear to allow for adequate clearance. The temple earpiece should allow some play behind the ear for minimal slippage and to relieve pressure on the bridge of the nose, which may cause a frontal headache. Once the temples make contact anterior to the ears, there should be constant contact all the way to the end of the earpiece, providing even distribution of the pressure by the temples.

Adding Adjustable Nose Pads

It is difficult to achieve a proper bridge fit on children who have flat noses and large cheeks. A good fit is especially important if a bifocal or progressive addition lens is to be prescribed. Without adequate support from the bridge, frames will continue to slip regardless of how the temples are adjusted.

Adding adjustable nose pads is a simple procedure that can be done in the office with the following equipment: nose pads arms, a hand drill, a felt-tipped marker, Super Glue, wide-jawed pliers, and clip-on nose pads (Figs. 8.3–8.6).

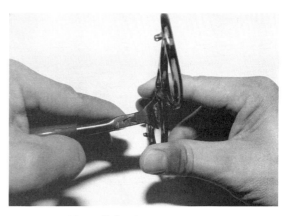

Figure 8.3 Clip off the fixed nose pads.

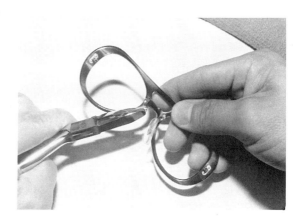

Figure 8.4 Clip on nose pads.

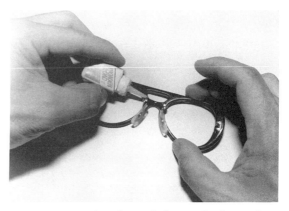

Figure 8.5 Touch a drop of glue to the base of the pad arm.

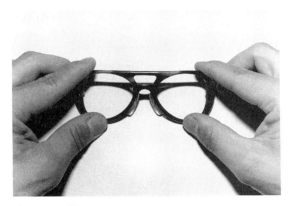

Figure 8.6 Front view.

Procedure

1. Decide where to position the frame. Lift the frame off the patient's nose or cheek and bring it slightly forward and upward. This allows you to approximate the location of the nose pads and the fit of the frame after the nose pads have been added.
2. Mark the location of the holes with a felt-tipped pen or the drill tip. Pick a flat area on the bridges or eyewire. If the nose pad arms will be drilled into the eyewire, the fixed nose pads may need to be clipped off. File the rough edges with a file and smooth sandpaper and polish with a buffing wheel. Be sure the top holes are exactly aligned with each other.
3. Use the prongs of the nose pad arms to gauge the depth of the holes. Adjusting the drill bit to the exact length prior to drilling may help prevent drilling too deep. Drill the holes to the exact depth.
4. Push the pad arms into the frame with pliers that have wide jaws. Protect the front of the frame with a cloth to avoid marring it.
5. Touch a drop of Super Glue to the base of the nose pad arm and dry for 5 to 10 minutes. Do not attempt to put the glue in the holes before the pads are inserted as this will prove quite messy. Do not allow wa-

ter to touch the glue while it is still wet, as this will make the glue turn white and become visible.
6. After the glue has dried, clip on the nose pads with wide-jawed pliers. Do not clip the pads too tightly. Pads should have some play for self-adjustment as the glasses slide up and down the nose.
7. Allow the glue to dry for a minimum of 20 minutes before putting the frame on the patient. This permits any residual fumes, which can cause some stinging to the patient's eyes, to dissipate.

Add-A-Pads

Add-a-pads are used to fill gaps between the frame and the nose. They lift the frame and increase the vertex distance, or they can also be used to increase the surface area contact. They come in three thicknesses: heavy, medium, and light. One end of the add-a-pad is thicker than the other, so the support can be distributed evenly. The pad can be used with the thicker portion on either the top or the bottom of the eyewire, depending on which area of the bridge needs the added support. If the upper portion of the bridge needs more surface area contact, the thicker portion of the pads is positioned on the top and the thinner portion on the bottom. If the lower portion of the bridge needs more surface area contact, the pad is simply inverted.

The following materials are used: add-a-pads, Super Glue, acetone, and tape.

1. Determine areas of support.
2. Position the pads by taping the add-a-pads to the eyewire.
3. This step is only for zyl and proprionate frames. After determining the correct position of the pads, remove one of the pads and dab the eyewire with acetone. While the acetone is still wet, push the pad onto the eyewire. This conforms the eyewire to the pad and will help reduce the number of bubbles when the pad is finally glued on. Be sure to do this step one pad at a time, so there is a landmark by which to position the second pad.

4. Remove the pad, add a drop of glue, and press the pad back onto the eyewire.
5. Repeat with the other pad.

Modifying Fixed Nose Pads

The contour of the fixed nose pads on plastic frames sometimes do not approximate the contour of the child's nasal bridge. In most cases the bridge of the nose is too flat for the angle of the nose pads. This angle can easily be widened by heating the nose pads and rolling the pads wider to follow the contour of the child's bridge. If a thermal jet warmer is used, the heat can be applied directly to the nose pads. If only a salt pan or glass bead frame warmer is available, use a tablespoon to scoop some of the salt out of the pan and immerse the nose pad in the salt.

Hidden Hinge Repair

On occasion, a hidden hinge may be pulled out of the frame front or the hinge barrels may be damaged. A hinge repair may be quite handy in an emergency. A 12-volt soldering iron, clipper pliers, a screwdriver, a probe, a replacement hinge, and Super Glue are needed.

Technique Before removing the old hinge, be sure to have an adequate replacement. The hinge plate should approximate the size of the old hinge plate. The barrels of the new hinge should be able to interlock with the barrels of the old temple.

1. With a 12-volt soldering iron, heat the broken hinge until it begins to loosen.
2. Quickly use clipper pliers to pull the hinge out by the remaining part of the barrel. If just the plate remains, use a screwdriver to uproot the plate and then clipper pliers to pull it out.
3. Place the new hinge in the crevice. Put a probe in the barrel holes to hold the hinge in place.
4. Heat the hinge with the soldering iron.
5. As the plastic softens, gently press the hinge into the frame.
6. After the hinge is in place, use Super Glue around the edges of the hinge plate to secure the hinge. Use glue sparingly. One drop is usually all that is needed.
7. After the glue is dry, mount the temple.
8. Remember not to allow water to come into contact with the glue while it is drying, as this will turn it white.

CONCLUSIONS

Spectacles for children may raise a number of complex points. On one hand, eyeglasses may expose children to social criticism, or, on the other hand, they may improve their social acceptance. There is a need for research on the social and cosmetic implications of glasses.

Children demand special spectacles. It is not enough to consider only the optical properties of glasses. One must also take into account comfort, durability, safety and protection, and appearance. To complicate matters, sometimes one set of criteria may conflict with another equally important set.

We conclude this chapter with a number of practical suggestions drawn from the material presented above.

Select Materials Carefully Children's eyeglasses demand special attention to materials to ensure comfort, durability, safety, and good appearance as well as visual acuity.

Fashion and function are two independent selection criteria. It probably makes sense to have different frames for different clothes and different occasions. For example, it may pay to have dress frames, for which appearance is a major selection criterion, and athletic frames, for which durability and protection are the major selection criteria.

Spectacles that are uncomfortable are probably not going to be worn by a child. The child's small face, flat nose, and full cheeks cause special problems with evenly distributing the pressure of the frames. Uneven pressure is likely to result in sore spots, which must be prevented.

The child's life style also dictates materials. Because children are so physically active, their frames and lenses must be selected for durability and safety. Synthetic materials are generally preferred over metal and glass.

Be Sensitive Getting the first pair of glasses does not have to be a stressful occasion for a child (or the parents). The child can be helped to feel special if a separate waiting area is provided with appropriate furniture, decor, toys, and activities. This will make the office less intimidating.

There may be considerable fear of physical and social discomfort. Taking time and using effective measures to alleviate this apprehension will produce future gains. The child should be encouraged to ask questions and answers should be given in terms that the child can understand. The child, not the parent, is the patient and must be included in all discussions and decisions. A child who is allowed a say in frame selection is more likely to comply with wearing them.

When feasible, children's frames are displayed separately so children will feel special. How the frames are displayed can play an important role in the success of the glasses. A range of frames in various styles and colors should be offered, but only two or three at a time, to avoid overwhelming and confusing the child.

Emphasize the Positive The optometrist should be positive during the dispensing session and should let children know that eyeglasses make them look more intelligent. Little girls, especially, should know that looking intelligent is a good thing. It is very important to reassure young patients of their social appeal with comments on the child's good looks. It is helpful to point out how attractive and grown up the child looks. The child must feel good about the eyeglasses in order to feel good about himself or herself.

Wearing glasses is a new experience for a child. If the dispenser and the parent show enthusiasm toward the glasses, the child is less likely to be intimidated. Pointing out that the glasses are special and were made especially for the child may make the child feel better about wearing them.

Use Sympathy Judiciously Do not "catastrophize" by commenting on "you poor, poor child". The child may become sensitized to the negative implications of such sympathy and come to think that something is wrong. It is useful to emphasize that the child may wear glasses or is entitled to, not that he or she is forced to wear them or must. If it is not possible to be matter-of-fact about wearing eyeglasses, it is good to emphasize instead how fortunate the child will be to have better vision rather than how unfortunate it is that the child has visual problems.

It is best to stress the positive aspects of the glasses, to explain that an eyeglasses prescription is a step to improve vision rather than to correct a visual defect. If the child asks why he must wear glasses the answer should be couched in terms of "So you will see things clearly" rather than "Because your eyes are not very good" or "You can't see well."

Reward Achievement The improved vision stemming from eyeglasses is often reflected in improved scholastic and athletic performance. It is essential that the child's higher achievement be attributed to the eyeglasses and that it be generously rewarded. Be alert to valued activities that are now permitted by the new glasses.

Teach Eye Care The child who is old enough should be taught correct cleaning techniques, but simply. One method of cleaning and one set of products is enough. The child should rinse the glasses with water and wipe them with a soft facial tissue. (Although some practitioners fear that facial tissue is too abrasive, it is better than running the risk of the child using a more abrasive napkin or dirty cloth.)

The child must be taught how to put the glasses on and take them off. Some children try to put the glasses on by bringing them over the top of their head. This will cause the glasses to get out of adjustment sooner than if they are put on and removed from the front. The child who wears skull temples must be encouraged to use both hands. If the child has comfort cables, the temples should be put on and removed one at a time. This should be demonstrated and the child should repeat the maneuver.

Child and parent should be clearly fore-warned about some of the common problems and discomforts glasses can cause. They should be assured that such experiences may be expected and that the child is not at fault. The child should inform the parents when there is discomfort or a vision problem. If the parents cannot deal with the problem, the optometrist should be contacted. It is better that the child overreport problems than underreport them.

Follow-up examinations should be scheduled. An examination a week or two after dispensing may serve to reinforce the early establishment of eye care habits. This exam may also reassure the child that support and assistance are indeed close at hand and convince the parents that their child is receiving professional care.

Utilize Role Models Young children tend to imitate; this stems in part from their moldable body image. Young patient can be helped to identify positive role models (idols) who wear eyeglasses. Photographic models, athletes, entertainers, and other valued people who wear glasses can be pointed out.

To the extent possible, the child should associate with peers who also wear glasses. If "everyone" is wearing glasses, the child will feel less conspicuous and will be less likely to define herself or himself in terms of the glasses.

Maintain Perspective We must be careful not to create such a strong expectation of social rejection or criticism that it operates as a kind of self-fulfilling prophecy. Much of the research documenting negative social reactions to eyeglasses may be discountable. Some of it is quite old, and it may no longer be replicable. There are now highly attractive frames and lenses, which may reduce some of the social stigma. And there has been virtually no systematic research on young child patients. The typical research participant is a late adolescent college freshman; it might very well be that we cannot generalize from this research to young children and infants. Finally, perhaps our society is becoming more egalitarian and less concerned with physical appearances (though there remains a very strong mandate to conform to social standards of attractiveness).

Consider Contact Lenses Unless they are optometrically or medically contraindicated, contact lenses should be seriously considered (10, 13). New generations of soft daily wear extended wear contact lenses are making them an increasingly appealing alternative for children. Even very young children are proving that they can adapt nicely to contact lenses (see Chap. 9). When spectacles must be prescribed for optical or functional reasons, the optometrist should counsel the parents as well as the patients.

Acknowledgment

The authors are grateful for the material on psychosocial aspects on spectacles and contact lenses contributed by Roger L. Terry, Ph.D., Professor of Psychology, Hanover College, Hanover, Indiana.

REFERENCES

1. Barrineau HG, Berg AJ, Terry RL: Eyeglasses and interaction distance. Optom Mon 72:22, 1981.
2. Classé JG: Legal aspects of sports-related ocular injuries. Int Ophthalmol Clin 28:211, 1988.
3. Davis JK: Perspectives on impact resistance and polycarbonate lenses. Int Ophthalmol Clin 28:215, 1988.
4. Eakin RS: Designing and adjusting spectacles for children. In Hirsch MJ, Wick R (eds): Vision of Children: An Optometric Symposium. Philadelphia, Chilton, 271, 1963.
5. Edwards K: Effects of sex and glasses on attitudes toward intelligence and attractiveness. Psychol Rep 60:590, 1987.

6. Elman D: Physical characteristics and the perception of masculine traits. J Soc Psychol 103:157, 1977.

7. Jacob JL, Beaulieu Y, Brunet E: Progressive-addition lenses in the management of esotropia with a high accommodation/convergence ratio. Can J Ophthalmol 15:166, 1980.

8. Smith JB: Progressive addition lenses in the treatment of accommodative esotropia. Am J Ophthalmol 99:56, 1985.

9. Terry RL: Anxiety induced by visual correctives and role reversal. Optom Mon 72:18, 1981.

10. Terry RL: The psychology of visual correctives: Social and psychologic effects of eyeglasses and contact lenses. Optom Mon 73:137, 1982.

11. Terry RL: Psychological considerations of visual correctives for children. Cont Lens Forum 14:70, 1989.

12. Terry RL: Judgments of persons who wear eyeglasses: Mediating effects of gender. Cont Lens Spectrum (in press).

13. Terry RL, Brady CS: Effects of framed spectacles and contact lenses on self-ratings of physical attractiveness. Percept Mot Skills 42:787, 1976.

14. Valentino JA: Clinical use of progressive addition lenses on non-presbyopic patients. Optom Mon 73:513, 1982.

Chapter 9

Contact Lenses for Children

Barry A. Weissman

Paul B. Donzis

Children, even those only days or weeks old, can successfully wear contact lenses. We define success as both being able to physiologically tolerate a contact lens for a substantial part of the day and benefit from the use of such a device during that period of time. Such contact lens wear can be both safe and effective for the majority of young patients.

Indications for use of contact lenses in the younger age group, under 5 years of age, are principally extreme refractive errors. Aphakia, high myopia, irregular astigmatism (often following trauma or corneal grafting secondary to some disease process), and aniseikonia are definite indications. Patching for management of amblyopia is another form of therapy that might alternatively be considered for opaque contact lens application, as is the use of a contact lens as a prosthetic to mask some ocular disfigurement.

We do not believe that it is in the best interest of *most* children to wear contact lenses for the correction of modest refractive errors. Contact lens wear has certain complications and risks as well as benefits. Young children often cannot articulate problems. Thus, much contact lens care becomes the responsibility of the parents or guardians, and this can become a burden. Furthermore, children's eyes change rapidly with growth, both in refractive error and corneal topography, necessitating more frequent professional evaluation and contact lens changes for both fit and power, which may involve some expense. If children do not return for professional care, a contact lens may become inappropriate in power, fit, or both. Without good care, compliance with proper hygiene, and appropriate lens fit, contact lens wear may become hazardous. Complications of contact lens wear can range from slight irritation and red eyes to neovascularization of the cornea and perhaps corneal infection and secondary loss of vision (2, 11).

Our clinical experience documents the feasibility of applying contact lenses in the care of the pediatric patient when the benefits clearly outweigh the potential risks and when good contact lens care is available.

REFRACTIVE APPLICATIONS

Aphakia

The primary indication for contact lens wear in very young children (under 1 year of age) is unilateral or bilateral cataract extraction (9, 16). Cataract development may be due to inheritance with proven pedigree, rare events such as persistent hyperplastic primary vitreous (PHPV), which often results in microophthalmia and congenital cataract, or disease in utero such as rubella. Postpartum trauma may

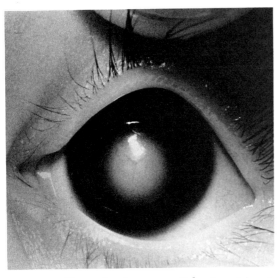

Figure 9.1 Example of a congenital cataract in an infant only days old; note the Y sutures evident within the lens. (Courtesy of JB Bateman)

also result in cataract formation. Once a cataract interferes with vision of a very young child, neurologic visual development may be compromised (1, 15, 25–28), with secondary development of amblyopia. Prompt cataract extraction and subsequent optical correction become essential to maximize the potential for vision rehabilitation and proper neurologic development (1, 15) to establish binocular vision.

Optical correction of pediatric aphakia presents numerous challenges to both the ophthalmic professional and the child's family. Spectacles may theoretically be used, especially when aphakia is bilateral, but there are several sources of problems with spectacles, including both optical distortion and magnification, as well as difficulties in obtaining pediatric spectacle frames that will be tolerated and will stay in place during an infant's activity. Unilateral aphakia almost universally generates aniseikonia (14) when corrected with spectacles; this precludes proper visual development.

For optical correction of pediatric aphakia alternatives to spectacles and contact lenses are intraocular lens implantation and epikeratophakia. Intraocular lenses theoretically give the least optical distortion and magnification (8), but normal ocular growth may quickly make any stable power correction obsolete. Some form of overcorrection or secondary invasive surgery will almost undoubtedly be necessary, perhaps several times as the eye grows. There is also concern about potential unknown long-term adverse effects of such implants being lodged within the eye for periods in excess of 20 to 40 years. Epikeratophakia offers some advantages in that it is a less invasive surgical procedure and affords lenticle removal and replacement. Although there have been some problems in children under 1 year of age undergoing this procedure, such as inaccurate lenticle power, epikeratophakia has shown much promise (12). The principal advantage of both procedures is that they require no substantial commitment of parental time and effort.

Contact lens correction offers advantages

and disadvantages of its own. The major advantage of contact lens wear is that the practitioner can quickly change optical correction in response to ocular growth without additional surgery. Retinoscopy allows accurate and simple assessment of refractive requirements. Difficulties include lens care, maintenance, and handling, which must be performed by parents or guardians. Some parents have a psychological reluctance to using contact lenses. Lens loss, breakage, and obsolescence may cause interruptions in vision therapy, possibly complicating amblyopia management. Frequent lens replacement can be expensive. Frequent professional supervision is essential, both to monitor and prescribe changes in fit and power as needed and to observe physiologic tolerance. Clinicians often have difficulty providing such professional care to infants and young children, who are often less than fully cooperative with the examiner. Contact lenses to treat pediatric aphakia are often expensive and difficult-to-obtain custom-made devices, often with optical power between +20 and +40 D.

Rigid contact lenses have been used for many years with relative success (9, 15, 18, 20). Advantages of this modality include availability even in extreme prescriptions, optical performance (in most cases neutralizing both spherical and astigmatic ametropias), ease of handling, and decreased unit expense. Disadvantages include occasional lens breakage and loss, and some initial discomfort anticipated by the parent for the child. The literature reports good physiologic tolerance with polymethylmethacrylate (PMMA) lenses; one can only anticipate improved physiology with new rigid gas-permeable materials. Many aphakic infants are currently fitted with flexible silicone lenses. Advantages are superior corneal oxygenation and reported decreased lens loss (7, 10, 13). Disadvantages include the expense of the lenses, inability to obtain full optical correction due to limited parameters, rapid soilage of the lens, and occasional abrasions of the cornea. Hydrogel lenses have been used almost from the inception of this therapy (9,

21), and improved availability of custom lenses from several manufacturers allows the clinician to obtain almost any needed parameters readily (see Table 9.1). Disadvantages include the fragility of these devices, poor correction of residual astigmatism, and occasional instances of rapid lens loss.

Most clinicians and parents agree that, theoretically, extended wear lenses would be ideal for children with aphakia; however, owing to the increased incidence of severe complications (e.g., acute red eye reactions, giant papillary conjunctivitis, neovascularization, abrasion, infective keratitis) associated with use of current contact lens designs and materials for extended wear (23), daily wear is recommended for all lens types at present. Use of contact lenses on a daily wear basis initially demands a substantial investment of time and patience from doctor and parents. During the first several weeks of care, the process of lens handling and care must be taught to and mastered by the parents, but after that period, in most instances, lens care procedures become familiar and convenient for most families. Any extended wear (with high water content hydrogels, silicone elastomers, or highly transmissible rigid gas-permeable lenses) might be "easier" on all concerned—doctor, parents, and child—but may be anticipated to increase the risk of physiologic compromise. In our opinion, therefore, extended wear lenses should only be considered when daily wear lenses cannot be employed.

Results are mixed. In our experience, most children with some vision potential obtain some benefits, even if only a stable (i.e., not nystagmic), relatively straight eye. Children with bilateral aphakia as a rule do better than those with unilateral aphakia; some in our patient group have achieved Snellen acuities in the 20/40 range and others report similar results (15). It is true, however, that even with the best care and proper lens application and patching, some patients do not attain usable vision, although it is usually those with unilateral aphakia who have surgery after 3 to 4 months of age or nonaggressive patching and follow-up care.

Table 9.1 MANUFACTURERS OF FLEXIBLE CONTACT LENSES WITH POWER >+20 D

Manufacturer (Telephone)	Lens Name	Material	Available Powers
American Hydron (800-645-7544)	Hydron custom[a]	Hydrogel 38% water	+20 to +30
Bausch & Lomb (800-828-9030)	Silsoft	Silicone elastomer	+23 to +32
Danker (800-237-9641)	Sila-Rx[b]	Silicone	+20 to +35
Flexlens (800-223-3539)	Flexlens	Hydrogel 45% water	−50 to +50
Optech (800-525-7465)	Fre-flex	Hydrogel 55% water	−40 to +40
Strieter (800-851-4557)	Accugel	Hydrogel 47% water	+21 to +36
VisionTech (800-221-1108)	VT 79 pediatric aphakic	Hydrogel 79% water	+20 to +35
	VT 45 pediatric aphakic	Hydrogel 45% water	+20 to +35

[a] Personal communication with American Hydron.
[b] Product communication from Danker Laboratories.
Data compiled from Reference 24.

Myopia

Substantial amounts of myopia (approaching and exceeding 10 D) are also an indication for contact lens wear in the pediatric group (especially if unilateral, to prevent amblyopia). Although it is encountered less commonly than pediatric aphakia, occasional young children may present with this type of refractive error. Contact lens correction will result in image magnification and decreased peripheral distortion compared to spectacle correction. Because of magnification, even modest amounts of astigmatism may be masked by simple spherical hydrogels, and visual acuity with lenses on the eyes may easily be better than that attained with spherocylindrical spectacles. Rigid lenses would be expected to improve visual acuity much more than hydrogels when the refractive state is compound myopic astigmatism.

Documentation is equivocal regarding the therapeutic role of contact lenses in retarding progression of simple myopia (6).

One school firmly believes in the therapeutic efficacy of rigid contact lenses, without real documentation of mechanisms or success, whereas others suggest that this is a clinical observation based on the usual age of contact lens dispensing (late teens and early twenties) when myopic progression would be expected to slow even without contact lens wear. Because of this controversy the astute clinician might offer, but not encourage, rigid contact lens correction for the young child with about 5 D of myopia, presenting all opinions to the parents in an effort to allow them to decide on an informed course of action.

Astigmatism

In children most normal degrees of astigmatism are most easily treated with spectacles. This is not true, however when astigmatism is extreme or irregular, as in cases of trauma, disease, or surgery. Occasionally very young children may present to the clinician with keratoconus or with irregular corneas secondary to penetrating wounds or infections. Often, simple spherical rigid contact lenses will dramatically improve visual acuity, eliminating the need for surgical intervention (in the form of a corneal graft or Ruiz-type procedures).

Other more sophisticated contact lenses may also be considered when indications suggest. Such lenses include spherical power effect, cylindrical power effect, front surface toric rigid lenses (22), and toric hydrogels as well.

Aniseikonia

Rarely, a child presents with developmental or acquired (i.e., unilateral aphakia or high myopia as above, or following corneal graft) aniseikonia. In most instances, use of a contact lens on at least one eye is advisable. It minimizes pure retinal image size differences which may be related to retinal element dispersion (3), as well as to axial length and corneal power and is difficult to quantify in adults and children. Contact lenses also reduce the unwanted prismatic differences between the eyes, especially in vertical gaze which exists when anisometropic spectacle lenses are used.

Accommodative Esotropia

Young children with uncorrected hyperopia may develop accommodative esotropia. If full optical correction will allow for binocularity (i.e., if a concomitant prism is not needed), it is possible that contact lenses may be used to improve cosmesis, decrease the weight of the spectacle correction, and improve optics through minimization of distortion and magnification. Contact lenses thereby enhance patient compliance and are therefore themselves therapeutic to some degree. Optometrists have noted, moreover, that plus power acceptance may be enhanced by the hyperopic patient using contact lenses instead of spectacles; one proposed classical mechanism is the expectation of decreased

accommodative demand (19) under such conditions, and another more recently proposed hypothesis is that of neurosensory feedback (17).

PROSTHETIC APPLICATIONS

Amblyopia

Patching an eye to manage amblyopia is a common part of pediatric ophthalmic practice. Children often object to this treatment, in the younger groups because it reduces their vision in the better eye and in the older more peer pressure–conscious groups because of cosmesis. Contact lens patches are more difficult for a younger child to learn to remove and more acceptable cosmetically for an older child to tolerate, so ideally they should improve compliance in both groups.

It has been said that the failure of occlusion is the failure to totally occlude, so the only patches expected to really be effective would be those that occlude all light transmission in the optical zone. It has been determined clinically that for occlusion to occur, not only must light be prohibited but the diameter of the occluding "optical zone" must be quite large (10 or 11 mm), thus effectively eliminating the potential use of rigid lenses, which are commonly less than 10 mm in overall diameter. Tinted American and European hydrogels are available that allow for this application.

On the other hand, clear lenses offer some distinct advantages. High plus, and possibly high minus, lenses may blur the retinal image enough to function as a patch. Advantages include ease of application (they are even easier to prescribe than normal lenses as power need not be precise), decreased expense (when compared to blackened custom hydrogels), and improved availability. Rigid lenses or hydrogels may be used. The mechanical fit and physiologic tolerance may be clinically assessed with normal techniques. Finally, but perhaps most important, cosmesis is substantially enhanced as the eye under treatment appears normal rather than blackened. One of us (BAW) treated at least two amblyopic patients who showed definite visual acuity improvement in the amblyopic eye while using such a clear lens to occlude the nonamblyopic eye.

Similarly, clinical situations may arise in which it is necessary to occlude the eye that has *poorer* visual acuity because it is interfering with vision of the better fellow eye. A clear high-power occluder should be considered before a total (black) occluder lens, for the reasons stated above.

Ocular Disfigurement

Many conditions may disfigure an eye. Congenital microcornea is easily noticed. Inoperable cataracts can produce leukocoria. Trauma can lead to obvious corneal scars or lesions in the iris-pupil plane. When a child is so afflicted, peer pressure can be devastating. Restoration of a normal appearance can dramatically improve a child's social situation and self-image. Early methods involved scleral lenses, which were often difficult to tolerate for long periods of time and quite expensive, owing to the art and skill involved in fitting them. Most children do not tolerate the fitting and wearing of a scleral contact lens.

The first consideration in applying prosthetic contact lenses must be the clinical goal. Does the eye under consideration have vision potential? If it could attain usable visual acuity, the clinical goals are vision primarily and cosmesis secondarily. If, on the other hand, the eye is effectively blind, the clinician can consider the lens to be totally prosthetic.

Rigid corneal lenses (11 mm in diameter) with painted iris have been used with some success to mask corneal scars in the past and offer the advantage of looking much like the better eye. When there is vision potential, the clinician can first attain a good contact lens design with clear lenses of the proper *fit*, providing both proper visual acuity and physiologic response; then a lens of duplicate optical and mechanical parameters may be ordered with a painted iris and a clear pupillary zone. Unfortunately, children are often intol-

erant of these rigid lenses. They are not yet readily available in a gas-permeable plastic, and it is not clear whether such a lens would remain gas permeable after being painted. Thus, rigid lenses almost certainly compromise corneal physiology in some manner.

Prosthetic hydrogels offer many advantages. Comfort is almost universally assured. Currently approved tints—both the "cosmetic enhancing" transmitting variety and the dot matrix type—are often adequate, especially for masking a small corneal leukoma. Both of these types of lenses are FDA approved and are available in stock parameters, physical, optical, and tint, from several manufacturers. Patients with vision potential can usually be accommodated with these devices.

Both American and European custom prosthetic lenses are also available, and are especially useful for dealing with an essentially blind eye. We have found it useful to stock custom hydrogel devices of approximately 8.6- and 8.9-mm base curve, 14.0-mm diameter, with 11.0-mm iris (blue, brown, and green)/4.0-mm black pupil tints. These lenses are all nominal power of +3 to +5 D, to allow for improved lens manipulation by patient or family member. Clear pupillary zones and various physical and tint parameters are available, but a good proportion of patients may be accommodated from about 10 lens designs with darkened pupillary zones. Alternately, the clinician might obtain a clear hydrogel lens with a central 3 or 4 mm diameter black spot to position, with manipulation of base curve and diameter, before an inoperable cataract to obtain remarkable cosmetic improvement (Fig. 9.2). Patients and families should be cautioned that although there will be a cosmetic improvement, the results probably will not be absolutely perfect and lenses will still need to be replaced and cared for appropriately. In the example above, such a lens would still move slightly with the blink, and the new "pupil" would not respond to illumination or accommodation as its normal mate would. For matching purposes it is occasionally necessary to fit both the subject eye and the good eye with

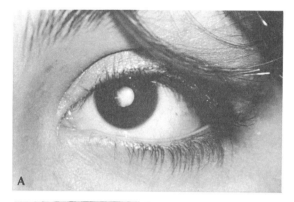

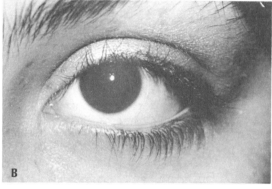

Figure 9.2 The cosmetic improvement made possible by use of a black-dotted hydrogel to mask an inoperable cataract (**A**) in a 15-year-old girl. (**B**) Note slight inferior position of lens and blackened dot.

similar devices. The clinician should also remember to prescribe safety spectacles (polycarbonate) to one-eyed patients to protect the better eye.

Nystagmus, Albinism, and Aniridia

Patients with congenital structural abnormalities of the eye may also benefit from the use of specialized types of contact lenses. Albinism and aniridia may be associated with extreme light sensitivity. Darkly tinted contact lenses or those with an opaque periphery and small central clear zone may be of great benefit to such patients. Furthermore, since large refractive errors may be associated with both

conditions, the contact lens can incorporate the appropriate refractive correction.

Nystagmus is the term used to describe the condition of rhythmic oscillatory movements of the eyes. It may be congenital or may be acquired from a number of causes and is often accompanied by extreme refractive errors. Contact lens correction is believed to afford improved visual acuity for nystagmic patients with usable vision by centering the optics of the refracting lens over the pupil, thus reducing prism and spectacle distortion encountered during eye movements behind spectacles.

CLINICAL ASPECTS OF CONTACT LENS APPLICATION

A contact lens prescription consists of several separate parameters. Base curve, power, diameter, color, central, edge, and junction thickness are only the beginning. Other elements include anterior and posterior peripheral curves and bevels (radii and widths) and material properties: oxygen permeability (Dk); specific gravity; optical index and so forth. Criteria for a good fit in the pediatric group are no different, we believe, then those desired for the adult group, namely:

1. Optimal optical correction when applicable
2. Good centering, movement, and alignment of the lens with the corneal surface
3. Adequate comfort to allow wear for at least 10 hours per day
4. No evidence of physiologic distress on repeated progress evaluations.

Achieving the good fit is often a greater challenge with a child than it would be with an adult because the child cannot be the final judge of whether the device will be used. Also, amblyopia may be induced if the power of the lens is inappropriate. Some children will report irritation with optimum correction—for psychological gain or perhaps because they wish to avoid using the device. Other children will staunchly wear a poorly fitting lens in the face of physiologic distress, to please their parents or because it makes them feel adult. Very young children often have no choice in the matter, so more responsibility lies with the clinician and the parents or guardians.

Power

Power is probably the easiest parameter to establish, especially when the child is aphakic. Retinoscopy is the clinician's best tool, aided by correcting for vertex distance. When cooperation is poor and the cornea less than perfectly clear, a good approach for aphakic children may be to calculate power from measurements of corneal curvature and axial length. Initially very high plus power is expected to decrease some 10 D over the first 12 to 18 months of life. When children reach 3 or 4 years of age they usually begin to give the clinician subjective information that can be used to assess visual acuity and refine optical correction.

Prosthetic hydrogel lenses used on blind eyes, as discussed above, are usually about +3 to +5 D in power to aid lens manipulation, and clear occluder lenses are usually +20 D to promote maximal blur while maintaining the cost and stock availability advantages. Other types of lenses require optical power as needed.

Corneal Curvature and Base Curve

Once they are old enough to sit up on a parent's lap, cooperative children may assist the clinician and allow keratometry to assess corneal curvature. Younger or less cooperative children must be examined by other techniques. Rigid lenses are perfect for this task. A series of rigid trial lenses of 10.0 mm diameter and varying base curves may be used as templates (4), with the assistance of sodium fluorescein and a hand-held cobalt blue light source, to define corneal curvature. Such examination may be performed on a squirming child in the office or in the operating room under anesthesia immediately prior to cataract extraction, or later if, for example, the surgeon requires an examination for addi-

tional reasons after surgery. Operating room keratometers may be used alternatively, but the template technique is probably preferable as it gives the clinician a better impression of the topography of a greater portion of the corneal surface.

Choice of Lens

Once corneal curvature and required power have been estimated, the clinician can decide whether to use a rigid, hydrogel, or silicone lens and can design an initial lens. Silicone lenses are available only in limited parameters and should be applied with the aid of fluorescein to attain a light apical touch relationship with the corneal apex. Aphakic infants often require high plus powers (+20 to +40 D or more), especially when microophthalmia is involved. The 1-month-old child fitted with a hydrogel lens usually requires a steep base curve (7.00 to 8.00 mm, usually about 1 mm flatter than the corneal curvature determined by rigid lens templates above) and a modest lens diameter (13.0 to 14.0 mm) to attain sagittal depth alignment with the eye's anterior segment and to fit in the palpebral aperture. As the child grows slightly, however, diameter must usually be increased to 15.0 mm to fit the lens as a semiscleral design and thereby decrease or prevent lens loss. The clinician should bear in mind that while these children's eyes are indeed all smaller than adults', corneal curvature is not universally steep. Children over 3 years old can usually be approached with adult type parameters unless there is obvious microophthalmia or trauma.

Rigid lenses should be fitted as adult lenses are, usually to obtain light apical alignment as defined by fluorescein examination, good centration, movement, and tear venting. When attempting visual correction of traumatized corneas, a rigid lens is the lens of choice. It should be fitted so that approximately one third of the back surface is in alignment with the anterior corneal surface and two thirds shows pooling as defined by fluorescein evaluation, while still maintaining adequate centration and tear venting. The fluorescein pattern itself may be quite irregular.

These initial lenses then become an "optical platform" upon which to further define power, by retinoscopy and subjectively, when possible, to allow maximum vision. If the ordered power is vastly different from power in the trial lens the clinician may anticipate some change in the fit of the lens.

Evaluation

The initial lens can be inserted with the child awake in the office. Younger children are usually restrained on a pediatric table. The lenses are examined for further refinements by the usual clinical techniques, which may be somewhat modified depending on the cooperation of the child. Such examination consists of first observing the movement and centration of the lens on the cornea as much as is possible. If the child cooperates, a hand-held biomicroscope or magnifying light is ideal; if not, perhaps the only view the clinician sees is with a penlight. If the lens appears to be adequately centered on the cornea, retinoscopy, often assisted by a lens bar, allows estimation of residual power error, if any. Use of a hand-held slit lamp (with fluorescein if the lens is rigid or silicone elastomer) permits observation of alignment, centration and movement, and physiologic response.

If the lens appears relatively close to optimum, it can be dispensed (see below for training and dispensing). One note of caution, especially in dealing with the very young aphakic children: even if the original lens initially appears perfect, a period of adaptation (at least a half hour) should be allowed. Many hydrogel lenses initially seem to perform adequately then loosen in the office or later, during the first week of wear. This may be due to an initial response of the child squeezing the lids, which slowly relax, or perhaps the tissues become less edematous with recovery from surgical procedures.

Small improvements can be noted and new lenses can be ordered that incorporate the changes. It is important for both clinician and family dealing with pediatric aphakia to recognize that such contact lens therapy is a process and that it is not completed when one contact lens is fitted. Changes in fit and power and lens loss will necessitate replacement about 9 or 10 times per eye during the first year (1) to 18 months of life. Nonetheless, especially in the case of pediatric aphakia, if the original lens is close and usable, it is important that it be dispensed and worn—both to afford the child visual input as early as possible and to help the family learn the lens care process.

LENS CARE PROCEDURES

Contact lenses require maintenance—insertion, removal and recentering, and cleaning. Care of contact lenses for young children is totally the responsibility of a parent guided by a clinician. Daily wear is indicated whenever possible and extended wear, at this date, is only a last resort.

An inexperienced clinician might predict that most children would prove to be difficult patients. Actually, in our experience, the reverse is true. Some children, especially between the ages of 2 and 3 years, are difficult, but most, even those who initially were somewhat rowdy, quickly calm down, tolerate lens wear and care, and cooperate well in clinical examinations.

Some children at age 3 or 4 begin to assume some aspects of lens care themselves. Commonly, in our experience, the first task learned is that of lens removal; lens insertion and recentering may also be mastered by some young children quite readily. If the parents consider the child responsible, these small tasks should probably be encouraged; lens cleaning and disinfecting, however, should be the parent's task until the child's teen years.

Hydrogels

Several approaches are discussed in the literature for inserting hydrogels on young children, but we feel our technique is effective and nontraumatic. The child is positioned on soft flooring or a convenient sofa. One parent restrains the child from above by resting the elbows on either side of the child's head and using the remainder of the arms to restrain the child's body. This approach should be gentle but firm. The other parent washes his or her hands then uses two fingers of the dominant hand to make the clean and rinsed hydrogel lens into a fan, and with the other hand, aided by a paper tissue to improve grasp, controls the child's upper lid. A slight gap is created between the globe and the upper lid, and the leading edge of the lens is slid up, under and into this space. If it is done correctly, the lens will slide down into position under the lower lid as well. Occasionally the lower lid must be moved over the lower edge of the lens. The parents should observe the lens carefully to make certain it is properly on the cornea and did not wind up on the floor or fold during the insertion process, as it could then easily dislodge and become lost. If the lens appears to be properly on the eye and the child calms quickly, all is fine. If the child continues to cry for more than a couple of minutes or the eye reddens, the lens must be removed and inspected for foreign material or defects. If the problem occurs twice in a row without resolution the clinician must be consulted.

Hydrogel lens removal is equally simple. The parents must first be certain the lens is on the eye and did not get lost during the wearing period. If the lens is properly in place, after washing hands, with the child in the same restrained position as described above, the lens is gently pinched off the eye.

We believe at this time that careful daily lens cleaning with heat disinfection is best for patients of this age group. This is the most likely method to ensure that the lens is not contaminated with microorganisms prior to insertion, and lenses usually do not last long enough for soiling to become an issue. When the child is wearing the lens for some time and is over the initial hurdles, weekly enzyme cleaning should be added. Peroxide cleaning is an additional option which can be considered should complications arise with a heat system or should there be need to prescribe a hydrogel lens with a medium to high water content (55 percent or greater). We usually use low–water content (38 to 45 percent) hydrogel lenses for these patients; hydrogels of 55 percent water or higher should be peroxide cleaned and sterilized and the parents should be warned not to get any of the peroxide solution directly into the eyes.

Rigid Lenses

Rigid contact lens insertion, removal, and recentering follow normal clinical techniques, even for very young patients. Insertion and removal may be assisted in the very young group by the restraint technique described above, but a rigid lens is inserted directly onto the cornea and almost always is removed with a suction cup. The authors believe that gas-permeable materials should be used for all children (and perhaps for all patients who are not already successfully wearing PMMA). Lens care should be appropriate to clean and disinfect the material used, and good hygenic procedures should be emphasized.

PROGRESS EVALUATIONS

Frequent professional evaluations are vital for continued contact lens success, especially in children. As described above, changes in both corneal topography and refractive state may be rapid and erratic in children (5), and very often they do not report a change to parents. We suggest that children under 18 months of age be seen every week initially and then at least every 1 to 2 months. Beyond this, if all appears stable, the child should be seen every 2 to 3 months until age 5 or 6 years, and then at least every 4 months until into the teen years.

The clinician must observe and document vision progression (both parental impressions of acquisition of vision skills and objective visual acuity with techniques for specific ages, including, perhaps, preferential viewing, visual evoked potentials, pictographs, tumbling S, and Snellen letters), binocularity, optical refraction (retinoscopy solely in younger patients and retinoscopy with subjective refraction when possible), lens fit (movement, alignment, and fluorescein evaluation when applicable), and physiologic tolerance. In addition, the overall health of both eyes must be evaluated periodically. It is important to remember the vision needs of the other eye as well as the fitted eye when caring for patients who need only one contact lens.

CONCLUSIONS

The application of a contact lens to a 1-month-old aphakic infant can be very challenging. It begins a process that continues for many months, and perhaps years. It demands patience, skill, and care from all concerned. Nonetheless, it can be the most rewarding clinical experience of a career when the child obtains useful vision because of the combination of surgical and optical intervention, even if the vision is only in the 20/100 range. The use of a tinted prosthetic hydrogel lens to normalize the appearance of a small child's eye with microcornea or a large scar can also be quite clinically satisfying to both clinician and patient and has more immediate impact. Children are quite adaptable and quickly adjust to using a lens. Although risks are increased and responsibility is shared with parents, the benefits of this form of contact lens application may be quite substantial.

REFERENCES

1. Beller R, Hoyt CS, Marg E, et al: Good visual function after neonatal surgery for congenital monocular cataracts. Am J Ophthalmol 91:559, 1981.

2. Brennan NA: Current thoughts on the aetiology of ocular changes during contact lens wear. Aust J Optom 68:8, 1985.

3. Bradley A, Rabin J, Freeman RD: Nonoptical determinants of aniseikonia. Invest Ophthalmol Vis Sci 24:507, 1983.

4. Enoch JM: Fitting parameters which need to be considered when designing soft contact lenses for the neonate. Contact Lens Intraocular Lens Med J 5:310, 1979.

5. Gordon RA, Donzis PB: Refractive development of the human eye. Arch Ophthalmol 103:785, 1985.

6. Goss DA: Attempts to reduce the rate of increase of myopia in young people—A critical literature review. Am J Optom Physiol Opt 59:828, 1982.

7. Harris M: Correction of pediatric aphakia with silicone contact lenses. CLAO J 11:343, 1985.

8. Hiles DA: The need for intra-ocular lens implantation in children. Ophthalmic Surg 8:162, 1977.

9. Levinson A: Comparative study of the fitting of hard and Soflens contact lenses on infants and children. Optician 171:10, 1976.

10. Matsumoto E, Murphree AL: The use of silicone elastomer lenses in aphakic pediatric patients. Int Eyecare 2:214, 1986.

11. Mondino BJ, Weissman BA, Farb MD, et al: Corneal ulcers associated with daily-wear and extended-wear contact lenses. Am J Ophthalmol 102:58, 1986.

12. Morgan KS, Arffa RC, Marvelli TL, et al: Five year followup of epikeratophakia in children. Ophthalmology 93:423, 1986.

13. Nelson LB, Cutler SI, Calhoun JH, et al: Silsoft extended wear contact lenses in pediatric aphakia. Ophthalmology 92:1529, 1985.

14. Ogle K, Burian H, Bannon R: On correction of unilateral aphakia with contact lenses. Arch Ophthalmol 59:639, 1958.

15. Parks MM: Visual results in aphakic children. Am J Ophthalmol 94:441, 1982.

16. Parks MM, Hiles DA: Management of infantile cataracts. Am J Ophthalmol 63:10, 1967.

17. Paugh JR, Matoba R, Matoba ENY: Plus acceptance in hard contact lens wearers. Am J Optom Physiol Opt 64:703, 1987.

18. Pratt-Johnson JA, Tillson G: Hard contact lenses in the management of congenital cataracts. J Pediatr Ophthalmol Strabismus 22:94, 1985.

19. Robertson DM, Ogle KN, Dyer JA: Influence of contact lenses on accommodation. Am J Ophthalmol 64:860, 1967.

20. Sauders RA, Ellis FD: Empirical fitting of hard contact lenses in infants and young children. Ophthalmology 88:127, 1981.

21. Weissman BA: Fitting aphakic children with contact lenses. J Am Optom Assoc 54:235, 1983.

22. Weissman BA, Chun MW: Use of SPE bitoric rigid contact lenses in hospital practice. J Am Optom Assoc 58:626, 1987.

23. Weissman BA, Remba MJ, Fugedy E: Results of the extended wear contact lens survey of the Contact Lens Section of the American Optometric Association. J Am Optom Assoc 58:166, 1987.

24. White P, Scott C: Contact lenses and solutions summary. Contact Lens Spectrum August 1989.

25. Wiesel TN, Hubel DH: Effects of visual deprivation on morphology and physiology of cells in the cat's lateral geniculate body. J Neurophysiol 26:978, 1963.

26. Wiesel TN, Hubel DH: Single cell responses in striate cortex of kittens deprived of vision in one eye. J Neurophysiol 26:1003, 1963.

27. Wiesel TN, Hubel DH: Comparison of the effects of unilateral and bilateral eye closure on cortical unit responses in kittens. J Neurophysiol 28:1029, 1965.

28. Wiesel TN, Hubel DH: The period of susceptibility to the physiological effect of unilateral eye closure in kittens. J Physiol 206:419, 1970.

Chapter 10

Issues in the Clinical Management of Binocular Anomalies

Merton C. Flom

Chapters 10, 11, and 12 deal with the clinical management of binocular anomalies. Here the focus is on *issues* involved in determining *whether or not to treat* a binocular anomaly; it ends with a model for estimating the probability of obtaining functional correction of strabismus. Chapter 11 starts from the premise that treatment will be undertaken; it discusses the various treatment options available for managing binocular anomalies and lays out a model for considering, in sequence, different treatment procedures for different types of binocular anomalies. Chapter 12 presents details for providing vision therapy using orthoptics (vision training), particularly for infants and preschool children.

One approach to viewing the universe of binocular anomalies is to start with the oculo-motor deviation for distance fixation, which derives from the tonic innervation. When the tonic innervation is very low, an exodeviation results; high tonic innervation leads to distance esodeviation. In general, the larger the exodeviation or esodeviation, the more likely it is that the oculomotor deviation will be a strabismus; that is, bifoveal fixation will be totally absent (constant strabismus) or absent at least at some distance, in some field of gaze, or under some circumstances (occasional strabismus). There are exceptions: clinically one sees small-angle strabismus, especially esotropia, and large-angle phorias, especially exophorias. Strabismus and phoria can be considered to lie along a continuum, strabismus being a more severe form of heterophoria because the angle of deviation is typically larger in strabismus, and the associated anomalies, such as suppression and amblyopia, are more common and more severe in strabismus than in heterophoria (Table 10.1).

The anomalies associated with strabismus and heterophoria determine the prognosis of treatment as well as the selection of specific treatment options. Certain of these anomalies can limit the likelihood of correcting the strabismus. For heterophoria, on the other hand, the associated anomalies are generally fewer and less severe; for this reason treatment of the problems associated with heterophoria is characteristically successful. Before contemplating treating a strabismus, it is vital to determine what factors influence the prognosis (see below). Before doing so, we look at the problems encountered by persons who have strabismus or heterophoria; then we discuss the criteria for establishing functional and cosmetic correction of strabismus and the successful treatment of phoria patients. An appreciation of the problems of squinters and phoria patients and an understanding of what constitutes a functional and

Table 10.1   ANOMALIES ASSOCIATED WITH STRABISMUS AND HETEROPHORIA

Associated Anomaly	Strabismus	Heterophoria
Monocular fixation	Eccentric with amblyopia or anomalous retinal correspondence (ARC)	Foveal unless anisometropic amblyopia; then unsteady and perhaps slightly eccentric
Noncomitance	Significant in about 13% of squints	Significant in only a small portion (anisophoria)
Amblyopia (20/40)	About 14% of all squinters have amblyopia with 20/40 or worse acuity (mean acuity 20/74).	About 0.4% of phoria patients have amblyopia; 2.8% of all phorias are associated with anisometropia and 14% of these have amblyopia; mean acuity 20/60
Suppression	Common, especially with NRC; can be deep, preventing fusion	Foveal common in anisometropia
Anomalous correspondence	Affects most constant esotropes	Absent or inconsequential
Poor sensory fusion	Common lack of sensory fusion	Sometimes poor stereopsis
Poor motor fusion	Fusional vergence usually slow or absent	Fusional amplitudes may be reduced as well as facility of accommodation
Nystagmus	Monocular often seen in amblyopia; congenital nystagmus usually has strabismus.	Not usually visible in amblyopic eye; congenital nystagmus rare
Torticollis	Frequent with oblique involvement and lateral rectus fibrosis or palsy.	Rare; may be head tilt with involvement of oblique muscle
Diplopia	Common if of recent origin and sometimes after treatment; may be monocular in ARC	Binocular is rare; monocular sometimes with irregular astigmatism
Horror fusionalis	Associated with ARC	Rarely seen

cosmetic correction of strabismus and successful treatment of phoria patients will be a good basis for analyzing, one by one, the factors that affect the prognosis for functional correction of squint.

PATIENTS' VISION PROBLEMS

Strabismus Patients: Abnormal Binocular Vision and Conspicuous Deviation

Strabismus (squint, heterotropia) is an anomaly of binocular vision in which the visual axis of one eye fails to pass through the point of regard. It can be constant (continual) or occasional (intermittent). Although it can result from trauma or disease, squint is considered to be a developmental defect with a strong hereditary basis that occurs during early childhood and affects in the neighborhood of 4.8 percent of children (20), and perhaps a somewhat larger percentage of adults. When the deviation of the nonfixating eye is so large as to be conspicuous (20Δ horizontally, 10Δ vertically), the functional impairment of binocular vision is compounded by the problem of cosmesis. Interestingly, it is the appearance of the eyes of such children and not their symptoms or performance that usually prompts their parents to bring them in for professional attention. This fact has led many optometrists, ophthalmologists, pediatricians, and family practitioners to view strabismus mainly, if not entirely, as a cosmetic problem, like a large nose, baldness, or freckles.

This view is unnecessarily restrictive and not in the best interest of patients. Many strabismus patients can obtain functionally straight eyes with normal binocular vision. When functional correction is achieved, the cosmetic appearance of the eyes is satisfactory. When the squint is merely reduced to provide an acceptable appearance of the eyes, normal functional use of the eyes is not present. Because acceptable cosmesis accompanies functional correction of squint, but not the reverse, it is reasonable to consider first the chances of obtaining normal binocular vi-

sion. If the prognosis is poor or if treatment directed toward functional improvement is not advisable for some other reason, the prognosis for improved cosmesis should be considered. Often, improved cosmesis is all that can reasonably be expected from any form of treatment; however, to view strabismus only as a cosmetic problem is to deny some children the opportunity of obtaining normal binocular vision. On the other hand, to offer all strabismus patients the hope of functional correction is unrealistic and impractical. The reward—normal binocular vision—must be weighed against the time, effort, and expense required to obtain it. Knowing the factors that influence successful functional correction of strabismus (one of which is the skill of the professional) and being able to estimate the chances of obtaining functional correction are vital for giving the optometrist a sense of balance when deciding whether to treat strabismus to obtain normal binocular vision or to settle for improved cosmesis.

Phoria Patients: Ocular Discomfort and Impaired Performance

Phoria patients' eyes are straight all the time, so eye turn is not a problem. The binocular problems of adult phoria patients are usually ocular discomfort and impaired performance. These problems are typically related to the presence of one or more of the anomalies associated with heterophorias (see Table 10.1), the most common being central suppression, reduced stereopsis, and poor facility of fusional vergence and accommodation. It is usually difficult to get a child to acknowledge or describe discomfort associated with use of the eyes. Aside from shyness, language limitations, and restricted introspective abilities, the child may not have experienced long enough periods of comfort against which to compare discomfort. Would a child who has always had a significant vertical phoria and continual ocular discomfort have a basis for complaining about discomfort? Without basis for comparison, the child might believe that discomfort is the norm. There is a similar problem in establishing the role of vision in *impaired performance* in children. In the formative years children are learning to perform in so many new ways and so many factors are involved with each performance that it is difficult to identify the reason for any particular performance deficit. It is therefore necessary to rely largely on the variance of visual functions from average as determined by clinical tests. While such tests have merit, they cannot detect discomfort. At a minimum, abnormal clinical measures of visual functions can prompt the optometrist to alert the parents to watch for possible discomfort or impaired performance. In the best circumstances, the clinician would know or strongly suspect discomfort or impaired performance, in which case treatment would likely be undertaken because it is so successful in phoria patients (with the possible exception of cyclodeviations and incomitant phorias).

EVALUATION OF TREATMENT RESULTS

Criteria for Functional Correction of Strabismus

In an evaluation of the treatment of 61 cases of esotropia and 40 cases of exotropia, I (17) used the following criteria:

"Functional Cure" Clear, comfortable, single binocular vision must be present at all distances up to the near point of convergence, which is normal itself. There must be stereopsis and normal ranges of motor fusion. An occasional turning of the eyes may occur (up to about 1 percent of the time), providing diplopia is experienced whenever this happens. Correction lenses and small amounts of prisms ($\leq 5\Delta$) may be worn if necessary.

"Almost Cured" In this category a patient may lack stereopsis, may exhibit strabismus with diplopia up to 5 percent of the time, and may need larger amounts of prism to maintain comfortable binocular vision. In all other respects the patient must meet the criteria for functional cure.

These criteria for functional correction of

strabismus have been referred to as Flom's criteria and have been used in some studies (7, 14, 15, 31, 35, 36, 48).

In 1963 I proposed that the definition of the functional cure of strabismus should be maintenance of bifoveal fixation in the ordinary situations of life. Loss of bifixation should not occur more often than 1 percent of the time, i.e., at most, about 5 to 10 minutes a day. Vision should be clear and generally comfortable. The range of bifixation should include all fields of gaze and extend from very great viewing distances to only a few centimeters. Corrective lenses and reasonable amounts of prism may be worn if necessary (19).

In this later definition I dropped the requirements of stereopsis, of diplopia when the eyes rarely turn, and of normal ranges of motor fusion. Limiting the amount of prescribed prism to 5Δ was replaced by "reasonable amounts of prism." And added to the criteria was the requirement that bifixation be present in all fields of gaze (albeit with a possibly noncomitant phoria).

In seeking reasonable and appropriate criteria for the functional correction of strabismus, it is crucial to remember that *strabismus is an oculomotor anomaly characterized by a lack of bifoveal fixation in everyday situations of life.* Although it is true that strabismics typically have certain other defects that are associated with the strabismus, such as suppression, amblyopia, and poor stereopsis, it is necessary to realize that these associated defects are not the principal anomaly and that some persons who never squint have these defects. Nonetheless, some studies (13) include a criterion of stereopsis (say, 70 arc seconds) as indicative of bifoveal fusion; the problem with this indirect measure of bifoveal fixation is that many patients with small-angle esotropia and anomalous correspondence exhibit fairly good stereoscopic threshold angles.

Logically, then, any definition of functional correction of strabismus must have as its overriding criterion the *maintenance of bifoveal fixation in everyday situations of life.* It is inappropriate to consider as a criterion the fact that a squinter can, for example, maintain fusion for second-degree targets with the tubes of a major amblyoscope set at zero; such an accomplishment is merely a measure of the patient's ability to execute fusional vergence for two similar transilluminated targets presented dichoptically in separate tubes. It is also inappropriate to include criteria such as being able to control the squint without wearing glasses or without asthenopia, because many nonsquinters wear glasses, including bifocals, and have asthenopia.

Some day a professional organization, hopefully an interprofessional one, will adopt criteria for evaluating the treatment of strabismus for functional and cosmetic correction. In the meantime, we need to strive for uniformity of criteria in our search for answers about effective treatment.

In evaluating factors that influence the prognosis for functional correction of strabismus (see below), studies have been limited to those in which the criteria are specified and are in accord with the general principles discussed here.

Cosmetic Correction of Strabismus

When contemplating improved cosmesis in strabismus, either alone or in conjunction with achieving functional correction, a number of factors must be assessed and taken into account. It is unfortunate that so few practitioners take the time to identify these factors and evaluate the conspicuousness of the strabismus.

When a horizontal strabismus is less than 15 to 20Δ, it is usually not conspicuous, but persistent epicanthal folds, small interpupillary separation, and negative angles Kappa can make esotropia more noticeable and exotropia less so. On the other hand, an especially well-formed inner canthus, wide interpupillary separation, and positive angles Kappa tend to exaggerate exotropia and mask esotropia. A deviated nasal septum and other facial asymmetries can make a squint more or less obvious.

Vertical deviations of more than 10Δ usu-

ally present a cosmetic problem, as the eyes and lids appear to be out of alignment. Observers get the impression of a unilateral ptosis when there is a large hypotropia and of a one-eyed look of surprise when there is a large hypertropia. In other words, the vertical dimensions of the palpebral apertures appear to be noticeably unequal.

For both horizontal and vertical deviations, intermittency, alternation of fixation, and prominence of the eyes, as in proptosis or exophthalmos, make a squint more noticeable. Contrariwise, a constant unilateral squint in a person with deep-set eyes and a prominent brow is relatively less noticeable. If a strabismus is markedly noncomitant, as in complete paralysis of an extraocular muscle, the inability of the eyes to move conjugately within the field can be obvious and disconcerting to an observer.

With very large deviations and some noncomitant ones (e.g., Duane's retraction syndrome), the eye may be retracted into the orbit, giving the appearance of a small eye (enophthalmos) or of a drooping lid (pseudoptosis). The habitual head turn (seen commonly in Duane's retraction syndrome) or head tilt (seen frequently with involvement of one of the oblique muscles) can be more of a cosmetic problem than the ocular deviation; indeed, treatment of the strabismus can be directed to correcting abnormal head position (see Chapter 11).

The clinical examination of a squinter should include assessment of the conspicuousness of the squint and inspection for factors that affect cosmesis (Table 10.2).

Successful Treatment of Heterophoria Patients

As I pointed out above, the binocular problems of phoria patients are primarily ocular discomfort and impaired performance. Logically, then, the criteria for successful treatment of phoria patients ought to relate to alleviation of ocular discomfort and improvement in performance.

Assessing change in ocular discomfort relies almost exclusively on the patient's evalu-

Table 10.2. FACTORS THAT INFLUENCE THE CONSPICUOUSNESS OF STRABISMUS

Factor	Esotropia	Exotropia	Vertical
Deviation >10Δ	——	——	Worsens
Deviation >15 to 20Δ	Worsens	Worsens	Worsens
Persistent epicanthal folds	Worsens	Improves	——
Inner canthus especially well formed	Improves	Worsens	——
Small interpupillary distance	Worsens	Improves	——
Large interpupillary distance	Improves	Worsens	——
Positive angle Kappa (nasalward reflex)	Improves	Worsens	——
Negative angle Kappa (temporal reflex)	Worsens	Improves	——
Nose deviated toward squinting eye	Worsens	Improves	——
Nose deviated away from squinting eye	Improves	Worsens	——
Intermittency	Worsens	Worsens	Worsens
Constancy	Improves	Improves	Improves
Alternating squint	Worsens	Worsens	Worsens
Unilateral	Improves	Improves	Improves
Prominent eyes, minimal brow	Worsens	Worsens	Worsens
Deep-set eyes, prominent brow	Improves	Improves	Improves
Marked noncomitance	Worsens	Worsens	Worsens
Comitance	Improves	Improves	Improves
Large eyeglass frames	Worsens	Improves	Improves
Small eyeglass frames	Improves	Worsens	Worsens

ation of the change in symptoms, and children are not particularly adept at doing this. When children undertake treatment, improvement is usually desired and expected. Assessing change is very subjective and is often influenced by the patient's investment in the treatment. Bias is usually present, but careful questioning by the optometrist can yield useful information about alleviation of discomfort. Improvement in performance can be quantified objectively if actual performance can be closely simulated in the clinical setting. For example, impaired ability to look from the chalkboard to the desk, and vice versa, and to quickly see clearly can be simulated satisfactorily in the office. Speed of performance on an assembly line is difficult to simulate in the office, but sometimes it can be quantified in the workplace before and after treatment.

The difficulties notwithstanding, improvement of symptoms and performance must be assessed as objectively and concretely as possible. Support, but not confir-

mation, can be derived from improvement in clinical test results.

FACTORS THAT AFFECT PROGNOSIS FOR FUNCTIONAL CORRECTION OF STRABISMUS

We have already discussed the functional correction of strabismus, pointing out that the main criterion is maintenance of bifoveal fixation in the ordinary situations of life in all fields of gaze and extending from great viewing distances to a few centimeters. To obtain this bifixation, lenses and reasonable amounts of prism may be worn. To predict whether a strabismus patient can obtain such functional correction with treatment (lenses, prisms, occlusion, orthoptics, surgery) is to determine the prognosis for functional correction. The optometrist and the parent need to know the child's chances of obtaining functional correction of the squint. How is this done in practice? Most clinicians who treat strabismus learn through experience which squinters with which combinations of associated conditions achieve the best and worst results. For these practitioners, prognosis is determined by their experience with different kinds of strabismus. Another approach that can be used in conjunction with the first is to review clinical reports of functional results of treating strabismus associated with different conditions.

This approach is used here. Selected for analysis are factors associated with strabismus that are known or believed to influence the prognosis for functional correction. The studies reported here are intended to be illustrative, not exhaustive. They are studies that (1) had a described and reasonably representative sample, (2) used one or more specified treatment procedures, (3) indicated the criteria for functional correction of strabismus, and (4) analyzed the results in terms of one or more factors associated with strabismus.

Constancy of Strabismus

Everyone who works with strabismus recognizes that functional correction is easier when it is occasional (present only some of the time) than when it is constant (present all the time). The factor of constancy accounts in large part for the greater success in treating exotropia than esotropia, as about 80 percent of exotropias are occasional and about 75 percent of nonaccommodative esotropias are constant (17, 22, 37). Table 10.3 clearly shows that persons with constant strabismus, both esotropic and exotropic, obtain functional correction significantly less often than those whose disorder is occasional.

It is interesting to note that if a squint is occasional, the chances of obtaining functional correction are about the same in esotropia and exotropia. On the other hand, when the squint is constant, functional correction is somewhat more likely in exotropia than in esotropia. Because the element of constant or occasional is so important to the prognosis for functional correction, it is necessary to mention the value of the unilateral cover test for making this determination. The Worth Dot

Test is not satisfactory for this purpose, as fusion can be reported by a constant squinter with anomalous correspondence.

Several results shown in Table 10.3 merit comment. Ludlam's 1961 results are considerably higher than mine (19, 35); after a 4-year follow-up (36), the results approximate mine for the combined occasional squinters (55 percent and 56 percent) and become closer for the combined constant squinters (14 percent and 37 percent). In both studies, optometry students provided the treatment; more faculty supervision probably occurred in Ludlam's study. The substantially poorer results observed by Daum (12) in a retrospective study of patient records in an optometry school are probably attributable to the very stringent criteria for improvement that included a phoria with twice the fusional reserve and no asthenopia or amblyopia. The high success rates of Hoffman et al can be attributed in part to their treating only exotropia with normal correspondence. The functional results of Sanfilippo and Clahane (39) with exotropia (25 percent for constant, 78 percent for occasional) were achieved by patients who were able to do intensive orthoptics at home. Mulberger and McDonald (38) treated exotropia primarily with surgery but included some orthoptics before and after surgery and obtained straight eyes with fusion for only 7 percent of those with constant exotropia and only 32 percent of those with the occasional type. Altizer (1), on the other hand, compared surgical and nonsurgical treatment of exotropia; treating constant exotropia she obtained better results with surgery (31 percent vs 10 percent) and treating occasional exotropia she got better results with nonsurgical treatment (69 percent vs 44 percent). Hardesty et al (29) first operated on 100 persons with occasional exotropia, and 26 percent of them wound up with no squint; of the remaining 74 who were then treated by nonsurgical means, 69 percent were relieved of their squint.

All the studies cited here—using different samples, different treatment methods, and different criteria for functional correction—support the conclusion that the occa-

Table 10.3 FUNCTIONAL CORRECTION OF CONSTANT AND OCCASIONAL STRABISMUS

		Esotropia	Exotropia	Combined
Flom (19)[1]	Constant	6/55 = 11%	3/11 = 27%	9/66 = 14%
	Occasional	18/36 = 50%	29/49 = 59%	47/85 = 55%
Mulberger and McDonald (38)[2]	Constant		7/104 = 7%	
	Occasional		8/25 = 32%	
Ludlam (35)[3]	Constant	33/60 = 55%	14/20 = 70%	47/80 = 59%
	Occasional	10/11 = 91%	52/58 = 90%	62/69 = 90%
Ludlam and Kleinman (36)[4]	Constant			0.62 × 0.59 = 37%
	Occasional			0.63 × 0.90 = 56%
Hoffman et al (31)[5]	Constant		18/30 = 60%	
	Occasional		24/25 = 96%	
Sanflippo and Clahane (39)[6]	Constant		2/8 = 25%	
	Occasional		18/23 = 78%	
Altizer (1)[7]	Constant (no surgery)		1/10 = 10%	
	Occasional		9/13 = 69%	
	Constant (surgery)		4/13 = 31%	
	Occasional		7/16 = 44%	
Hardesty et al (29)[8]	Occasional (surgery)		26/100 = 26%	77/100 = 77%
	Occasional (nonsurgical after)		51/74 = 69%	
Etting (15)[9]	Constant	21/34 = 62%	12/15 = 80%	33/49 = 67%
	Occasional	9/9 = 100%	13/15 = 87%	22/24 = 92%
Daum (12)[10]	Constant		0/3 = 0%	
	Occasional		16/43 = 37%	

[1] Unselected cases treated by all methods (prisms, added lenses, occlusion, orthoptics, surgery). Used "cured" and "almost cured" categories.

[2] Exotropia was treated with surgery and orthoptics before and after. Criterion for result was "eyes are straight and fusion is present."

[3] Treated by orthoptics only; used Flom's "cured" and "almost cured" categories.

[4] Follow-up of same patients 3 to 7 years after treatment.

[5] Treated by orthoptics only; excluded patients with anomalous correspondence and previous surgery. Used Flom's "cured" criterion.

[6] Patients selected to be able to do intensive orthoptics at home. Occlusion if necessary. Criteria for result: Phoria at all distances, relative convergence >14Δ, unlimited convergence nearpoint, no suppression, and no asthenopia.

[7] Occlusion, prisms, and orthoptics, for one group; surgery for a second group. Criterion for success: Controlled phoria <20Δ.

[8] 100 occasional exotropes received surgery; the 74 who did not have a successful result received nonsurgical treatment (miotics, occlusion, prisms, and orthoptics). Functional cure: no tropia and some stereopsis.

[9] Referred patients, at least 6 years old, received lenses and/or orthoptics in office and at home. Used Flom's "cured" criterion.

[10] Primarily home orthoptics; retrospective study. Criteria for result: Phoria with twice the fusional reserve; no asthenopia, amblyopia, eccentric fixation, or anomalous correspondence.

sional quality of a strabismus is a favorable prognostic factor and that constancy is an unfavorable factor that substantially reduces the prognosis for functional correction.

Anomalous Retinal Correspondence

Anomalous correspondence is present in about 50 percent of all esotropia and about 20 percent of all exotropia. It is more likely to be present when the squint is constant than when it is occasional, especially in esotropia. In occasional strabismus, anomalous correspondence manifests itself only when the deviation is present; when fusional vergence overcomes the deviation and the eyes become straight, the angle of anomaly (of anomalous correspondence) becomes zero through a phenomenon called covariation (28).

Only about 25 percent of all esotropias are occasional; even when precautions are taken to disrupt fusion and cause the eye to go to its deviated position, only a very small percentage of occasional esotropia patients exhibit anomalous correspondence. Thus, studies reporting the rates of functional correction of esotropia with anomalous correspondence are providing treatment results primarily for constant esotropia; rates of correction for esotropia with normal correspondence represent a mixture of constant and occasional esotropia.

About 80 percent of exotropias are occasional, and perhaps 15 percent of these cases have associated anomalous correspondence when the deviation is manifest. Among the 20 percent of exotropia patients with constant squint, about 40 percent have anomalous correspondence, so reports of functional cure rates for exotropia with anomalous correspondence include a fairly equal mix of occasional and constant exotropia. This situation for exotropia differs sharply from that for esotropia, where anomalous correspondence represents mainly constant squinting and may account for why exotropia, even with anomalous correspondence, has a better prognosis for functional correction than esotropia.

Table 10.4 shows results of studies on the rate of functional correction of esotropia and exotropia according to the type of retinal correspondence before treatment. The clinical determination of anomalous retinal correspondence is usually made with the Bielschowsky Afterimage Test (the two foveal afterimages are perceptually displaced) or the major amblyoscope (objective measure of the angle of deviation differs significantly from the subjective angle of directionalization). In England, when a patient attempts to put the lion in the cage at an angle different from the objective angle of deviation but cannot do so because of suppression, the performance is referred to as a lack of normal retinal correspondence. Although some writers have speculated on a causal connection between suppression and anomalous correspondence (23, 43), the fact is that each can be present without the other.

After distinguishing between abnormal (anomalous) retinal correspondence and lack of normal correspondence, two English investigators reported no functional correction of 89 (9) and 28 (34) cases of esotropia with anomalous correspondence, and 16 percent (9) among 174 cases of esotropia lacking normal correspondence. In the United States, Ludlam (35) considered as one of five tests of anomalous correspondence a lack of fusion at the angle of deviation; this would presumably include subjects having no simultaneous foveal perception resulting from suppression. Thus the relatively high rate (23 percent) of functional cures among Ludlam's esotropic patients who exhibited anomalous correspondence on any one of the five tests may be due to the fact that some of these patients had suppression that obscured the fact that the two foveas actually corresponded. This interpretation is strengthened by the fact that, of the 39 squinters (esotropic and exotropic) Ludlam considered to have anomalous correspondence, thirteen showed *normal* correspondence on three of the five different tests he employed. Considering only his subjects who showed anomalous correspondence on at least three of the five tests, only 26 (instead of 39) squinters had anomalous correspondence, and only four of them (15 percent) achieved a functional correction. Ludlam and

Table 10.4 FUNCTIONAL CORRECTION OF STRABISMUS ACCORDING TO TYPE OF RETINAL CORRESPONDENCE PRESENT BEFORE TREATMENT

Reference		Esotropia	Exotropia	Combined
Cashell (9)[1]	Normal	347/856 = 41%		
	Anomalous	0/89 = 0%		
	Lack of normal	27/174 = 16%		
Flom (19)[2]	Normal	23/58 = 40%	27/47 = 57%	50/105 = 48%
	Anomalous	1/33 = 3%	5/13 = 38%	6/46 = 13%
Bedrossian (5)[3]	Normal	8/19 = 42%		
	Anomalous	0/19 = 0%		
Levinge (34)[4]	Anomalous	0/28 = 0%		
Cooper (10)[5]	Normal	94/289 = 33%		
	Anomalous	10/93 = 9%		
Swan (44)[6]	Normal		42/70 = 60%	
	Anomalous		0/17 = 0%	
Ludlam (35)[7]	Normal	37/45 = 86%	58/65 = 89%	45/58 = 78%
	Anomalous	6/26 = 23%	8/13 = 62%	14/39 = 36%
Ludlam (35)[8]	Normal			55/71 = 77%
	Anomalous			4/26 = 15%
Ludlam and Kleinman (36)[9]	Anomalous			0.33 × 0.15 = 5%
Etting (14)[10]	Normal	9/12 = 75%	16/18 = 89%	25/30 = 84%
	Anomalous	1/10 = 10%	1/2 = 50%	2/12 = 17%
Etting (14)[11]	Normal	25/25 = 100%	24/29 = 83%	49/54 = 91%
	Anomalous	5/18 = 28%	1/1 = 100%	6/19 = 32%
Wick and Cook (48)[12]	Anomalous	28/53 = 53%		

[1] Treated by all methods.

[2] Unselected cases treated by all methods (prisms, added lenses, occlusion, orthoptics, surgery). Used "cured" and "almost cured" categories.

[3] Treated by surgery and postoperative occlusion. Excluded amblyopia worse than 20/40.

[4] Treated by orthoptics and surgery.

[5] Treated by surgery, occlusion, and orthoptics. The 10 patients with anomalous correspondence who obtained a functional result had normal correspondence just before surgery, four following occlusion, and six following orthoptics.

[6] Exotropia was corrected with surgery and occasional orthoptics. Sensory status was determined by: correspondence tests, prisms, red-green and Polaroid filters, amblyoscope, afterimage, and anaglyphic tests.

[7] ARC considered if one or more tests showed anomaly. Treated by orthoptics only. Used Flom's "cured" and "almost cured" categories.

[8] Same study but considered ARC only if three or more tests showed anomaly.

[9] Follow-up of same patients (as in 7 above) 3 to 7 years after treatment.

[10] Patients from private optometric practice of Dr. Donald Getz were given orthoptics in office and at home. Used Flom's "cured" criterion.

[11] Patients were referred and treatment was begun after 6 years of age. Treatment included lenses and/or orthoptics in office and at home. Used Flom's "cured" criterion.

[12] Patients from private optometric practice were given occlusion, orthoptics, biofeedback, prism overcorrection, and surgery as indicated. Used Flom's "cured" and "almost cured" criteria.

Kleinman (36) reexamined the patients 4 years after completion of treatment; from their follow-up data it appears that of the four anomalous correspondence patients who originally attained functional correction, only one patient's correction persisted after 4 years. This amounts to a long-term cure rate of only 4 percent (or perhaps 5 percent), which is somewhat less than the 13 percent functional cure rate of all strabismus cases with anomalous correspondence that I found (19) up to a year after treatment.

In two different studies, Etting (14, 15) reported using nonsurgical treatment methods and obtained functional cures for 17 percent of squinters with anomalous correspondence in the first study and 32 percent in the second study. A high rate of functional correction of squinters having anomalous correspondence was reported by Wick and Cook (48); using nonsurgical methods on 53 squinters in his practice and referring eight of them for subsequent surgery, Wick obtained "cured" or "almost cured" status for 28 (52 percent) patients. For 16 patients who had deviations less than 15Δ, he instituted divergence training using the Flom swing technique; nine (56 percent) of these 16 cases of small-angle esotropia were functionally corrected. The Wick and Cook (48) paper states that, ". . . for esotropic patients with anomalous correspondence and large angles (>16Δ), many times the extra effort required on the part of the patient and doctor/therapist is disproportionate to the gain when Flom cure was the desired result. 'Nearly cured' results (including microtropia) and cosmetic cures were much easier to obtain."

In reviewing the literature on surgery leading to a change in correspondence from anomalous to normal, Wick and Cook (48) report on five studies in which the average normalization of correspondence was about 20 percent. The issue under discussion here, however, is the rate of functional correction of strabismus in patients with anomalous correspondence. In separate studies, Bedrossian (5) and Levinge (34) found no functional correction in a total of 47 cases of esotropia with anomalous correspondence when surgery

was the principal form of treatment. Swan (44), similarly, obtained no functional results among 17 cases of exotropia with anomalous correspondence treated primarily with surgery. Cooper (10) obtained 9 percent functional cures in 93 patients with esotropia with anomalous correspondence, but all the patients obtained normal correspondence by occlusion or orthoptics before surgery. In spite of the low success rate of surgery for functional correction of squint with anomalous correspondence, and even though surgery often fails to normalize an anomalous correspondence, it is important to recognize that surgery can change the *angle of anomaly.* My colleagues and I (24) reported on a patient with intermittent exotropia of 54Δ who had harmonious anomalous correspondence (angle of anomaly of −54Δ) when squinting and normal correspondence (angle of anomaly of 0) when bifoveally fixating. After surgery, the bilateral surgical patches were removed and binocular vision was allowed for the first time since the operation 6 hours earlier; the angle of anomaly was momentarily −54Δ, then it shifted instantly to −7Δ and 0, even though the angle of deviation was fairly constant at about 11Δ *esotropia.* A second operation was performed 4 days later; 2.5 months hence there was exophoria of 3Δ with normal correspondence when fusing and harmonious anomalous correspondence (angle of anomaly of −3Δ) when fusion was disrupted to exhibit a 3Δ exodeviation.

In summary, there is little doubt that anomalous correspondence generally hinders functional correction of strabismus. Nonsurgical methods of treatment such as vision training seem to normalize anomalous correspondence and provide functional correction better than surgery does. Anomalous correspondence is less of a deterrent to functional correction of exotropia than esotropia and of an occasional than a constant strabismus. And, anomalous correspondence is easier to treat in esotropia when the deviation is less than 15Δ. In any case, treatment of an anomalous correspondence is easiest when motor fusional vergence can be activated to overcome the ocular deviation, at which time the retinal correspondence becomes normal. This approach to treating anomalous correspondence applies to all exotropia (occasional or constant, and small- or large-angle), to all occasional esotropia, and to constant esotropia with deviation less than 15Δ. For constant esotropia with large angles of deviation, a different treatment for anomalous correspondence is required, forced elimination. It is time consuming and difficult, and for most practitioners the probability of functional correction of the strabismus is low.

Amblyopia and Eccentric Fixation

Amblyopia is most commonly defined as a nonoptical and nonpathologic loss of visual acuity to 20/40 or worse. By this criterion, amblyopia has a prevalence among school children of about 1 to 2 percent (21). Interestingly, more than half of these children had acuity in the affected eye of 20/40, 20/50, or 20/60; acuity of 20/200 or worse was observed in only about 20 percent of the amblyopes. When amblyopia is observed in clinical practice, it is almost always associated with anisometropia or strabismus. Occasionally it is seen in association with unilateral childhood cataract or ptosis. About one third of amblyopic children have anisometropia only; a third have strabismus only; and approximately a third have both anisometropia and strabismus (20). About 20 percent of anisometropic persons with at least 1.0 D of interocular refractive difference in corresponding meridians have amblyopia (20). Among all squinters (esotropic, exotropic, constant, and occasional), amblyopia is found about 14 percent of the time. It is this group that concerns us here. We ask, "When amblyopia is present in a squinter, how does it affect the chances of obtaining functional correction of the strabismus?" Table 10.5 shows the results of several studies.

Costenbader (11) found that surgery for congenital esotropia produced a functional correction for only 4 percent, regardless of whether they had amblyopia. Etting (15) found an approximately equal functional cure rate (>80 percent) among patients with exo-

tropia with and without amblyopia. Table 10.5 shows that, except in Costenbader's and Etting's series, the functional cure rates for both esotropia and exotropia were lower when amblyopia was present. Amblyopia appears to be less of a deterrent to functional correction with exotropia than with esotropia. This result may be due partly to the higher prevalence of occasional squint in exotropia, and to the generally better acuity found in amblyopic persons with exotropia than with esotropia.

Strabismic amblyopic persons tend to fixate eccentrically by an amount that is correlated with the degree of amblyopia: $r = +0.94$ (22); $r = +0.62$ (30). The worse the acuity, the larger the degree of eccentric fixation. Kirschen and I (32) demonstrated that in eccentrically fixating strabismic amblyopia patients acuity is maximum at the fovea, even though it is less than normal there. Generally, the reduced acuity in an eccentrically fixating strabismic amblyopic eye results partly from the normally reduced acuity at an eccentric locus and partly from a sensory (amblyopia) deficit that extends from the fovea out to 10 degrees or so. Hess (30) found that three of 10 strabismic amblyopic eyes had letter acuity that was consistent with that expected from the eccentric retinal locus they used for fixation. Kirschen and I (32) refer to this phenomenon as the retinal locus effect in amblyopia. These three patients would be expected to attain normal acuity if they could be trained to master foveal fixation. Three of Hess's other strabismic amblyopic patients had foveal fixation, so their acuity loss would be attributed to what Kirschen and I (32) called the sensory deficit in amblyopia. In anisometropic amblyopia, this sensory deficit is believed to be primarily a resolution loss (23); in strabismic amblyopia, on the other hand, the deficit is believed to be primarily spatial uncertainty and distortion (2, 4, 23) or spatiocortical undersampling (33). In any case, for strabismic amblyopia with central fixation and a sensory deficit, training would need to be directed toward improving spatial localization across the central retina without concern for the locus of fixation or resolution,

Table 10.5 FUNCTIONAL CORRECTION OF STRABISMUS ACCORDING TO THE PRESENCE OF AMBLYOPIA

Reference	Amblyopia	Esotropia	Exotropia	Combined
Flom (19)[1]	Yes	3/31 = 10%	6/16 = 37%	9/68 = 13%
	No	21/60 = 35%	26/44 = 59%	47/104 = 45%
Cooper (10)[2]	Yes	25/190 = 13%	7/20 = 35%	32/210 = 15%
	No	79/192 = 41%	65/84 = 80%	144/276 = 52%
Sternberg and Bohar (43)[3]	Yes			22/156 = 14%
Costenbader (11)[4]	Yes	7/189 = 4%		
	No	12/311 = 4%		
Sanfilippo and Clahane (39)[5]	Yes		1/6 = 17%	
	No		19/25 = 76%	
Etting (15)[6]	Yes	9/18 = 50%	6/7 = 86%	15/25 = 60%
	No	21/25 = 84%	19/23 = 83%	40/48 = 83%

[1] Unselected cases treated by all methods (prisms, added lenses, occlusion, orthoptics, and surgery). Criterion for amblyopia: Greater than one line acuity difference between eyes.
[2] Amblyopia considered absent when acuity equal in two eyes and free alternation present. Used surgery, orthoptics, and occlusion.
[3] Sample included patients with esotropia and exotropia having eccentric fixation associated with the amblyopia. Treated by occlusion of good eye, orthoptics, and surgery.
[4] Infantile esotropia was corrected surgically. Criterion for amblyopia was acuity of 20/40 or worse. Criterion for success was stereopsis of 50% or more by Wirt stereopsis test.
[5] Patients were selected for ability to do intensive orthoptics at home. Occlusion if necessary. Criteria for result: Phoria at all distances, relative convergence >14Δ, unlimited convergence near point, no suppression, and no asthenopia.
[6] Patients treated after 6 years of age. Criterion for amblyopia: One line or more difference between the eyes with 20/30 at best. Received lenses and/or orthoptics in office and at home. Used Flom's "cured" criterion.

both of which can be essentially normal. Hess' remaining four patients with strabismic amblyopia had a combination of retinal locus effect and sensory deficit. Interestingly, successful training of spatial localization in these patients tends to result in monocular fixation becoming more central along with improvements in acuity, making specific training to centralize fixation unnecessary.

We know a lot about the eccentric fixation that frequently occurs in strabismus. The question is, "Does eccentric fixation influence the prognosis for correcting the amblyopia or for obtaining functional correction of the strabismus?"

Girard et al (27) treated 72 patients for anisometropic and strabismic amblyopia with either central or eccentric fixation; they used spectacles, occlusion, pleoptics, orthoptics, drugs, and surgery. They found a final acuity of 20/30 or better in 15 of 20 (75 percent) central fixators and in 27 of 52 (52 percent) eccentric fixators. While these results implicate eccentric fixation as a deterrent to obtaining good acuity, it is worth noting that the central fixators tended to have better acuity than the eccentric fixators, many of whom had quite profound amblyopia. This suggests that the degree of the amblyopia, and not eccentric fixation, may be the principal determinant. The same thing can be said for the eight other studies cited by Girard et al (27), in which 78 percent of centrally fixating amblyopic patients obtained 20/40 to 20/30 acuity or better and only 39 percent of eccentric fixators did.

The presence of amblyopia reduces the chances for functional correction of strabismus. From clinical experience we observe that the acuity of severely amblyopic eyes must be improved to 20/100 to 20/60 before binocularity can be demonstrated and the strabismus corrected. Thus, it may be that severe amblyopia, perhaps in conjunction with eccentric fixation, further worsens the prognosis for functional correction of strabismus; but this is only conjecture.

Although this section deals with amblyopia and the eccentric fixation that accompanies it in strabismic amblyopia, it is important to point out that eccentric monocular fixation can occur in nonamblyopic eyes. This sounds impossible: how could acuity be normal at an eccentric retinal locus? In a study of eccentric fixation in strabismus and amblyopia, Weymouth and I (22) measured the position of an entoptic image of the macular pigment (Maxwell's spot) with respect to a fixation mark that subjects were told to "look right at." Among our 117 subjects were a subset of 11 strabismus patients with anomalous correspondence who exhibited no amblyopia. Nine of them had eccentric fixation. Three of the nine were recalled for further examination; all perceived Maxwell's spot to be displaced from the fixation dot when told to "look right at the fixation mark," and in each case, when instructed to "observe the small figure scratched out within the fixation mark," they perceived it to be centered. These squinters (with anomalous correspondence and no amblyopia) apparently have two retinal fixing loci: one, the fovea, is used for acuity or resolution tasks; the other, the eccentric fixation locus, is used for directionalization and referencing of monocular eye movements. If such dual retinal fixation occurs in the deviating nonamblyopic eyes of strabismus patients with anomalous correspondence, it seems reasonable that it occurs in deviating *amblyopic* eyes of such patients also. Indeed, clinicians frequently encounter amblyopic patients who can read more letters, albeit not the smallest ones, on the acuity chart when they report looking with the amblyopic eye to one side of each letter and not right at it. If these amblyopes have dual retinal fixing points associated with anomalous correspondence, as do the 9 nonamblyopic subjects reported by Weymouth and me

(22), then one wonders whether the prognosis for functional correction of such anomalously corresponding amblyopic strabismus is determined less by the amblyopia and eccentric fixation than by the anomalous correspondence (which was noted above to be a serious deterrent among those with constant esotropia whose deviation is greater than 15Δ).

Suppression and Sensory Fusion

A large proportion of strabismic persons— and many others—fail to perceive some part of one ocular image when tested under certain binocular conditions, but the differences in depth and extent of this suppression are large and they depend greatly on the test situation. Suppression in nonsquinters tends not to be very deep and to be confined to the foveal region of one eye; it is usually associated with anisometropia, amblyopia, or large heterophoria. When suppression is present in squinters, on the other hand, it usually extends from the image point to the fovea of the deviating eye and tends to be deeper than in nonsquinters.

It is important to recognize that squinters who deny experiencing diplopia do not necessarily have suppression. Squinters with harmonious or nearly harmonious anomalous correspondence will have the image of the fixated object fall on a peripheral retinal area of the deviating eye that corresponds to the fovea of the fixating eye. Thus these squinters may experience a form of binocular "fusion" without suppression. On the other hand, the absence of diplopia in strabismus with normal correspondence can be taken as evidence of suppression.

The role of suppression in obtaining functional correction of strabismus is difficult to determine because suppression is affected so much by the stimulus conditions of the testing situation. Moreover, the extent and intensity of suppression are difficult to quantify. In light of these problems, most clinicians employ a favorite test or two and learn through experience to grade suppression as slight, moderate, or marked.

In 1963 I reported on a study in which the level of sensory fusion was assessed before treating 91 patients with esotropia and 60 with exotropia; with one exception, I found that obtaining functional correction did not depend much on the degree of sensory fusion exhibited before treatment (Table 10.6). The exception appears to be esotropes who suppressed second-degree (fusible) targets of subtense 6° or 2°. Of 62 such suppressing esotropes, only 11 (18 percent) obtained functional correction of the strabismus. In contrast, 45 percent of the esotropic patients (13 of 29) who demonstrated sensory fusion for both targets achieved functional correction after treatment. In accord with this result is the report by Cashell (9) on 1,119 esotropic patients: a "binocular result" was obtained by 71 percent of those with good "fusion," but by only about 15 percent who had deep or extensive suppression.

Logically, one would think that the higher the degree of sensory fusion the better the chances for functional correction of strabismus. The unexpected results of Table 10.6 may simply indicate that other factors, such as constancy and state of retinal correspondence, generally outweigh the influence of grades of sensory fusion in predicting functional correction of strabismus, except in esotropia where fusion or suppression of small (2°) and large (6°) second-degree targets still affects prognosis.

Comitance

The degree of phoria or strabismus is specified by the angle of deviation measured in straight-ahead or primary gaze. If the ocular muscles are functioning properly, a target moved into different directions of gaze will elicit accurately conjugated eye movements so that the two eyes move equally; consequently, any oculomotor deviation present in the primary position will be present to the same degree in an eccentric direction of gaze. Such phorias or squints are said to be concomitant or comitant; they are characterized by an angle of deviation that is approximately equal in all directions of gaze. A significant change in angle of deviation with change in gaze defines a nonconcomitant, noncomitant, or incomitant deviation.

Incomitant deviations result from under- or overaction of one or more of the oculorotary muscles. Underaction of an oculorotary

Table 10.6 PREVALENCE OF FUNCTIONAL CORRECTION OF SQUINT ACCORDING TO TYPE OF SENSORY FUSION PRESENT BEFORE TREATMENT*

	Esotropia	Exotropia
Large (5°) first-degree		
Suppression	5/22 = 23%	8/17 = 47%
Sensory fusion	19/69 = 18%	24/43 = 56%
Large (6°) and small (2°) second-degree†		
Suppression with either target	11/62 = 18%	26/48 = 54%
Sensory fusion with both targets	13/29 = 45%	6/12 = 50%
Detailed third-degree		
No stereopsis	18/69 = 26%	23/40 = 58%
Stereopsis	6/22 = 27%	9/20 = 45%

* Unselected cases treated by all methods (prisms, added lenses, occlusion, orthoptics, surgery).
† For second-degree targets, differences are significant by chi-square test at the 0.05 level.
(From Flom MC: The prognosis in strabismus. In Hirsch MJ, Wick RE (eds): Vision of Children. Philadelphia, Chilton, 214, 1963.)

muscle is most commonly produced by partial paralysis or paresis (due to reduced neural activity to the muscle); less common causes of muscle underaction are complete paralysis (as in sixth nerve palsy), muscle malinsertion (behind its normal insertion), muscle fibrosis (as in Duane's retraction syndrome), and space-occupying orbital lesions (e.g., tumors). Muscle overaction is most often produced by a muscle being malinserted in front of its normal insertion; rarely is an irritative lesion seen that causes an extraocular muscle to overact.

In 1963 I reported significant incomitance in 16 percent of 179 squinters, with about equal prevalence in esotropia and exotropia. The most common incomitance was overaction of one or both inferior oblique muscles, which produced an increasing hyperdeviation of the adducting eye on upgaze to the right or left and a relative divergence of the eyes on straight upgaze. This type of incomitance is now called the V syndrome or pattern, to describe relative divergence on upgaze and relative convergence on downgaze. The opposite is the A pattern. Von Noorden (47) cites a number of prevalence studies of A and V patterns and concludes, "It is clear that one out of every three or four patients with strabismus may be expected to have an A or V pattern" (p. 335). Based on data from Costenbader, von Noorden showed the relative breakdown of 421 squinters who had an A or V pattern (Table 10.7). A or V pattern incomitance was about twice as likely to be associated with esotropia as with exotropia (66 percent vs 34 percent) and the incidence of V pattern incomitance was twice that of A pattern (64 percent vs 36 percent). Relatively more V than A patterns occurred among the exotropic patients (23/11 = 2.1) than among the esotropic ones (41/25 = 1.6). Although no single cause (innervational or structural) explains the A and V patterns, underaction or overaction of one or more of the oblique muscles is the most common clinical finding.

A and V patterns notwithstanding, paresis of the vertical eye muscles occurs about four times as often as paresis of the horizontal muscles (37). Indeed, truly comitant vertical deviations are rare (6), and nearly all significant cyclodeviations are noncomitant and involve an oblique muscle.

When considering how noncomitance might affect the prognosis for functional correction of squint, an important place to start is to recognize that many noncomitant squinters have bifoveal fixation in some field of gaze—making them occasional squinters, whose prognosis is better than that of constant squinters. In combination with constant strabismus, marked noncomitancy makes attainment of functional binocular vision extremely unlikely (37).

Disregarding constancy, noncomitancy worsens the prognosis for functional correction. Cooper (10) obtained a "fusional result" four times as often (32 percent) treating comitant esotropia as vertically incomitant esotropia (8 percent). Scobee's (41) functional results were about twice as good when the esotropia was uncomplicated by a noncomitant vertical deviation (47 percent and 24 percent).

Management of markedly incomitant squint usually involves surgery; the functional outcome depends on several presurgical factors (comitance, constancy, state of retinal correspondence, and amblyopia). When an ocular muscle is completely or largely paralyzed, normal ocular motility usually cannot be obtained with surgery; in these cases an attempt is made to obtain bifoveal fixation in the central portion of the field, or, if this is impossible, simply to improve the cosmesis.

Table 10.7   BREAKDOWN OF COSTENBADER'S 421 STRABISMUS PATIENTS WITH A OR V PATTERN INCOMITANCE

	V	A	Total
Esotropia	41%	25%	66%
Exotropia	23%	11%	34%
Total	64%	36%	100%

(Data from VonNoorden [47].)

Age of Onset and Duration of Strabismus

Conventional wisdom says that the earlier the onset of a strabismus, the poorer is the prognosis for its functional correction. The underlying idea is that a squint that appears very early in life (say, before 6 months) affords little opportunity for the visual system to develop the neurophysiological substrate for binocularity. Conversely, if strabismus occurs at an age when the system is reasonably well developed (say, after 2 years), the chances of recovering binocularity with subsequent treatment ought to be quite good.

Studies relating age of onset to obtaining functional correction are fraught with difficulties, not the least of which is confirming when the squint actually started. Information about onset usually comes from parents who are reporting when they remember first noticing the child's eye turn. They may interpret an infant's early random convergence movements or epicanthal folds as strabismus. Costenbader (11) found that about 50 percent of children reported by parents to have squint did not have it; he also analyzed age-of-onset data obtained from parents of strabismic children. He concluded that onset-information obtained from parents is questionable. Flawed as onset studies might be, they generally indicate that the percentage of functional corrections increases with age of onset. To ascertain the rate of change of functional correction per year of age at onset, a straight line was fitted to the linear portion of the data obtained from four studies (see Fig. 10.1).

The slopes of the fitted lines for the Ludlam (32) and the Cashell (9) studies are quite steep and have similar values of about 12 percent per year. This means that, for these investigators, the success rate of functional correction is 12 percent greater for strabismus with onset at 1.5 years than with onset at age 6 months. For Ludlam's patients this amounts to an increase in functional correction from 50 to 62 percent, and in Cashell's study from 10 to 22 percent. On the other hand, the slopes of the lines fitted to the data of Fletcher and Silverman (16) and to my data (19) are fairly shallow, being approximately equal at about 3 percent per year. For the patients in the Fletcher and Silverman study, this rate represents a change in functional correction from about 37 percent at 6 months to about 40 percent at 1½ years; the corresponding values for my study are 18 percent and 21 percent. Clearly, the 3 percent rates indicate that age of onset of squint is not a major determinant of successful functional correction. The 12 percent rate suggests that age of onset has an influence on functional correction.

What is an optometrist to do? Given the disparate results of these (and comparable) studies and the acknowledged lack of validity of parents' dating of the onset of their child's strabismus, it seems imprudent to place much importance on age of onset as a predictor of functional correction. Costenbader, whose 1961 data on surgical correction of infantile esotropia are plotted in Figure 10.1 for comparison, asked (11), "If the history is not reliable, of what value is the presumed age of onset as a prognostic criterion?"

Costenbader's question also applies to the duration of the squint, the time from the onset of a squint to the beginning of treatment. To the extent that age of onset is invalid, so is duration of strabismus. Nonetheless, some studies show that longer duration worsens the prognosis for functional correction. Cashell's (9) data are representative: 76 percent of his 21 patients treated within 5 years of onset of the squint obtained a functional result and only 28 percent of 25 patients treated after 5 years duration obtained this result. Since duration would be expected to have its greatest effect on early-onset strabismus, it is revealing to look at Costenbader's 1961 study (11) of infantile esotropia, all cases with onset before age 11 months (Table 10.8). Posttreatment fusional data are provided for 360 esotropic children; the percentage who attained stereopsis (gross or refined) is highest for durations of 3 to 4 years and not for the shortest durations, as Costenbader expected. One could speculate that children 4 to 6 years old can cooperate better in the di-

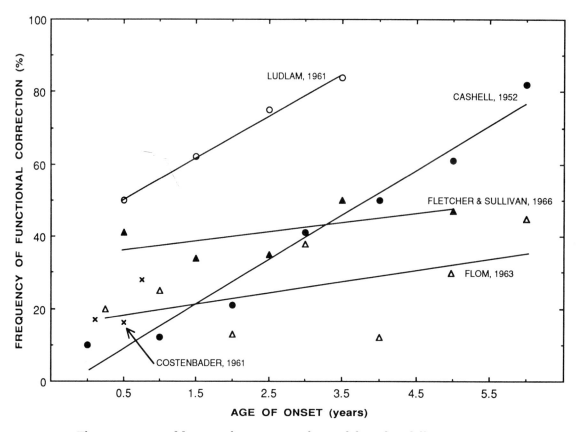

Figure 10.1 The percentage of functional corrections obtained from five different studies are plotted as a function of the reported age of onset of the strabismus. Ludlam's 1961 study included data for onsets at 5, 6, 7, and >7 years; the average percentage of functional corrections for these onsets was about 85 percent. The slope of the line fitted to the plotted Ludlam (35) data is about 12 percent per year, as is the slope for the Cashell (9) data. The slopes of the lines fitted to the data of Fletcher and Silverman (16) and of Flom (17) are approximately equal, about 3 percent per year. These four studies employed all forms of treatment (lenses, prisms, occlusion, orthoptics, and surgery), except the Ludlam study in which all patients received extensive orthoptics and few received surgery. The data of Costenbader (10) are plotted for comparison; he treated all infantile esotropia with surgery primarily.

Table 10.8 INCIDENCE OF STEREOPSIS IN INFANTS WITH ESOTROPIA FOLLOWING TREATMENT STARTED AT DIFFERENT INTERVALS AFTER ONSET OF STRABISMUS

	Interval Between Onset and Initial Treatment						
	<1 yr	1–2 yr	2–3 yr	3–4 yr	4–5 yr	5–6 yr	>6 yr
Number of Subjects	25	38	73	78	62	42	42
Stereopsis							
Present (%)	12	16	18	29	24	21	20
Absent (%)	88	84	82	71	76	79	80

(From Costenbader FD: Infantile esotropia. Trans Am Ophthalmol Soc 59:397, 1961.)

agnostic and management phases than younger children, thereby contributing to better treatment results. And, because parents' observations are unreliable, some of the reported 3- and 4-year durations may be invalid: some children might not have had infantile esotropia but rather a later onset esotropia, for which the prognosis may be better.

When a child is old enough to perform tests that provide information about the important conditions associated with squint—about 3 or 4 years—then information about age of onset and duration of squint have little predictive value for treatment outcome.

Fixation Preference

When a squint is present, most patients use the same eye to fixate objects of interest in the vast central portion of the visual field (unilateral squint). The preferred eye is usually, but not always, the eye with better acuity, less suppression, smaller refractive error, or nonparetic muscle. Other squinters change fixation from one eye to the other for no apparent reason and usually without realizing it (alternating squints). Patients with alternating squint usually prefer to fixate with one eye, even though they switch fixation from one eye to the other inadvertently, without instruction, and for no apparent reason.

The terminology of alternating and unilateral strabismus is sometimes confused with equality or inequality of visual acuity, refractive error, or suppression in the two eyes. This confusion has resulted in some misleading implications about laterality of squint and prognosis for functional correction. For example, Cooper (10) assumed a direct relationship between equal acuity and alternation of fixation; he found a higher proportion of functional cures for esotropia with equal acuity (41 percent) than esotropia with "monocular fixation preference" (13 percent). His results more likely reflect the influence of amblyopia on functional correction.

For many patients the distinction between unilateral and alternating strabismus rests largely on the clinician's criterion and

judgement. Laterality is usually assessed from the Unilateral Cover Test and Hirschberg Test; when the deviation is large (say, greater than 25 to 30Δ), direct observation can be the determinant. Table 10.9 shows the occurrences of functional corrections among unilateral and alternating squinters reported in six studies. Although different samples were used and somewhat different criteria for alternation and functional correction were employed, it is remarkable how similar the percentages are in each study for unilateral and alternating squinters. The evidence is strong: the unilateral or alternating nature of a squint has no demonstrable influence on its functional correction.

Family History of Strabismus

A genetic basis for some strabismus has been well-established (42). It seems that functional correction should have a higher success rate for acquired strabismus than for inherited strabismus. In a sample of esotropia patients, Cashell (9) obtained a slightly higher percentage of functional corrections when there was a family history of strabismus (35 percent) than when there was not (30 percent); the difference was not statistically significant by chi-square test at the .05 level (Table 10.10). My (19) results for esotropia indicate significantly better functional results when there was a family history of squint (42 percent as opposed to 15 percent); corresponding differences for exotropia (63 percent and 49 percent) were not significant statistically. How might a family history of squint improve the chances for functional correction of esotropia? A parent who had a squint or knew a family member who did might recognize the esotropia earlier and might be prompter in seeking professional attention and more diligent in following the optometrist's instructions. Such factors would enhance the probability of functional correction. Since most exotropias are occasional, family history of squint should have little effect on an already good prognosis. Whatever the explanation for the investigative results, it is clear that a family history of

Table 10.9   FUNCTIONAL CORRECTION OF STRABISMUS WITH UNILATERAL AND ALTERNATING FIXATION

Investigator	Fixation	Esotropia	Exotropia	Combined
Flom (19)[1]	Unilateral			43/121 = 36%
	Alternating			13/30 = 43%
Ludlam (35)[2]	Unilateral			59/81 = 73%
	Alternating			50/68 = 74%
Ludlam (35)[3]	Unilateral			$0.90 \times 0.73 = 65\%$
	Alternating			$0.90 \times 0.74 = 67\%$
Hoffman et al (31)[4]	Unilateral	10/15 = 67%	4/4 = 100%	14/19 = 74%
	Alternating	7/14 = 50%	21/22 = 95%	28/36 = 78%
Taylor (45)[5]	Unilateral	18/26 = 69%		
	Alternating	12/24 = 50%		
Etting (15)[6]	Unilateral		35/51 = 69%	
	Alternating		26/35 = 74%	

[1] Unselected cases treated by all methods (prisms, added lenses, occlusion, orthoptics, surgery). There was no significant difference between esotropia and exotropia.
[2] Treated by orthoptics only; used Flom's "cured" and "almost cured" categories.
[3] Treated by orthoptics only; used Flom's "cured" and "almost cured" categories. Patients were reexamined 3 to 7 years after treatment.
[4] Treated by orthoptics only and excluded patients with anomalous correspondence and previous surgery; used Flom's "cured" criterion.
[5] Patients with infantile esotropia were surgically corrected; criterion for result is conversion of tropia to phoria with sensory fusion.
[6] Patients were referred and treatment was begun after age 6 years. Treatment included lenses and/or orthoptics in office and at home; used Flom's "cured" criterion.

strabismus is not an unfavorable factor for functional correction of esotropia or exotropia, and it may indeed contribute favorably to the prognosis for esotropia.

Size of the Angle of Deviation

It might seem logical that it would be more difficult to achieve functional correction of larger angles of deviation than of smaller angles. On the other hand, the prevalence of anomalous correspondence substantially decreases for angles of esotropia larger than 25 to 30Δ (8, 19), suggesting that the prognosis ought to be better for larger angles because there is less chance of anomalous correspondence. Yet, the frequency of occasional strabismus is greater for small angles of deviation

Table 10.10   FUNCTIONAL CORRECTION OF SQUINT ACCORDING TO FAMILY HISTORY OF SQUINT

		Esotropia	Exotropia	Combined
Cashell (9):	Family history	138/393 = 35%		
	No family history	127/430 = 30%		
Flom (19):	Family history	16/38 = 42%	12/19 = 63%	28/57 = 49%
	No family history	8/53 = 15%	20/41 = 49%	28/94 = 30%

than for large angles, suggesting that prognosis ought to be better for smaller angles because the occasional type has a much better prognosis than the constant type, especially with esotropia.

Relevant studies lead to a fairly consistent conclusion. Costenbader (11) found the rate of functional correction of infantile esotropia to be more or less uniform at 2 to 6% for presurgical angles up to more than 50Δ. In another sample of infantile esotropia, Taylor (45) reported functional correction of 64 percent for esotropias less than 50Δ and 58 percent for larger angles. Ludlam (35) obtained 50 to 79 percent functional cures for all angles of esotropia and exotropia, except esotropia greater than 30Δ, where the cure rate dropped to 9 percent. As his treatment program emphasized orthoptics and did not rely on surgery, one wonders whether the cure rate would have been greater among the 11 cases of large-angle esotropia if surgery had been performed. I (19) found a fairly uniform rate of functional correction for deviations up to 30Δ for both esotropia (24 percent) and exotropia (56 percent); only a small number of my strabismic patients had angles greater than 30Δ.

Altogether, these studies tend to indicate that angle of deviation alone is probably not a major determinant of prognosis for functional correction of strabismus. Other factors such as constancy and retinal correspondence are probably more important.

Summary of Factors That Affect Prognosis for Functional Correction of Squint

Because the optometrist and the parents need to know before treatment is undertaken what the chances are for functional correction of squint, we have looked at numerous factors to determine how each individually affects the prognosis for functional correction. The results of this analysis are summarized in Table 10.11. What is immediately apparent is that only two factors are definitely favorable for both esotropia and exotropia: occasional squint and normal correspondence. Further,

only three factors are definitely unfavorable for both esotropia and exotropia: constancy of squint, deep amblyopia, and marked incomitance. Anomalous correspondence is definitely an unfavorable factor only for large-angle esotropia.

Factors for which the evidence is uncertain or for which the effect on prognosis is not strong have been listed in Table 10.11 as perhaps being favorable or unfavorable. For example, having no amblyopia is perhaps favorable with both esotropia and exotropia; perhaps favorable for esotropia only are having fusion for small and large second-degree targets, having a family history of squint, and having a small angle of deviation. Factors that are perhaps unfavorable are: anomalous correspondence in exotropia and small-angle esotropia, eccentric fixation for esotropia and exotropia, and suppressing small and large second-degree fusion targets only for esotropia. Factors that are probably not important in predicting functional correction of squint are listed in the central column of Table 10.11.

Another way to look at the prognosis situation is to observe how each factor by itself influences the overall percentage of functional corrections obtained for esotropes and exotropes. I have used this approach (19), and it is the basis for the revised analysis shown in Table 10.12. The figures derive from the results obtained from a sample of esotropic and exotropic patients treated by senior students under supervision of a preceptor in an optometry school clinic. Because of the teaching clinic setting and the students' limited experience in the management of strabismus, the probabilities of functional correction are surely lower than they would be for an experienced optometrist. Still, the listed probabilities are useful for showing how different factors affect the prognosis for functional correction of squint. Consider all the esotropias treated by the optometry students; 30 percent of them were functionally corrected; the indicated probability of functional correction for all esotropes is therefore 0.30. Similarly, the probability of functional correction for occasional and constant eso-

Table 10.11   INFLUENCE OF FACTORS ON FUNCTIONAL CORRECTION OF STRABISMUS

	Definitely Favorable	Perhaps Favorable	Probably Unimportant	Perhaps Unfavorable	Definitely Unfavorable
Constancy					
Constant					Esotropia & exotropia
Occasional	Esotropia & exotropia				
Correspondence					
Anomalous			Occasional squint	Exotropia & small esotropia	Large esotropia
Normal	Esotropia & exotropia				
Amblyopia					
Deep					Esotropia & exotropia
Moderate			Esotropia & exotropia		
None		Esotropia & exotropia			
Fixation					
Eccentric				Esotropia & exotropia	
Foveal			Esotropia & exotropia		
Second-degree targets					
Suppress			Exotropia	Esotropia	
Fused		Esotropia	Exotropia		
Incomitance					
Marked					Esotropia & exotropia
None			Esotropia & exotropia		
Squint					
Age at onset			Esotropia & exotropia		
Duration			Esotropia & exotropia		
Squint type					
Unilateral			Esotropia & exotropia		
Alternating			Esotropia & exotropia		
Family history of squint					
Positive		Esotropia	Exotropia		
Negative			Esotropia & exotropia		
Angle of deviation					
Small		Esotropia	Exotropia		
Large			Esotropia & exotropia		

Table 10.12. RELATIVE PROBABILITY OF OBTAINING FUNCTIONAL CORRECTION OF ESOTROPIA AND EXOTROPIA WHEN ONE OF LISTED FACTORS IS PRESENT

Esotropia	Factor	Exotropia
0.50	Occasional squint	0.60
0.40	Normal correspondence	0.60
0.40	Good 2nd-degree fusion	——
0.40	Family history of squint	——
0.35	No amblyopia	0.60
0.35	Comitant deviation	0.55
0.35	Deviation <16Δ	——
0.30	Direction of squint	0.50
0.20	Marked suppression	——
0.15	Marked incomitance	0.30
0.15	Constant squint	0.30
0.10	Deep amblyopia	0.40
0.10	Anomalous correspondence	0.45

tropes are, respectively, 0.50 and 0.15. According to these data, whether an esotropia is occasional or constant results in a difference in probabilities of 0.35 (0.50–0.15) or a ratio of probabilities of 3.3 (0.50/0.15), both of which reflect the influence of frequency of an esotropia on prognosis for functional correction. Using this same analysis it is seen that frequency of the squint affects exotropia less (difference in probabilities = 0.30; ratio = 2.0). Some other observations worth noting are that retinal correspondence is an important prognostic factor for all squinters, being more important for esotropes than exotropes, and that having a family history of squint is a slightly favorable factor for esotropes while not having this history does not act negatively.

The data in Tables 10.11 and 10.12 give us an idea of how various factors influence functional correction of squint and which are the most important. Still, we need some way to determine the probability of functional correction of an individual child's strabismus. Table 10.13 provides a model for estimating the probability on the basis of the

type of strabismus a patient has plus different associated factors. This model derives from my earlier (19) schema, which was based on treatment results obtained by optometry students. The present model takes into account the data of other investigators and the experience of practicing optometrists.

The use of the prognosis model is illustrated by a sample case. Consider an 8-year-old child with constant, unilateral 25Δ esotropia and anomalous correspondence; there is a family history of strabismus, deep amblyopia (acuity 20/200), and complete paralysis of the right lateral rectus muscle. To estimate the prognosis, one first finds the basic probability for functional correction, in this case 0.10. The only positive factor is the family history, which adds 0.10. Two negative factors (marked incomitance and deep amblyopia) are present; subtract 0.10 for each. The unilateral nature of the squint is irrelevant. The estimated probability of functional correction of this child's esotropia is therefore 0.10 + 0.10 − 0.2 = 0. Given this dismal prognosis, most parents and optometrists would not pursue treatment directed at a functional correction. In spite of the prognosis, some optometrists might undertake treatment aimed at functional correction because of their own exceptional skills, high motivation of the parents and child, and unusual abilities of the child. The option of cosmetic correction by prisms (see Chapter 11) or surgery is usually considered when the prognosis for functional correction is poor.

Consider a second child, age 10 years, who has an intermittent, alternating, comitant exotropia of 15Δ and normal correspondence; she has good second-degree fusion, slight to moderate suppression, a family history of squint, and no amblyopia. The estimated probability of functional correction of this child's exotropia is calculated by starting with the basic probability of 0.80. Good second-degree fusion, a family history of squint, a small angle of deviation, and alternation are irrelevant. No amblyopia contributes +0.10. As none of the negative factors is present, the estimated probability is 0.80 + 0.10 = 0.90. Because of the high probability of success,

Table 10.13 A MODEL FOR ESTIMATING THE PROBABILITY OF FUNCTIONAL CORRECTION OF DIFFERENT TYPES OF SQUINT AND ASSOCIATED FACTORS

	Esotropia				Eight Basic Squint Types	Exotropia			
	Occasional NRC	Occasional ARC	Constant NRC	Constant ARC		Constant ARC	Constant NRC	Occasional ARC	Occasional NRC
Basic Probabilities	0.60	0.50	0.30	0.10		0.40	0.50	0.70	0.80
					+ Factors (add 0.1)				
					Good second-degree fusion				
					Family history of squint				
					No amblyopia				
					Deviation <16Δ				
					− Factors (subtract 0.1)				
					Marked suppression				
					Marked incomitance				
					Deep amblyopia				
					Estimated probability				

treatment for functional correction should probably be undertaken.

This model is presented as a guide to estimating prognosis. Individual optometrists may have experiences and results with certain types of squint or associated conditions that allow them to substitute their own probabilities in the model. No matter; the objective is for the optometrist to know, and to be able to inform the parents of, the likely outcome of treatment for functional correction of the child's strabismus.

REFERENCES

1. Altizer LB: The nonsurgical treatment of exotropia. Am Orthoptic J 22:71, 1972.

2. Bedell HE, Flom MC, Barbeito R: Spatial aberrations and acuity in strabismus and amblyopia. Invest Ophthalmol Vis Sci 26:909, 1985.

3. Bedell HE, Flom MC: Monocular spatial distortion in strabismic amblyopia. Invest Ophthalmol Vis Sci 20:263, 1981.

4. Bedell HE, Flom MC: Normal and abnormal space perception. Am J Optom Physiol Opt 60:426, 1983.

5. Bedrossian EH: Anomalous retinal correspondence in alternating strabismus. Arch Ophthalmol 52:669, 1954.

6. Bielchowsky A: Lectures on Motor Anomalies, 2nd ed. Hanover, NH, Dartmouth Publications, 59, 1956.

7. Borish IM: Clinical Refraction. Chicago, The Professional Press, 1323, 1970.

8. Burian HM, Luke NE: Sensory retinal relationships in 100 consecutive cases of heterotropia. Arch Ophthalmol 84:16, 1970.

9. Cashell GTW: Long-term results of treatment of concomitant convergent strabismus in terms of binocular function. Trans Ophthalmol Soc UK, 72:367, 1952.

10. Cooper EL: Muscle surgery and orthoptics. Am J Ophthalmol 40:883, 1955.

11. Costenbader FD: Infantile esotropia. Trans Am Ophthalmol Soc 59:397, 1961.

12. Daum KM: Characteristics of exodeviations: 1. A comparison of three classes. Am J Optom Physiol Opt 63:237, 1986.

13. Dickey CF, Scott WE: The deterioration of accommodating esotropia: Frequency, characteristics, and predictive factors. J Pediatr Ophthalmol 25:172, 1988.

14. Etting GL: Visual training for strabismus—Success rate in private practice. Optom Week 64:1172, 1973.

15. Etting GL: Strabismus therapy in private practice: Cure rates after three months of therapy. J Am Optom Assoc 49:1367, 1978.

16. Fletcher MC, Silverman SJ: Strabismus: Part I. A summary of 1,110 consecutive cases. Am J Ophthalmol 16:86, 1966.

17. Flom MC: University of California Strabismus and Orthoptics Study: A preliminary report prepared for the Research Projects Committee of the American Academy of Optometry (unpublished). September 29, 1954.

18. Flom MC: The prognosis in strabismus. Am J Optom Arch Am Acad Optom 35:509, 1958.

19. Flom MC: Treatment of binocular anomalies of vision. In Hirsch MJ, Wick RE (eds): Vision of Children. Philadelphia, Chilton, 214, 1963.

20. Flom MC, Bedell HE: Identifying amblyopia using associated conditions, acuity, and non-acuity features. Am J Optom Physiol Opt 62:153, 1985.

21. Flom MC, Neumaier RW: Prevalence of amblyopia. U.S. Public Health Reports 81:329, 341, 1966. Reprinted in Am J Optom Arch Am Acad Optom 43:732, 1966.

22. Flom MC, Weymouth FW: Centricity of Maxwell's spot in strabismus and amblyopia. Arch Ophthalmol 66:260, 1961.

23. Flom MC, Bedell HE, Barbeito R: Spatial mechanisms for visual acuity deficits in strabismic and anisometropic amblyopia—Developmental failure or adaptation? In Keller EL, Zee DS (eds): Adaptive Processes in Visual and Oculomotor Systems. New York, Pergamon Press, 45, 1986.

24. Flom MC, Kirschen DG, Williams AT: Changes in retinal correspondence following surgery for intermittent exotropia. Am J Optom Physiol Opt 55:456, 1978.

25. Frandsen AD: Occurrence of squint; A clinical-statistical study . . . in different groups and ages of the Danish population. Acta Ophthalmologica [Suppl] (Copenh) 62:1960.

26. Giles GH: The Practice of Orthoptics. London, Hammond, Hammond, 1947.

27. Girard LJ, Fletcher MC, Tomlinson E, et al: Results of pleoptic treatment of suppression amblyopia. Am Orthoptic J 12:12, 1962.

28. Halldén U: Fusional phenomena in anomalous correspondence. Acta Ophthalmologica [Suppl] (Copenh) 37:1952.

29. Hardesty HH, Boynton JR, Keenan JP: Treatment of intermittent exotropia. Arch Ophthalmol 96:268, 1978.

30. Hess RF: On the relationship between strabismic amblyopia and eccentric fixation. Br J Ophthalmol 61:767, 1977.

31. Hoffman L, Cohen AH, Feuer G, et al: Effectiveness of optometric therapy for strabismus in a private practice. Am J Optom Arch Am Acad Optom 47:990, 1970.

32. Kirschen DG, Flom MC: Visual acuity at different retinal loci of eccentrically fixating functional amblyopes. Am J Optom Physiol Opt 58:144, 1978.

33. Levi DM, Klein SA: Sampling in spatial vision. Nature 320:360, 1986.

34. Levinge M: Value of abnormal retinal correspondence in binocular vision. Br J Ophthalmol 38:332–344, 1954.

35. Ludlam WM: Orthoptic treatment of strabismus. Am J Optom Arch Am Acad Optom 38:369, 1961.

36. Ludlam WM, Kleinman BI: The long range results of orthoptic treatment of strabismus. Am J Optom Arch Am Acad Optom 42:647, 1965.

37. Lyle TK, Foley J: Prognosis in cases of strabismus with special reference to orthoptic treatment. Br J Opthalmol 41:129, 1957.

38. Mulberger RD, McDonald FR: Surgical management of nonparalytic exotropia. Arch Ophthalmol 52:664, 1954.

39. Sanfilippo S, Clahane AC: Effectiveness of orthoptics alone in selected cases of exodeviation: The immediate results and several years later. Am Orthoptic J 20:104, 1970.

40. Schlossman A, Boruchoff SA: Correlation between physiologic and clinical aspects of exotropia. Am J Ophthalmol 40:53, 1955.

41. Scobee RG: Esotropia: Incidence, etiology, and results of therapy. Am J Ophthalmol 34:817, 1951.

42. Sorsby A: Genetics in Ophthalmology. St. Louis, CV Mosby, 1951.

43. Sternberg AR, Bohar: A study on the occlusion therapy of eccentric fixation; Report on 109 cases. Ophthalmologica 141:229, 1961.

44. Swan KC: Surgery for exotropia: Fusional ability and choice of procedure. Am J Ophthalmol 50:1158, 1960.

45. Taylor DM: Is congenital esotropia functionally curable? Trans Am Ophthalmol Soc 70:529, 1972.

46. Travers T a'B: Suppression of vision in squint and its association with retinal correspondence and amblyopia. Br J Ophthalmol 22:577, 1938.

47. Von Noorden GK: Burian-Von Noorden's Binocular Vision and Ocular Motility: Theory and Management of Strabismus. St. Louis, CV Mosby, 1985.

48. Wick B, Cook D: Management of anomalous correspondence: Efficacy of therapy. Am J Optom Physiol Opt 64:405, 1987.

Chapter 11

A Model for Treating Binocular Anomalies

Merton C. Flom

Bruce Wick

The previous chapter made the point that the primary question in the clinical management of binocular anomalies is whether or not to treat, and if so, what treatment procedures to consider and in what order. Further, it was mentioned that strabismic and nonstrabismic anomalies of binocular vision can be considered to lie along a continuum and that a general plan of treating binocular anomalies can include both strabismic and nonstrabismic patients.

The rationale for this approach is that strabismus can be viewed as a more severe form of heterophoria, as the angle of deviation (tonic innervation) is typically larger in strabismus and the associated complications, such as suppression and amblyopia, are more common and more severe in strabismus than in heterophoria. Using this rationale, the se-

quence of procedures for treating strabismus and heterophoria are similar and many of the treatment procedures are the same. Surely there are other approaches to the clinical management of binocular anomalies. What we propose here is an approach that we have found to be useful in clinical practice and readily accepted by students and practitioners. It is a logical, organized, practical clinical model for treating patients with binocular anomalies.

In the model, four kinds of strabismus are identified on the basis of constant or occasional squint and normal or anomalous correspondence. Additionally, three kinds of heterophoria are identified on the basis of a low, normal or high accommodative convergence/ accommodation (AC/A) ratio. These four kinds of strabismus and three kinds of heterophoria require sufficiently different treatment sequences to preclude a single, standardized treatment approach. The model proposed here takes into account these differences and directs treatment to the specific needs of a patient with one of these binocular anomalies. In short, the model is problem oriented.

Before describing the model for treating specific binocular anomalies, we discuss each of the available treatment options in their usual order of implementation in practice: optical correction of ametropia, added lenses, prisms, occlusion, vision training, and surgery.

OPTIONS FOR TREATING BINOCULAR ANOMALIES

Optical Correction of Ametropia

Refractive anomalies are common in strabismus (12). About 75 percent of esotropes and 60 percent of exotropes have a significant refractive anomaly. Among persons with esotropia, 65 percent have hyperopia (>1D) and only 10 percent have myopia (>0.75 D). With exotropia (constant or occasional), a reverse picture is seen: only 10 percent have hyperopia and 50 percent have myopia. Anisometropia (>1 D) is more common (25 percent, typically myopic) with exotropia than with esotropia (15 percent, typically hyperopic). Because of the early onset of hyperopia and esotropia (usually before 4 years), it seems logical to assume that they are either concurrent (genetic?) events or that the hyperopia resulting from uncorrelated growth of the eye leads to development of esotropia through the (AC/A) ratio. Of later onset are exotropia and myopia; exotropia (usually intermittent) typically precedes myopia. Compared to the general population, not only are refractive anomalies more common in strabismic persons (suggesting some link) but the prevalence of myopic anisometropia with exotropia (25 percent) is remarkably higher, again suggesting a possible link.

Neutralizing a refractive anomaly with lenses sharpens the retinal image or alters the vergence posture of the eyes, or both. These effect are so important and fundamental in the management of binocular anomalies that they should be considered first in any program of treatment.

The change in vergence that occurs upon neutralizing a refractive anomaly with lenses is well illustrated by the elimination or reduction of an esotropia or esophoria when convex lenses are prescribed for a moderate amount of hyperopia in a young person (e.g., +3.50 D). In this case the lenses permit relaxation of accommodation, which produces a decrease in the esodeviation through the accommodation-vergence synkinesis. In a similar way, correcting the myopia of a young patient with exophoria or exotropia at near distances results in increased near accommodation, which may cause an increase in accommodative convergence and a consequent reduction in the exodeviation at near distances. In addition to affecting accommodative vergence, corrective lenses can also facilitate fusional vergence by providing equally sharp retinal images, lessening suppression, and enhancing sensory fusion. Correcting even a small unilateral refractive anomaly in a patient with intermittent exotropia, for example, can substantially reduce the frequency of the strabismus. With bilateral refractive anomalies that produce blurred retinal images, such as astigmatism in both eyes, optical correction can enhance fusional vergence to overcome, for example, a small strabismus at distance. When correcting these bilateral refractive anomalies, the sharpened retinal image also facilitates accuracy of accommodation for near distances with resulting changes in accommodative vergence. The multiple effects of corrective lenses—on image sharpness, accuracy of accommodation, accommodative vergence, and fusional vergence—justify their initial consideration for managing binocular anomalies.

A curious feature about optical correction of anisometropia associated with strabismus is that, in spite of the presence of aniseikonia with the lenses, the strabismus may now be improved or eliminated, but it is possible that large amounts of aniseikonia may preclude binocular vision and cause strabismus (3). Aniseikonia is difficult to measure in children, especially if strabismus is present. Even if aniseikonia were measured or were suspected from the origin of the refractive anomaly (for example, unequal corneal astigmatism or refractive anisometropia),* it is nonetheless useful clinically to prescribe the full anisometropic correction and then to observe over time the effects on binocular vision. Initially disregarding the possibility of aniseikonia more often leaves clinicians pleasantly surprised than discouraged with the results. The implication from these results is that equally sharp retinal images are more important for facilitating binocular vision than unequal ocular images are for hindering it.

A common clinical approach is optical "fogging" of eyes with esodeviations—with excessive plus lens power prescribed if there is hyperopia or too little minus power if there is myopia. The underlying idea is to provide maximum relaxation of accommodation for distance with the goal of reducing the angle of deviation. In a young child with constant esotropia, this fogging procedure has some merit; the child sees near objects clearly with

---

* Ogle (42) reported that placing spectacle lenses at the anterior focal points of a pair of eyes whose ametropias differed primarily because of different ocular optical powers (refractive anisometropia) leads to retinal image size differences (aniseikonia) of 1.5 percent per diopter of difference in corneal powers and 2.0 percent per diopter of difference in crystalline lens powers. For axial anisometropia, on the other hand, spectacle lenses placed at the anterior focal point lead to no image size difference. If anisometropia is left uncorrected, no aniseikonia occurs if it is refractive in origin, but if the anisometropia is axial aniseikonia of 1.4 percent per diopter is expected. From a clinical standpoint, it seems that to avoid aniseikonia axial anisometropia should be corrected optically; spectacle lenses may perform better than contact lenses from an image size standpoint. Further, to avoid or minimize aniseikonia when correcting refractive anisometropia, contact lenses are preferable to spectacles. When the anisometropia is large (say, 5D), contact lenses may be preferable to spectacle lenses for both refractive and axial anisometropia because of the more nearly equal stimuli for binocular (conjugate) movements that contact lenses provide.

less accommodation than if only the manifest hyperopia were corrected. Through the accommodative convergence synkinesis, the esodeviation at near is reduced and, in the rare instance in esotropia, bifixation occurs at some close distance. The difficulty with this procedure is that the blurring of distant objects may be sufficient to cause the child to refuse to wear the glasses. This is often the problem when hyperopic children rebel at having to wear their glasses. Generally there is limited value in prescribing such excessive amount of plus power that distance acuity is significantly reduced. Blurring of the retinal image for distance seeing is not conducive to binocular vision. Moreover, some subjects react to fogging lenses by increasing their accommodation at distance (44, 60) and show increased esodeviation (13). Studies of this unexpected effect of fogging lenses indicate that it is unlikely to occur with small amounts (<1 D) of added plus power. Prescribing fogging lenses is not a panacea for correcting esodeviations; it should be used intelligently, not indiscriminately. More accommodation can be relaxed at near distances without reducing distance acuity by prescribing added plus power in the form of a bifocal lens.

A corollary philosophy to prescribing small amounts of fogging power to reduce accommodation (and vergence) in patients with esodeviations is prescribing full minus or least plus lenses for exodeviations. The idea is to provide maximal acuity at distance and optimal accommodation for near vision, both of which facilitate fusion.

Spectacles can influence the appearance (cosmesis) of strabismus. A frame with a large eye size and wide bridge tends to make esotropia more noticeable and exotropia less so. A thick eyewire tends to cast shadows on the eyes; that and leaving lenses without antireflective coating both make the eyes and the strabismus less visible. Frame color influences conspicuousness of strabismus; a narrow and clear bridge can improve cosmesis in esotropia, for example. Prism prescriptions used in the management of either strabismus or heterophoria need to be evaluated, both in terms of their functional effects in facilitating fusion and in terms of their optical effects on the appearance of the eyes. For example, base-out prisms prescribed to provide fusion for an esotropic patient, or comfort to one with esophoria, will make the eyes appear to be deviated more nasalward, giving the appearance of esotropia. Countering optical effects can be utilized to overcome the appearance of strabismus.

Added Lens Power

If there is no amblyopia or if it is only slight to moderate (acuity better than 20/100), added lenses should be considered next. It is often possible to alter the oculomotor deviation by prescribing lenses that differ in power from the refractive correction. More plus lens power or less minus power constitutes a plus lens addition or simply a "plus add," which may be prescribed as a single-vision lens or a multifocal lens. Similarly, less plus power or more minus power is called a "minus add." The change in vergence with added lens power is a function of the change in accommodation and the size of the AC/A ratio.

With the ametropia corrected, the AC/A ratio can be calculated quickly in a clinical situation using the following formula:

$$(AC/A)(\Delta/D) = PD \text{ (cm)} + \text{Near distance (m)}$$
$$\times \{\text{Near angle } (\Delta) - \text{Distance angle } (\Delta)\}$$

One simply subtracts the angle of deviation at distance from the angle at near (eso is +, exo is −); multiplies this difference by the near fixation distance, in meters; and adds the interpupillary distance in centimeters. From this formula it can be seen that when the distance and near angles of deviation are equal, their difference is zero, and the AC/A ratio equals the PD in centimeters. Further, when the near angle is more eso or less exo than the distance angle, the AC/A ratio is greater than the PD. And, when the near angle is less eso or more exo than the distance angle, the AC/A is less than the PD.

Suppose a youngster with an interpupillary distance of 60 mm (6.0 cm) had 20Δ of esotropia at 6 m and 30Δ at 40 cm (0.4 m). The calculated AC/A ratio would be 6.0 + 0.4 (30 − 20) = 10Δ/D. One would, therefore, expect a decrease in the esodeviation at near of 10Δ for each diopter of added lens power that relaxed accommodation. With a +2.50 D addition, the esodeviation at 40 cm would be expected to decrease by 25Δ, to 5Δ esodeviation. Because of proximal convergence and the fact that the accommodative response is usually less than the accommodative stimulus, this calculated value of the AC/A predicts a change in vergence with added lenses that is somewhat greater than is actually obtained. For this patient, instead of the expected 5Δ esodeviation at 40 cm with a +2.50 D add, one would probably find about 10Δ of esodeviation. From experience it has been found that multiplying the calculated AC/A ratio by 0.8 produces a better indicator of the actual change in vergence per diopter of added lens power.

Whenever a +2.50 D add does not fully reduce the esodeviation at 40 cm, it is interesting to know the plus add and the viewing distance at which the angle of deviation can be reduced to zero. This can be calculated from the following simple formula:

Plus add (D) =

$$\frac{\text{Angle of deviation at distance } (\Delta)}{\text{Interpupillary distance (cm)}}$$

The reciprocal of the added lens power designates the viewing distance. For the present example, the formula indicates that a +3.33 D add would reduce the esodeviation to zero. This could be checked quickly in the examining room with trial lenses of +3.50 D and a detailed target placed at approximately 30 cm. It is interesting to note that the plus add that reduces the esodeviation to zero is related only to the size of the deviation at distance and the interpupillary distance; it is independent of the AC/A ratio. Two patients with a 6 cm PD and 20Δ of esotropia at distance, one with a low AC/A ratio and another with a high one, would both require a +3.50 D add to be ortho at about 30 cm; this add would reduce a small near esodeviation for the low AC/A patient and would reduce a larger near esodeviation for the high AC/A patient.

Patients with constant esotropia and anomalous correspondence usually do not bifixate with any amount of added plus power. They may often be seen to make a disjunctive "fusional" movement with added lenses (30) to maintain "fusion" with the same corresponding retinal points. In sum, added lenses work consistently well in changing the angle of deviation when retinal correspondence is normal and inconsistently, if at all, when correspondence is anomalous.

With esotropia, the alternate and unilateral cover tests (15) are helpful in deciding how much added plus power to prescribe. It is important to use a detailed target so that accommodation will be active. If bifixation seems to be indicated by the unilateral cover test, confirmation can be obtained by quickly placing before the preferred eye a loose prism of about 5Δ and noting whether a disjunctive movement of 5Δ occurs. In very young children, it may be necessary to employ the Hirschberg test or perhaps only direct observation without a corneal light reflection.

When there is binocular vision and added plus is being considered to alleviate symptoms associated with a near esophoria, subjective measures of the dissociated phoria and fusional vergence can be used to apply some criterion such as that of Sheard (47). Or plus lens power can be added until the fixation disparity is reduced to near zero. Also the Worth Dot Test can be used to note the smallest plus add for which sensory fusion is promptly recovered in a dark room upon removal of the cover before one eye.

Near point esophoria in myopic patients who formerly have been undercorrected in minus should not be of much concern, at least initially. In most instances this esophoria is reduced or eliminated with continuous wear of the full minus prescription (14). If it is not eliminated or if binocular symptoms persist, a short regimen of negative vergence and accommodative accuracy training should be undertaken.

Added plus lenses for the treatment of esodeviations are usually prescribed as bifocals so that good distance acuity can be obtained through the major portion of the lenses. Children generally need to have the bifocal segments set higher, because they are not nearly so inclined as adults to move their eyes to use the segment, and they seem to be less bothered by a high-placed segment when walking. For preschool children it is a good routine to place the top of the segment at or above the center of the pupil with head erect and eyes straight ahead. Children at these ages do much of their seeing at close range and do not appear to be disturbed by lowering the head to look above the segment to observe distant objects. Flat-top segments have the advantage of providing a wider field of view through the segment with minimal downward gaze. These bifocals can be provided with fused or optically ground segments or with Fresnel Press-On segments (19). If the deviation is noncomitant so that either the horizontal or vertical deviation increases on down gaze, it is especially important to use a flat-top bifocal that is set high in the lens. For patients with a distant esodeviation and a high AC/A ratio, progressive addition lenses can be helpful in providing a range of added powers as the patient views at different intermediate distances.

Added plus lenses can be viewed as training lenses to improve binocular vision (5) and they can be considered corrective in the same sense that ophthalmic lenses correct ametropia. When reduction of the added plus power is made and comfort is maintained, improved quality of sensory fusion and a greater amplitude of relative divergence are present. It is not known whether the AC/A ratio changes.

Added minus lenses have been prescribed to correct exotropia at least since the turn of the century (10), and there has been much interest in this method (6, 7, 35, 52).

These lenses are also effective in reducing the symptoms associated with exophoria.

Added minus lenses can also be used to reduce constant exotropia to a cosmetically acceptable deviation. More often they are prescribed as training lenses to be used in conjunction with occasional occlusion to eliminate suppression and orthoptics to improve the quality of fusion. Kennedy (35) found that 19 percent of his 153 exotropic patients obtained a good cosmetic result with added minus lenses; 12 percent obtained constant binocular vision, 36 percent obtained improved but occasional binocular vision, and 33 percent did not respond to the treatment.

Added minus lenses are probably effective in three different ways. (1) The angle of deviation can be reduced through accommodative vergence by an amount sufficient to provide comfort or allow the residual angle to fall within the range of motor fusion. (2) Added minus lenses can also be effective in exotropia by initiating accommodative vergence movements as the eyes clear the "over-minused" blurred retinal image. Once the eyes are in disjunctive motion, reflex positive relative convergence is more readily utilized. This phenomenon is akin to blink vergence facilitating fusional vergence (49). (3) Blurred distance vision from overaccommodation is made clear with added minus lenses. This overaccommodation results either from accommodative convergence to facilitate motor fusion or through positive fusional vergence stimulating accommodation (convergence accommodation).

The following is an effective method of determining the added minus power that will control an exotropia or alleviate the symptoms of exophoria: The patient looks at a fixation object and is told to relax the eyes and let them do what they want to do. Unobtrusively, the nonpreferred eye is uncovered and the quality of the fusional recovery movement is noted. Increasing powers of added minus are placed before the eyes until the nonpreferred eye is seen to move immediately and with acceleration upon being uncovered. The usual range of added minus

lenses prescribed for exotropia is between 1 and 3 D (1.75 D is average).

An advantage of added minus lenses over base-in prisms for the correction of exodeviations is that a more acceptable amount of vertical prism can be determined. A larger vertical prism correction is frequently indicated when base-in prisms are used. This result occurs because the base-in prisms permit the eyes to diverge toward the field of action of the superior and inferior rectus muscles, where an imbalance between them frequently occurs. If, instead, minus lenses are added, the eyes are brought away from the field of action of the vertical recti muscles. Indeed, if sufficient minus power is added for diagnostic purposes to eliminate the horizontal deviation (measured with the Alternate Cover Test), then any vertical movement observed should represent the vertical deviation present when the eyes are bifixating. Correction of this vertical deviation with prisms should be optimal.

Some children are unable to obtain clear vision with added minus lenses, presumably because of an inability to accommodate sufficiently. Headaches and other ocular symptoms may temporarily occur when these lenses are used. Only rarely is it necessary to abandon the use of the added minus lenses because of reduced distance acuity or symptoms. With continued use of minus lenses, most children soon obtain good acuity and comfort, although a small number may require training to improve accommodative facility and fusion. Following functional success, it is usually better to have the child reduce the wearing time of the added lenses gradually (discontinuing use starting in the morning) than to reduce the power gradually.

Ophthalmic Prisms

Light emerging from a prism has a direction different from that of the incident light. It is this feature of a prism that makes it optometrically valuable. When a prism is placed base-out before one eye of a subject who is bifoveally fixating a target, the image of the target is displaced onto the temporal retina of the eye behind the prism. If this displacement were within the motor fusion range the eye would then rotate nasalward (converge) to place the fovea under the displaced image. For a patient with esophoria larger than the value of this prism, the convergent movement of the eye comes from a decrease in the negative relative vergence being employed to maintain bifixation. If the esophoria and prism power were equal, the eye would converge to its heterophoria position and bifoveal fixation would be possible without the use of relative vergence. If the esophoria were less than the power of the prism, the convergence of the eye would derive partly from a decreased negative relative vergence and increased positive vergence (relative or accommodative). A similar analysis can be applied for base-in prisms. Thus, when bifixation is present initially and the displaced images are within the range of motor fusion, the addition of prisms base-out before the eyes results in convergence, and base-in prisms produce divergence.

Suppose a base-out prism of 12Δ were placed before the deviating eye of a patient who has a constant, comitant, unilateral esotropia of 15Δ with normal correspondence, no amblyopia, slight suppression, good second-degree fusion, and occasional diplopia. The image of the target of regard would now lie 3Δ nasal to the fovea of the deviating eye; it is probable that the squinting eye would make a (temporalward) fusional divergence movement of 3Δ to place the fovea under the image.

A prism placed before a blind, deeply amblyopic, or markedly suppressing eye will still displace the image of the target on the retina, but reflex fusional movement of the eye is unlikely; the eye may not rotate in response to any amount or direction of prism. If a prism were placed before the other (seeing) eye, this fixating eye would rotate in response to the prism and the nonseeing eye would rotate conjugately.

In addition to displacing the image of a target across the subject's retina, prisms have another effect. People looking at a subject wearing prisms see the subject's eyes through the prisms; each eye and its orbit appear displaced in the direction of the apex of the prism.

From the preceding discussion it should be concluded that ophthalmic prisms can be used in several ways in the management of binocular anomalies: to relieve symptoms of heterophoria, to improve binocular vision in squint, and to improve cosmesis in squint.

Prism prescriptions are surprisingly successful at alleviating the symptoms of heterophoria in children. Prismatic distortion and ghost images are not as annoying to children as they are to adults, but selection of the proper base curve (43) and use of antireflective coating can obviate these difficulties. Weight can be minimized by keeping the glasses as small as is practical and by using plastic lenses. By and large, the clinical methods for prescribing added lenses can also be used to prescribe prisms. Particularly useful with children are the Cover Test, observation of the fusional recovery movements, measures of the associated phoria, and the Worth Dot Test (see Added Lenses above).

The increase in heterophoria sometimes observed after adults wear a prismatic prescription also occurs in children. This so-called prism adaptation should not be alarming as the original symptoms usually do not reappear; if they do, only a conservative increase in the prismatic prescription is generally necessary. For children with a significant and approximately equal esophoria at distance and near, base-out prisms tend to be more satisfactory than bifocals. With normal angles kappa and inner canthi, prescribing moderate amounts of horizontal prism (up to 10Δ) for heterophoria usually creates no cosmetic problem.

The use of ophthalmic prisms for functional correction of squint is too often overlooked. For angles of squint less than 25Δ, a prism prescription in conjunction with occlusion and orthoptics may lead to functional correction without surgery. Surgery is usually necessary for larger deviations, but the chances of obtaining a functional cure after surgery are immensely better if constant binocular vision can be achieved with prism glasses before surgery. This may require occlusion, orthoptics, and large amounts of prism; but if a functional cure is a likely outcome the effort is justified. With care, glasses with a total of 20Δ can be made cosmetically and optically acceptable; for larger amounts of prism, Fresnel Press-On (membrane) prisms are useful (19).

Prescribing prisms for improved cosmesis of squint is based on the ideas outlined earlier in this section. Thus, placing a base-in (reverse) prism before a blind esotropic eye, for example, will make the eye appear to be more temporalward, in the head. If this constantly converged eye had fairly good acuity and there was anomalous retinal correspondence, a base-in prism might also stimulate a divergence fusional movement (quite slow with ARC) that results in an actual reduction in the angle of deviation. Such a reverse prism can provide a purely cosmetic effect through perceived displacement of the eye and orbit and an actual slow vergence response associated with anomalous correspondence—hence a dual effect. Hirsch (31) reported prescribing a base-out prism before a constantly exotropic, poorly seeing eye, which markedly improved the appearance of the strabismus.

Ocular torticollis (head tilt) and head turn are cosmetic problems associated with noncomitant strabismus that merit consideration; the guiding principle is to prescribe prisms that correct for the oculomotor deviation and, insofar as possible, direct the nonaffected eye away from the field of action of the affected muscle. This means not splitting the prescribed prisms equally between the two eyes as is the custom when prescribing for ordinary phorias. Consider a patient with a moderate paresis of the left superior oblique muscle, 15Δ of left hypertropia with the head in the primary position, and a habitual head tilt to the right (where fusion is possible because of the decreased vertical and cyclodeviations). Base-down prism before the left eye would permit bifoveal fixation with the head in a more erect position; base-up prism before the right eye would correct the oculo-

motor deviation somewhat less, since this prism directs the nonaffected eye to downward gaze, where the left hypertropia increases. It would be desirable to prescribe as much of the necessary prism before the left eye and as little as possible before the right eye. Figures 11.1 through 11.5 show the patient used in the present example. The head tilt to the right was present from early childhood. Base-down prisms of 6Δ before the left eye and 4Δ base-up before the right eye were prescribed; this corrected the torticollis (Fig. 11.5). In some patients with superior oblique paresis, correction of the head tilt is less successful with vertical prisms because of a large cyclodeviation and limited cyclofusional amplitude.

When prescribing prisms for noncomitant deviations, as mentioned, more of the prism should be applied before the eye with the underacting muscle. The greater the degree of muscle underaction, for both phorias

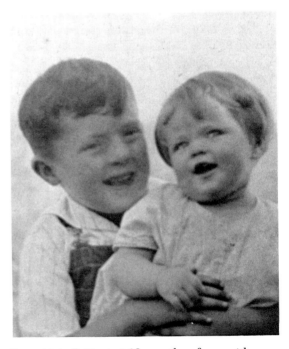

Figure 11.1 Patient at 18 months of age with older brother (possibly having similar head tilt); no glasses worn.

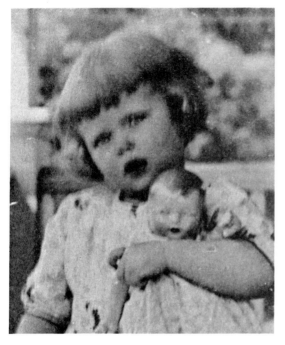

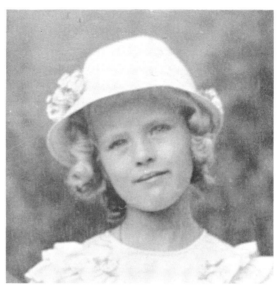

Figure 11.3 Patient at 10 years; had glasses that did not correct head tilt, but removed them for photograph.

Figure 11.2 Patient at 3 years; no glasses worn.

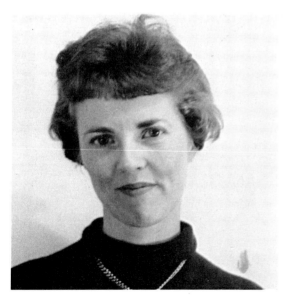

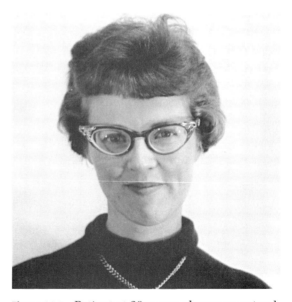

Figure 11.4 Patient at 30 years; had glasses that did not correct head tilt, but removed them for photograph.

Figure 11.5 Patient at 30 years; glasses contained 6Δ base-down before left eye and 4Δ base-up before right eye, which nearly corrected the right head tilt. With additional 2Δ base-down left eye, there was no head tilt.

and squints, the more of the total prism power should be placed before the affected eye. For complete paresis or paralysis, the full amount of the prism prescription before the affected eye may be indicated. With fibrosis of the right lateral rectus muscle and no demonstrable abduction from that muscle (Duane's retraction syndrome), the resulting right esotropia in primary gaze and the usual right face turn are typically corrected with a base-out prism (of 15 to 25Δ) prescribed before the affected right eye. Placing base-out prism before the left eye directs the gaze into the right field, where the angle of deviation increases, thereby negating part or all of the effect of the prism.

Occlusion

Diagnostically, occlusion can be used to determine whether symptoms are associated with binocular use of the eyes (45), expose latent heterophoria (38), and stabilize variable heterophoria. The most fruitful therapeutic results of monocular occlusion occur in treating amblyopia with central fixation and suppression. Occlusion may have value when used in conjunction with orthoptics to break down ARC, but the efficacy of treating anomalous retinal correspondence (ARC) solely with occlusion is questionable. The elimination of one image for patients (usually adults) with insuperable diplopia is a special application of occlusion.

Occlusion may be constant or occasional with respect to time, and total (complete) or partial (graded or incomplete) with respect to the degree of retinal image obscuration. Constant total occlusion generally yields greater improvement in a shorter time than does occasional total occlusion or constant partial occlusion. The choice of these variables in prescribing occlusion depends on the character of the anomaly and the activities of the child; as a rule, the more severe the anomaly the greater the need for constant and total occlusion. Generally, constant total occlusion is used only for patients who have constant strabismus. Practical considerations such as school work and personal safety may limit the objective of constant total occlusion for these patients. For occasional strabismus or phoria patients with suppression or anisometropic amblyopia, occlusion should be either occasional and total or constant and partial. (Partial occlusion, providing incomplete obscuration of the retinal image, can be accomplished with clear lacquer or translucent tape on the lens or with a graded occluder lens.) Occasional partial occlusion (e.g., part-time wearing of a stippled lens) has limited application and value.

Rarely is a child pleased to wear an occluder. The child's activities may be curtailed because of having to use the nonpreferred eye; and there is the problem of social acceptance of the patch. It is imperative that the optometrist take account of these problems during instructions and discussions with the child and parents.

The greatest cause of failure in occlusion is the failure to occlude! The most common causes of failure to occlude are incomplete or unconvincing instructions, instructions to occlude too infrequently, parents' failure to understand instructions, incomplete parental support of the child, and insufficient interest and follow-up by the doctor. If occlusion is worth considering as a treatment, then it should be prescribed with professional confidence and human understanding; instructions should be explicit (e.g., written) and the occlusion should be frequent and complete enough to be effective in a reasonable length of time. The parents under all circumstances and the child if at all possible should be made to understand the purpose of the occlusion, how it works, and the expected results. The optometrist's enthusiasm and expectation (not guarantee) of success can indeed be contagious. A positive approach ("The patching will make your eyes strong!") is more effective than a negative approach ("If you don't patch, your weak eye will get worse.") and, importantly, provides the child with the kind of information and assurance he or she needs when someone asks about the occluder. Guarding against humiliation is the best insurance against the development of a social problem.

Occlusion requires special instructions and attention when the acuity of the uncovered amblyopic eye is so poor (worse than 20/400) that the child may be endangered and in the rare instance when there is a known psychological problem that might be aggravated by occlusion. There is also some risk that constant total occlusion in heterophoria or occasional squint can precipitate constant squint (8, 46, 53).

Once occlusion is begun, it should be continued for at least 6 to 8 weeks to give ample opportunity for improvement. If no improvement occurs, occlusion may be discontinued; with improvement, occlusion should be continued for about 6 to 8 weeks beyond the last measurable change. Sometimes amblyopia recurs after successful occlusion therapy, even if binocular vision has been obtained. When this happens, it is most likely that anisometropia is present; in any case, reinstituting occlusion for a short time is usually sufficient to restore the acuity.

The preferred eye is usually occluded (direct occlusion) for either suppression or amblyopia. If there is no amblyopia and the suppression switches with alternation of fixation, then occlusion may be alternated daily. When the child is very young or when the acuity is worse than about 20/70, occlusion is best accomplished with an adhesive patch (e.g., Elastoplast) on the face. For older children and those with less deep amblyopia, the occluder may be attached to the spectacle lens or frame. Occlusion is generally considered to be a passive form of treatment; it is, however, much more effective when the affected eye must be used in critical vision tasks such as reading, coloring, and doing puzzles.

How effective is direct occlusion in treating amblyopia in general? Fulton and Mayer (23) used only direct, total, constant occlusion in conjunction with glasses to treat the amblyopia of 30 patients with congenital and acquired esotropia between ages 3 and 10 years whose initial acuity in the amblyopic eye ranged from about 20/400 to 20/40. The duration of occlusion ranged from 2 to 9.5 months (average <4 months). At the cessation of full-time patching, the authors report that 25 of the 30 children (83 percent) were not amblyopic and presumably had 20/20 acuity. Four of the five failures had improvement in acuity but refused further patching. The final patient complied with the occlusion regimen for 1 year but achieved a final acuity of only 20/30, from an initial 20/100. No mention was made in this report of the presence of eccentric fixation in these esotropic amblyopic children; presumably most of them would have nasal eccentric (nonfoveal) fixation.

How effective is direct occlusion in treating amblyopia when eccentric fixation is known to be present? Urist (58) found that all 21 of his eccentrically fixating amblyopic patients under 4 years of age obtained central fixation and equal visual acuity in the two eyes; 62 percent of 37 children over 4 years of age showed this degree of improvement. Sternberg and Bohar (51) found that with direct occlusion 74 percent of their 73 eccentrically fixating amblyopic patients under 6 years of age obtained improvement in acuity to at least 20/40. None of their 66 children between 6 and 10 years got such improvement; in part, this may be due to the fact that older children are less likely to comply in wearing the patch, as was also the case for most of Fulton and Mayer's failures.

When there is an associated eccentric fixation, patching the amblyopic eye (inverse occlusion) has been used separately in the very young and in conjunction with pleoptics in older children (1, 24, 27). The idea is to lessen the preference for fixation in the peripheral retina and to encourage foveal fixation. If successful, the change in fixation alone can result in improved acuity. Direct occlusion and orthoptics (if the child is old enough) are then prescribed.

What results are obtained with inverse occlusion? Barnard (2) reported that inverse occlusion alone improved fixation in 84 percent and acuity in 39 percent of his eccentrically fixating amblyopic patients who were too young to receive pleoptics. Greater improvement in acuity was obtained when direct occlusion was also used. Graham (28) gave inverse occlusion to 31 young amblyopes with various degrees of eccentric fixation. Fixation improved for three of the 13 children who had large eccentric fixation, but not for those with paracentral or unsteady fixation. Subsequent direct occlusion led to central fixation in seven of the children with paracentral or unsteady fixation.

Should inverse or direct occlusion be used to treat amblyopia associated with eccentric fixation? There are no data to support the contention that direct occlusion intensifies eccentric fixation, especially in older children (27). The uniformly good results obtained with direct occlusion, even for strabismic amblyopia, which characteristically is associated with eccentric fixation, argues strongly for the initial use of direct occlusion for virtually all patients with amblyopia. If direct occlusion is properly carried out and there is failure, consideration can be given to indirect occlusion, especially if the eccentric fixation is large and fixed.

Although constant total direct occlusion is the most common form of occlusion, it is sometimes appropriate to consider some special occlusion method. Part of one lens can be covered to provide occlusion only when the suppression or squint is present; for example, covering the upper half of one bifocal lens for occasional esotropia with squinting at distance. Occlusion of the nasal portion of each lens has been used in esotropia and when there is suppression of an eye on abduction (10). Swenson (54) has occluded the temporal part of the lens before the eccentrically fixating amblyopic eye with esotropia; this procedure prevents stimulation of the nasal retina and is essentially a form of inverse occlusion. The analogous scheme has been used for exotropia by occluding the nasal part of the lens (50).

For hygiene purposes it is sometimes advisable to dispense with total constant occlusion every seventh day; there is more advantage, however, in transferring the occluder to the other eye on the seventh day. For infants whose acuity is still developing, occlusion of the preferred eye to overcome amblyopia in the strabismic eye can lead to reduction of acuity in the preferred eye (56). For this rea-

son, occlusion regimens for infants and preschoolers must take into account the loss of acuity that can result from continuous occlusion of the preferred eye. A recommended regimen for occluding amblyopic infants and preschoolers who have constant strabismus is to occlude the preferred eye for a number of consecutive days equal to the age in years, and then to occlude the amblyopic eye for one day before beginning the cycle again.

There is no doubt that occlusion has value in treating certain binocular anomalies in children. Its proper use requires an idea of the known or probable results that can be expected from treatment of different binocular anomalies with various methods of occlusion.

Vision Training

Orthoptics (vision training) is an active training process that can improve certain sensory and motor aspects of binocular vision in children. Vision training is most commonly used to reduce amblyopia, eliminate suppression, correct anomalous correspondence, improve sensory fusion including stereopsis, and increase the facility and range of accommodation and vergence responses. Some additional uses of vision training are to improve perceptual responses (e.g., speed of perception), to permit further testing to aid in the diagnosis, and to assist in a patient's adaptation to a new lens prescription. If the child cooperates, the success rate of vision training for phoria is very high. For strabismus, orthoptics is usually employed in hope of producing normal binocular vision. If the prognosis for functional cure is significantly improved following surgery, orthoptics can be considered at that time.

Before proceeding with orthoptics, the purpose of the training should be explained to the child and parents. They should understand what is expected of them, the frequency and duration of treatment, possible inconveniences or problems, the cost, and the likelihood of success. It should be stressed that orthoptics is an active training process and that instruments will not correct the condition; they only help the child learn to use the eyes better. The possibility that it will be necessary to occlude, wear special training lenses, and do orthoptics at home should also be pointed out. It is imperative that the parents understand the role that surgery can play in the management of strabismus and large phorias.

Many orthoptic procedures are used; as different as they may seem initially, their similarities are striking. The following brief outline is offered as a guide to the orthoptic treatment of binocular anomalies in children. Specific methods of treatment will not be discussed, as they are described in several textbooks (25, 26, 29, 32, 37, 48) and in Chapter 12. Before instituting any training procedure, it is always worth considering spectacles that provide or enhance binocular vision and other procedures such as occlusion.

Amblyopia

For normal, comfortable, binocular vision, monocular foveal fixation and good acuity are required of each eye. The orthoptic treatment of amblyopia essentially involves monocular training of foveal fixation and resolution by altering the brightness, contrast, color, on period, position, and size of the target. Simultaneous kinesthetic and auditory stimulation is effective. When training monocular fixation, the goal is to obtain steady and accurate foveal fixation of a stationary target or one that moves smoothly or abruptly (good pursuit and saccadic tracking). In conjunction with the fixation training, resolution targets are used that are above threshold size and continual recognition is encouraged as the size is decreased. Monocular accommodational facility should be practiced in conjunction with the acuity training. When acuity is as good as 20/60 to 20/100, attempts should be made to introduce some binocular training.

Suppression

Orthoptic treatment of suppression is a binocular procedure that essentially involves changing the stimulus parameters of the target before the nonpreferred (suppressing) eye. If suppression is extensive, it is attacked initially in the peripheral field with dissimilar targets and later in the central (foveal) field with dissimilar and then similar targets. The treatment encourages the appreciation of physiological diplopia for phoria patients, and pathological diplopia for squinters with normal correspondence.

Anomalous Correspondence

Different kinds of strabismus require different approaches to treating anomalous retinal correspondence (ARC). For occasional strabismus, constant exotropia, and constant esotropia less than 15 to 20Δ, the treatment consists primarily of vergence training. The idea is that as the oculomotor deviation is overcome by fusional vergence, the retinal correspondence (angle of anomaly) changes synchronously, so that it becomes normal (angle of anomaly becomes 0) when the eyes are straight or bifoveally fixating (covariation) (30). This vergence technique of "treating" anomalous correspondence is very successful for occasional strabismus and constant exotropia. For small-angle esotropia with ARC, a special method (61) must be used to drive the slow divergence system; response to this treatment typically occurs very quickly or not at all. The success rate with this method is good enough to warrant at least an attempt at treatment.

For the other squints—namely large-angle constant esotropias—the treatment method (called forced elimination) is aimed at eliminating the anomalous correspondence (between the fovea and a peripheral locus) by stimulating the two foveas simultaneously and developing binocular perception in a single egocentric direction. Binocular stimulation is achieved in a haploscopic device, the deviating eye's target being larger and more intense and being made to pulse and move. When correspondence is anomalous and not simply impossible to determine because of suppression (lack of correspondence is discussed in Chapter 10), establishing normal correspondence through the forced elimination technique is very difficult. When surgery for a large-angle constant esotropia with ARC reduces the deviation to less than 15 to 20Δ, vergence training of the anomalous correspondence should be attempted afterward—even if the ARC is decidedly unharmonious—if functional correction is desired.

Sensory and Motor Functions

This phase of training is directed at identifying and overcoming deficits in sensory unification of foveal images, stereopsis, accommodation, and fusional vergence. Treatment consists of first using dissimilar targets of decreasing size followed by similar (fusible) targets of decreasing size. Stereopsis training is then given using targets with large amounts of horizontal disparity (to improve the upper stereoscopic threshold) and targets with minimal disparities (to increase stereoacuity).

An interesting observation is that the accommodative and vergence responses are often greatly improved simply as a result of successfully treating the amblyopia, suppression, and sensory functions. If further motor improvement is needed, training should be directed at changing accommodation and vergence abruptly, emphasizing speed and quality of response over maximum amplitudes of response. It is important to transfer the motor abilities acquired through training to ordinary visual situations; such transfer is facilitated by using nonaperture devices as much as possible.

Surgery

The principal function of surgery of the oculorotary muscles is to change their mechanical advantage to produce a change in the relative position of the eyes with minimal limitation of their motility. Obtaining motility that is well conjugated (comitant) is especially important when functional correction of the squint is a goal. Postsurgical comitance seems to be more likely when there is symmetrical surgery (e.g., recession of medial rectus and resection of lateral rectus of the same esotropic eye) of one or both eyes than when a large operation is performed on one muscle.

There is great interest in the advantages of early surgery. Most of the data seem to suggest a greater proportion of functional results when esotropia patients undergo surgery within 4 years of the onset (41), but some results fail to support an advantage to early surgery (4). For early-onset (congenital) esotropia, Fisher et al (11) analyzed the surgical results of Ing et al. (33), Taylor (55), and their own data and found that surgery performed between 12 and 24 months of age gave results as good as surgery performed between 6 and 12 months. Maruo et al. (39) reported no difference in long-term results (after 4 years) for congenital esotropia when surgery was performed at less than 1 year, 12 to 18 months, 18 to 24 months, or after 24 months of age. Surgical results for children with exotropia appear to be the same regardless of age at surgery (22, 39).

For strabismus, the type and amount of surgery depend on many features, only one of which is the distance angle of deviation. Noncomitancy, the size of the AC/A ratio, the refractive state, state of correspondence, and presence of amblyopia are but a few factors involved. The experience and skill of the surgeon cannot be overemphasized. The chances for good results from surgery are maximal when there is close cooperation between optometrist and ophthalmic surgeon.

Surgery is not recommended for phoria patients unless optical and training measures fail (57, 59). When surgery is performed it is specifically for the angle of deviation, independent of other factors such as significant noncomitancy, retinal correspondence, and amblyopia, because these factors typically are not at issue. Because angles of phoria are generally smaller than angles of strabismus, the surgery for phorias tend to be less extensive. When the AC/A ratio is very low or very high (conditions associated with a very different phoria angle at near than at distance) the surgeon is specially challenged to avoid creating diplopia at one distance or the other.

THE TREATMENT MODEL: RATIONALE AND USE

In developing a model for treating binocular anomalies, we considered strabismus first. We relied heavily on the schema of Table 10.13 that was developed to estimate the prognosis for functional correction of strabismus. In that prognosis schema, two main factors affect prognosis for both esotropia and exotropia; constancy (constant or occasional strabismus) and retinal correspondence (anomalous or normal). In the prognosis schema are eight basic squint types, each with its own probability for functional correction.

In the proposed treatment model, constancy and retinal correspondence are the two most important factors for determining the sequence of the different treatment options. There are four combinations of constancy and retinal correspondence: occasional strabismus and normal correspon-

dence (best prognosis), constant strabismus and normal correspondence, occasional strabismus and anomalous correspondence, and constant strabismus and anomalous correspondence (worst prognosis). For treatment sequencing, esotropia and exotropia patients can be considered together. It is the four combinations of constancy and retinal correspondence that define the four kinds of strabismus cases that require somewhat different sequences of treatment considerations.

Table 11.1 illustrates the elements of the treatment model. The first four column headings identify the defining characteristics of the four basic kinds of squint cases. The fifth column, Treatment Options, lists the various treatments used in strabismus in the sequence they should generally be considered. No one of the basic case types exactly follows this sequence, but the recommended sequences for occasional strabismus (columns 1 and 2) are close.

Table 11.1   SEQUENCE OF TREATMENT CONSIDERATIONS FOR STRABISMUS (ESOTROPIA AND EXOTROPIA)

Four Basic Squint Types				
Occasional NRC	Occasional ARC	Constant NRC	Constant ARC	
Sequence of Treatment Considerations				Treatment Options
1	1	1	1(a)†	Optical prescription
2	2	5	8	Added lenses
3	3	6	2(c)	Prisms*
4	4	2	3(b)	Occlusion
—	—	3	4(b)	VT‡: Amblyopia
5	5	4	5	VT: Suppression
—	6	—	6	VT: ARC
6	7	7	7	VT: Sensorimotor Functions
7	8	8	9(d)	Surgery

* Vertical prisms are often useful to neutralize a vertical deviation that is present in the fused position. Base-in prisms for exotropia and base-out prisms for esotropia can be helpful for functional correction if the correspondence is normal; this is usually not the case with anomalous correspondence. If functional correction is not under consideration but cosmesis is, base-in prisms can be used to improve the appearance of constant esotropia with anomalous correspondence of deviations up to 35Δ; base-out prisms can be similarly used for cosmetic purposes with exotropia.
† Letters in parentheses designate the treatment sequence if cosmesis is the main goal.
‡ VT stands for vision training or orthoptics.

For these two kinds of occasional strabismus (those with normal correspondence and those with anomalous correspondence), the model indicates the following sequence of treatment considerations: 1) lenses to neutralize the refractive error; 2) added lenses to facilitate fusion (plus for esotropia, minus for exotropia); 3) vertical prisms (horizontal prisms if NRC); and 4) occlusion for the small degree of amblyopia that may be present in occasional strabismus. Vision training for the slight amblyopia of occasional strabismus is not a necessary consideration, so columns 1 and 2 in Table 11.1 indicate no consideration of orthoptics for amblyopia. Instead, the fifth treatment option to consider is vision training to break down suppression. The sixth treatment consideration for occasional strabismus with anomalous correspondence is vergence training for the ARC; occasional squinters with normal correspondence do not need such training, so the sixth consideration for them is sensory and motor fusion training. The last treatment option for both types of occasional squint is surgery.

The approach to treating constant strabismus is very different. If retinal correspondence is normal, occlusion to treat any amblyopia is the second consideration (third column). If, on the other hand, correspondence is anomalous, prescribing vertical prism is the second consideration if functional correction is sought (numbers in fourth column); if improved cosmesis is the main goal, then the second consideration should be occlusion and active training to improve the amblyopia sufficiently to permit prescribed inverse prisms to stimulate a vergence movement opposite to the direction of the deviation (letters *b* in the fourth column). Elaboration of how to treat squinters and phoria patients is provided in the following sections.

For nonsquinters, the prognosis for functional correction typically is high; the main determinant in the sequence of treatment is the magnitude of the AC/A ratio, which in conjunction with the tonic vergence (distance phoria) determines the near phoria. Thus, three basic kinds of nonsquint or pho-

ria cases result: low, normal, and high AC/A ratios. And each basic case includes persons with low, normal, and high tonic vergence, correspondingly, distance exophoria, orthophoria, and esophoria.

The basic cases are as follows:

1. Low AC/A ($<3\Delta/D$) with:
   a. Low tonic vergence (distance exophoria $>5\Delta$
   b. Normal tonic vergence (distance phoria between 3Δ esophoria and 5Δ exophoria)
   c. High tonic vergence (distance esophoria $>3\Delta$)
2. Normal AC/A (3 to $7\Delta/D$) with:
   a. Low tonic vergence (distance exophoria $>5\Delta$
   b. Normal tonic vergence (distance phoria between 3Δ esophoria and 5Δ exophoria)
   c. High tonic vergence (distance esophoria $>3\Delta$)
3. High AC/A ($>7\Delta/D$) with:
   a. Low tonic vergence (distance exophoria $>5\Delta$
   b. Normal tonic vergence (distance phoria between 3Δ esophoria and 5Δ exophoria)
   c. High tonic vergence (distance esophoria $>3\Delta$)

The sequence of treatment is different for these three case types. Table 11.2 shows that the differences in treatment sequence center about when one should consider use of added lenses and prisms.

To use the model as a guide in treating a specific strabismus or phoria case, it is first necessary to ascertain from the clinical diagnosis whether the strabismus is constant or occasional and whether it is associated with normal or anomalous correspondence; for phoria patients it is necessary to know whether the AC/A is low, normal, or high. Once this information is known, the appropriate column in Table 11.1 or 11.2 is used to determine the sequence in which the different treatment options should be *considered*. For example, the model indicates that the fourth step to consider in treating occasional

Table 11.2   SEQUENCE OF TREATMENT CONSIDERATIONS FOR NONSQUINTING PATIENTS
(ESOPHORIA AND EXOPHORIA)

Low AC/A Low, Normal, High Tonic	Normal AC/A Low, Normal, High Tonic	High AC/A Low, Normal, High Tonic	Treatment Options
1	1	1	Optical prescription
7	3	2	Added lenses
2	2	3	Prisms*
3	4	4	Occlusion
4	5	5	VT†: Amblyopia
5	6	6	VT: Suppression
—	—	—	VT: ARC
6	7	7	VT: Sensorimotor Functions
8	8	8	Surgery

* Vertical prisms are often useful for vertical deviations in fused position (associated phoria); base-out prisms are helpful for esophorias especially at distance; for exophorias, base-in prisms at near should be considered if vision training is impractical or unsuccessful.
† VT stands for vision training or orthoptics.

strabismus with normal correspondence is occasional occlusion to reduce amblyopia and suppression; in the absence of amblyopia and with little suppression, this step would be skipped and the practitioner would proceed to consider orthoptics to break down the central suppression, with emphasis on diplopia awareness. The model serves as a guide to thinking about the order in which different treatment procedures should be considered for efficient and successful management of a specific kind of binocular anomaly.

TREATMENT SEQUENCES FOR STRABISMUS

Esotropia and Exotropia Compared

In the clinical management of strabismus, it is worth remembering that the prognosis for functional correction is generally better for exotropia than for esotropia. The reason stems from the fact that 80 percent of all cases of esotropia are occasional and that they exhibit fairly normal binocular vision at least occasionally, whereas 75 percent of all cases of esotropia are constant and these patients have only rudimentary aspects of normal binocular vision. A corollary of this fact is that patients with exotropia generally have few major deterrents to normal binocular vision whereas those with esotropia typically have deterrents such as anomalous correspondence, substantial amblyopia, and deep suppression. As a result, the treatment of exotropia is usually directed at solidifying and improving the existing sensory and motor fusion, whereas the challenge in treating esotropia is to overcome the deterring conditions and to establish fusion, often a difficult task that reduces the prognosis for functional correction of esotropia. In spite of the observation that esotropia is generally different from exotropia, there is marked similarity in the treatment sequence of esotropia and exotropia when they have the same combination of constancy and retinal correspondence. In other words, a person with occasional esotropia with normal correspondence should, in our treatment model, receive the same sequence of treatment considerations as a person with occasional exotropia with normal correspondence. The point here is that the direction of the strabismus does not influence the order in which the different treatment options are considered; the direction does, however, determine certain specifics of the treatment, such as whether a plus or minus added lens power or a base-out or base-in prism should be used. The following sections amplify this point.

Treating Occasional Strabismus with Normal Correspondence

The preponderance of occasional squinters fuse most of the time at near and squint more often at distance. The consequence of this fact is that management of these squinters, particularly with vision training, is best implemented by capitalizing on the fusion at near, thus employing optics or training that enhances vision abilities that are already developed.

It is often surprising how much optical correction of seemingly trivial refractive anomalies affects fusion. Commonly, correction of 0.50 D of astigmatism or anisometropia substantially increases the percent time of fusing for a person with occasional exotropia or esotropia. After correcting the refractive anomaly (optimum plus for esotropia, optimum minus for exotropia) to provide sharp retinal imagery that facilitates sensory and motor fusion, added lens power should be considered. A plus add for esotropia and a minus add for exotropia is a logical second consideration, because it facilitates motor fusion and actively reduces the angle of deviation through the AC/A ratio.

When prescribing added lens power, vertical prism should be considered to neutralize any vertical deviation present when the eyes are in the fused position. Horizontal prism, a passive treatment that permits the eyes to deviate toward the squinting position but reduces the demand on fusional vergence, should be considered next primarily when the squint is present more of the time than not. For persons with occasional strabismus who rarely squint, horizontal prisms are less useful than an active treatment.

Occasional squinters usually do not have much amblyopia; when it is present, occasional occlusion, especially for distance, should be considered next. This passive form of amblyopia treatment is facilitated by an active program of vision training directed at decreasing central suppression, which is often present. Awareness of diplopia when an ocular deviation is precipitated is an ideal outcome of this treatment, as it serves as the provocation for a fusional vergence recovery movement.

Training of sensorimotor functions logically comes next; training the sensory aspects of fusion (such as stereopsis) typically results in improved motor fusion. If any motor fusion training is necessary, it is needed less for amplitude than for facility of fusional vergence. Optical and orthoptic management of occasional strabismus usually result in functional correction.

Surgery typically is not necessary unless the angle of deviation is large and discomfort is present. Surgery is sometimes performed with an adjustable suture and tends to be conservative to avoid onset of a vertical deviation or noncomitancy. Optical and orthoptic follow-up immediately after surgery can be helpful.

Treating Occasional Strabismus with Anomalous Correspondence

Most of what we know about treating occasional strabismus with anomalous correspondence comes from experience with exotropia, where this combination of conditions is fairly common. Nonetheless, the treatment principles apply to the rare case of occasional esotropia with anomalous correspondence. When treating occasional squinters with anomalous correspondence it is important to recall that when these patients are not squinting (fusing) they have normal retinal correspondence (zero angle of anomaly). The anomalous correspondence that manifests itself when the strabismus is present becomes normal as fusional vergence is exercised to straighten the eyes. This covariation between fusional vergence and the angle of anomaly (30) forms the basis for treating this type of strabismus. Treatment is directed at enhancing existing fusional vergence, which allows the squint and the anomalous correspondence to be overcome simultaneously.

Since most of these patients have exotropia, about half have significant refractive errors. About 25 percent of exotropic patients have bilateral myopia and another 25 percent have myopic anisometropia. Correcting the refractive error of these patients produces results much like those for occasional squinters with normal correspondence; that is, correcting seemingly trivial refractive errors produces substantial increases in the frequency of fusion. Added lenses are useful for some of these patients, but they do not produce the straightforward results that occur in occasional squinters with normal correspondence. Added lenses change accommodative vergence, but this vergence rarely if ever (9, 36) produces associated changes in the angle of anomaly. When added minus lenses, for example, are applied clinically to occasional exotropia with anomalous correspondence, small amounts seem to facilitate fusional vergence and enhance bifixation and correspondence becomes normal. Larger added lens powers seem to interfere with covariation and can result in bifixation with diplopia or blurred vision from lack of accommodative response to the added lenses. Cavalier use of added lenses for occasional squinters with anomalous correspondence should be avoided, and judicious use should be encouraged.

Like added lenses, horizontal prisms can be troublesome for occasional squinters with anomalous correspondence. Prescribing base-in prisms for intermittent exotropia with anomalous correspondence, for example, will probably result in the eyes diverging to the prisms in order for the retinal images to continue to fall on (anomalously) corresponding retinal points. Prisms need to be considered early in treating these patients, principally to neutralize any vertical deviation that may be impeding fusion. Usually, but not always, anomalous correspondence is not present vertically in occasional squinters; so vertical prisms are effective in neutralizing vertical deviation and enhancing fusion for these patients.

Patients with occasional strabismus usually do not have much amblyopia, so treatment of the amblyopia can usually be accomplished with occasional occlusion. This passive treatment can be facilitated by antisuppression training, but there is typically little if any suppression coexisting with the anomalous correspondence. These patients usually need antisuppression orthoptic training only to break down small areas of central suppression, not to create diplopia (when the eyes deviate) as a stimulus to fusion, as for occasional squinters with normal correspondence.

As was pointed out earlier, motor fusion training gets the eyes straight and when that is accomplished, correspondence becomes normal. The challenge is to train fusional vergence when diplopia cannot be used as a stimulus for such vergence when the eyes are deviated because the anomalous correspondence with the eyes deviated prevents diplopia. Patients with occasional strabismus and anomalous correspondence can be trained to sense when the eye deviates (sometimes through the increased visual panorama) and to straighten the eye by executing a *reflex* fusional vergence movement. Training facility of fusional vergence and the sensory aspects of fusion (such as stereopsis) helps these patients develop the necessary reflex fusional vergence.

Surgery for these patients is not usually necessary unless the angle of deviations is large or there is discomfort. It is not clear what effect anomalous correspondence has on the outcome of surgery. Germane to this issue is a report by Flom and associates (21) on intermittent exotropia with anomalous correspondence. Measures of retinal correspondence were made before and immediately after surgery, and some time later. The patient had intermittent exotropia of 54Δ with harmonious anomalous correspondence; 6 hours after surgery the angle of anomaly shifted abruptly by as much as 54Δ, with some fluctuations; ultimately the angle was 3Δ exophoria with an angle of anomaly of −3Δ (harmonious). Clearly, correspondence can change quickly after surgery and in ways not associated with covariation; prompt evaluation of postsurgical status can help determine the need for additional surgical management (including adjusting the original suture) or in giving postsurgical vision training or optics.

Treating Constant Strabismus with Normal Correspondence

The main point in treating persons with constant esotropia or constant exotropia with normal correspondence is to recognize that they do not fixate bifoveally at any time. Many patients who appear to have constant exotropia on initial examination are found subsequently to be able to fuse at some distance (usually extremely close) or under some circumstances (with voluntary effort). Such persons technically have occasional exotropia, and their prognosis is considerably better and treatment considerably easier. The challenge in treating true constant strabismus with normal correspondence is initially to reduce suppression and any amblyopia to the point that fusion can be obtained at some distance (usually near) at least some of the time. To this end, occlusion therapy and vision training for the amblyopia and suppression usually precede the use of optics (added lenses or prisms) or vision training to obtain fusion.

Occlusion to reduce the amblyopia and suppression is facilitated by first correcting the refractive state fully to provide the sharpest possible retinal image and to maximize the potential for fusion. Generally, the most effective occlusion for constant strabismus is constant and total. It must be monitored frequently. When the amblyopia is deep or rapid progress is sought, orthoptic training is beneficial to break down the amblyopia and suppression.

The training consists initially of monocular fixation training, with feedback, if the eccentric fixation is greater than about 4Δ; the amblyopia is treated by direct stimulation of

the fovea with resolution targets presented under monocular conditions followed by dichoptic stimulation, which breaks down the suppression. Moving the antisuppression targets from periphery to the central field is effective. Target size and element separation are gradually reduced. Other stimulus parameters that can be manipulated in the treatment are brightness, contrast, color, on period, and movement. The orthoptic training goal is foveal fixation, normal acuity, and pathological diplopia when the eyes deviate and physiological diplopia when they are fused.

When the acuity and suppression improve to the point where sensory fusion can be demonstrated, occlusion can be reduced over time as sensory fusion increases correspondingly. The level of acuity that just permits sensory fusion is quite variable among patients; few can fuse with monocular amblyopia of 20/200, and almost all can fuse, at near points with the aid of optics, with amblyopia of 20/40. For most patients the threshold for sensory fusion is in the 20/60 to 20/100 range. When acuity reaches the threshold level where sensory fusion is possible, added lenses and prisms become a major factor in treatment.

For constant squinters, the angle of deviation tends to be large; so fairly large amounts of added lens power are often needed as training lenses (up to 4 or 5 D plus or minus). Prisms that correct a vertical deviation that remains when the eyes are fused should be considered in conjunction with added lenses. Although a plus add can be very effective in reducing an esotropia at near points, it does nothing for the distant angle.

When the esotropia is about the same magnitude at distance and near points (when the calculated AC/A ratio equals the PD in centimeters), base-out prisms approximating the angle of deviation should be considered instead of an add, to provide fusion at the angle of deviation. For AC/A ratios greater than the PD (esotropia larger at near than at distance), added plus power can be prescribed to neutralize the near-point esotropia that remains after prescribing base-out prism that nearly equals the distance angle.

The large amounts of base-out prism initially needed to provide fusion for constant esotropia can be reduced as orthoptic training successfully improves sensory and motor fusion. Sensory fusion training needs to precede fusional vergence training. Traditionally, one thinks about gaining amplitude of fusional vergence, but fusional vergence and accommodative facility, as well as transfer of training responses to free space, are probably more important than fusional amplitude in obtaining functional cure of strabismus. For persons with exotropia the rapid improvement in fusional vergence with orthoptics tends to eliminate the need for large amounts of base-in prisms; therefore, orthoptics should be considered for constant exotropia after or in conjunction with the added minus lenses and before or in place of base-in prism.

If the optics necessary to provide constant fusion are large or unwieldy, or if fusion is not maintained well, surgery should be considered. It needs to be controlled, possibly with an adjustable suture, to avoid onset of a vertical deviation or noncomitancy. Postsurgical follow-up with optics and orthoptics can be important in dealing with resulting vertical deviations, noncomitancy, or diplopia.

Treating Constant Squinters with Anomalous Correspondence

About 75 percent of all esotropias are constant, but only 20 percent of exotropias are. Somewhat more than half of all cases of constant esotropia are associated with anomalous correspondence, as are somewhat less than half of all cases of constant exotropia. Thus, most of the patients with constant strabismus and anomalous correspondence have esotropia. Constant strabismus with normal correspondence typically is associated with suppression; anomalous correspondence fairly often accompanies amblyopia. For constant squinters with normal correspondence, the treatment sequence was directed at eradicat-

ing suppression (see previous discussion of treating constant squinters with normal correspondence). For constant squinters with anomalous correspondence the treatment consists of either fusional vergence training for exotropia and for small-angle (<15 to 20Δ) esotropia (for both of which the prognosis is fairly good) or establishing normal (fovea to fovea) correspondence with the eyes in the deviated position for large-angle (>20Δ) esotropia (for which the prognosis is poor). Before either treatment is begun, acuity must usually be in the neighborhood of 20/60 and second-degree fusion must be demonstrated for targets of 5 degrees subtense. The poor prognosis for functional correction of constant ARC esotropia with squint angles greater than 20Δ means that cosmetic management is frequently a consideration.

The preponderance of esotropia among constant strabismus patients with ARC dictates that hyperopia will be the most common refractive anomaly, necessitating attention to latent hyperopia. Such attention is required for either functional or cosmetic correction, as maximum plus correction will relax accommodation and reduce the esodeviation, which is desirable for functional or cosmetic treatment. After correcting the refractive anomaly, treating for functional correction is very different from treating for cosmetic correction.

In attempting to get functional correction, it is necessary to neutralize any vertical deviation with prisms. Such prisms are usually effective because the anomalous correspondence typically does not exhibit itself vertically. Manifestation of anomalous correspondence in the horizontal dimension, however, leads to the problem of horizontal prisms inducing a horizontal fusional vergence response. Thus, prescribing base-out prisms for esotropia with anomalous correspondence characteristically produces an increase in fusional vergence, the angle of squint, and the angle of anomaly (covariation). (Cosmetically, the result is doubly bad, because the angle of squint actually increases and additionally through the base-out prisms the eyes appear to be displaced nasalward.)

Putting base-in prisms before the eyes of an esotropic patient with anomalous correspondence produces fusional divergence and associated reduction in the angle of anomaly. Unfortunately, with base-in prisms the divergence response is limited to a few prism diopters. The strong vergence stimuli available on the major amblyoscope permit larger fusional divergence responses than with prisms, so esodeviations up to 20Δ can be overcome with a simultaneous decrease in the angle of anomaly through covariation.

Occlusion is used for these patients in much the same way as it is for constant squinters with normal correspondence. Occlusion tends to be most effective when it is constant and total. When the amblyopia or suppression is deep or when rapid progress is sought, orthoptics is beneficial. Amblyopia may be more common among constant squinters with anomalous than with normal correspondence; but its management is the same (see previous section on treating amblyopia and suppression in constant squinters with normal correspondence). The purpose of occlusion and orthoptic treatment of amblyopia and suppression in constant squinters with ARC is to obtain sufficiently good acuity and sufficiently little suppression to permit regular and systematic changes in fusional vergence in response to the more powerful vergence stimuli that can be generated in a major amblyoscope. Thus, the initial treatment of the amblyopia and suppression need continue only until the desired fusional vergence responses can be obtained, regardless of the degree of amblyopia or suppression. Indeed, if fusional vergence can be appropriately driven at the outset, in spite of the presence of amblyopia or suppression, then treatment of these conditions can be deferred.

As stated at the start of this section, treatment for functional correction of constant squinters with ARC centers around either orthoptic training of fusional vergence to overcome the deviation and angle of anomaly or (for large-angle esotropia) orthoptic training to break down the anomalous correspondence directly. The essential elements of the fusional vergence training to overcome the angle of deviation and angle of anomaly are to use second-degree, or preferably third-degree, targets that are large, detailed, and have high contrast and to change the vergence disparity slowly enough (perhaps 1Δ per minute) to drive the slow vergence (and maybe the tonic vergence system). For esotropic deviations less than 20Δ, this training is conveniently accomplished with a major amblyoscope using third-degree "swing" targets (set at the subjective angle of directionalization) that are flashed rapidly while the instrument arms are slowly diverged and the patient continues to see the target singly, without suppression, and ideally with stereopsis, until the eyes are physically straight and can be maintained so when the patient sits back from the instrument, first in a dark room and then as the illumination is slowly increased to normal (61). Although this technique also works for constant exotropia, it is usually simpler and quicker for them to train by initiating convergence outside an instrument, for example as when looking from a distance to very close, detailed, accommodative targets. With both methods, the angle of anomaly goes to zero when the vergence overcomes the oculomotor deviation.

The main idea underlying training methods that attempt to eliminate the ARC directly is to stimulate the two foveas simultaneously with sufficient vigor (especially the deviating eye's fovea) to "reestablish" the presumably dormant normal fovea-to-fovea correspondence. When this occurs in the presence of the anomalous correspondence, binocular triplopia, and sometimes monocular diplopia, results, indicating the simultaneous presence of normal and anomalous correspondence. Quite a few cases of constant large-angle esotropia with ARC can be treated to this point. The difficulty in this orthoptic method occurs at this point, when one attempts to eliminate the anomalous correspondence between the fixating eye's fovea and the associated peripheral area in the deviating eye.

If orthoptic treatment of the ARC succeeds, it should be followed by training that improves the qualitative aspects of sensory and motor fusion, and perhaps by surgery. If treatment of the ARC fails, cosmetic improvement by optical methods (described above) or surgery should be considered.

Constant squinters who achieve functional correction with optics and orthoptics

Table 11.3 SUMMARY OF KEY POINTS IN TREATING STRABISMUS

Type of Strabismus	Sequence of Treatments
Occasional with NRC	Refractive correction Added lens power and prisms Suppression treatment Sensorimotor training
Occasional with ARC	Refractive correction Limited, cautious use of prisms and added lenses Suppression treatment Fusional vergence training (covariation)
Constant with NRC	Refractive correction Suppression (and any amblyopia) treatment Aggressive use of prisms and added lens power Sensorimotor training
Constant with ARC	Functional Refractive correction Amblyopia (and any suppression) treatment Fusional vergence training (covariation) or ARC treatment for esotropia >20Δ Limited, cautious use of prisms and added lenses Cosmetic Refractive correction Amblyopia treatment Reverse prisms

may need surgery if the deviation cannot be completely controlled, if maintaining control is uncomfortable, or if the (vertical) prism required to maintain fusion is excessively large and unsightly. If optics and orthoptics fail, surgery can be considered primarily for cosmetic purposes, although in some cases there is a postsurgical change in correspondence sufficient to effect a cure or to justify follow-up orthoptics aimed at a functional cure. According to von Noorden (59), patients who have "deep-seated" anomalous correspondence without functional potential require less surgery, because postsurgically a cosmetically acceptable residual angle of deviation is desired so that later the eyes do not drift to a large angle of the opposite type (e.g., esotropia into exotropia).

The discussion above on the treatment of strabismus is summarized in Table 11.3.

TREATMENT SEQUENCES FOR PHORIA PATIENTS

Esophorias and Exophorias Compared

As we already mentioned, the prognosis for functional correction of phoria is generally very good. Functional correction of phorias involves different parameters than in strabismus, where the principal goal is overcoming the turning of the eye and establishing good binocular vision. For phorias the chief concern of the patient is overcoming symptoms or some visual performance deficiency (such as limited ability to maintain clear vision while reading or reduced stereoacuity), and the goal of the optometrist is usually to improve certain visual functions in some measurable way. Relieving symptoms and improving vision functions do not always go hand in hand. Possibly for this reason, the criterion that practitioners use to define functional correction of phoria cases usually involves some combination of decrease in symptoms and improvement in measured visual functions.

It is widely believed that better results are obtained treating exophoria than esophoria, but this may result from the fact that some optometrists are more reluctant to prescribe base-out than base-in prisms or to prescribe the larger amount of prisms needed for eso-phorias than exophorias. It may also result from the fact that divergence training for eso-phoria usually takes longer than training con-vergence for exophoria. The reluctance of some practitioners to prescribe bifocals for esophoric children adds to the belief that they have better success treating exophoria than esophoria. When all treatment methods are fully utilized, the prognosis is remarkably good for both esophoria and exophoria.

Accommodative problems are frequently associated with both esophoria and exopho-ria. Differences do occur. Exophoric patients often have a problem looking from a near task to a distant one: the distant object is slow to clear or a blurred binocular image may per-sist. One explanation for this effect is that ac-commodation is stimulated to promote sin-gleness through accommodative vergence and it is slow to be released. Another expla-nation, not incompatible with the first, is that convergence accommodation brought about by the continually required positive fusional vergence is likewise not easily inhibited. Conversely, esophoric patients tend to see near objects blurred, often when looking from distance to near and sometimes when sustaining near fixation. In their case, the ex-planation is inhibition of accommodation at near points to facilitate fusion or fusional di-vergence that reduces accommodation. Ac-commodative insufficiencies in these phoria patients may stem from the binocular oculo-motor problem (or conversely); regardless, the concomitant poor accommodative facility is clearly evident in these patients. Often it is exhibited in monocular vision, and it can be quickly remedied with added lens power—or more effectively with accommodative fa-cility training. For unknown reasons, some patients without significant phoria exhibit similar accommodative difficulties; on a purely pragmatic basis optometrists are quite successful in improving accommodation and alleviating the symptoms with training.

Amblyopia in phoria patients is almost al-ways associated with anisometropia (20). Even though anisometropia is about equally common in hyperopia and myopia, amblyo-pia is more common and tends to be deeper when associated with hyperopia than with myopia in anisometropia (34). The degree of amblyopia appears to be directly correlated with the amount of hyperopic anisometropia, starting with as little as 1 D or so of anisome-tropia. With myopia, however, significant am-blyopia (20/40 or worse) does not appear to occur very often until the difference in myo-pia is quite large, say more than 6 D. Optom-etrists have the impression that esophoria is more often associated with hyperopia than exophoria and that the opposite is true of my-opia, but we are unable to find research data to support this opinion. To the extent that hyperopia is more common with esophoria, and myopia with exophoria, amblyopia is more common and deeper with esophoria than with exophoria. Patients who have an-isometropic amblyopia have an average acu-ity of 20/60 (20), and most are hyperopic. Re-gardless of whether more patients with anisometropic amblyopia have esophoria or exophoria, the treatment of the amblyopia and any associated suppression always must be considered immediately after prescribing prism to compensate for a vertical phoria. Oc-clusion needs to be either part-time and com-plete or full-time and partial to avoid the pos-sibility of precipitating strabismus. Active treatment (orthoptics) can be mainly binocu-lar to break down suppression and improve acuity simultaneously.

Based on epidemiological data of Morgan (40), the prevalence of significant distance phorias in the population is in the neighbor-hood of 5 percent (about the same as that of strabismus); the prevalence of significant near point phorias is considerably higher because of the additional large variance in AC/A ra-tios in the population. In our system for treat-ing phorias, the direction of the distance phoria (eso or exo) does not determine the sequence of treatments. It is the size of the AC/A ratio (low, normal, high) that estab-lishes the treatment sequence. The direction of the distance phoria determines certain particulars of treatment, such as whether base-out or base-in prism should be prescribed given that prism treatment is under consideration.

Treating Phoria Patients Who Have a Low AC/A Ratio

Phoria patients who have a low AC/A ratio will have more exophoria at near than at distance or less esophoria at near than at distance. In the former case the problem is worsened in near viewing; in the latter, it is reduced. In either case, added lens power does not greatly change the near phoria because of the low AC/A ratio (that is, each diopter of lens power produces a unit change in accommodation that is associated with only a small amount of accommodative vergence).

Thus, after correcting the refractive anomaly to improve sensory and motor fusion, one needs to consider not added lens power but vertical prisms (that neutralize any vertical deviation present with the eyes in the fused position) for further improvement of sensory and motor fusion. Prisms prescribed to neutralize even small amounts of vertical phoria can overcome symptoms and enhance horizontal fusion.

Whether to consider prescribing lateral prisms at this point depends on the distance phoria. For the rare patient with *esophoria at distance* and a low AC/A ratio, base-out prisms are characteristically helpful at distance but may overcorrect at near points, requiring two pairs of glasses or specialty base-in prism segments. Measures of the associated phoria (prism power that reduces fixation disparity to zero) usually indicate that nearly the full amount of any (disassociated) vertical phoria or esophoria needs to be corrected with prism. For the low AC/A-ratio patient who has *orthophoria at distance*, base-in prisms for near viewing can be considered either in a single-vision form or as a prism-controlled segment with a low-power add. Measures of associated exophoria usually indicate that only small amounts of base-in prism need be prescribed. For the common patient with *distance exophoria* and a low AC/A ratio, lateral prisms can be deferred until after fusion training, which is generally successful and produces results that can be viewed as better than those achieved with prisms (that is, binocular vision is more stable, especially when glasses are removed). Prescribing base-in prisms for low AC/A patients with exophoria is usually considered when fusion training is impractical or unsuccessful.

Any amblyopia should be treated with passive occlusion or active training, primarily under binocular conditions. Suppression, which is usually slight and confined to the central retina, must also be treated, whether or not amblyopia is present. The ultimate goal here is to eliminate any amblyopia and suppression so that sensory and motor fusion training can be maximally effective, however sensory and motor fusion training can be introduced as the amblyopia and suppression are eliminated. Indeed, fusion training can be additionally effective in breaking down suppression and amblyopia. As is the case for all phoria patients, both of the vergence functions and accommodative facility must be trained. Even though accommodative facility is readily achieved by esophoric and exophoric patients, overall clinical success through training is more often achieved by the latter group, because convergence is more readily improved than divergence.

Surgery is rarely recommended for low AC/A patients, even those with distance exophoria. The reason is that optical and training procedures so often produce long-term success and further that surgical procedures for the patient with exophoria at near (bilateral medial rectus resection) frequently result in overcorrection with ensuing diplopia for several weeks or even months (59).

Treating Phoria Patients Who Have Normal AC/A

When the AC/A ratio (in prism diopters of vergence per diopter of accommodation) numerically equals the patient's interpupillary distance (P.D.) in centimeters, the angle of oculomotor deviation (phoria or squint) is the same at all distances up to the near point of convergence. (This assumes the AC/A ratio is linear, which is not exactly correct, but it is adequate for most patients) (16). The average adult interpupillary distance is in the neighborhood of 6.4 cm, and the average *calculated* AC/A ratio for 24 normal control subjects was found to be about 5.2Δ/D (17). From Morgan's (40) expected clinical values, the calculated AC/A ratio (assuming an average PD of 6.4 cm) is 5.6Δ/D. Thus, for patients with average P.D.s and AC/A ratios, the distance and near phorias will be about the same, the near angle being perhaps a little more exo or less eso. The importance of this situation is that these patients tend to have the same kinds of symptoms or vision problems during distance and near viewing and treatment tends to be equally effective for both distances. For example, a patient with 6Δ esophoria at all distances (AC/A equals P.D.) would probably benefit at distance and near with a single-vision lens prescription of, say, 4Δ base out. When the AC/A ratio is very low (1Δ/D) or very high (9Δ/D), the distance and near angles are so different that a single prism prescription is not likely to be effective for distance and near vision. When the AC/A differs from the P.D., the distance and near angles will differ by approximately 2.5Δ for a 1Δ/D change in AC/A. So, a patient with a 4Δ/D. AC/A ratio will have about 5Δ more exodeviation or less esodeviation for near (i.e., 40 cm) than distance viewing. For both esodeviation and exodeviation cases, a single prism prescription would probably work because people tend to need less prism for near viewing than for distance viewing. We have accepted the average range to be from 3 to 7Δ/D., which range has a mean value of 5Δ/D. For patients with such AC/A ratios, vision training of fusional vergence is typically equally effective for distance and near viewing.

A second and important consequence of having a normal AC/A ratio is that added lenses produce significant changes in vergence. Thus, added plus lenses can be used effectively for near esophoria, and added minus lenses can be considered as a treatment for exophoria at all distances. Of course, the change in vergence per diopter of added lens power depends on the AC/A ratio. In our experience, the calculated AC/A gives a better indication of the ultimate vergence change than does the gradient AC/A ratio.

As mentioned earlier, the difference in the sequence of treatment for phoria patients with low, normal, and high AC/A ratios consists mainly of when to consider the use of added lenses and prisms. For phoria patients with a low AC/A (discussed in the previous section) added lenses were considered either very late in the treatment or not at all because of the small change in vergence per diopter of added lens power. For phoria patients having a normal AC/A ratio (3 to 7Δ/D) (considered in this section), added lenses are a useful treatment to be considered after deciding on the refractive correction. In the model, we have indicated considering prisms before added lenses mainly because of the important effect vertical prisms can have in the treatment. Lateral prisms and added lenses can be about equally effective for these phoria patients; the advantages and disadvantages of both should be considered for an individual patient. Some factors that influence the decision are: (1) large distance esophorias usually require vision training even if added minus lenses or prisms are prescribed; (2) large distance esophorias often require base-out prisms even after training; and (3) near esophorias are quickly aided with a plus add.

Once the optical considerations have been dealt with in the format described here for normal AC/A patients, the other treatment considerations are similar for all phoria patients. Treatment of amblyopia and suppression and training fusion and accommodation are considered as for low and high AC/A patients. Surgery is not the problem for normal AC/A patients as it is for the low and high AC/A patients. Even so, surgery is considered in the occasional instance of a very large phoria when optical and training management are unsuccessful.

Treating Patients Having High AC/A Ratio

Phoria patients who have a high AC/A ratio have more eso (or less exo) during near viewing than at distance. With esophoria, the problems are usually worse during near viewing; with exophoria, they typically are less severe. In both cases, added lenses are especially effective in changing vergence because of the high AC/A ratio.

Immediately after assessing how the correction of the refractive state facilitates sensory and motor fusion, consideration should be given to prescribing added lens power, either added minus power for a distance and near exophoria or added plus power for a near-point esophoria. The high AC/A ratio dictates prompt attention to the benefits of added lenses, which are different for patients with low and normal AC/A ratios. The calculated AC/A ratio gives a good indication of the actual vergence change that can be expected.

Next prisms are considered, especially for any vertical deviation indicated on the associated phoria test. Although horizontal prisms are generally less effective than added lenses for high AC/A patients, there are circumstances where prisms are clearly indicated, the most common instance being distance esophorias alleviated by base-out prisms. Often both added lenses and horizontal prisms are necessary; for the high AC/A-ratio patient with distance esophoria, base-out prisms can ameliorate the distance problem, and a plus add may be needed to handle the greater esophoria at near. In this case, the added plus power prescribed for near vision will be less if base-out prisms are prescribed to manage the distance esophoria than if no prisms are prescribed. Because of the high AC/A ratio, only a relatively small change in add will result from prescribing a fairly large amount of prism. For a patient with a 10Δ/D AC/A ratio, prescribing 5Δ of base-out prism for a distance esophoria would result in a reduction of the near add by only 0.5 D. These points about added lenses and prisms notwithstanding, it is necessary to recognize that in the management of high AC/A patients *large* distance exophorias usually require vision training in addition to optics and distance esophorias usually require base-out prisms even after vision training.

After considering the various optical options for managing these high AC/A patients, further management is like that for all phoria patients. (Treatment of amblyopia and suppression and training fusion and accommodation are discussed above, Treating Phoria Patients Who Have a Low AC/A Ratio).

Surgery is rarely recommended for high AC/A phoria patients because of the problem of postsurgical diplopia at one distance or the other. It is rarely undertaken because optical and training methods are so successful for these patients. On the rare occasion when they fail, controlled surgery with prompt follow-up for possible optics and training may be considered.

REFERENCES

1. Bangerter A: Amblyopie Behandlung. Basel, S Karger, 1955.

2. Barnard W: Treatment of amblyopia by inverse occlusion and pleoptics: A review of the results in 144 cases. Br Orthop J 19:19, 1962.

3. Bielschowsky A: Lectures on Motor Anomalies. Hanover NH, Dartmouth Publications, 59, 1956.

4. Bonsor A: Some comments on the question of early operation. Br Orthop J 16:114, 1959.

5. Burian HM: Use of bifocal spectacles in the treatment of accommodative esotropia. Br Orthop J 13:3, 1956.

6. Caltrider N, Jampolsky A: Overcorrecting minus lens therapy for treatment of intermittent exotropia. Ophthalmology 90:1160, 1983.

7. Costenbader FD: The physiology and management of divergent strabismus. In Allen JH (ed): Strabismus Ophthalmic Symposium (I). St Louis, CV Mosby, 1950.

8. Dal Fiume E, Cardi G: Clinical study of acute strabismus due to occlusion (in Italian). In Abstr Am J Ophthalmol 51:194, 1961. From Arch Ottalmol 64:87, 1960.

9. Daum KM: Covariation in anomalous correspondence with accommodative vergence. Am J Optom Physiol Opt 59:146, 1982.

10. Duke-Elder WS: Textbook of Ophthalmology, vol 4. St Louis, CV Mosby, 4024, 1949.

11. Fisher NF, Flom MC, Jampolsky A: Early surgery of congenital esotropia. Am J Ophthalmol 65:439, 1968.

12. Flom MC: University of California strabismus and orthoptics study: A preliminary report. Prepared for the Research Projects Committee of the American Academy of Optometry (unpublished). Sept 29, 1954.

13. Flom MC: Variations in convergence and accommodation induced by successive spherical lens additions with distance fixation; an investigation (with a description of a clinical method for testing the validity of the refractive correction). Am J Optom Arch Am Acad Optom 32:111, 1955.

14. Flom MC, Takahashi E: The AC/A ratio in undercorrected myopia. Am J Optom Arch Am Acad Optom 39:305, 1962.

15. Flom MC: A minimum strabismus examination. J Am Optom Assoc 27:642, 1956.

16. Flom MC: On the relationship between accommodation and accommodative convergence, part I: Linearity. Am J Optom Arch Am Acad Optom 37:1, 1960.

17. Flom MC: On the relationship between accommodation and accommodative convergence, part III: Effects of orthoptics. Am J Optom Arch Am Acad Optom 37:619, 1960.

18. Flom MC: Treatment of binocular anomalies of vision. In Hirsch MJ, Wick RE (eds): Vision of Children. Philadelphia, Chilton, 214, 1963.

19. Flom MC, Adams AJ: Fresnel optics. In Safir A (ed): Refraction and Clinical Optics. Hagerstown MD, Harper & Row, 1976.

20. Flom MC, Bedell HE: Identifying amblyopia using associated conditions, acuity, and non-acuity features. Am J Optom Physiol Opt 62:153, 1985.

21. Flom MC, Kirschen DG, Williams AT: Changes in retinal correspondence following surgery for intermittent exotropia. Am J Optom Physiol Opt 55:456, 1978.

22. Folk ER: Surgical results in intermittent exotropia. Arch Ophthalmol 55:484, 1956.

23. Fulton AB, Mayer DL: Esotropic children with amblyopia: Effects of patching on acuity. Graefes Arch Clin Exp Ophthalmol 226:309, 1988.

24. Gerard LJ, Fletcher MC, Tomlinson E: Results of pleoptic treatment of suppression amblyopia. Am Orthoptic J 12:12, 1962.

25. Gibson HW: Textbook of Orthoptics. London, Hatton Press, 1955.

26. Giles GH: The Practice of Orthoptics. London, Hammond, Hammond, 1947.

27. Gortz H: The corrective treatment of amblyopia with eccentric fixation. Am J Ophthalmol 49:1315, 1960.

28. Graham PA: Recent developments in the treatment of amblyopia. Br Orthop J 18:1, 1961.

29. Griffin JR: Binocular Anomalies: Procedures for Vision Therapy. Chicago, Professional Press, 1976.

30. Hallden U: Fusional phenomena in anomalous correspondence. Acta Ophthalmol (Copenh) [Suppl] 37: 1952.

31. Hirsch MJ: Prism in spectacle lenses for cosmesis. Am J Optom Arch Am Acad Optom 45:409, 1968.

32. Hugonnier R, Clayette-Hugonnier S, Veronneau-Troutman S (trans): Strabismus, Heterophoria, Ocular Motor Paralysis. St Louis, CV Mosby, 1969.

33. Ing M, Costenbader FD, Parks MM, et al: Surgery for congenital esotropia. Am J Ophthalmol 61:1419, 1966.

34. Jampolsky AJ, Flom BC, Weymouth FW: Unequal corrected visual acuity as related to anisometropia. Arch Ophthalmol 54:893, 1955.

35. Kennedy JR: The correction of divergent strabismus with concave lenses. Am J Optom Arch Acad Optom 31:605, 1954.

36. Kerr K: Accommodative and fusional vergence in anomalous correspondence. Am J Optom Physiol Opt 57:676, 1980.

37. Kramer ME: Clinical Orthoptics. St. Louis, CV Mosby, 1953.

38. Marlow FW: The technique of the prolonged occlusion test. Am J Ophthalmol 15:320, 1932.

39. Maruo T, Kubota N, Iwashige H, et al: Long-

term results after strabismus surgery. Graefes Arch Clin Exp Ophthalmol 226:414, 1988.

40. Morgan MW: Analysis of clinical data. Am J Optom Arch Am Acad Optom 21:477, 1944.

41. Nordlow W: Permanent convergent squint— Early operation and long-term follow-up. Arch Ophthalmol 55:87, 1956.

42. Ogle KN: Researches in Binocular Vision. New York, Hafner Publishing, 262, 1950.

43. Ogle KN: Distortion of the image by ophthalmic prisms. Arch Ophthalmol 47:121, 1952.

44. Reese EE, Fry GA: The effect of fogging lenses on accommodation. Am J Optom Arch Am Acad Optom 18:9, 1941.

45. Roper KL, Bannon RE: Diagnostic value of monocular occlusion. Arch Ophthalmol 31:316, 338, 1944.

46. Sanchez Agesta R, Galvez Montes J: La oclusion monocular como factor desencadenante del estrabismo concomitante. Arch Soc Optalmol Hisp-Am 20:318, 1960.

47. Sheard C: Zones of ocular comfort. Am J Optom 7:9, 1930.

48. Smith W: Clinical Orthoptic Procedure. St Louis, CV Mosby, 1954.

49. Stella SL: The association of blinks and refusion in intermittent exotropia. Am J Optom Arch Am Acad Optom 45:465, 1968.

50. Stelzer AJ: Practical aspects of temporal and nasal occlusion in treatment of strabismus. Am Orthoptic J 5:53, 1955.

51. Sternberg AR, Bohar: A study on the occlusion therapy of eccentric fixation. Report on 109 cases. Ophthalmologica 141:229, 1961.

52. Sugar HS: Intermittent exotropia. Treatment. Am Orthoptic J 2:18, 1952.

53. Swan KC: Esotropia following occlusion. Arch Ophthalmol 37:444, 1947.

54. Swenson A: Temporal occlusion in concomitant convergent strabismus. Am Orthoptic J 3:48, 1953.

55. Taylor DM: Congenital strabismus. The common-sense approach. Arch Ophthalmol 77:478, 1967.

56. Thomas J, Mohindra I, Held R: Strabismic amblyopia in infants. Am J Optom Physiol Opt 56:197, 1979.

57. Trevor-Roper PD, Curran PV: The Eye and Its Disorders. Boston, Blackwell Scientific Publications, 1984.

58. Urist MJ: Eccentric fixations in amblyopia ex anopsia. Arch Ophthalmol 54:345, 350, 1955.

59. Von Noorden GK: Burian-Von Noorden's Binocular Vision and Ocular Motility: Theory and Management of Strabismus. St Louis, CV Mosby, 312, 1985.

60. Ward PA, Charman WN: An objective assessment of the effect of fogging on accommodation. Am J Optom Physiol Opt 64:762, 1987.

61. Wick B: Vision therapy for small-angle esotropia. Am J Optom Arch Am Acad Optom 51:490, 1974.

Chapter 12

Vision Therapy for Preschool Children

Bruce Wick

In the immediately preceding chapters two important areas of the management of patients with strabismus and amblyopia were presented; in Chapter 10 the prognosis for management was discussed and in Chapter 11 a treatment rationale was developed that suggests a hierarchical approach to the management of any type of binocular anomaly. The management considerations presented in Chapter 11 did not detail vision therapy management, present vision therapy strategies, or consider the modifications that may be required in vision therapy programs for preschool children.

Chapters (24) and books (7, 10) have been written about vision therapy for older children and adults. Many of these suggest that it is difficult or impossible to begin active vision therapy programs until a child is approximately 5 years of age (15). As a result, management of infants and toddlers has generally been considered to be limited to passive therapies such as lenses, prisms, and occlusion. With proper design of the therapy program, however, active vision therapy can be provided to surprisingly young children, in many instances even to infants.

In writing this chapter I assumed that the reader is generally familiar with vision therapy techniques and emphasized the factors that must be considered when planning management for the preschool patient, including occlusion and vision therapy programs. Thus, guidelines for occlusion and early vision therapy management are presented along with a brief discussion of certain techniques that can be used for vision therapy treatment of preschool patients with binocular visual dysfunction. Specific techniques for many types of binocular problems are discussed, highlighting the areas where either different techniques or modifications of commonly used techniques must be used to achieve satisfactory results with younger patients. Management and techniques are illustrated using representative case reports that detail diagnosis and treatment.

BACKGROUND CONSIDERATIONS

Although binocular vision evaluation and care are considered fundamental parts of optometry, surveys have demonstrated that fewer than one third of optometrists offer vision therapy as part of their service to preschool patients (15). Apparently, many optometrists do not feel comfortable managing preschool patients with binocular vision dysfunction. Care of preschool children can enable practitioners to increase their practice and at the same time provide visual readiness for reading and learning.

Preschool children who need binocular vision care generally have problems such as strabismus and amblyopia. In addition, when children reach school age, it has been estimated that one in five (20 percent) needs some form of therapy for binocular vision or accommodative dysfunction. The majority of such school-aged patients have heterophoria or accommodative problems (21). Fortunately, both preschool and school-aged patients with binocular dysfunction can be managed by following the management strategy outlined in Chapter 11. When an active vision therapy program becomes necessary, it often can be devised by using or modifying a few simple therapy procedures. Therapy programs can be used to eliminate amblyopia through active therapy, followed by vision therapy for suppression, anomalous correspondence, and sensorimotor functions.

GENERAL SEQUENCE OF MANAGEMENT

Diagnosis

Accurate diagnosis is essential to proper management of binocular dysfunction (6). Lens prescription, management, and vision therapy procedures can be planned for all nonstrabismic patients from data obtained from standard optometric tests. After appropriate lens and prism management, heterophoria, near point of convergence, and accommodative problems that continue to require remediation can be treated with vision therapy. Patients with these conditions respond rapidly and have approximately a 90-percent chance of successful elimination of symptoms (9). Diagnosis of strabismic patients also requires assessment of comitance, status of fixation (in the presence of amblyopia), suppression, stereopsis, and state of retinal correspondence.

Older Children

The diagnosis is based on the results of binocular refraction techniques (4), an accurate careful cover test (5, 19), thorough accommodative assessment, and fixation disparity tests (8, 13) in addition to standard tests of vergence range and facility. These tests also provide the basis for decisions concerning management of binocular vision dysfunctions. Optometric evaluation of learning problems in school-aged children includes careful binocular and accommodative evaluation as well as the perceptual evaluations discussed in Chapter 21. Referral to other professionals for management of certain learning problems is indicated after the vision function has been maximized.

Preschool Diagnosis

Because of the unreliable responses often given by preschool children, diagnostic testing must emphasize tests that do not require subjective responses. Often retinoscopy is used for lens prescription purposes because subjective refraction techniques do not yield reliable results. Although an accurate careful cover test is preferred for determining eye alignment, many times an uncooperative preschool patient can only be diagnosed initially using a Hirschberg or another test of alignment. Tests of simultaneous perception (e.g., Worth Dot) and stereopsis must be simplified so that the preschool child can respond adequately. Additional diagnostic techniques for preschool children include developmental assessment and visual and auditory perceptual evaluations. These evaluations confirm that the preschool child has an adequate visual and perceptual system for reading and learning readiness. Developmental assessment and visual and auditory perceptual diagnostic techniques are described in other chapters in this book.

Signs and Symptoms

The most common problems of the preschool child who needs binocular vision therapy are strabismus and amblyopia. Common symptoms reported by school-aged children who have uncompensated heterophoria or accommodative problems are listed in Table 12.1.

Sequential Management Considerations

The general considerations for management of binocular vision dysfunction in a preschool child are similar to those presented in Chapter 11 for older patients. Optimal lens correction, the first consideration, is followed by added lens power, prism correction, and management of amblyopia using passive occlusion therapy. Detailed use of occlusion will be discussed here, because this form of passive therapy is frequently an integral part of management and is often included in pro-

Table 12.1   COMMON SYMPTOMS OF HETEROPHORIA

Blurring
Burning
Car sickness[a]
Diplopia
Eye strain
Fatigue
Headaches associated with use of the eyes
Loss of place when reading[a]
Print swimming[a]
Usually clear vision but intermittent blurring
   associated with looking to a new location

----

[a] Frequently associated with vertical heterophoria and aniseikonia.

grams of active vision therapy. When a vision therapy program is needed it can be used to eliminate amblyopia through active therapy, followed by vision therapy for suppression, anomalous correspondence, and sensorimotor functions.

Some preschool children have angles of deviation so large that surgery needs to be considered as part of the overall treatment. Surgery may be required for angles greater than 20 PD esotropia and 30 PD exotropia. In these instances, pre- and postsurgical optical correction and vision therapy can be helpful. Careful postsurgical management enables sustained eye alignment during the immediate postsurgical period, which ordinarily enhances the surgical result.

VISION THERAPY

Vision therapy is an active process that can be used "to improve fixation ability, reduce amblyopia, eliminate suppression, correct anomalous correspondence, improve sensory fusion (including stereopsis), and increase facility and range of accommodative and vergence responses" (6). Active vision therapy is not necessary for many patients. When the considerations for management of binocular dysfunction outlined in Chapter 11 are followed binocular vision can often be enhanced solely through proper use of lenses and prisms. Additional techniques are required to treat visual perceptual problems (see Chapter 21).

General Considerations

Assuming the cooperation of the child and parents, the success rate of vision therapy in providing normal binocular vision is very high, but for some strabismic children, vision therapy is initially deferred in preference to surgical management. When the prognosis for functional cure is significantly improved following surgery, vision therapy is reconsidered.

Before proceeding with therapy the purpose of the therapy should be explained to the parents—and to the child if she or he is old enough to understand. The optometrist should explain what is expected, frequency and duration of treatments, possible inconveniences or problems, cost, and the chances of success. It is important to stress that vision therapy is an active process and that instruments do not correct the condition; they only help the child learn to use his eyes better. The possibility of needing to occlude and wear special therapy lenses in addition to home and office therapy should also be emphasized.

Vision therapy procedures for symptomatic school-aged children with heterophoria or accommodative problems can be programmed on a home therapy basis with office visits weekly to assess progress. Most patients with heterophoria or accommodative problems achieve complete relief of symptoms and improve clinical measures of the quality of binocular vision to within normal limits in 4 to 8 weeks (21). Strabismic or amblyopic children and some children with perceptual dysfunction that interferes with learning may require a longer course of treatment. For example, vision therapy for strabismic or amblyopic children often requires approximately 3 to 4 months for total reeducation of binocular vision.

When active therapy is required for the preschool child, care must be taken to structure therapy programs so that they are not too complicated. The principal emphasis of therapy for a child this young is to keep the program simple and game like, so that it can be done long enough each day to be effective. For this reason it is frequently advisable to break therapy sessions down into several short sessions rather than one long one each day, so that the child's attention span is not taxed and high levels of interest and response are maintained. For maximum success, the child should perform active therapy techniques 20 to 30 minutes per day. In many instances this can mean that the techniques must be practiced 20 or more times for 1 minute each.

Occlusion

Amblyopia is virtually always associated with strabismus, anisometropia, or both. Recent research indicates that amblyopia associated with anisometropia has different characteristics than amblyopia associated with strabismus (12a). As a result, the occlusion and treatment modes need to be somewhat different for the two types of amblyopia. These important distinctions are considered below.

Occlusion Schedule for Anisometropic Amblyopia

Because the anisometropic amblyopic patient usually already has partial binocular vision, full-time occlusion is contraindicated, as it may precipitate constant strabismus. As a result, only *part-time,* and not full-time, direct occlusion should be used to treat anisometropic amblyopia in patients with peripheral binocularity and no strabismus. When combined with binocular enhancement therapy, 2 to 4 hours of occlusion of the good eye per day is sufficient. Passive therapy of occlusion should be combined with active vision therapy procedures designed to enhance monocular acuity under binocular as well as monocular conditions and to reduce or eliminate suppression.

Occlusion Schedule for Strabismic Amblyopia

Patients with strabismic amblyopia can also be treated at any age, but patients with amblyopia and constant strabismus often have eccentric fixation, and diagnosis in depth using special equipment may be necessary to determine which course of eccentric fixation treatment and what occlusion schedule will be most successful (17). In general, the schedules listed below will be appropriate for most patients.

One of the most dramatic differences in treatment of preschool children and adults or older children is the prescription of occlusion schedules. Occlusion sustained too long on one eye of a preschool child can be detrimental instead of helpful if it causes occlusion amblyopia. So careful consideration must be given to the guidelines described below when prescribing occlusion for the preschool child. Table 12.2 describes these differences.

Table 12.2   DIRECT OCCLUSION FOR AMBLYOPIA

	Anisometropic	Strabismic
Daily duration	2–4 hours/day	Constant
Number of days	Every	1 day per week for each year of age, on successive days
Duration of occlusion	6–8 weeks after last measured improvement	6–8 weeks after last measured improvement

Direct Occlusion

When the amblyopic patient has a constant strabismus, full-time direct occlusion (patching the good eye) is the initial treatment of choice (11). Direct occlusion for young patients with a constant strabismus should be constant and alternated on a schedule based on the age of the patient: the good eye is occluded 1 day per year of age, the other eye is patched for 1 day, and then the cycle is repeated. For a 1-year-old child this would mean alternating the patch each day. For older patients the "good" eye is patched more of the time, so that the amblyopic eye is used more. Occlusion on such a schedule generally affords rapid improvement in acuity and lessens the chances of occlusion amblyopia occurring in the covered, sound eye (1, 12). In addition to constant occlusion, vision therapy procedures should be given to enhance monocular acuity by reducing eccentric fixation magnitude, eliminating crowding effects, and increasing fixation accuracy and steadiness.

Inverse Occlusion (Occluding the Amblyopic Eye)

Direct occlusion is almost always the initial treatment of choice, especially for preschool children. Occasionally even 6 to 8 weeks of direct occlusion is not successful for older patients with large-magnitude steady

eccentric fixation. When direct occlusion fails, a 6- to 8-week trial of inverse occlusion should be considered, which may cause the eccentric fixation to become more unsteady so that improvement can be realized when direct occlusion is reinstituted. When inverse occlusion is used, daily therapy emphasizing foveal fixation should be continued. This includes therapy that enhances monocular acuity (by using smaller tasks) and eliminates crowding effects (by moving tasks closer together). After the trial of inverse occlusion is completed, resuming direct occlusion often allows continued improvement of the amblyopic eye's acuity.

Occlusion for Strabismic or Anisometropic Amblyopia

Daily Period   To be effective occlusion must be maintained for a certain minimum amount of time. Two hours per day is generally considered to be the minimum for effective occlusion. Anything less is not effective for most patients, but sometimes preschool patients need to start out with shorter periods and to gradually increase the time to an effective amount per day, especially if compliance is initially a problem.

Duration of Occlusion Therapy   Occlusion must be used correctly for a reasonable amount of time before the possibility of further improvement in acuity is ruled out. Six to 8 weeks is the minimum period for initial occlusion. If it is done properly for this length of time and no improvement in acuity is observed it is unlikely that continued occlusion will bring any improvement. It is always wise to carefully question the parent about compliance. More often occlusion fails because of noncompliance than because an eye is incapable of improvement.

During amblyopia therapy visual acuity often does not improve steadily; frequently there are plateaus—the patient remains at the same acuity level for a substantial period. For this reason, 6 to 8 weeks is also used as a guideline for continuing occlusion beyond the last measured improvement. When occlusion continues with no measured acuity improvement for this length of time there is generally no advantage in continuing the occlusion.

Amblyopia

Amblyopia therapy can be considered to consist of passive therapy (various forms of occlusion) and active therapy. Active amblyopia therapy can be conveniently divided into two sections, monocular and binocular.

Monocular

Monocular therapy, which is used to increase monocular responses of the amblyopic eye in strabismic *and* anisometropic amblyopia, involves patching combined with monocular stimulation. Monocular acuity therapy is almost always beneficial as part of the management of anisometropic amblyopia, whereas both monocular acuity and fixation enhancement therapy usually are needed to manage strabismic amblyopia.

Hand-Eye Coordination Most types of unsteady or eccentric fixation can be treated in conjunction with acuity improvement programs. Large (>2 to 4 PD) steady eccentric fixation should ordinarily be treated as an oculomotor problem. To treat preschool patients with these conditions, stimulate foveal fixation using rapid pointing techniques (Fig. 12.1). Have the child point rapidly at small toys; gradually include motion of the target.

Pointing, tracing, and coloring exercise hand-eye coordination to improve fixation and visual acuity of the amblyopic eye. As acuity improves, tasks are made more difficult. These tasks are appropriate for treating anisometropic and strabismic amblyopia. Preschool children especially like to spear Cheerios floating in milk with a straw. This is an excellent procedure because it combines specific fixation improvement therapy with a high-interest task.

Foveal Tagging and Alignment When the child is over 3 years old the success of foveal stimulation can be increased using alignment

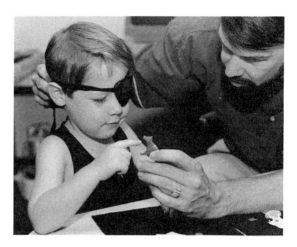

Figure 12.1 Having the child point rapidly to details on small targets can help enhance central fixation and reduce the time of occlusion therapy.

of entoptic imagery. These techniques, which are generally best for older patients with strabismic amblyopia, include alignment of foveal entoptic images (Maxwell Spot or Haidinger's Brush) (3) and afterimage transfer (2, 22). Both can be used successfully with older preschool children (over approximately 3½ years) but are difficult for very young children. When the patient cannot see the entoptic image or the afterimage does not transfer well, pleoptic procedures may be used, or direct occlusion can be relied on, even though progress may be slower.

Binocular

Binocular therapy is used for patients with anisometropic amblyopia and for strabismic patients as binocularity develops. Many amblyopic patients begin to develop rudimentary binocular skills when the acuity level in the amblyopic eye approaches 20/70. As soon as binocularity can be established in the amblyopic patient, more rapid acuity improvement can be obtained with therapy programs that include stimulation of the fovea under binocular conditions (i.e., antisuppression therapy) in order to improve simultaneous perception and resolution.

Binocular therapy involves antisuppression emphasis, with the amblyopic eye being given tasks increasingly closer to threshold. Active therapy can include playing with small figures while wearing red-green anaglyphs or tracing small figures with red-green anaglyphs; these techniques often work well because they hold the child's attention during the therapy. Alternatively, active therapy can include stereograms, either in office or at home. Attention is drawn to simultaneous perception of suppression clues and clearness of the clues seen by the amblyopic eye. Vectograms and Tranyglyphs can be used in similar fashion.

For preschool children it is best to design any type of active therapy to be as enjoyable as possible so that a maximum time can be spent doing therapy each day with the full cooperation of the child. The initial starting level for all active therapy for preschool children is determined empirically by evaluating whether the child can perform the task and then the distance at which the child can achieve satisfactory responses. As performance improves the tasks are made more difficult by increasing the distance, using lenses or prisms, or reducing the contrast. As the child reaches age 4, video games containing detailed visual tasks (binocularly using anaglyphs) can be introduced. These procedures work well because they keep the child's attention during the therapy task.

Suppression

Active treatment involves binocular (dichoptic) stimulation of peripheral retinal areas followed by gradual encroachment upon central areas. For young children, real anaglyphic targets are used in tasks, such as a flannel board (Fig. 12.2). When the child is over age 2 and office therapy is contemplated, therapy is structured using dissimilar targets (first-degree, e.g., soldier and house in troposcope) initially, then similar targets (second-degree, e.g., snowman in troposcope). Other valuable techniques that can be used for preschool children include Polaroid or anaglyphic TV trainers, anaglyphic coloring activities, and

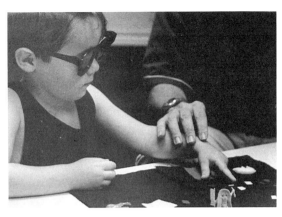

Figure 12.2   The flannel board consists of a black felt background combined with red, green, and yellow figures. The child wears red-green glasses and separates the figures or otherwise locates the appropriate figure.

Tranyglyphs or Vectograms. Finally, therapy for physiologic and pathologic diplopia is added.

For occasional strabismics with normal correspondence, the ideal goal is awareness of pathologic diplopia when an eye deviates. Stimulus parameters that can be modified to reduce or eliminate suppression include brightness, contrast, color, size, on period, position, and movement of targets. Therapy should be reinforced with kinesthetic, auditory, and visual feedback.

Anomalous Correspondence

The approach taken when managing a patient with anomalous correspondence depends on the type of strabismus. In general, the treatment consists primarily of vergence therapy for occasional strabismus, constant exotropia, and constant angle esotropia less than 15 to 20 PD. The concept is that, when the oculomotor deviation is overcome by fusional vergence, retinal correspondence changes synchronously so that correspondence becomes normal when the eyes are fixating bifoveally.

Based on the argument presented above, vision therapy for anomalous correspondence is best directed at expanding fusional vergence until the patient can align the eyes bifoveally. The vergence technique for treating anomalous correspondence is the most successful form of therapy and works well for all children with exotropia and when an esotropic angle is less than 20 PD. The therapy goal for these strabismics is to increase the fusional vergence response so that binocular alignment can be maintained for longer periods.

Thus, appropriate therapy for the very young child with exotropia, intermittent exotropia, and some with small angle esotropias involves fusional vergence initiation therapy. For the exotropic patient a small, detailed target is held within 4 inches of the child, whose eyes are closed. After the eyes are opened a fusional vergence movement is encouraged to fuse and clear the target. The motive is to improve fusional convergence responses and increase the time that alignment can be maintained (Fig. 12.3). Many different interesting targets can be constructed that will maintain the child's interest. This excellent technique, which works well even for very young exotropic children, occasionally also works when the esotropic child has an angle that allows the target to be held within the centration point.

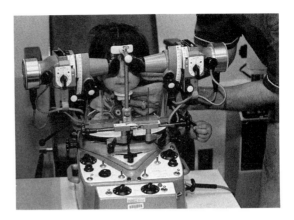

Figure 12.4 The time-consuming process of eliminating anomalous correspondence at the angle of deviation often needs to be done in office with special equipment such as a synoptophore. Most children must be at least 2½ years of age before such therapy is instituted.

For patients who have large-angle constant esotropias, therapy involves simultaneous stimulation of the foveas until the correspondence between them is restored. This treatment is difficult, time consuming, and has a poor prognosis; generally it must be done in office (Fig. 12.4). As a result, it is difficult to initiate before the child is 2½ years of age.

Sensorimotor Functions

For all preschool children with strabismus or amblyopia sensory fusion should be maximally developed before motor fusion therapy begins. In either condition, however, facility is more important than magnitude. It is essential to achieve facility and accuracy of accommodation during the treatment of heterophoria and strabismus. Transference to free-space situations must be recognized by designing programs that utilize the most natural environment possible that is consistent with controlling the therapy so that improved binocularity is achieved. This can be done by using red-green or Polaroid procedures (i.e., Tranyglyphs or Vectograms) as soon as possible in the therapy program.

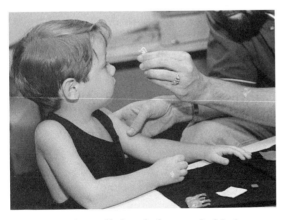

Figure 12.3 A small detailed target held close to the child makes an excellent convergence task. Many targets may be needed to hold the child's interest. At least 20 1-minute sessions should be arranged every day.

Generally, when treating constantly strabismic patients, the optometrist attempts to improve grades of fusion in order of difficulty by using first-degree (dissimilar) targets first and then going to second-degree (fusible) targets. Treatment of any patient, however, should begin with training at the distance or with a technique the child can perform moderately easily; gradually the tasks are made more difficult as the condition improves. After suppression is minimized, stereothresholds are trained to increase the ability of previously strabismic patients to recognize stereopsis and to "use" it to maintain fusion.

Sensorimotor therapy generally involves programs designed to modify either vergence or accommodation or to utilize procedures that affect their interactions.

Vergence

An interesting observation is that accommodation and vergence are often significantly improved as a result of successful treatment of amblyopia and suppression. When additional motor improvement is necessary, therapy should be directed at making abrupt changes, emphasizing speed and quality of response over maximum amplitudes of response. It is important to transfer the motor abilities acquired through therapy to ordinary visual situations; such a transfer is facilitated by programs that utilize the most natural environment possible consistent with controlling the therapy so that maximal binocularity improvement occurs.

Many vision therapy procedures can be used to improve vergence ability in very young children; as different as they may seem initially, their similarities are striking. The primary emphasis is the improvement of magnitude and especially facility of vergence responses. To this end many of the following techniques can be used.

Office Therapy

Troposcope The optometrist should use targets that are interesting to the child and that incorporate either second-degree or stereoscopic contours. The advantage of the tro-

poscope is that the parameters of the target can be varied (by brightness, flashing) to eliminate suppression and anomalous responses. Vergence can be varied by moving the tubes (Fig. 12.5). Other instruments, discussed below, can be used for therapy in the office or at home.

Office and Home Therapy

Stereoscope It is best to use targets that are interesting to the child and that have second-degree fusion or stereoscopic contours. With a stereoscope the parameters of the target can be varied in the same manner as with the troposcope to eliminate suppression and anomalous responses. Vergence can be varied using split stereograms or by tromboning the targets (Fig. 12.6).

Cheiroscope Again, targets that are interesting to the child and contain second-degree fusion or stereopsis tasks should be used. To eliminate suppression the child is asked to point at details of the target and the parameters of the target are varied by altering the brightness, making it flash, or changing the size. Vergence can be varied by moving the

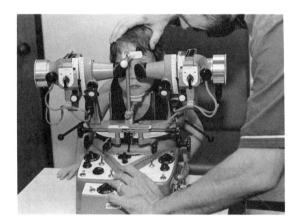

Figure 12.5 A Troposcope can be used to vary the stimulus parameters in ways that are difficult to effect with any other combination of instruments. A disadvantage of using this instrument, aside from the expense, is that transfer of training to normal situations is sometimes difficult.

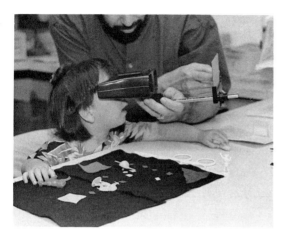

Figure 12.6 Many of the targets available for the stereoscope can be adapted to make it an excellent device for home or office therapy for preschool children.

targets as the child maintains a fusion response. The child draws or traces the targets to increase fusion and eliminate suppression.

Stripe Therapy When an infant has large-angle esotropia it is often difficult to design a therapy program that gives eye alignment for a significant period. Even though large amounts of prism often can be used, it is difficult to be certain that normal fusion develops. To attempt to establish fusion a "sheet" of vertical half-inch black and white stripes can be draped across the infant's crib for 15 to 20 minutes per day while the child is awake. The principle is to arrange conditions so that a minimum vergence movement is sufficient to stimulate corresponding retinal points.

Convergence and Accommodative Facility Procedures

Appropriate therapy for preschool children with exodeviations or accommodative dysfunction includes the following:

Convergence Initiation Therapy A small, detailed target is introduced about 4 inches in front of the child. The child closes the eyes then opens them and converges to fuse and clear the target.

The goal is to improve convergence responses and time that alignment can be held (Fig. 12.7). This is an excellent technique, even for very young children, as many different interesting targets can be used that will hold the child's interest.

Push-Ups After vergence ability has developed, targets are moved between 40 cm and the near point of convergence, keeping the target *single* or watching to be sure the eyes stay aligned as long as possible. This technique is appropriate for children with eso- or exotropia.

Vergence Change Therapy The child alternates fixation between two targets, one a detailed target at the near point of accommodation and the other a more distant target. It is not always easy for a young child to recognize diplopia, and a parent's observation and encouragement to make the correct vergence eye movement may be all that can be done (Fig. 12.8).

Anaglyphs and Prism Tranyglyphs or a flannel board (Fig. 12.9) are inexpensive versa-

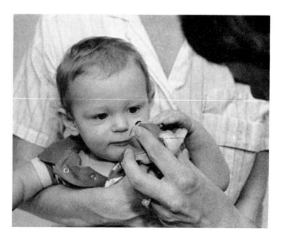

Figure 12.7 Convergence initiation therapy can even be done by infants, as this photo of a child who is not quite a year old demonstrates.

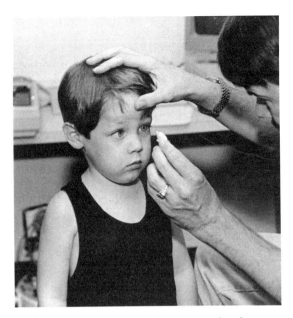

Figure 12.8 Convergence therapy can be done quite successfully by having the child look from a distance to a near point.

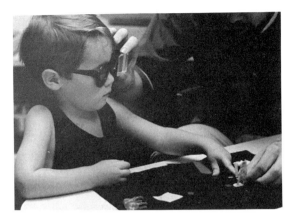

Figure 12.9 A flannel board can be modified with loose prisms or lenses to increase the difficulty of the task.

tile devices for therapy for motor and sensory fusion that work well with preschool children. Step vergence changes can be achieved using a prism bar (19) or loose prisms.

Vergence Therapy for Older Children or Adults

The following vergence therapy techniques work very well but they are generally too difficult for all but the most advanced preschool children. They generally work best for children in late grade school or older.

Single- or Double-Aperture Rule Trainer   This is an excellent instrument for home and office once the patient is over 9 or 10 years of age. Younger children often have difficulty learning the required responses. Fusion, step, and jump vergences can be done depending on the techniques used. An Ortho-fusor or Vectograms can be used in a similar manner to develop convergence ability and accommodative facility.

Free-Fusion Stereo Rings (Opaque or Transparent Eccentric Circle Cards) or Red-Green Circles   The patient must be instructed in what he or she should see during this procedure because it is possible to do the techniques backward (i.e., diverge instead of converge and get negative therapy). When the outside circles are fused, the inside circles fall on noncorresponding points but within Panum's fusional areas and are seen in depth. The direction of the disparity determines whether a bucket or a stool shape is apparent. *Sliding vergences* can be done by slowly separating the cards laterally. *Jump vergences* can be done in the same manner as the free fusion circles. This requires more vergence control than the sliding method.

Lenses can be used to alter the accommodative demand initially so that the task is easier to perform; as responses improve the lenses can be changed to increase the difficulty.

Accommodative Therapy

Accommodative therapy can be done for young children by combining red-green or Polaroid techniques (i.e., Tranyglyphs or Vectograms) with lenses as early as possible in the therapy program. Plus and minus lenses or prisms are used to modify the accommodative or vergence demand (Fig. 12.10). When patients with exodeviations perform the procedures binocularly the fusional vergence demand is decreased with minus lenses and increased with plus lenses.

Perceptual and Learning Dysfunctions

Before a perceptual or learning dysfunction is managed, the child's binocularity and accommodation should be made maximally efficient with lenses, prisms, or vision therapy. When the visual system is maximally efficient, therapy for perceptual and learning problems can be most effective. Subsequent therapy can be designed to modify visual memory, sequencing, and gross and fine motor development.

Management

Management of the most common preschool conditions requiring vision therapy is considered in the ensuing sections. These conditions (amblyopia and strabismus, exotropia and esotropia) have specific characteristics that require individual management sequences, as outlined in Chapter 11. Following is a discussion of the management, including occlusion and vision therapy, which is different for preschool children and for older children and adults.

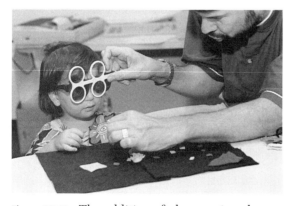

Figure 12.10 The addition of plus or minus lenses to therapy is a simple method of increasing the therapy demand while keeping the tasks interesting to the child.

MANAGEMENT OF AMBLYOPIA

Amblyopia is defined as a condition in which reduced visual acuity is not correctable by refractive means and is not attributable to obvious structural or pathologic anomalies. It is assumed in this definition that the best lens correction is worn for the viewing distance. In general, a reduction of acuity to less than 20/30 or 20/40 in one eye or a two-line difference between the eyes is considered to represent amblyopia.

For young children or older ones with anisometropic amblyopia, the general sequence of therapy is similar to that outlined for esophoric patients in Chapter 11: optimal plus lens correction, added lenses, prism, occlusion, and vision therapy as needed. Certain areas require additional attention.

Refraction and Lenses Because the underlying basis for many amblyopias is anisometropia, the full correction is needed to achieve maximal improvement; partial correction often leads to frustration because it allows only minimal or very slow improvement. Correction can be effected with spectacles or contact lenses, although contact lenses become more desirable when there is significant anisometropia. As visual acuity improves in the amblyopic eye, there may be need for refinements in what was originally thought to be the optimal and full correction. Thus, refraction should be re-evaluated on a regular basis (at least every 2 to 3 weeks) and lens changes that improve acuity and minimize aniseikonia should be made when needed.

Occlusion Proper occlusion is one of the most important factors in successful treatment. Provided the guidelines discussed previously in this chapter and outlined in Table 12.2 are followed, direct occlusion (good eye covered) can be used safely with young patients. Part-time occlusion is used for anisometropic amblyopia with binocularity, and constant occlusion is used for constant strabismus patients.

Vision Therapy   Monocular acuity therapy is almost always beneficial as part of the management of anisometropic amblyopia, whereas both monocular acuity and fixation enhancement therapy are usually needed to manage strabismic amblyopia. Vision therapy consists of techniques that are sequenced to improve eye movement ability and focusing accuracy and eliminate suppression. Vision therapy procedures can be conveniently grouped into two categories—those that monitor and attempt to improve monocular fixation (foveal tagging and alignment procedures) and those that require eye-hand coordination and reduce suppression when done under binocular conditions (pointing, tracing, coloring). As amblyopia therapy progresses, binocular vision therapy is used to establish peripheral and central sensory fusion without suppression. For preschool children it is best to structure therapy so that it is as enjoyable as possible, so that maximum time can be spent doing therapy each day with full cooperation of the child.

Case Report 1

A 4-years-and-1-month-old girl was referred by an ophthalmologist for treatment of amblyopia. He had seen her and prescribed lenses. Her eye health was within normal limits. Her refractive state and lens prescription were the same:

R + 6.75 − 0.75 × 180   20/80 line, 20/70
                                                       + 1 single letter

L + 1.75 − 1.00 × 178   20/20

There was unsteady central fixation of the right eye (Projectoscope, Haidinger brushes). There was no strabismus, but a 2-Δ esophoria was present at 6 m and 40 cm. There was suppression of the right eye on fixation disparity tests and no measurable stereopsis (Titmus at 40 cm).

Part-time direct occlusion (good eye covered) was started 3 hours per day 7 days per week. Home therapy consisted of specific amblyopia procedures of pointing and Haidinger Brush alignment. In 4 weeks, acuity improved to 20/25 in the right eye. A recheck of retinoscopy and refraction of the right eye indicated no correction change was required. Diagnostic testing now indicated intermittent suppression. Binocular therapy

was instituted for 30 minutes per day using a TV trainer, flannel board with anaglyphic toys (Fig. 12.11), and stereoscope.

Four more weeks of therapy (with 2-week progress reports) developed 20/25+2 acuity in the right eye, but the patient was noticing occasional vertical diplopia. Fixation disparity tests indicated a need for 2Δ down (left eye) to reduce fixation disparity to zero and eliminate diplopia. This was prescribed, and home vision therapy continued for 6 months with monthly progress reports. The final lens correction and visual acuities were as follows:

R + 7.00 − 1.00 × 179   1Δ up   20/20 + 2

L + 2.50 − 1.00 × 180   1Δ down   20/20 + 4

There was no fixation disparity, suppression, or evidence of aniseikonia when the patient wore her correction. Stereopsis was 60 arc seconds at 6 m (AO Vectographic) and 40 arc seconds at 40 cm (Titmus).

Special Features of Therapy for Young Patients   Therapy for this anisometropic amblyopic patient was very similar to what would be used for an older person. The primary difference was the simplicity of the active therapy techniques that were used, which made them appropriate for the very young patient. Essentially this means that pointing, drawing, and tracing can still be done as long

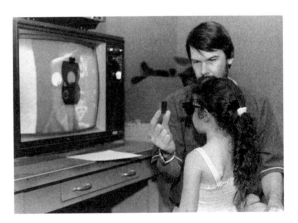

Figure 12.11   The TV trainer is an excellent device for home therapy. As the child's binocularity improves the TV trainer can also be used with lenses or prisms to increase the demand of therapy.

as the material is not too detailed. Other therapy that could have been used for this child includes spearing Cheerios, playing catch, and coloring small letters in the paper or coloring books, either with the amblyopic eye alone (monocular therapy) or with both eyes using anaglyphs (binocular/anti-suppression therapy).

MANAGEMENT OF EXODEVIATIONS

Exotropia is a divergent deviation of the eyes from the position of bifoveal fixation requiring use of fusional convergence to maintain single binocular vision (18). Overall management sequences for exodeviations are listed in Chapter 11; they include optimum minus correction, added minus lenses, amblyopia therapy if needed, vertical prism correction, and vision therapy. Most (80 percent) exotropias are intermittent, and when the parent is responsible and can carry out instructions accurately, home therapy is often very effective after optimal lens and prism management. If the parent cannot or will not perform therapy at home it will be necessary to manage the exotropic preschool patient with office-based therapy or to refer the patient for surgical care.

Constant Exotropia

When there is constant strabismus, constant occlusion is used to eliminate the need for the patient to suppress and to avoid reinforcing anomalous strabismic adaptations. Because there is already a constant strabismus sensory and motor fusion is either abnormal or absent. Vision therapy emphasizes developing convergence responses and eliminating suppression. Small near targets are shown to the patient, who is encouraged to converge the eyes to fuse (see details of therapy below). This therapy may need to be carried out 30 minutes per day for up to 8 weeks before adequate convergence responses are achieved. When convergence responses are possible, the patient will be able to maintain binocular alignment briefly and can then be treated as one who has intermittent exotropia.

Intermittent Exotropia and Exophoria

Because peripheral sensory and motor fusion are present at times, the emphasis in therapy is placed on quality and facility of motor responses; sensory fusion is enhanced with targets that contain central fusion cues. Full-time occlusion is contraindicated for patients with intermittent strabismus because of the risk of precipitating constant strabismus; however, occlusion may be considered late in the day (when the patient with an intermittent exotropia usually has difficulty maintaining fusion), usually on the distance vision portion of one lens.

During vision therapy procedures clearness and singleness are stressed so that the accommodative response is appropriate to the stimulus and not an overcompensation to induce convergence. The total convergence response includes tonic, accommodative, fusional, and proximal vergence. Deficiencies of accommodative convergence may compound the ocular problem. Specific accommodative therapy may be as important to the successful treatment of patients with exodeviations as convergence therapy. The ultimate goal of therapy is to increase the patient's convergence responses so that they can maintain binocular alignment for longer periods.

Case Report 2

The patient was a 3-years-and-4-months-old boy. At the time of the examination his parents complained that he had an intermittent outward eye turn that had been present for at least 18 months. They felt that the right eye was the one that usually turned, although they also noticed the left one turn at times. The eye turn was more frequent late in the day and when the boy was tired.

Examination revealed normal ocular tissues and fundus. Refractive state and binocular status were:

R Plano   20/15 − 1
L + 0.25 D − 0.25 DC × 180   20/15 − 1

Eye alignment:

   15Δ intermittent right exotropia at 6 m
   20Δ intermittent right exotropia at 40 cm
     Exotropia present about 45 percent of the
     time
   Comitant in all fields of gaze
   Near point of convergence, 11 cm

Stereopsis (when fusing):
   Could not accurately assess at 6 m
   50 arc seconds (Titmus) at 40 cm

Retinal correspondence:
   Troposcope: ARC when eyes deviate
   Afterimages: ARC when eyes deviate

Accommodative status:
   Amplitude: R 15 D
           L 15 D
   Facility: could not accurately assess
   Lag of accommodation: 0.62 D (by MEM reti-
   noscopy)

Primary lens or prism management was not appropriate for this patient, although an overminus distance correction, possibly with a near addition, could be a future consideration. Home therapy for intermittent concomitant exotropia with anomalous correspondence was prescribed. Therapy consisted of convergence initiation, push-up convergence, and antisuppression procedures (as described above, Fig. 12.12) to be done 5 minutes at a time, 6 to 10 times per day.

Two-week progress reports over the next month indicated that exotropia occurred less frequently. The vision therapy program was made more difficult by adding base-out prism jumps with concurrent antisuppression procedures (TV trainer, red-green anaglyphs with 10Δ base-out prism).

Special Features of Therapy for Young Patients
Therapy for this patient was similar to that for an older patient. The anomalous correspondence was treated indirectly (through covariation by convergence therapy). Treating exotropia with ARC and NRC is similar in that convergence responses need to be developed in both instances; the major difference is that pathologic diplopia awareness is not trained in the ARC patient, rather accuracy of convergence and stereopsis are stressed.

The major difference in exotropia therapy for the preschool patient described above is that simple active therapy techniques were used because a complicated technique would have been too dif-

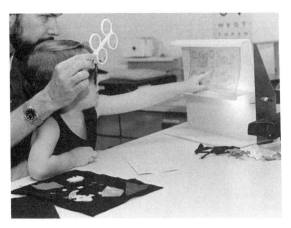

Figure 12.12 Convergence and antisuppression therapy can easily be done by young children at home or in the office using Tranyglyph slides. Lenses and prisms are useful additions that increase the demand.

ficult for the child to follow. Therapy was provided in a number of brief sessions every day to ensure that enough time was spent in therapy to be successful while keeping the child's interest and concentration keen during the sessions.

Convergence therapy can easily be done, even with very young children, using simple inexpensive equipment. If this child had been older (i.e., aged 10 instead of 2 years) a single-aperture rule trainer or eccentric circles could have been used. Unfortunately, these procedures are too difficult for the preschool child. Tranyglyphs or Vectograms combined with a base-out prism bar to vary the vergence demand could also be used if the child's interest can be maintained with them.

MANAGEMENT OF ESODEVIATIONS

Esotropia is a manifest convergent deviation of the eyes from the orthoposition (18). Management sequence considerations for esodeviations are presented in Chapter 11. These include full plus corrections, base-out prism (often a significant amount), and near plus corrections in addition to vision therapy for amblyopia, suppression, anomalous correspondence, and fusion. In general, the more rapidly binocularity can be established the better; often this requires large amounts of base-out prism initially. After binocularity is established, vision therapy can be used to increase fusion responses and reduce the need for prism or near additions.

As with treatment of exotropia, when the parent of an esotropic preschool child is responsible and can carry out instructions accurately, home therapy is often very effective. If the parent cannot or will not perform such therapy it will be necessary to manage the patient in the office. When the angle of deviation is large (>20Δ) surgery is often a necessary part of the total therapy program.

Esotropia

Constant Esotropia

When there is constant strabismus and anomalous sensory or motor fusion (or none), constant occlusion is used to eliminate the need for the patient to suppress and to prevent reinforcing any anomalous strabismic adaptations. In the vision therapy, emphasis is placed on eliminating amblyopia and subsequently developing divergence responses by eliminating suppression. When binocularity begins to develop the patient will be able to sustain binocular alignment briefly and can be treated as are those who have intermittent esotropia.

Intermittent Esotropia and Esophoria

Peripheral sensory and motor fusion are already present at some distance or time of day. As a result, vision therapy emphasizes quality and facility of motor responses and aims at enhancing existing sensory fusion using targets containing central and peripheral stereopsis and fusion cues. During vision therapy procedures clearness and singleness are stressed so that the accommodative response that is trained is appropriate to the stimulus and not an undercompensation to induce divergence.

Constant occlusion is generally contraindicated for patients with intermittent strabismus because of the risk of precipitating constant strabismus. Fortunately, when amblyopia exists in patients with intermittent esotropia or esophoria it is usually relatively slight, and occasional occlusion (2 to 4 hours per day) can be used successfully for treatment.

To enhance fusion, stereoscopic targets with differing disparities are often placed initially at the angle of deviation in instruments such as a Troposcope, stereoscope, or cheiroscope. As soon as possible, tasks are changed to free space instrumentation. Ability to perform stereoscopic fusion tasks in free space often relaxes excessive accommodation and convergence responses, stimulates divergence, and allows easier transfer of learned visual skills to everyday vision tasks. When the parent is responsible and can carry out instructions accurately, home therapy can be done, but it is often simpler and more successful to manage the esotropic preschool patient with office-based therapy.

Case Report 3

A 2-years-and-9-month-old boy was seen for his first examination. According to the parents he had a constant esotropia for the last 6 months and seemed to be slightly clumsy. His development was normal. He had measles 6 months earlier, and the parents thought that the eye turn began about then. There was no other family or personal history of illness.

External and internal ocular conditions within normal limits. Retinoscopy showed:

$$R + 2.75 - 0.50 \times 90 \quad 10/10- (20/20-)$$

(Sheridan Gardiner; matching)

$$L + 4.75 - 0.25 \times 85 \quad 10/30 \ (20/60)$$

Cycloplegic evaluation revealed only 0.50 D more sphere for each eye.

Eye alignment (with retinoscopic correction):

25Δ constant left esotropia at 6 m

35Δ constant left esotropia at 40 cm

Comitant by Hirschberg and cover test in all fields of gaze

Calculated AC/A equals 10Δ/1 D or with lag 12.5Δ/1 D

Stereopsis:

None measurable at 6 m or 40 cm

Retinal correspondence:
Troposcope, apparently NRC
Afterimages, no valid response

Fixation: approximately 1 to 2Δ unsteady nasal EF (eccentric fixation) left eye
Accommodative status:
Amplitude: R 16 D
L ~14 D
Facility: Could not accurately assess
Lag of accommodation: 0.50 (MEM retinoscopy)

Spectacle lens correction was prescribed in the full cycloplegic correction with 24 base-out (12-Δ Fresnel base-out before each eye) and a +1.75 add. With the lens and prism correction there was peripheral fusion and the patient could see through both portions of a TV trainer at 2 to 3 feet.

Constant occlusion was prescribed: right eye 2 days, left eye 1 day, and so forth. In addition to the passive amblyopia therapy of constant occlusion, active monocular amblyopia therapy (pointing, Cheerios) was done 5 minutes twice a day. The active therapy involved pointing at small features on toys, spearing Cheerios floating in milk, and a TV trainer. The TV trainer was used to watch *Sesame Street* (one half hour per day). At all other times there was constant occlusion following the schedule above.

At the 2-week progress evaluation the parents reported that the child seemed to be able to see better with the left eye over the past week. His left eye acuity was 10/15 with unsteady central fixation. He was able to move further from the TV (out to 5 feet) before suppressing. Without the patch the eyes were always aligned with the prism spectacle correction. The same home therapy was continued, but because the eyes were aligned with the lenses, the patch was worn only afternoons. Within 3 more weeks visual acuity had improved to 10/10 (20/20).

Patching was further decreased and therapy was instituted to improve divergence ability. This consisted of a TV trainer with base-in prism jumps and playing with anaglyphic toys while different amounts of base-in prism were interposed by the parent. Progress visits continued over the next 3 months as the constant esotropia and amblyopia disappeared and the child maintained fusion at all times.

Final pertinent clinical tests were as follows:

Lens correction:

R + 3.75 − 0.75 × 95   3Δ BO   10/10 (20/20)
L + 5.00 − 0.50 × 80   3Δ BO   10/10 (20/20)
Add: +2.00

Phoria (through correction):

10 PD esophoria at 6 m   Near point of convergence, nose

17 PD esophoria at 40 cm

Stereopsis:

Not easily assessable at 6 m
40 (Titmus) at 40 cm

Worth Dot four dots at distance and near; cover test, no movement
Accommodative responses within normal limits through the near addition.

Three- and 6-month follow-up examinations revealed virtually the same findings. There has been no recurrence of the esotropia, although a moderate esophoria remains.

Special Features of Therapy for Young Patients
Therapy for this patient was similar to that for an older patient. The major difference is that simple active therapy techniques were used because a complicated technique would have been too difficult for this young child to follow. This child was fortunate to have a parent who could work with him at home. Many times this is not possible. Then office-based therapy using the Troposcope, stereoscope, or vectographic or anaglyphic techniques would probably have been necessary.

As evidenced by the therapy program for this patient, divergence therapy can be done as long as the instruments are not too complicated. If this child had been older (i.e., aged 9 years instead of 2) a double-aperture rule trainer or eccentric circles could have been used. Unfortunately, these techniques are too difficult for preschool children. Tranyglyphs or Vectograms combined with a base-out prism bar to vary the vergence demand could also be used if the child's interest can be sustained with them.

SUMMARY

Many preschool children need some form of management for problems related to binocularity. This management can include lenses, prisms, and added lens power in addition to occlusion and vision therapy. Fewer than one third of optometrists emphasize binocular vision therapy care for preschool children in their practice. A philosophy of the order of considerations for management for patients with binocular anomalies was covered in Chapter 11. This chapter expanded that philosophy to include the design of vision therapy programs for the preschool child.

APPENDIX

The therapy procedures selected for discussion in this chapter are those that work well and require a minimum of inexpensive equipment.

Stereoscopes, cheiroscopes, and free-fusion stereo rings are available from Keystone View, 2212 East 12th Street, Davenport, IA 58803.

Stereoscopes, cheiroscopes, rule trainers, and Vectograms are available from Bernell Corporation, 422 East Monroe Street, South Bend, IN 46601.

Ortho-fusor is available from Bausch and Lomb, Rochester, NY 14602.

REFERENCES

1. Burian HM: Occlusion amblyopia and the development of eccentric fixation in occluded eyes. Am J Ophthalmol 62:853, 1966.

2. Caloroso E: After-image transfer: A therapeutic procedure for amblyopia. Am J Optom Arch Am Acad Optom 49:65, 1972.

3. Duke-Elder S (ed): System of Ophthalmology, Ocular Motility and Strabismus, vol VI. St Louis, CV Mosby, 173, 1973.

4. Eskridge JB: A binocular refraction procedure. Am J Optom Arch Am Acad Optom 50:490, 1973.

5. Eskridge JB: The complete cover test. J Am Optom Assoc 44:602, 1973.

6. Flom MC: Treatment of binocular anomalies of vision. In Hirsch MJ, Wick RE (eds): Vision of Children. Philadelphia, Chilton, 225, 1963.

7. Griffin JR: Binocular Anomalies: Procedures for Vision Therapy, 2nd ed. Chicago, Professional Press, 1989.

8. Grosvenor T: Clinical use of fixation disparity. Optom Weekly Dec 18:31, 1975.

9. Hoffman L, Cohen A, Feuer G: Effectiveness of non-strabismic optometric vision training in a private practice. Am J Optom Arch Am Acad Optom 50:813, 1973.

9a. Hoffman MG, Rouse MW: Vision therapy revisited: A restatement. J Am Optom Assoc 58:7, 1987.

10. Hugonnier R, Clayette-Hugonnier S: Strabismus, Heterophoria, Ocular Motor Paralysis. St Louis, CV Mosby, 247, 1969.

11. Hurtt J, Rasicovicci A, Windsor C: Orthoptics and Ocular Motility. St Louis, CV Mosby, 105, 1972.

12. Levi D: Occlusion amblyopia. Am J Optom Physiol Opt 53:16, 1976.

12a. Levi DM: The Glenn A Fry award lecture: The "spatial grain" of the amblyopic visual system. Am J Optom Physiol Opt 65:767, 1988.

13. Ogle KN: Researches in Binocular Vision. New York, Hafner Publishing, 64, 1965.

14. Parks M: Ocular Motility and Strabismus. Hagerstown MD, Harper & Row, 158, 1975.

15. Patient management: How do you measure up? Opt J Rev Optom 8:20, 1976.

16. Schwerscharf W, Springer K: A Set of Materials for Patients in Orthoptics. Doctor of Optometry Thesis. Berkeley, University of California, 1976.

17. Shapiro M: Amblyopia. Philadelphia, Chilton, 139, 1971.

18. Cline D, Hofstetter HW, Griffin JR: Dictionary of Visual Science. Radnor, PA, Chilton, 1989.

19. Sloan P: The cover test in clinical practice. Am J Optom Arch Am Acad Optom 31:3, 1954.

20. Smith W: Clinical Orthoptic Procedure. St Louis, CV Mosby, 9, 1954.

21. Vodnoy B: The basis for the practice of orthoptics. Optom Weekly June 22: 15, 1972.

22. Wick B: Anomalous after-image transfer—An analysis and suggested method of elimination. Am J Optom Physiol Opt 51:862, 1974.

23. Wick B: A fresnel prism bar for home visual therapy. Am J Optom Physiol Opt 51:576, 1974.

24. Wick B: Lateral deviations. In Amos J (ed): Clinical Management. Butterworths, 1987.

Chapter 13

Pediatric Pharmacology

Siret D. Jaanus

Use of pharmaceutical agents for diagnosis and therapy of ocular conditions in the pediatric age group often requires special considerations. Children, particularly those with certain systemic conditions, may be more sensitive to certain classes of drugs. When prescribing topical ocular drugs—but particularly in systemic therapy—it may be necessary to adjust the dose or to select a more appropriate drug. Despite FDA requirement for proof of safety and efficacy, relatively few drugs are currently available in children's dose forms and few have been tested and proven safe for children (1, 2). Whereas proper utilization of drugs for diagnostic purposes depends on the knowledge and experience of the clinician and usually takes place in an office or hospital setting, adherence to therapeutic drug regimens outside such confinements requires an informed parent, a cooperative child, and a prescriber willing to instruct in proper drug use.

This chapter is a brief overview of some general pharmacologic principles as they relate to child patients. Individual classes of drugs commonly used in the pediatric population will be considered in terms of their pharmacology, clinical uses, side effects, and contraindications. This discussion is not meant to be exhaustive and the interested reader is referred to additional references listed at the end of this chapter.

ASPECTS OF DRUG DOSAGE FOR CHILDREN

The cardinal rule of effective drug use in the pediatric population is that the dosage of drug selected should provide the desired clinical effect for the patient without producing undesirable secondary effects. Selecting the correct dose for a child is complicated, because even within a given age group, children vary widely in body size and developmental stage. The child is not a miniature adult, and pediatric dosages may not be extrapolated from available adult dosage recommendations since other developmental changes must be taken into account (1, 3). Thus, the recommended dosage for any drug should be carefully evaluated for the individual child. For neonates, in particular, dosages estimated from adult concentrations may not be reliable. Beyond the neonatal period, dosages for children can be calculated on the basis of age, body weight, or body surface area.

Age and Weight

Several methods have been devised for estimating dosage by the body weight or age of a child.

Young's rule is based on the age of the child. It would seem to be the least useful, as children of a given age vary widely in body weight and development (3).

Young's rule:

$$\text{Child dose} = \frac{\text{Age}}{\text{Age} + 12} \times \text{Adult dose}$$

Young children have a greater proportion of fluid in their bodies than adults. For such children a dosage based on weight, as in *Clark's rule*, could be too low, as a given amount of drug will be dissolved in a relatively greater amount of fluid (3).

Clark's Rule:

$$\text{Pediatric dose} = \frac{\begin{array}{c}\text{Child's weight}\\ \text{(kg or lb)}\end{array}}{\text{(70 kg or 150 lb)}} \times \text{Adult dose}$$

Augsberger's rule, also based on weight, is used for children under 2 years of age (4).

Augsberger's Rule: Pediatric dose

$$= \frac{(\text{Child's weight in kg} \times 1.5) + 10}{100}$$

A 5-kg child would receive 17.5 percent of the adult dose:

$$\frac{(5 \times 1.5) + 10}{100} = .175.$$

Body Surface Area

Body surface area is considered a more accurate parameter of a child's developmental state than compared weight or age (3). Tables are available (Table 13.1) that give the relationship between body weight and surface

Table 13.1   CALCULATION OF PEDIATRIC DOSAGES BASED ON WEIGHT OR BODY SURFACE AREA

Weight kg (lb)	Surface Area (m^2)	Approximate % of Adult Weight	Approximate % of Adult Surface Area
6 (13)	0.30	10	15
10 (22)	0.45	15	25
20 (44)	0.80	30	45
30 (66)	1.05	45	60
40 (88)	1.30	55	75
50 (110)	1.50	70	85
60 (132)	1.65	85	95
70 (154)	1.75	100	100

(Adapted from Apt L: Pediatric aspects of drug therapy. In Leopold IH (ed): Symposium on Ocular Therapy. St Louis, CV Mosby, 92, 1968.)

area as percentages of adult weight and surface area. For premature and newborn infants during the first few weeks of life, one-half or less of the calculated child's dose is recommended (3, 5).

Body Fluid Composition

The volume and distribution of total body fluid are different in infants and adults (3, 6). Approximately 75 to 80 percent of total body weight of the newborn infants is fluid. The ratio decreases with age to about 50 to 60 percent in adults (3). The plasma and interstitial fluid compartments, which constitute the extracellular fluid, represent about 50 percent of the total fluid in infants but only 20 percent in adults (3). As most drugs are distributed throughout the extracellular fluid in order to reach their site of action, the size of this compartment is an important determinant of the final drug concentration (6). The concentration of a drug administered as a fixed proportion of the adult dose would be lower in a child. Fluid turnover is also more rapid, about three times as fast in infants. One half of an infant's extracellular fluid volume is replaced every 24 hours but only one seventh of an adult's. Blood volume is also relatively greater in infants (approximately 80 ml/kg body weight as compared to 65 mg/kg for adults). These factors explain in part why a relatively larger dose of drug in proportion to body weight may be required by a child to achieve the same blood levels or therapeutic effect as an adult patient (3, 6).

Kidney Function

Renal function does not approach adult levels until a child is about 2 years old, so drugs that are eliminated by glomerular filtration or renal tubular secretion may exhibit reduced renal clearance and their half-life may be greatly prolonged (6). Drugs that are eliminated from the body by renal excretion, such as the antibiotics penicillin, tetracycline, and kanamycin, must be administered in low concentrations and at greater intervals between doses (3).

Liver Function

Quantitatively, the most important organ for drug metabolism is the liver. Enzymes involved in drug inactivation and detoxification may be age dependent. For example, production of enzymes involved in glucuronide conjugation and acetylation reactions, two major mechanisms for drug transformation in the liver, is slow or even absent in newborns, so drugs such as barbiturates, corticosteroids, salicylates, and certain antibiotics that are metabolized in the liver by these pathways may be eliminated more slowly by young children. Because of potentially serious complications, these drugs should be used with extreme caution and avoided if possible (3, 6).

Miscellaneous Factors

For reasons that are not well understood, children may respond differently than adults to certain drugs (the phenomenon of altered sensitivity) (3). In general, children appear to be more sensitive to central nervous system—stimulatory effects of such drugs as antihistamines, phenothiazines, salicylates, and atropine. In contrast, the sedative effect of the barbiturates is greater than one would expect from dosages calculated on the basis of adults' and children's weights.

In addition, plasma protein binding of drugs may be a factor. Data for drugs studied thus far indicate that certain drugs bind less avidly in infant's blood (6). This includes salicylates, some penicillins, phenobarbital, and phenytoin (Dilantin). In contrast, diazepam (Valium) and digoxin (Lanoxin) bind similarly to infants' and adults' serum (2).

ROUTES OF ADMINISTRATION AND FORMULATIONS

Proper drug utilization can be considered both a science and an art. When the patient is a child, the responsibility for ensuring compliance rests with the person who administers the medication. The best results are generally obtained, particularly with home use of drugs, when this effort is one of cooperation between the prescriber and the person responsible for administration of the medication. That person should be instructed in the technique of administration, the reason for prescribing the drug, and the possible adverse effects on the child. Although the ideal scenario is one of cooperation, the prescriber has the ultimate responsibility of seeing that the orders given are carried out properly. Written instructions worded in layman's language are recommended, especially for drugs that have the potential to cause serious adverse effects (1).

Oral Route

For systemic administration, giving drugs by mouth is preferred (1). Effective use of medication by this route is easier if the child is cooperative. The aim should be to gain the child's confidence with techniques appropriate to his or her level of development. Professionals and parents should demonstrate empathy and compliment the child on positive aspects of behavior. They should explain, if possible, the benefits of the medication. Juice or water should be offered after the medication, but not candy or other special treats that suggest that a reward is in order. For children under 5 years of age, crushing pills and dissolving them in syrup or nonessential foods like applesauce can make them more palatable. Although most children will take solid medications, children under the age of 5 years may find it easier to swallow liquid formulations if they are available. Plastic measuring devices can be useful for measuring proper doses of liquids for oral use (1). Oral medications should not be forced because of the hazard of aspiration.

Topical Route

When possible, topical administration for ocular drugs is preferred. In most instances, distinctions between adult and pediatric dosages are not made in the clinic setting and the child receives the adult dose. In recent years,

experimental evidence has shown that tear production and nasolacrimal drainage rapidly wash drug from the eye into the systemic circulation (7, 8). Up to 80 percent of the instilled dose is available systemically through drainage within the first 2 minutes (8). As neonates and children have a tear turnover rate similar to that of adults, the rates of drainage of drug following topical instillation are similar (9). If the systemic level of a drug is the same for children and adults, the relative smaller size of the child can lead to serious systemic toxicity with certain topical ocular drugs (see below).

Patton and associates (10) developed a pharmacokinetic model to determine topical children's doses as a fraction of the adult dose. Factors that contribute to drug distribution and movement in the ocular structures, such as ocular surface area, tear and instilled solution drainage rates, and ratio of aqueous volumes in children and adults were taken into account in their considerations. Their calculations indicate that, from birth to 2 years of age, one half the adult dose should produce equivalent drug concentrations in children. Between 2 and 3 years, about two thirds the adult dose is recommended and after 3 years, the adult amounts should be used. Although the validity of the investigators' assumptions may be questioned, the calculations can serve as guidelines for practitioners in situations where risk for ophthalmic drug toxicity may be high.

Solutions

Solutions remain the most common formulation for topical ocular drugs. A medication that has been refrigerated should be warmed to room temperature prior to instillation. Care must be taken with the eye dropper tip to prevent injury should the child suddenly move. Attention can be drawn away from the dropper by asking the child to place the hands on the forehead. This reinforces upward gaze. The palpebral aperture can be widened for drop instillation by instructing the child to open the mouth (11). If resistance is expected, the help of assistants may be necessary to restrain the child. Following instillation the hands may be held to prevent rubbing the eyes. Small children may be swaddled in a blanket (1).

Another recommended method is for the parent to sit on the floor, with the child's head placed firmly between the parent's thighs (12). The child's arms are placed beneath the thighs, and the parent's legs are crossed over the child's lower trunk and legs. The parent's hands thus remain free to administer the drops.

Diversion can be useful—asking the child to recite the alphabet or count, playing music, or setting a toy in motion. Talking to the child can also help, as can explaining, whenever possible, the benefits of the medication. At least 3 to 5 minutes should pass between instillation of each drop, to avoid a washout effect of the first drop. Eye drops administered to a crying child are washed out quickly.

The individual clinician usually feels comfortable with a particular technique of drop instillation; however, in recent years the "pouch" method has been advocated. The lower lid is pulled away from the globe at right angles to the plane of the head and the drop is placed in the inferior conjunctival sac (13). The lids are then gently closed, and the patient is asked to gaze downward to bring the cornea into maximum contact with the instilled drop. This method allows the topical solution to remain in contact with the cornea for a somewhat longer period. Regardless of the method of instillation, closure of the lid following instillation markedly increases drug contact time with ocular tissues.

Systemic absorption via nasolacrimal drainage can be minimized by applying pressure with the fingertips to the lower puncta and canaliculi for at least 1 minute. Punctal occlusion is particularly useful in a cooperative child but is difficult to employ in all children. Punctal occlusion is highly recommended when drugs with potential systemic effects, such as atropine or beta-blockers such as timolol, are instilled (8, 13).

Another possibly useful method of drop instillation is to instruct the child to close both eyes. Children usually cooperate and so, do not see the clinician approach with the dropper. By gently pulling the lower lid of the closed eye to a small opening, the drop can be instilled (11). A modification of the eye closed technique is to have the child either lying supine or sitting in a chair with the head tilted as far back as possible. A drop is placed on the inner canthus of both closed eyes, then the child is asked to open the eyes. After the solution has entered the eye, the patient is asked to close the eyes again and excess solution is gently wiped with a tissue. It is important to keep the dropper tip at least 2 cm from the eye to avoid contact contamination.

Ointments

Solutions are most commonly used, but ointments can be a very effective formulation for ocular drug for children. Ointments afford longer ocular contact time and drain more slowly through the nasolacrimal system (14). Moreover, the frequent complaint of blurred vision following instillation of ointment in adults is usually less of a problem with children.

Ointment is properly instilled in the inferior conjunctival sac as a $\frac{1}{4}$- to $\frac{1}{2}$-inch ribbon. Then the eyes are closed and the lids are gently massaged to distribute the drug evenly across the ocular surface. An alternative method is to place the ointment on a cotton-tipped applicator and apply it to the upper lid margin and lashes and the medial and lateral canthi. This method allows the ointment to act as a drug reservoir and also minimizes blurring of vision and possible drug irritation (11).

Because ointments are characterized by prolonged ocular contact, contact dermatitis of the lids can occur (14). Ophthalmic ointments currently in use do not significantly inhibit corneal wound healing and may be used for superficial corneal abrasions. They are generally contraindicated for jagged or flaplike corneal lacerations, for eyes with impending corneal perforations, and for open conjunctival lacerations (11).

Sprays

Application of ophthalmic drugs as topical sprays has proven useful, particularly for mydriatic or cycloplegic examination of children (11, 15). Sharp and associates (15) compared various mydriatic and cycloplegic agents applied to the eyes as conventional drops and as spray on open and closed eyes. No significant difference in pupil diameter was observed with drops and spray, whether eyes were open or closed. (See Fig. 13.1.)

Bartlett (11) has used a combination of mydriatic and cycloplegic agents for routine cycloplegia in children. The spray is administered from a sterilized refillable perfume atomizer. The unit is held 5 to 10 cm from the eye and the solution is sprayed on the eyelids along the lash margins. There is usually an initial startle reaction if the spray is administered to an open eye (15). An advantage of the spray method is that the drug can also be de-

livered to a closed eye. The child does not see the drug approaching the face and usually resists less rigorously. Following application of the spray the patient is instructed to blink several times. Excess solution surrounding the eyes can then be wiped off. A mild stinging sensation is an indication that the drug reached the precorneal tear film. If the patient's lids are tightly closed, the spray may be prevented from reaching the eyelid margin and a second application may be necessary. The clinician should provide an opening while gently applying upward traction to the upper lid (15).

In general, sprays have been found to be a rapid, effective, and often less irritating method for drug delivery to children. Less drug solution flows down the face, and the child does not have to assume an awkward position to receive the spray. No adverse effects except for transient mild stinging when the medication reaches the precorneal tear film have been reported (11, 15).

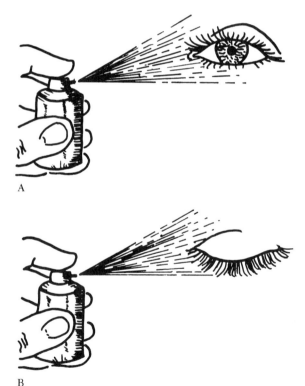

A

B

Figure 13.1 Opthalmic spray delivered to an open (A) or closed (B) eye. Adapted from: Sharp J, Wallace T, Hanna C: J Pediatr Ophthalmol 12:119, 1975.

DRUGS FOR DIAGNOSTIC EXAMINATION

Dilation of the pupil and paralysis of accommodation are often necessary procedures for examination of ocular health and refractive status. Careful choice of available drugs, dosage, and proper administration often determines the success of the clinical procedure that is to follow.

Mydriatics

Drugs that dilate the pupil are classified pharmacologically according to their mechanism of action. Adrenergic agonists produce their effect by stimulating the iris dilator muscle; they have little or no effect on ciliary muscles. Thus, near-point visual acuity usually is not affected. Cholinergic antagonists inhibit the actions of both the constrictor fibers of the iris and the longitudinal muscle of the ciliary body. Dilation of the pupil and inhibition of accommodation (cycloplegia) result from use of these agents (16, 17).

Adrenergic Agents

Currently available drugs include phenylephrine and hydroxyamphetamine (Table 13.2).

Phenylephrine Following topical application on the eye, phenylephrine dilates the pupil and constricts blood vessels by alpha-adrenergic receptor stimulation. In normal eyes, effects on intraocular pressure and accommodation are minimal. Phenylephrine is available commercially in two concentrations, 2.5 and 10 percent; use of the 10 percent concentration, particularly for children and elderly patients, has been discouraged by several investigators owing to the risk of a sudden rise in systemic blood pressure (17–19). Although the 2.5-percent concentration seems safe for most children (17), preterm infants have demonstrated increased blood pressure and heart rate in response to mydriatic solutions containing 2.5 percent phenylephrine (20–22). Administering smaller-volume drops of phenylephrine solution has been suggested as a means of reducing possible systemic side effects. Lynch and associates (23) found that 8-μl drops (versus 30-μl commercial size drops) produced nearly equivalent dilation in neonates and infants. Systemic absorption with 30-μl drops was more than twice the level achieved with the 8-μl drop. Reducing drop size may be one way to improve the risk-benefit ratio of topical ocular medications for children and adults.

Hydroxyamphetamine Hydroxyamphetamine, an indirectly acting adrenergic agent, has been less extensively studied as a mydriatic agent in children and neonates. No serious adverse effects have been reported with use of the commercially available 1-percent concentration (24).

Cycloplegics and Mydriatics

Drugs that paralyze accommodation have been used for over 100 years to better estimate the refractive status of the eye. A clinically useful cycloplegic drug should possess several characteristics, including a rapid onset and sufficient duration of action to allow for completion of refractive procedures (24, 25). Agents in current use include atropine, homatropine, cyclopentolate, and tropicamide (Table 13.3). These agents exert their pharmacologic effects by inhibiting the action of acetylcholinesterase on ocular smooth muscle, including the ciliary body and the constrictor fibers of the iris sphincter (26).

Atropine

Atropine, a naturally occurring alkaloid, is the most potent of the currently available cycloplegic agents (25, 27). It has remained the drug of choice for cycloplegic retinoscopy of infants and children up to age 4 to 6 years who are suspected to have accommodative esotropia (25, 27). It is used not only to produce cycloplegia for refraction but also as adjunctive therapy for uveitis, and for amblyopia and strabismus with latent nystagmus. Available as a solution and an ointment, the latter is usually preferred for refraction because the ointment decreases systemic absorption, which tends to minimize systemic side effects (25). Atropine traditionally has

Table 13.2 MYDRIATIC AGENTS

Drug	Concentration (%)	Onset of Maximum Effect (minutes)	Duration of Effect (hours)	Comments
Phenylephrine	2.5	40–60	2–6	10% is contraindicated
Hydroxyamphetamine	1:0	40–60	2–4	

Table 13.3 CYCLOPLEGIC MYDRIATIC AGENTS

Drug	Concentration (%)	Maximum Cycloplegic Effect (minutes)	Recovery (days)	Comments
Tropicamide	0.5, 1.0	25–35	0.25	Residual accommodation may average >2.00 D
Cyclopentolate	0.5, 1.0, 2.0	25–60	0.5–1.0	Black patients may need multiple instillations
Homatropine	2.0, 5.0	60–90	1–3	Residual accommodation can vary
Atropine	0.25, 0.5	60–180[a]	7–12[a]	Ointment is preferred. Two drops of 0.5% solution is near toxic dose for infants.

[a] Duration of action based on one instillation of 1% solution.

been instilled two or three times for 3 days at home prior to the office visit for refraction. No drug is instilled on the day of refraction, as the cycloplegia is complete and the ointment tends to interfere with the refractive procedure. The 3-day regimen is considered excessive, as maximum cycloplegia is usually achieved by the second day, but it does allow for missed instillation and therefore is preferred by some practitioners. It is strongly recommended that written instruction on the dosing procedure and possible adverse effects be given to the parent or guardian when atropine is used at home (26). In addition to its prolonged mydriatic and cycloplegic effects, the concern with ocular use of atropine is the development of adverse ocular or systemic side effects. Allergic reactions (usually of the lids), photophobia, thirst, fever, urinary retention, restlessness, and tachycardia are all possible toxic reactions to topical ocular atropine (25–27, 28). Deaths have been attributed to its use (27, 28). Caution is indicated, particularly in infants, and in children with Down's syndrome, spastic paralysis, brain damage, and lightly pigmented skin (29).

Because adverse effects are a possibility with atropine, its use should be reserved for infants with suspected accommodative eso-

tropia or when complete cycloplegia is considered essential. Treatment of atropine overdose can include both physostigmine (Eserine) and diazepam (Valium). Physostigmine, given by slow intravenous infusion, counteracts atropine's systemic effects. It may also be administered intramuscularly or subcutaneously. Diazepam can be effective in treating any accompanying agitation, hallucinations, and convulsions (24, 26).

Homatropine

Homatropine is about one-tenth as potent as atropine (26). Instillation of a 1-percent solution produces maximum mydriasis and cycloplegia in about 40 to 60 minutes. Full recovery takes about 3 days. Much less cycloplegia is produced than with atropine, particularly in darkly pigmented irides (24). It is not a reliable drug for ophthalmoscopy or cycloplegic refraction in children and its use has been discouraged (24).

Cyclopentolate

Cyclopentolate has become the drug of choice for cycloplegic refraction for older children with strabismus and for nonsquinters of any age (25, 26). Available as a 0.5-, 1-, or 2-percent solution, one drop of a 1-percent solution produces maximal mydriasis and cycloplegia within 40 to 60 minutes. The cycloplegia may last 8 to 24 hours. Recovery from mydriasis occurs within 24 hours (24–26). Residual accommodation is usually below the desired 2.00 D for refractions in Caucasians (26). Black patients may require additional instillations for reliable suppression of accommodation. The 2-percent solution should be avoided when possible because of increased risk of systemic side effects (26, 31, 32). For neonates, the lowest possible dose, 0.5-percent or less, has been recommended.

Ocular side effects with cyclopentolate are rare. The most common complaint is transient stinging and lacrimation following instillation (25, 26). Systemic side effects with cyclopentolate usually involve the central nervous system. Incoherent speech, disorientation, restlessness, visual hallucinations and drowsiness have been reported. Symptoms are more common with the 2-percent concentration, but multiple instillations of the 1-percent solution have also caused these effects (31, 32). Treatment of cyclopentolate toxicity is the same as for atropine.

Tropicamide

Tropicamide, available commercially in 0.5- and 1-percent solutions, is a useful mydriatic agent with relatively fast onset (25 to 30 minutes) and short duration of action (6 to 8 hours) (33). The cycloplegic effect of tropicamide is transient. Merrill and associates (34) reported an average residual accommodation of 1.60 D at 30 minutes and 2.40 D at 40 minutes with the 1-percent solution. Unless additional drops are instilled, the clinically effective cycloplegia can be maintained only up to 35 minutes following instillation of a single drop. The magnitude of the effects is also related to age, and usually 2.5 D or more of accommodation remains in patients under 40 years of age (33, 34). Thus, tropicamide alone does not produce the desired degree of cycloplegia in children. Clinically it is also important to remember that tropicamide has a greater mydriatic than cycloplegic effect, and mydriasis does not necessarily indicate adequate cycloplegia for refraction (25, 26),

as it does when cyclopentolate or another cholinergic blocking agent is used.

Side effects with tropicamide are rare. Transient stinging upon instillation has been reported by some patients. Wahl (35) has reported a reaction in a 10-year-old Caucasian boy who became unconscious following instillation of 1 drop of 0.5-percent tropicamide into each eye. He regained consciousness within a few minutes but remained drowsy and weak for the next hour; subsequently his vital signs became normal and he recovered fully.

It is generally agreed that toxic reactions to topical mydriatic-cycloplegic agents are more likely to occur in neonates and in children with a history of central nervous system disease; however, for all children, multiple instillations of drugs into the cul-de-sac should be made with much care and caution. An adequate amount of time should be allowed for the drug to take effect, especially with repeated instillation of eye drops (16).

Combination Preparations

For maximum mydriatic and cycloplegic effect and for ease of administration, "single-encounter" formulations have been advocated, particularly for children. Caputo and Lingua (36) recommended a combination of cyclopentolate, 1.3 percent, tropicamide, 0.16 percent, and phenylephrine, 1.6 percent. After instillation of 3 drops the patient is ready for ophthalmoscopy within 45 to 60 minutes. In 80 percent of eyes the cycloplegic effect is similar to that achieved with atropine. Another formulation, consisting of 3.75 ml of 2-percent cyclopentolate, 7.5 ml of 1-percent tropicamide, and 3.75 ml of 10-percent phenylephrine (final concentrations: cyclopentolate, 0.5 percent; tropicamide, 0.5 percent; phenylephrine, 2.5 percent) has also proven useful in children. One drop was found to produce adequate dilation, with the pupil size remaining 7.0 mm on exposure to light (37). Bartlett (personal communication) has found this combination useful as a spray formulation for cycloplegic refraction of young children. For dilated fundus examination a similar combination formulation can be prepared by substituting 3.75 ml of saline for the cyclopentolate.

DRUGS FOR PEDIATRIC GLAUCOMAS

Management of infantile and pediatric glaucoma is a complex process and usually involves surgical intervention, but adjunctive drug therapy may be possible. Anatomic and physiologic characteristics peculiar to children and compliance with the prescribed drug regimen present special challenges to the clinician. Regardless of the differences, drug treatment of children with open-angle glaucoma is similar to that for adults, but the lowest possible concentrations of drug are used. Most drugs currently in use have not been rigorously tested or approved for pediatric use.

Miotics

When a miotic is indicated, pilocarpine (Table 13.4) is usually the drug of choice (38). A direct-acting cholinergic agonist, pilocarpine lowers intraocular pressure by enhancing aqueous outflow. It is administered topically to the eye one to four times a day as a 1- to 4-percent solution.

Side effects are relatively rare with pilocarpine (38). Allergic reactions involving the conjunctiva and lids and miotic cysts following long-term use have been observed. The cysts are not of clinical significance and can be eliminated by adding 2.5-percent phenylephrine to the drug regimen. Pilocarpine is not recommended for patients with obstructive airway disease (24).

Carbachol (see Table 13.4), also a direct-acting cholinergic agonist, is used when resistance or sensitivity to pilocarpine develops. It does not penetrate the intact cornea as well as pilocarpine, and side effects are more common, especially in patients with bronchial asthma (24).

Among the available miotics (see Table 13.4), the anticholinesterases are used less frequently. Echothiophate iodide (Phospholine) is used when tolerance develops to a direct-acting cholinergic agonist. Echothiophate is available in 0.6-, 0.125- and 0.25-percent concentrations and must be refrigerated to maintain its effectiveness during use (24).

Table 13.4   DRUGS FOR PEDIATRIC GLAUCOMA

Drug	Available Preparations	Dosing Schedule; Comments
Pilocarpine	0.25, 0.5, 1, 2, 4%	Every 4–6 hr. Higher concentrations not recommended.
Carbachol	0.75, 1.5, 3%	Every 4–8 hr.
Echothiophate	0.03, 0.06, 0.125, 0.25%	Every 12–24 hr. One dose per day may be satisfactory.
Epinephrine HCl	0.25, 0.5, 1, 2%	Every 12–24 hr.
Epinephrine bitartrate	1%	Use as infrequently as possible.
Epinephrine borate	0.5, 1, 2%	
Dipivefrin	0.1%	Every 12–24 hr
Timolol	0.25, 0.5%	Every 12–24 hr
Levobunolol	0.5%	Every 12–24 hr
Betaxolol	0.5%	Every 12 hr
Acetazolamide	125-mg, 250-mg tablets	Children 2 yr and up: 10–30 mg/kg Children under 1 yr: 5–10 mg/kg (4)
Methazolamide (Neptazane)	25-mg, 50-mg tablets	2–8 mg/kg/24 hr. (4)

The lowest possible concentration of echothiophate is recommended; both ocular and systemic side effects can occur (38). Iris cysts, which may occur due to proliferation of the pigmented epithelium, almost always disappear when the drug is discontinued. Addition of a few drops of phenylephrine, 2.5 percent, to the echothiophate solution seems to prevent the formation of the cysts (24).

Systemic side effects of anticholinesterase use manifest themselves as excessive stimulation of the cholinergic nervous system. Diarrhea, excessive salivation, general weakness, and a slow heart rate are among the more common symptoms. Systemic absorption of these agents can also significantly lower serum levels of cholinesterase and pseudocholinesterase. This is of particular concern if surgery with general anesthesia is contemplated and succinylcholine is used for muscle relaxation. Low levels of cholinesterase enzyme prevent hydrolysis of succinylcholine to succinate and acetate, and prolonged apnea can result (38). It is recommended that echothiophate therapy be discontinued for at least 2 weeks prior to general anesthesia (4).

Adrenergic Agents

Among the adrenergic agonists both epinephrine and its prodrug dipivefrin (Propine) have been used (see Table 13.4). Epinephrine hydrochloride is available in 0.5-, 1-, and 2-percent concentrations. As the solution is acid (pH 3.5), a burning sensation occurs upon instillation of the drops, which may interfere with compliance. Epinephrine in the bitartrate formulation, with a pH of 7, may be less irritating (38). The usual dosage is once or twice a day. Since the safety of topical epinephrine in children has not been fully tested, dipivefrin is generally the drug of choice when use of an adrenergic agent is desired.

Epinephrine can cause side effects that are severe enough to cause discontinuation of use. Allergic conjunctivitis and blepharitis are common. Melanin-like deposits can occur in the conjunctiva and cornea following pro-

longed use of the drug. Cystoid macular edema is a possibility in aphakic patients (24).

Propine in 0.1-percent solution is generally considered to produce fewer side effects and better patient compliance (39).

The beta-adrenergic blocking agent timolol has been used to treat childhood glaucoma. Available as 0.25- and 0.5-percent solution, it blocks both beta$_1$ and beta$_2$ receptors and is thought to lower intraocular pressure by inhibiting production of aqueous (24). At present the FDA has not ruled on the safety or efficacy of timolol (or the other available ophthalmic beta-blockers) in children.

Several studies (40–43) have reported acceptable control of intraocular pressure in pediatric glaucoma and compliance with timolol therapy. All studies, however, caution of potential complications, and nasolacrimal obstruction following instillation is strongly recommended.

Side effects associated with ophthalmic timolol can involve the cardiovascular, respiratory, and central nervous systems (24). Bradycardia, asthmatic attacks, hyperactivity, dizziness, and light-headedness have occurred, particularly with the 0.5-percent concentration (40–43). It is recommended that children with a history of cardiac or respiratory disease be excluded from timolol therapy; if timolol must be used in such patients, extreme caution is imperative. It is also important that the instiller of the drug be made aware of potential side effects so that therapy can be discontinued immediately (44).

Carbonic Anhydrase Inhibitors

Carbonic anhydrase inhibitors are recommended for short-term use only in young patients (see Table 13.4) (38). Acetazolamide (Diamox) can suppress aqueous humor production by 40 to 50 percent when it is administered orally in maximum doses to adults (45). For children, doses are reduced according to the age of the child and the individual experience of the practitioner. Very young infants may be given up to 15 mg/kg body weight per day in divided doses. Older children may be given 5 to 10 mg/kg body weight every 4 to 6 hours. The dose may be doubled for older children (38). In addition to acetazolamide, methazolamide (Neptazane) is also available for oral administration (45).

Side effects associated with carbonic anhydrase administration can include gastrointestinal distress, skin eruptions, and genitourinary problems. Blood tests must be performed regularly during therapy to monitor for abnormalities in electrolyte balance, particularly acidosis, and for possible, though rare, occurrences of agranulocytosis and thrombocytopenia (45).

ANTIBIOTIC AGENTS

Ideally, selection of antimicrobial therapy should be based on knowledge of the causative pathogens and of the effect of drugs on the pathogens and the patient. In practice, treatment is usually started empirically. If the desired therapeutic response is not obtained, culture and sensitivity testing becomes necessary. Standard testing in vitro can give additional guidance about the organisms and their antibiotic sensitivity.

Antimicrobial therapy is generally more effective for bacterial than for viral or fungal infections. Because of their external location, superficial ocular infections such as blepharitis and conjunctivitis respond to topical application of antibiotics. More severe types of infections, such as chlamydial inclusion conjunctivitis and particularly those involving the posterior segment such as endophthalmitis, require systemic, periocular, or parenteral administration. High local concentration of drug can be obtained with frequent application of drops. Ointments are useful at bedtime but may also be used during the day, as often as necessary. An additional benefit of topical administration is that drugs that are too toxic for systemic use can be used with greater safety and therapeutic success in ophthalmic drop and ointment formulations. Moreover, owing to their chemical properties certain drugs do not penetrate well into intraocular tissue when they are administered by mouth. If the eye is inflamed, a higher con-

centration of drug may be obtained, because the blood-aqueous barrier is reduced in the presence of inflammation (46–49).

Choice of antimicrobial agent, route of administration, and dosage requires special consideration for children. In general, it is recommended that children up to the age of 12 years receive a fraction of the average adult systemic dosage. Certain drugs, such as tetracyclines, chloramphenicol, and the long-acting sulfonamides, are generally contraindicated in infants and young children (46, 48).

Tables 13.5 and 13.6 list antimicrobial agents currently in use for ocular infections. As use of antimicrobial agents for specific ocular infections are discussed in Chapter 14, only a brief overview of the pharmacologic properties of selected agents is presented.

Bacitracin and Gramicidin

Both antibiotics are effective against many gram-positive organisms, including *Staphylococcus aureus* and *S. epidermidis*. Bacitracin is also effective against some gram-negative species, including *Neisseria* species and *Haemophilus influenzae*. They are ideal for use in superficial eye infections because bacterial resistance seldom develops during therapy (50). Both of these agents are too toxic for systemic use.

Since bacitracin is unstable in solution, it is available as a single entity or fixed-combination product in ointment form only (see Table 13.6). Gramicidin is stable in solution and is used in place of bacitracin in some combination ophthalmic solutions (see Table 13.6) (51). Bacitracin is considered to be perhaps the most effective agent commercially available for the treatment of staphylococcal blepharoconjunctivitis (49).

Erythromycin

Similar to penicillin in its antibacterial activity, erythromycin is effective against gram-positive organisms and *Chlamydia* (49). It is available as an ophthalmic ointment (see Table 13.6) and is considered the least toxic of

Table 13.5 LIST OF SOME COMMERCIALLY AVAILABLE ANTIBIOTIC EYE-DROP FORMULATIONS

Drug	Available Preparations	Concentrations
Chloramphenicol	Chloramphenicol ophthalmic, Chlorofair, Chloroptic, Ophthochlor	5 mg/ml
Gentamicin	Gentamicin ophthalmic, Garamycin, Genoptic, Gentacidin, Gentafair, Gentak	3 mg/ml
Neomycin	A-K Spore, Neosporin	
	Neomycin	1.75 mg/ml
	Gramicidin	0.025 mg/ml
	Polymixin B sulfate	10,000 U/ml
	Statrol	
	Neomycin	3.5 mg/ml
	Polymixin B sulfate	16,250 U/ml
Sulfacetamide	Bleph 10 and Bleph 30	
	Sodium sulamyd	10% and 30%
	Sodium sulfacetamide	
Tetracycline	Achromycin ophthalmic	10 mg/ml
Tobramycin	Tobrex	3 mg/ml

Table 13.6 LIST OF SOME COMMERCIALLY AVAILABLE ANTIBIOTIC OPHTHALMIC OINTMENT FORMULATIONS

Drug	Available Preparations	Concentrations
Bacitracin	Bacitracin ophthalmic, AK-Poly-Bac, Polysporin	500 U/g
	Bacitracin zinc	500 U/g
	Polymixin B	10,000 U/g
Chloramphenicol	AK-Chlor, Chloromycetin, Chloroptic	10 mg/g
Erythromycin	Erythromycin, AK-Mycin, Ilotycin	5 mg/g
Gentamicin	Gentamicin ophthalmic, Garamycin, Gentak, Genoptic S.O.P.	3 mg/g
Neomycin	AK-Spore, Neosporin	
	Neomycin	3.5 mg/g
	Bacitracin	400 U/g
	Polymixin B	10,000 U/g
	Statrol	
	Neomycin	3.5 mg/g
	Polymixin B	10,000 U/g
Sulfacetamide	Sodium sulfacetamide, AK-Sulf, Bleph 10 S.O.P., Sodium sulamyd	10%
Tetracycline	Achromycin	10 mg/g
	Terramycin W/Polymixin B	
	Oxytetracycline	5 mg/g
	Polymixin B	10,000 U/g
Tobramycin	Tobrex	3 mg/g

the commercially available topical antibiotic preparations. Although it can be effective for staphylococcal infections, bacteria can develop a resistance to it. It is also used topically, as an alternative to silver nitrate, in prophylaxis of gonococcal ophthalmia neonatorum (52). Oral erythromycin may be used in combination with topical therapy to treat recalcitrant staphylococcal blepharitis, especially with recurrent chalazion not responsive to topical therapy (49).

Polymixin B

This antibiotic is primarily effective against gram-negative organism, including *Pseudomonas aeruginosa. Proteus* and *Neisseria* species are resistant. Polymixin B is rarely used systemically since it is very toxic to the kidneys and nervous system. It is frequently combined with antibiotics effective against gram-positive organisms, such as bacitracin and neomycin, for topical ocular use (51).

Aminoglycosides

The aminoglycosides in common ocular use include neomycin, gentamicin, and tobramycin (see Tables 13.5, 13.6). They exhibit a broad spectrum of activity against gram-negative bacteria, including *P. aeruginosa*, and some gram-positive organisms, such as *S. aureus* and *S. epidermidis*, are usually sensitive (49). Of all commercially available topical ophthalmic antibiotics, they are used most frequently (particularly gentamicin and tobramycin). They are seldom used systemically, as they are toxic to kidneys and nervous system (51).

Neomycin, available since 1949, is the oldest member of the group in ocular use. It is available as a combination ophthalmic product (see Table 13.6). Topical ocular use can result in punctate epithelial keratitis and hypersensitivity reactions involving the lids and skin (49, 53). Routine use of topical preparations containing neomycin generally is not recommended.

Topical ophthalmic gentamicin is commonly used to treat bacterial infections of the external eye and adnexa. For many years gentamicin has been the antibiotic of choice for initial treatment of bacterial corneal ulcers (54); however, some strains of *P. aeruginosa* exhibit resistance to gentamicin (55). Side effects of topical gentamicin can include minor irritation following instillation, pseudomembranous conjunctivitis, and delayed wound healing (54).

Tobramycin is comparable to gentamicin in its antibacterial activity, but it is more active against *P. aeruginosa*, including some gentamicin-resistant strains (55). It is available both in solution and ointment formulations for topical ocular use. Topical ocular use can cause tearing, photophobia, conjunctival hyperemia, and punctate epithelial erosions (55). Both gentamicin and tobramycin appear to be as efficacious in treating external ocular infection due to susceptible organisms in children as they are in adults (56).

Chloramphenicol

Chloramphenicol is active against gram-positive and gram-negative bacteria, including *Neisseria* species and *H. influenzae*. Because of its lipid solubility, it also penetrates ocular tissue well, following topical and systemic administration. Although topical ophthalmic use is effective against many bacterial infections of the external eye, toxic reactions can occur. Aplastic anemia, resulting in death, has been reported following topical ocular use in children (57). It is recommended that use of chloramphenicol be limited only to infections for which other antibiotics are ineffective (46, 51).

Tetracyclines

The tetracyclines have a broad spectrum of activity against gram-positive and gram-negative bacteria, including *Chlamydia, Actinomyces*, and *Mycobacteria* species (51). Available as an ophthalmic solution and ointment, the ointment formulation has been recommended as a possible alternative to silver nitrate or erythromycin for prophylaxis of gonococcal ophthalmia neonatorum (52). Its wide systemic use has resulted in bacterial resistance which also has limited its topical ophthalmic use. *P. aeruginosa* is rarely responsive to tetracyclines (52).

Tetracyclines can deposit in embryonic and growing bone tissue, temporarily depressing bone growth. They can also affect tooth development and cause discoloration of teeth (48). Phototoxicity can be a problem. Teratogenic effects have also been implicated with tetracycline administration. Due to these possible effects tetracyclines are contraindicated for pregnant and lactating women and for children under age 8 years (59).

Sulfonamides

Sulfacetamide is available for topical ophthalmic use both as a single entity (see Tables 13.5, 13.6) and in combination with corticosteroids. Its spectrum of activity can include gram-positive and gram-negative bacteria, including *Chlamydia* and *Nocardia* (51). Because resistance to sulfonamides appears to be a problem, other antibacterial agents are most commonly chosen for treatment of common external ocular infections. Use of these agents is primarily limited to treating ocular toxoplasmosis and chlamydial disease (49). With systemic administration, sulfonamides cross the placenta with ease and may sensitize the fetus. Immature renal function can also prolong the serum half-life of the drug (46).

The overall incidence of toxic reactions has been estimated at 5 to 10 percent. Common reactions include nausea, dizziness, headache, drug fever, and sensitization reactions manifesting as skin rashes (51).

Silver Nitrate

In 1881, Crede introduced the use of 1-percent topical silver nitrate solutions as prophylaxis against gonococcal ophthalmia neonatorum. This procedure has played a major role in the significant reduction of blindness due to neonatal gonococcal eye infections.

Silver nitrate exerts its antimicrobial effect by denaturing proteins in bacteria, but it can also affect human epithelial cells (60).

In addition to its possible toxic effect on human cornea and conjunctiva, prophylactic use of silver nitrate has other shortcomings. It does not provide certain protection against gonococcal neonatal conjunctivitis, nor does it prevent infection by *Chlamydia* species; for these reasons, the Centers for Disease Control (CDC) have issued guidelines suggesting alternative antibiotics. Both topical erythromycin, 0.5 percent, and tetracycline, 1 percent, have been recommended as alternatives to silver nitrate for prevention of gonococcal ophthalmia neonatorum. Erythromycin has the advantage of also being active against *Chlamydia* (61).

ANTIVIRAL AGENTS

Antiviral agents currently available for topical ocular use include idoxuridine, adenine arabinoside, and trifluridine. (Table 13.7). All three disrupt viral DNA synthesis by being phosphorylated by virus-specific kinases (51). They are used to treat herpes simplex infections of the eye, primarily herpes simplex virus (HSV). They have proven less effective with other DNA viruses that can affect the eye, including varicella zoster (VZV), Epstein-Barr (EBV), and cytomegalovirus (CMV) (62).

Idoxuridine

Because of its inability to penetrate the cornea, idoxuridine (IDU) use is limited to the treatment of superficial HSV epithelial keratitis. Treatment success rate has averaged about 75 percent (63). It does not eradicate the latent virus in the trigeminal ganglion, so the infection recurrence rate is high (64).

Because the drug can also affect DNA metabolism in normal cells, toxic effects involving the cornea, conjunctiva, and lids do occur. Superficial punctate keratopathy, follicular conjunctivitis, punctal occlusion, and lid margin effects have been reported with its

Table 13.7 COMMERCIALLY AVAILABLE OPHTHALMIC ANTIVIRAL AND ANTIFUNGAL AGENTS

Drug	Available Preparations	Concentrations	
	ANTIVIRAL		
Idoxuridine	Herplex, Stoxil	Solution	0.1%
	Stoxil	Ointment	0.5%
Vidarabine	Vira-A	Ointment	3%
Trifluridine	Viroptic	Solution	1%
	ANTIFUNGAL		
Natamycin	Natacyn	Suspension	5%

use. Corneal epithelial healing is slowed, and scarring may occur, particularly with prolonged therapy (51).

Adenine Arabinoside (Vidarabine)

This agent exhibits better corneal penetration and has shown some limited effectiveness in HSV stromal keratitis and IDU-resistant HSV epithelial keratitis (63). Vidarabine is somewhat more efficacious than IDU, having an 80- to 90-percent healing rate after 14 days of therapy. It is preferred for pediatric HSV epithelial keratitis because of its availability in ointment formulation (63).

The adverse effects observed with vidarabine can be similar to those of IDU. Follicular conjunctivitis, superficial punctate keratitis, punctal occlusion, and corneal scarring can occur with prolonged treatment (51, 63).

Trifluridine (Trifluorothymidine)

Similar to IDU, trifluridine exhibits greater water and lipid solubility. Like IDU and vidarabine, it is used to treat HSV keratitis. Clinical studies, however, indicate that it is a more potent topical antiviral agent, with a cure rate of 95 percent or greater in most studies (63). It is available only as a 1-percent ophthalmic solution, which can limit its usefulness in children.

Adverse effects with trifluridine can include corneal epithelial defects, conjunctivitis, lid effects including ptosis, punctal occlusion, and delayed hypersensitivity reaction with recurrent therapy (63).

ANTIFUNGAL AGENTS

Natamycin is currently the only commercially available antifungal drug for topical ophthalmic use (Table 13.7). Other available parenteral antifungal agents such as amphotericin B, nystatin, and miconazole can be used in dilute concentrations for topical therapy. Since all available agents penetrate the eye poorly, mycotic ocular infections are difficult to treat successfully (51).

Natamycin has proven effective in cases of keratomycosis caused by various fungi including *Acremonium* and *Fusarium* (51). Approximately 80 percent of patients obtain a clinical cure (63). Few adverse effects have been reported with topical therapy. Natamycin is commercially available as a 5-percent ophthalmic suspension (Natacyn).

CORTICOSTEROIDS

Since their introduction into clinical practice, corticosteroids have proven useful for controlling inflammatory and autoimmune disease. Although they are effective in protecting the ocular tissue from the deleterious effects of the inflammatory response, their use can be associated with adverse effects (65, 66). Coupled with the tendency to cause side effects is the need to use proportionately higher doses in children, particularly for conditions such as posterior uveitis (67).

Long-term systemic corticosteroid therapy can present problems for children that adults do not encounter. In addition to such side effects as Cushing's syndrome, increased susceptibility to infection, behavioral disturbances, and posterior subcapsular cataract, children experience growth retardation due to premature epiphyseal closure. Corticosteroids have also been shown to inhibit DNA synthesis in several cell types, including gastric mucosa and brain (66).

Corticosteroid toxicity can become evident not only during long-term high-dose therapy but also during the period of drug withdrawal. Since long-term systemic corticosteroid administration leads to suppression of adrenal and pituitary function, symptoms of adrenal insufficiency occur if therapy is discontinued abruptly. Withdrawal symptoms can include fever, myalgia, arthralgia, and malaise (65, 66, 68).

Long-term systemic corticosteroid therapy must use the lowest possible dose that controls the inflammatory reaction. With severe ocular inflammations such as peripheral uveitis, periocular injections rather than oral corticosteroids may be considered to minimize serious systemic side effects (67). It is important that proper withdrawal protocols be followed when discontinuing long-term systemic or topical ocular therapy (68).

BOTULINUM TOXIN

For the past decade, injection of botulinum A neurotoxin has proven valuable in managing selected cases of strabismus (69) (see Chapter 12). Botulinum A is one of eight immunologically distinct toxins produced by *Clostridium botulinum*, an anaerobic spore-forming bacterium. It is the most potent of the group and is composed of two polypeptide chains held together with interchain disulfide bonds (70). Botulinum toxin is the causative agent of cer-

tain cases of severe food poisoning characterized by progressive functional disturbances of the peripheral nervous system leading to flaccid paralysis (71). The toxin has been shown to act at the neuromuscular junction to prevent the release of acetylcholine. It binds to receptors on the surface of the nerve cell and, by a mechanism not well understood, interferes with transmitter release. The result is complete paralysis of the nerve fiber and atrophy of the associated muscles. The functional loss remains until a new protein end plate is formed (70).

Scott (69) pioneered the use of botulinum A toxin (also known as oculinum) as an alternative to strabismus surgery. He demonstrated—first in primates and later in human subjects—that a dilute solution was capable of weakening extraocular muscles when it was injected directly into the muscle. The method involves injection of a total volume of 0.1 ml saline, containing 0.5 to 10 ng toxin, into the muscle group to be weakened (72). The muscle weakens 24 to 36 hours following treatment.

Complications associated with the procedure include pain, subconjunctival hemorrhages, and induced diplopia and ptosis, which usually resolves within 8 weeks. The diplopia can be managed with a patch (71). The most serious complication associated with botulinum injection has been inadvertent perforation of the globe (71). Perhaps the most important consideration at present when use of botulinum toxin is contemplated is its effectiveness for long-term strabismus therapy.

BIBLIOGRAPHY

Bartlett JD, Jaanus SD (eds): Clinical Ocular Pharmacology. Boston, Butterworths, 1989.
Crawford JS, Morin JD (eds): The Eye in Childhood. New York, Grune & Stratton, 1983.
Marley RD: Pediatric Ophthalmology, vol. 1. Philadelphia, WB Saunders, 1983.
Shirkey HC (ed): Pediatric Therapy. St. Louis, CV Mosby, 1980.
Yaffe SJ (ed): Pediatric Pharmacology. Therapeutic Principles in Practice. New York, Grune & Stratton, 1980.

REFERENCES

1. Shirkey HC: Pediatric Therapy, 6th ed. St Louis, CV Mosby, 205, 1980.

2. Done AK, Cohen SN, Strebel L: Pediatric clinical pharmacology and the "therapeutic orphan." Ann Rev Pharmacol Toxicol 17:561, 1977.

3. Apt L: Pediatric aspects of drug therapy. In Leopold IH (ed): Symposium on Ocular Therapy, vol. 3. St Louis, CV Mosby, 88, 1968.

4. Lee PF: Congenital glaucoma. In Feman SS, Reinecke RD (eds): Handbook of Pediatric Ophthalmology, ch 5. New York, Grune & Stratton, 1978.

5. Glazko AJ: Simplified procedure for calculating drug dosages from body weight in infancy and childhood. Pediatrics 27:503, 1961.

6. Rane A, Wilson JT: Clinical pharmacokinetics in infants and children. Clin Pharmacokinet 1:1, 1976.

7. Mishima S: Pharmacology of ophthalmic solutions. Contact Intraocular Lens Med J 4:22, 1978.

8. Shell J: Pharmacokinetics of topically applied ophthalmic drugs. Surv Ophthalmol 26:207, 1982.

9. Apt L, Cullen BF: Newborns do secrete tears. JAMA 189:951, 1964.

10. Patton TF, Robinson JR: Pediatric dosing considerations in ophthalmology. J Pediatr Ophthalmol 13:171, 1976.

11. Bartlett JD, Cullen AP: Clinical administration of ocular drugs. In Bartlett JD, Jaanus SD (eds): Clinical Ocular Pharmacology, ch 2. Boston, Butterworth, 1989.

12. Diorio PC, Ober R: A method of instilling ophthalmic medication in a child's eye. J Pediatr Ophthalmol 2:123, 1975.

13. Fraunfelder FT: Extraocular fluid dynamics. How best to apply topical ocular medication. Trans Am Ophthalmol Soc 74:457, 1976.

14. Robin JS, Ellis PP: Ophthalmic ointments. Surv Ophthalmol 22:335, 1978.

15. Sharp J, Wallace T, Hanna C: Mydriasis using an aqueous spray of drugs on the closed eye. J Pediatr Ophthalmol 12:119, 1975.

16. Gettes BC: Choice of mydriatics and cycloplegics for diagnostic examination in children. In Apt L (ed): Diagnostic Procedures in Pediatric Ophthalmology. Boston, Little, Brown, 1963.

17. Caputo AR, Schnitzer RE: Systemic response to mydriatic eyedrops in neonates: Mydriatics in neonates. J Pediatr Ophthalmol Strabismus 15:109, 1978.

18. Borromeo-McGrail V, Bordiuk JM, Keitel H: Systemic hypertension following ocular administration of 10 percent phenylephrine in the neonate. Pediatrics 51:1032, 1973.

19. Fraunfelder FT, Scafidi AF: Possible adverse effects from topical ocular 10 percent phenylephrine. Am J Ophthalmol 85:862, 1978.

20. Rosales T, Isenberg S, Leake R, et al: Systemic effects of mydriatics in low birthweight infants. J Pediatr Ophthalmol Strabismus 18:42, 1981.

21. Lees BJ, Cabal LA: Increased blood pressure following pupillary dilation with 2.5 percent phenylephrine hydrochloride in preterm infants. Pediatrics 68:231, 1981.

22. Sindel BD, Baker MD, Maisels MJ, et al: A comparison of the pupillary and cardiovascular effects of various mydriatic agents in preterm infants. J Pediatr Ophthalmol Strabismus 23:273, 1986.

23. Lynch MG, Brown RH, Goode SM, et al: Reduction of phenylephrine drop size in infants achieves equal dilation with decreased systemic absorption. Arch Ophthalmol 105:1364, 1987.

24. Jaanus SD, Pagano VT, Bartlett JD: Drugs affecting the autonomic nervous system. In Bartlett JD, Jaanus SD (eds): Clinical Ocular Pharmacology, ch 3. Boston, Butterworth, 1989.

25. Beitel RS: Cycloplegic refraction. In Duane TD, Jaeger EA (eds): Clinical Ophthalmology, vol 1, ch 41. Hagerstown MD, Harper & Row, 1981.

26. Amos DM: Pharmacological management of strabismus. In Bartlett JD, Jaanus SD (eds): Clinical Ocular Pharmacology, ch 27. Boston, Butterworth, 1989.

27. North RV, Kelley ME: A review of the uses and adverse effects of topical administration of atropine. Ophthal Physiol Opt 7:109, 1987.

28. Morton HG: Atropine intoxication: Its mani-

festations in infants and children. J Pediatr 14:755, 1939.

29. Priest JH: Atropine response in eyes in mongolism. Am J Dis Child 100:869, 1960.

30. O'Conner PS, Mumma JV: Atropine toxicity. Am J Ophthalmol 99:613, 1985.

31. Simcoe CW: Cyclopentolate (Cyclogyl) toxicity. Arch Ophthalmol 67:406, 1962.

32. Bauer CR, Trottier MC, Stein L: Systemic cyclopentolate (Cyclogyl) toxicity in the newborn infant. J Pediatr 82:501, 1973.

33. Gettes BC: Tropicamide: Comparative mydriatic effects. Am J Ophthalmol 55:84, 1963.

34. Merrill DL, Goldberg B, Zavell S: Bis-tropicamide, a new parasympatholytic. Curr Ther Res 2:43, 1960.

35. Wahl JW: Systemic reactions to tropicamide. Arch Ophthalmol 82:320, 1969.

36. Caputo AR, Lingua RW: The problem of cycloplegia in the pediatric age group: A combination formula for refraction. J Pediatr Ophthalmol Strabismus 17:119, 1980.

37. Caputo AR, Schnitzer RE, Lindquist TD, et al: Dilation in neonates: A protocol. Pediatrics 69:77, 1982.

38. Kwitko ML: The pediatric glaucomas. In McAllister JA, Wilson RP (eds): Glaucoma, ch 5. London, Butterworth, 1986.

39. Theodore J, Leibowitz HM: External ocular toxicity of dipivalyl epinephrine. Am J Ophthalmol 88:1013, 1979.

40. McMahon CD, Hetherington J, Hoskins HD: Timolol and pediatric glaucomas. Ophthalmology 88:249, 1981.

41. DeLuise VP, Anderson DR: Primary infantile glaucoma (congenital glaucoma). Surv Ophthalmol 28:1, 1983.

42. Boger WP: Timolol in childhood glaucoma. Surv Ophthalmol 28:259, 1983.

43. Zimmerman TH, Kooner KS, Morgan KS: Safety and efficacy of timolol in pediatric glaucoma. Surv Ophthalmol 28:262, 1983.

44. Hoskins HD, Hetherington J, Magee SD, et al: Clinical experience with timolol in childhood glaucoma. Arch Ophthalmol 103:1163, 1985.

45. Becker B, Middleton WH: Long-term acetazolamide (Diamox) administration in therapy

of glaucomas. Arch Ophthalmol 54:187, 1955.

46. Ball AP, Gray JA: Antibacterial Drugs Today. Sidney, ADIS Health Sciences Press, 147, 1983.

47. Annable WL: Therapy of ocular infections. In Speck WT, Blumer JL (eds): Pediatr Clin North Am 30:389, 1983.

48. Eichenwald HF, McCracken GH: Systemic antimicrobial therapy. In Shirkey MC (ed): Pediatric Therapy, ch 29. St Louis, CV Mosby, 1980.

49. Baum JL: Antibiotic use in ophthalmology. In Duane TD, Jaeger EA (eds): Clinical Ophthalmology, vol. 4, ch 26. Philadelphia, J.B. Lippincott, 1988.

50. Bellows J, Farmer C: The use of bacitracin in ocular infections. Am J Ophthalmol 31:1211, 1948.

51. Yolton DP: Antiinfective Drugs. In Bartlett JD, Jaanus SD (eds): Clinical Ocular Pharmacology, ch 4. Boston, Butterworth, 1989.

52. Gonorrhea: CDC-recommended treatment schedules. Sex Transm Dis 6:38, 1979.

53. Wilson FM: Adverse external ocular effects of topical ophthalmic medications. Surv Ophthalmol 24:57, 1979.

54. Records RE: Gentamicin in ophthalmology. Surv Ophthalmol 21:49, 1976.

55. Wilhelmus KR, Gilbert ML, Osato MS: Tobramycin in ophthalmology. Surv Ophthalmol 32:111, 1987.

56. Timewell RM, Rosenthal AL, Smith JP, et al: Safety and efficacy of tobramycin and gentamicin sulfate in treatment of external ocular infections of children. J Pediatr Ophthalmol Strabismus 20:22, 1983.

57. Fraunfelder FT, Bagby GC, Kelley DJ: Fatal aplastic anemia following topical administration of ophthalmic chloramphenicol. Am J Ophthalmol 93:356, 1982.

58. Kucers A: Current position of chloramphenicol chemotherapy. J Antimicrob Chemother. 6:1, 1980.

59. Committee on Drugs, American Academy of Pediatrics: Requiem for tetracyclines. Pediatrics 55:142, 1975.

60. Wallace W: Diseases of the conjunctiva. In Bartlett JD, Jaanus SD (eds): Clinical Ocular

Pharmacology, ch 21. Boston, Butterworth, 1989.

61. Oriel JD: Ophthalmia neonatorum: Relative efficacy of current prophylatic practices and treatment. J Antimicrob Chemother 14:209, 1984.

62. Calasso GJ: Future prospects for antiviral agents and new approaches. J Antimicrob Chemother 14(Suppl):127, 1983.

63. Lass JH: Antivirals. In Lambert DW, Potter DE (eds): Clinical Ophthalmic Pharmacology, ch. 4. Boston Little, Brown, 1987.

64. Carroll JM, Martola EL, Laibson PR, et al: The recurrence of herpetic keratitis following idoxuridine therapy. Am J Ophthalmol 63:103, 1967.

65. Jaanus SD: Antiinflammatory drugs. In Bartlett JD, Jaanus SD (eds): Clinical Ocular Pharmacology, ch 5. Boston, Butterworth, 1989.

66. Chew E, McCulloch J: Ocular therapeutics.

In Crawford JS (ed): The Eye in Childhood. New York, Grune & Stratton, 527, 1983.

67. Giles CL: Uveitis in childhood. In Duane TD, Jaeger EA (eds): Clinical Ophthalmology, vol. 4, ch 56. Hagerstown MD, Harper & Row, 1987.

68. Byyney RL: Withdrawal from glucocorticoid. N Engl J Med 293:30, 1976.

69. Scott AB: Botulinium toxin injection of eye muscles to correct strabismus. Trans Am Ophthalmol Soc 79:735, 1981.

70. Simpson LL: Molecular pharmacology of botulinium toxin and tetanus toxin. Am Rev Pharmacol Toxicol 26:427, 1986.

71. Amos DM: Pharmacological management of strabismus. In Bartlett JD, Jaanus SD (eds): Clinical Ocular Pharmacology ch. 28. Boston, Butterworth, 1989.

72. Hoffman RO, Helveston EM: Botulinium in the treatment of adult motility disorders. Int Ophthalmol Clin 26:241, 1986.

Chapter 14

Ocular and Systemic Diseases of Infants and Children

Leonard Apt

David G. Kirschen

This chapter highlights ocular and systemic diseases that may be seen in infants and children and warns the reader of some diseases that may be sight- or life-threatening. Each section describes the disease, gives its clinical presentation, some background on its cause, likely clinical course, and available treatment modalities. Special emphasis is given to diseases that are true ocular emergencies and require immediate management.

THE EYELIDS

Congenital Anomalies

Palpebral coloboma is a cleftlike deformity that may vary from a small indentation or notch of the free margin of the lid to a large defect involving almost the entire lid. It can occur as an isolated defect or associated with other developmental abnormalities such as Goldenhar's or Franceschetti's (Treacher-Collins) syndrome. If the gap is extensive, xerosis, ulceration, and corneal opacities may result from exposure. Surgical repair is needed but may be delayed unless exposure keratitis occurs.

Ectropion (eversion of the eyelids) is a rare bilateral disorder most commonly seen in blacks and is due to orbital fat herniation. It may lead to overflow of tears (epiphora) and subsequent maceration of the skin of the lid, to inflammation of the exposed conjunctiva, or to superficial exposure keratopathy. Ocular lubricants provide corneal protection while spontaneous healing is taking place. Ectropion is also seen in children who have faulty development of the lateral canthal ligament, which may also occur in Down's syndrome. Surgical repair eventually may be necessary.

Blepharophimosis is a bilateral and symmetric disease affecting the size of the palpebral fissure. It is inherited as an autosomal dominant trait but may occur sporadically and may be associated with other lid anomalies including ptosis. This condition often requires surgical correction.

Epicanthus (epicanthal folds) is a common eyelid anomaly characterized by bilateral vertical semilunar folds arising in the upper lid, extending down the side of the nose to the lower lid, and covering the normal inner canthus. It is similar to the normal racial characteristic of many Asians and is a common finding in many chromosomal disorders. It is present to some degree in most young children and becomes less apparent with age. The folds may be sufficiently broad to cover the medial aspect of the eye, making the eyes appear crossed (pseudostrabismus). As the bridge of the nose becomes formed with development of the face, the folds eventually disappear.

Entropion (inward turning of the lid margin) may cause discomfort and corneal damage from the cilia (lashes) rubbing against the cornea (trichiasis). It may occur spontaneously with other congenital orbital abnormalities or may be secondary to large buccal pads of fat in babies. Surgical repair may be necessary if corneal damage ensues. Oculinum injections have been helpful in treating entropion in adults.

Distichiasis is an abnormal second row of lashes growing out of the meibomian gland orifice. It occurs as a dominant trait, usually without concomitant congenital anomalies; however, it may be associated with chronic lymphedema of the lower extremities (Falls-Kertesz syndrome). If keratitis or irritation occurs, surgical correction is effective.

Congenital *ptosis* or drooping of the upper lid is the most common anomaly of the eyelids. Blepharoptosis, which may be unilateral or bilateral, is secondary to defective development or absence of the levator muscle. It may be inherited as an autosomal dominant trait. Ptosis often is an isolated finding,

but it may occur with other local ocular anomalies such as superior rectus palsy on the same side, epicanthus, and strabismus or with systemic abnormalities such as Fabry's disease or Turner's syndrome. A child with unilateral congenital ptosis may raise the eyebrow and use the frontalis muscle to lift the lid, and one with bilateral ptosis may also tip the head backward.

Congenital ptosis can be corrected surgically; the age at which surgery is done depends on the amount of ptosis, its cosmetic and functional severity, the presence or absence of compensatory posturing, and the wishes of the parents. Unless the ptosis is extreme, surgery is usually deferred until the child is 4 to 5 years old, when adequate preoperative evaluation, including accurate measurement of levator function, can be performed. Children with ptosis may have associated strabismus, amblyopia, or astigmatism. Treatment of the associated conditions must begin promptly.

A peculiar form of ptosis occurs in Marcus Gunn jaw-winking syndrome. An anomalous connection between the external pterygoid muscle (innervated by the fifth cranial nerve) and the levator muscle (innervated by the third cranial nerve) leads to elevation of the ptotic lid when the mouth is opened or when the jaw is moved to the side opposite the ptosis. This condition often lessens with time, and surgery may not be required.

Differential diagnosis of acquired ptosis in childhood includes myasthenia gravis, progressive external ophthalmoplegia, progressive intracranial lesions affecting the third nerve, and inflammation or tumors affecting the levator, the orbit, or the lid. Ptosis may also be the result of trauma. Aberrant regeneration of the injured third nerve fibers may produce paradoxical lid and eye movements.

Infections

Blepharitis

Blepharitis is a common subacute or chronic recurrent inflammation of the eyelid margin associated with pain, itching, burning, and eyelid redness. It is most commonly bilateral, but it can be unilateral. The three most common forms are seborrheic, staphylococcal, and mixed.

Seborrheic blepharitis is characterized by yellow, greasy scales attached to the lashes. These scales are easily removed and are associated with seborrhea of the brow, scalp, and external ears. Conjunctivitis and keratitis are usually absent. Treatment is primarily lid hygiene and control of the general seborrheic condition. Hygiene consists of removal of the scales and crusts with hot moist compresses and scrubbing the eyelid margins with a gauze pad soaked in a specific eyelid cleanser or a dilute solution of baby shampoo. Sulfacetamide has antiseborrheic activity, but the commonly used antibiotics do not. It is important to treat the seborrhea that usually exists in other areas, such as the scalp, eyebrows, or ears.

Staphylococcal blepharitis is a local infection of the eyelid margin caused by pathogenic *Staphylococcus aureus* and *S. epidermidis*. This form of blepharitis is characterized by tenacious fibrinous collarettes or scales seen at the base of the lashes (they often look like an "impaled cornflake"). The lid margin can be ulcerated and the lashes are often broken, sparse, or absent (madarosis). If the infection spreads to the glands of Zeis, an external hordeolum (stye) can develop, and if the meibomian glands are involved, a meibomitis or internal hordeolum can develop. Conjunctivitis, superficial punctate keratitis, and marginal corneal ulceration can occur as a result of the exotoxins released by the staphylococcal organisms. Treatment involves both lid hygiene (scrubs to remove the crusts and scales) and the application of an appropriate antistaphylococcal preparation such as bacitracin, erythromycin, or sulfacetamide drops or ointment. Bacterial cultures and sensitivity tests are useful in guiding therapy. A topical corticosteroid-antimicrobial agent like sulfacetamide sodium (Blephamide) may be used in severe cases to reduce the inflammatory and hypersensitivity reaction. Treatment may be required over

a prolonged period because blepharitis often is a chronic problem, with frequent flare-ups. Tonometry is indicated if long-term corticosteroid therapy is used.

Mixed blepharitis occurs when a staphylococcal infection is complicated by seborrhea of the lids. This condition must be treated aggressively to prevent long-term structural damage to the lids and subsequent dry eye syndrome. The treatment is the same as for other forms of blepharitis.

Parasitic blepharitis results from infestation of the lids by the crab louse (*Pediculus pubis*) or the head louse (*P. capitis*), which cause excoriations and itching of the lid margins. The adult lice and their ova (nits), which are attached to the lids and brow, can be visualized with the slit lamp. Treatment consists of removing the parasite and the ova from the lashes with forceps and applying a smothering bland ophthalmic ointment two to four times a day for 1 week. Other areas of infestation such as the scalp or pubic area must be treated simultaneously with a delousing preparation.

Hordeolum

External hordeolum, also known as the common stye, is an acute staphylococcal infection of the ciliary follicles and the glands of Zeis (oil) and Moll (sweat) along the lid margin. The lesion begins as a circumscribed swelling at the lid margin, progresses to suppuration, and finally ruptures with resolution of the pain and tenderness. Treatment consists of warm, moist compresses applied for 20 minutes several times a day. Epilation of the affected lash is sometimes helpful in opening a drainage channel. Antibiotic ointment specific for staphylococcus should be applied. If topical treatment fails, systemic antibiotics such as erythromycin or ampicillin can be used. Occasionally the stye has to be incised to allow the pus to drain.

Internal hordeolum is an acute staphylococcal infection of the meibomian gland. There is localized swelling and redness, and the suppuration appears on the conjunctival surface of the lid corresponding to the location of the gland. Spontaneous rupture is less frequent than with the external hordeolum, but the treatment is the same.

Chalazion

Chalazion results from granulomatous inflammation of the meibomian glands. It may be difficult to distinguish from an internal hordeolum in the early stages; however, a chalazion does not drain spontaneously but quickly progresses to form a lipogranuloma, a slow-growing, mildly tender, firm round mass in the tarsus. The growth is usually painless, but it can affect vision if it is large enough to press on the cornea. It may gradually resorb within a month, but if it persists, it can be injected directly with a steroid such as triamcinolone acetonide (Kenalog) or can be surgically excised.

THE CONJUNCTIVA

Congenital Anomalies

Except for pigmentation, congenital conjunctival anomalies are rare. *Epithelial melanosis* appears clinically as patchy, flat, brown conjunctival pigment, mainly on the bulbar conjunctiva. *Melanosis oculi* is an inherited, unilateral disorder characterized by slate-blue mottled pigmentation of the conjunctiva and sclera. There may also be increased uveal pigment. *Oculodermal melanosis* (nevus of Ota) is seen before 1 year of age as unilateral slate-blue conjunctival and scleral pigment with associated pigmentation of the ipsilateral periorbital skin. There is a greater likelihood of oculodermal melanosis in Asians and blacks. None of these conjunctival anomalies has malignant potential and they do not disturb the function of the eye. However, patients with melanosis oculi and oculodermal melanosis may develop malignant melanomas of the uveal tract or pigmentary glaucoma. Therefore periodic examinations including ophthalmoscopy are indicated.

Epibulbar Tumors

Conjunctival nevi are the most common epibulbar tumors of childhood. They may be present at birth, but they frequently acquire increased pigment and first become noticeable at puberty. They usually occur at the limbus in the bulbar conjunctiva as well-circumscribed lesions of varying size and pigmentation. Because they have virtually no malignant potential in childhood, surgical excision is done only if the tumor is of cosmetic concern.

Epibulbar limbal *dermoids* and conjunctival nonlimbal dermolipomas are cream-colored tumors of the choristoma type. They are evident at birth and often increase in size with time. Approximately 30 percent of the patients with these tumors have associated ocular (e.g., lid coloboma, microphthalmos, aniridia) and systemic (e.g., Goldenhar's syndrome) anomalies.

Systemic diseases such as sarcoidosis, leukemia, and juvenile xanthogranuloma have conjunctival nodules or infiltrates. Orbital rhabdomyosarcoma may appear as a conjunctival mass in 7 percent of patients. The conjunctival infiltrates can be biopsied to help diagnose systemic disease.

Subconjunctival Hemorrhages

Subconjunctival hemorrhages from a capillary of the bulbar conjunctiva may occur with mild trauma, violent coughing, sneezing, vomiting, acute conjunctivitis, or the bleeding may be spontaneous (idiopathic). The appearance can be alarming to parents, but the condition is benign. It may, however, signify more serious intrabulbar damage, usually from trauma, that may not be volunteered in the history. The ophthalmic workup should include a detailed history, visual acuity, pupillary response, and oculomotility evaluations, a slit-lamp examination, and an ophthalmoscopic examination.

The blood usually resorbs within 1 to 2 weeks. Cool compresses (or ice) may be used initially several times a day for 2 days to ensure that the bleeding vessel has sealed, then warm compresses can be used to facilitate reabsorption of the pooled blood.

Conjunctivitis

Conjunctivitis is a common pediatric eye disorder. The visual signs are tearing, conjunctival injection, chemosis, papillae, and follicles. Membranes or pseudomembranes, regional adenopathy, and discharge also are often noted. Vision is usually not affected, and pain and photophobia are rare. If they are present, it should alert the clinician to suspect primary corneal disease. In the newborn the usual causes of conjunctivitis are chemical, bacterial, and chlamydial.

Appropriate bacterial and viral cultures of the conjunctival exudates or smears taken from the lower tarsal conjunctiva and microscopic studies of conjunctival scrapings are essential in cases of conjunctivitis that fail to respond to initial therapy within 48 hours. Determining the specific causative agent avoids the indiscriminate use of antibiotics and the risk of development of host sensitivity and resistance to the organism.

Topical antibiotics are used routinely in the treatment of conjunctivitis. Oral antibiotics are sometimes necessary in severe cases. In general, corticosteroids should be avoided when dealing with the pediatric population, because there is a significant danger of producing steroid-induced glaucoma. They also are contraindicated if corneal involvement is present (mainly herpetic lesions). For younger children, medication in ointment form may be preferred. It is easier to instill and there is less chance of overdose. For older children drops are used during the day and ointment at bedtime.

Ophthalmia neonatorum (acute conjunctivitis in the newborn) may be due to a chemical irritant, such as 1-percent silver nitrate instilled as prophylaxis against *N. gonorrhoeae*, or to a bacterial or viral agent acquired during or after delivery. Knowing the time of onset of the conjunctivitis is helpful in the diagnosis: silver nitrate conjunctivitis occurs in the first 24 hours after birth; *gonococcal conjunctivitis* occurs within 2 to 3 days after birth (but can be delayed up to 21 days if silver nitrate is used); other bacterial conjunctivitides occur 3 or more days after birth. *Chlamydial conjunctivitis* occurs 5 to 23 days after birth. Because the potential for blindness associated with gonococcus exists in all newborns with ophthalmia neona-

torum, the infection must be considered to be gonococcal until proven otherwise.

Chlamydia trachomatis has recently emerged as the most frequent cause of ophthalmia neonatorum. Clinically it produces a mucopurulent or purulent papillary conjunctivitis, occasionally with a pseudomembrane, usually in one eye. Premature infants are particularly susceptible. Chlamydia is resistant to silver nitrate, and therefore a new regimen for prophylaxis for ophthalmia neonatorum is being used. Acceptable prophylactic agents include erythromycin (0.5 percent) ointment or drops and tetracycline (1 percent) ointment or drops given as a single topical application to the eyes immediately postpartum. Both parents should be treated with systemic erythromycin for 3 weeks to avoid reinfecting the baby.

Of the various bacterial pathogens that can cause ophthalmia neonatorum *Neisseria gonorrhoeae* is potentially the most dangerous. Topical erythromycin or tetracycline may be used prophylactically in place of 1-percent silver nitrate to avoid the chemical conjunctivitis. It is characterized by a hyperacute, purulent bilateral conjunctivitis with substantial edema of the lids, chemosis, marked conjunctival injection, and copious discharge of pus. Because rapid corneal penetration may lead to perforation, panophthalmitis, and even septicemia or meningitis, proper treatment must be initiated immediately. Because the infection is highly contagious, all affected infants should be hospitalized and isolated for at least 24 hours after treatment begins. Medical care should be administered under the direct supervision of a pediatric ophthalmologist and a pediatrician (or neonatologist) and should include conjunctival smears and scrapings (looking for gram-negative intracellular diplococci), large doses of penicillin, and a drug such as cefotaxime for penicillinase-producing and chromosomal-mediated resistant *N. gonorrhoeae*. Systemic medication must be used for effective treatment. Topical medication alone is not adequate. The parents should also be treated with systemic tetracycline or oral penicillin.

S. aureus, Hemophilus influenzae, and other bacteria have been identified with ophthalmia neonatorum. Treatment is effective with topical broad-spectrum antibiotics such as Neosporin (bacitracin–neomycin–polymixin B). Conjunctival scrapings, cultures, and antibiotic sensitivity studies should be taken to guide therapy.

Acute Bacterial (Mucopurulent) Conjunctivitis (Pinkeye)

Acute bacterial conjunctivitis manifests with a sudden onset, mild to severe burning, an intensely injected conjunctiva, especially in the tarsal portion and fornices, and a mucopurulent discharge. The tarsal conjunctiva shows a papillary reaction that gives it a velvety appearance. It is highly contagious, spreads from one eye to the other, and may be transferred to another person by hands, towels, and other contact. The pathogens primarily responsible for bacterial conjunctivitis are staphylococcus, pneumococcus, *H. influenzae,* and beta-hemolytic streptococci. Petechial hemorrhages of the conjunctiva are common with pneumococcal and *H. influenzae* infections. Treatment consists of topical antimicrobial agents such as sulfacetamide, 10 percent, or erythromycin, 0.5 percent, drops or ointment four times a day. Precautions should be taken to avoid spreading the infection to other family members. Medications containing neomycin should be avoided if used longer than a week, because they tend to cause allergic reactions and toxic keratitis. Corticosteroids and patching are unnecessary. Although the infections may last from several days to 2 weeks, they are self-limiting.

Follicular Conjunctivitis

Follicular conjunctivitis is a condition in which follicles develop on the palpebral conjunctiva in response to a bacterial or viral infection of the conjunctiva. These fall into several categories:

Inclusion conjunctivitis is a viral infection most prevalent during the summer months and is often transmitted in inade-

quately chlorinated swimming pools. The prominent clinical feature is a significant follicular hypertrophy of the lower eyelid, and epithelial cell inclusions are rarely seen in conjunctival scrapings. It is important to differentiate this from an adenovirus infection. Inclusion conjunctivitis has a mucopurulent discharge that usually sticks the lids shut during the night and a large number of polymorphonuclear cells in the conjunctival scrapings. Adenovirus conjunctivitis has a more watery discharge and mainly mononuclear cells in the exudate. Scarring usually does not occur in children with inclusion conjunctivitis. Topical sulfacetamide can be used, but often systemic tetracycline or erythromycin is necessary.

Trachoma is still the greatest cause of impaired vision and blindness in the world, affecting approximately 400 million people. It occurs sporadically in all parts of the U.S.A., but is endemic in certain areas, notably on the reservations of the American Indian and in the Mexican-American population of the southwest. This is particularly true in families from or still living in rural areas. Trachoma usually starts in childhood and is associated with annual epidemics of bacterial conjunctivitis. With acute or subacute infections there is edema, hyperemia, papillary hypertrophy, follicles on the upper tarsal conjunctiva and upper limbus, superficial epithelial keratitis of the upper half of the cornea with associated pannus, Herbert's pits (small lucid depressions at the upper limbal border), and a small, tender preauricular lymph node. Limbal follicles and Herbert's pits in combination with pannus are pathognomonic of trachoma. Secondary bacterial infection is common and is the usual cause of severe corneal scarring with vision loss.

The conjunctivitis in trachoma can be treated effectively with a combination of local and systemic tetracycline or erythromycin. Erythromycin is used in pregnant women and children under 8 years old because of the detrimental effects of tetracycline on the teeth of infants and young children. Systemic therapy is given for 3 weeks and topical therapy for 6 weeks. Corticosteroids are contraindicated.

Epidemic keratoconjunctivitis (EKC) is a highly contagious viral infection of the conjunctiva and cornea caused most often by adenovirus types 8 and 19, but other serotypes also produce the disease. Infected persons are usually contagious for 2 weeks as they continue to shed active viral particles. Epidemics can occur by spread from contaminated fingers (poor hand washing), tonometers, and eye drops. The incubation period is approximately 7 to 10 days.

Clinically there is a rapid onset of severe follicular conjunctivitis, primarily in the lower fornix with serous discharge, chemosis, and a large, tender preauricular node. The second eye usually becomes infected—but less severely—by spread from the first. Subconjunctival hemorrhages may be present, and pseudomembranes form in about 30 percent of cases. Stage 1 begins 7 to 10 days after the onset, with a diffuse punctate epithelial keratitis. Stage 2 occurs from the 7th to 20th day and consists of a focal epithelial keratitis with subepithelial opacities. In stage 3, anterior stromal infiltrates appear and can persist for months. Infected children may demonstrate systemic signs, including fever, sore throat, and diarrhea.

EKC is a self-limiting disease lasting 2 to 3 weeks; however, the subepithelial opacities can persist for months or years. Scarring and entropion can occur from the membrane formation. Treatment may consist of topical antibiotics used prophylactically to prevent a secondary bacterial infection. In severe cases, topical corticosteroids in low concentrations may be used if herpes simplex infection is excluded.

Pharyngoconjunctival fever (PCF) is characterized by an acute, self-limiting follicular conjunctivitis that lasts 10 to 14 days in association with fever, malaise, pharyngitis (sore throat), and preauricular and cervical lymphadenopathy. Adenovirus types 3, 4, and 7 are classically associated, but all 31 serotypes may cause PCF. This is a highly contagious disease that is spread by direct contact or indirectly through contaminated swimming pools (even if they are chlorinated). Epidemics tend to occur in the late summer months.

The incubation period is 2 to 10 days with associated pharyngitis, conjunctivitis, and fever. The follicular conjunctivitis is often unilateral and usually involves the lower fornix. Acute symptoms are a serous discharge, hyperemia, discomfort, and photophobia. Corneal involvement is minor and resolves as the conjunctivitis subsides. Isolation precautions should be taken to prevent spread of the disease. Antivirals are ineffective, and corticosteroids are not indicated. Antibiotics can be prescribed prophylactically to prevent a secondary bacterial infection, especially if the cornea is involved.

Herpes simplex conjunctivitis is a primary viral infection in children 6 months to 5 years of age. Ninety percent of herpes infections are asymptomatic and involve the fellow eye 7 to 10 days after the onset. The clinical signs include follicular conjunctivitis with lymphadenopathy on the affected side. Ulcerative blepharitis may occur, and clusters of vesicles can erupt on the face and eyelids. The cornea, if involved, can show a punctate epithelial keratitis or dendritic keratitis.

The disease usually is self-limiting, lasting 2 to 3 weeks. Because dendritic keratitis can develop with potential loss of vision, treatment with topical antiviral agents, such as trifluridine (Viroptic) is indicated. Antibiotics are used to prevent a secondary bacterial infection.

Exanthematous Conjunctivitis

Many childhood exanthems like *measles*, *chicken pox*, and *smallpox* may be accompanied by an acute catarrhal conjunctivitis. Keratoconjunctivitis is a characteristic sign during the acute stages of measles. Ocular involvement may precede the skin eruptions by several days. A peculiar swelling of the plica semilunaris (Meyer's sign), a glasslike appearance of the conjunctiva, and Koplik's spots on the caruncle and semilunar fold can occur during the period of incubation. Epithelial keratitis then follows shortly. No specific treatment is necessary unless a secondary bacterial infection or corneal involvement occurs.

In *varicella* (chicken pox), small papular lesions may occur on the lid margin and the conjunctiva along with a mild catarrhal conjunctivitis. Superficial or deep keratitis may complicate the infection, but it usually resolves spontaneously.

Membranous Conjunctivitis

Membranes or *pseudomembranes* can occur in streptococcal infection or in severe conjunctivitis from any cause. The membrane forms on the conjunctiva from exudate; if it can be stripped off easily without bleeding it is known as a pseudomembrane. A true membrane adheres tightly to the conjunctiva and leaves a raw, bleeding epithelial surface when it is removed. True membranous conjunctivitis may result in severe damage to the conjunctiva and cornea; fortunately this inflammation is rare today.

Allergic Conjunctivitis

The conjunctiva, like other epithelial tissues, may develop a local hypersensitivity to a specific allergen. In acute hypersensitivity reactions, there is sudden vascular dilation with marked chemosis that disappears when the irritant is removed. In chronic allergy, cellular infiltration and newly formed connective tissue follow. Allergic conjunctivitis can be divided into four basic types: atopic, drug sensitivity, vernal, and phlyctenular.

Simple allergic or *atopic conjunctivitis* occurs in children with allergic disorders such as asthma and hay fever. It is caused primarily by pollens (hay fever), animal hair, fungi, dusts, and ingestion of some foods. A hyperemic reaction of the tarsal and bulbar conjunctiva is produced and edema of the lids and profuse lacrimation with itching follow. There may also be a scant, stringy mucoid discharge. For chronic forms of allergic conjunctivitis an attempt should be made to isolate the offending allergen and to eliminate contact with it. Desensitization to the allergen can be carried out if elimination of contact is not possible. Temporary sympto-

matic relief may be obtained by using cold compresses or ophthalmic solutions containing vasoconstrictors, antihistamines, or 4-percent cromolyn sodium (Opticrom). Rubbing the eyes should be discouraged. In severe cases corticosteroids may be used initially to control the reaction; then they are gradually withdrawn.

Drug sensitivity can produce a reaction in the conjunctiva similar to that of atopic conjunctivitis. In addition to the conjunctival reaction, contact dermatitis can form with intense hyperemia and eczematoid changes. Sensitivity to drugs usually occurs after repeated instillations. Topical neomycin is one drug that is a more common offender. Once developed, this sensitivity can last indefinitely and should become part of the child's drug history. Treatment consists of removing the offending agent and local use of corticosteroids on the skin for symptomatic relief.

Vernal conjunctivitis or spring catarrh is a bilateral, chronic, recurrent inflammation characterized by giant, polygonal, flat-topped papillae in the upper palpebral conjunctiva giving a typical cobblestone appearance. A ropy discharge, extreme itching, and photophobia are characteristic. Vernal conjunctivitis occurs during spring and summer and primarily is a disease of childhood, occurring most frequently in boys 5 to 15 years of age. A familial history of allergies is usual, but identification of specific allergens has been unsuccessful. Symptomatic relief consists of cold compresses and topical vasoconstrictors, antihistamines, or 4 percent cromolyn sodium (Opticrom). Corticosteroid therapy may be needed initially in severe cases to get the condition under control.

Phlyctenular conjunctivitis is characterized by one or more small, hard, red, elevated nodules surrounded by hyperemic vessels and appearing most commonly at the limbus and on the bulbar conjunctiva temporally. Microscopically the phlyctenule is a subepithelial infiltrate of lymphocytes. The apex of the phlyctenule turns gray and ulcerates, with healing in 10 to 12 days. The disease has been associated with a hypersensitivity reaction to the tubercle bacillus, to other bacteria such as the staphylococci, or to fungi. Today the disease is most commonly associated with *S. aureus* from marginal blepharitis. Corneal involvement is associated with severe photophobia and profuse lacrimation. Treatment should consist of an antibiotic-steroid combination to reduce the inflammation and be effective against *S. aureus*. A careful search should be made for a systemic disease such as tuberculosis.

THE CORNEA

Congenital Anomalies

Congenital anomalies of the cornea most often result in a defect of *transparency*. Congenital and infantile corneal opacification requires a total pediatric evaluation, because often a systemic abnormality is associated with the corneal defect.

Abnormalities of corneal size and shape require investigations for unusual refractive errors or other ocular defects. A corneal diameter, measured horizontally with a millimeter rule held on the bridge of the nose, of less than 10 mm in neonates and 11 mm in older infants and children is considered *microcornea*. If the microcornea occurs in an otherwise normal eye (e.g., normal axial length), there will be a significant myopic refractive error. If microphthalmos (e.g., shorter than normal axial length) accompanies the microcornea, no significant refractive error will occur. A frequent complication of microcornea is glaucoma. Less common associated anomalies are congenital cataracts, microphakia, coloboma, and small eyelids and orbits.

Megalocornea (horizontal diameter greater than 13 mm) is a nonprogressive condition in which there are large, clear corneas bilaterally, usually associated with high astigmatism. Enlargement of the cornea as part of buphthalmos in congenital glaucoma is easily differentiated. Megalocornea is associated with Lowe's syndrome, osteogenesis imperfecta, and Marfan's syndrome.

Cornea plana and keratoconus are anomalies in the curvature of the cornea. Cornea plana, a flat cornea, produces a pseudoptosis due to poor support of the upper eyelid, whereas keratoconus, a very steep cornea, can produce an irregular corneal surface resulting in high myopia and astigmatism and amblyopia if left untreated. It commonly appears in adolescence and with increased frequency in Down's syndrome. Vision can be improved with rigid contact lenses, but in selected cases a penetrating keratoplasty must be done.

Sclerocornea is a sporadically occurring bilateral anomaly in which scleral tissue with accompanying vessels extends into the otherwise normal cornea at the limbus. If the visual axis is affected, amblyopia, nystagmus, or strabismus may result. Sclerocornea may be associated with other ocular anomalies such as cornea plana, congenital glaucoma, or chromosomal abnormalities. In generalized sclerocornea, early keratoplasty should be considered to provide vision.

Corneal Inflammations (Keratitis)

Superficial punctate keratitis (SPK) is an inflammation of the corneal epithelium caused by a local ocular disease (conjunctivitis, exposure trichiasis) or an ocular manifestation of a systemic disease (familial dysautonomia, vitamin A deficiency). Slit-lamp examination with sodium fluorescein reveals fine punctate erosions of the epithelium that stain with fluorescein. Treatment is directed at the underlying cause.

Congenital syphilis is the most common cause of *interstitial keratitis* in children. Even though its incidence has dropped dramatically with the advent of penicillin, the disease still exists and is sight-threatening. Corneal changes appear between the ages of 5 and 15 years (rarely earlier) and consist of a diffuse corneal edema followed by vascularization of the posterior two thirds of the corneal stroma. The cornea assumes a ground-glass appearance with orange-red areas (salmon patches) due to the vascularization. Subjective symptoms accompanying the keratitis are decreased vision, intense photophobia, lacrimation, and pain. Associated uveitis is common. The keratitis regresses after several months, leaving deep stromal scarring and ghost vessels. Antisyphilitic medications are ineffective during the course of the disease. Local corticosteroids and cycloplegics can provide symptomatic relief. In patients with severe corneal scarring, penetrating keratoplasty can be performed after the inflammation has been quiescent for a number of years.

Herpes simplex keratitis is caused by the herpes simplex virus and is becoming a more common disease in children. The disease begins with a dendritic superficial ulcer. The dendrite has a branching, treelike pattern that is best demonstrated by fluorescein staining. Corneal sensitivity is reduced. The acute episode is accompanied by pain, photophobia, tearing, and conjunctival injection. Herpes simplex infections may occur in a baby born to a mother with genital (type 2) herpes. Two days to 2 weeks after birth keratitis appears either as an initial manifestation of the herpes infection or after skin or disseminated disease occurs. Prophylactic topical antiviral therapy is recommended for all newborns born to mothers who have genital herpes at the time of delivery.

Treatment of the superficial keratitis consists of débridement of the involved epithelium, short-term patching, and topical antiviral therapy such as trifluorothymidine, 1 percent solution (Viroptic). With stromal involvement these antiviral drugs are less effective. The eye is usually more comfortable if the pupil is kept dilated with 1-percent atropine or 5-percent homatropine. *Corticosteroids are contraindicated in the epithelial form of the disease because they accelerate the spread of the viral infection and can lead to rapid deterioration of the cornea.* They can be used in conjunction with antivirals in the stromal form of the disease to reduce the toxic or hypersensitive response to the virus or virus products.

Herpes zoster virus can affect the ophthalmic branch of the trigeminal nerve (fifth cranial nerve). Vesicular skin lesions are distributed in the sensory area innervated by the affected nerve. Those with vesicular eruptions on the tip of the nose (Hutchinson's sign) are most likely to have eye involvement. Zoster keratitis occurs in about 40 percent of patients. Keratitis and conjunctivitis usually occur during the acute phases of the skin eruptions. Corneal involvement begins as a superficial punctate keratitis and progresses to terminate in a large nummular stromal opacity. Corneal sensation is reduced or absent. Iritis always accompanies the keratitis and can be severe, with hypopyon, glaucoma, and hyphema.

The incidence of herpes zoster is highest in patients over 40 or under 14 years of age. Its presence in children should raise suspicion of underlying lymphoma, leukemia, or acquired immunodeficiency disease (AIDS). Treatment with topical corticosteroids, cycloplegics, and antivirals is indicated. Intravenous or oral acyclovir may reduce the incidence and duration of severe keratitis and anterior uveitis when given within the first 72 hours after onset.

Corneal Ulcers

Corneal ulcers are a serious ocular emergency that require *immediate* intensive therapy. Ulcers appear as a hazy or white spot on the cornea and can be identified most easily by instilling a drop of sterile fluorescein and observing the intense green staining. The release of proteolytic enzymes from the white blood cells or the invading organism causes severe destruction of the corneal tissue. The ulceration can spread quickly into deeper corneal layers, and without treatment it may cause perforation of the cornea. Infective corneal ulcers usually result from trauma of the corneal epithelium with subsequent invasion by bacteria. The incidence of various organisms causing corneal ulcers varies with geographic area and time, but the most commonly cultured pathogens are *Diplococcus pneumoniae*, *P. aeruginosa*, *Moraxella lacunata*, and *S. aureus*. *P. aeruginosa* produces an exceptionally destructive lesion, presumably because of its protease.

Antimicrobial therapy must be instituted immediately after smears and cultures of the ulcer are taken. Occasionally young children require general anesthesia for proper examination of the eye and adequate performance of scrapings and cultures. *It is prudent to assume that any infected corneal ulcer contains pseudomonas organisms or penicillin-resistant staphylococci until proven otherwise.* Therefore the initial therapy should consist of an antibiotic combination such as cefazolin or bacitracin plus gentamicin or tobramycin. The drops for the initial therapy are often formulated by the pharmacist in concentrations much greater than those available commercially. The fortified drops are administered every 15 to 30 minutes for 36 to 48 hours. Modification of this therapy should be made based on the culture and sensitivity tests. As the infection resolves, the dosing frequency and concentration of the drops are reduced.

Marginal infiltrates (sometimes called marginal ulcers) are usually benign and secondary to a hypersensitivity reaction of the cornea to bacterial antigens such as *S. aureus*. The infiltrates are in the superficial stroma and result in a loss of epithelium. This gives the characteristic appearance of a gray spot on the cornea separate from the limbus. These ulcers are considered sterile. Treatment usually consists of a topical antibiotic for the underlying blepharoconjunctivitis and a mild corticosteroid to heal the ulcer.

Fungal corneal ulcers usually occur following trauma or a foreign body, frequently plant or vegetative material. These ulcers have increased in frequency in recent years as a result of more widespread use of topical corticosteroids and antibiotics and the improper disinfection of extended-wear contact lenses. The diagnosis of a fungal infection should be considered in any persistent, slowly progressive corneal ulceration. Treatment consists of débridement and use of local antifungal agents such as natamycin, nystatin, miconazole, and ketaconazole. Refractory ulcers may require a conjunctival flap. A penetrating keratoplasty may be curative if the entire area of infection can be encompassed.

Corneal Drying

Xerosis (drying of the conjunctiva and cornea) can be caused by various ocular and systemic diseases. Keratoconjunctivitis sicca, in which tear production is decreased, can result from Still's disease, familial dysautonomia, or systemic lupus erythematosus in children. Exposure keratitis can be secondary to seventh nerve palsy and exophthalmos. Treatment of the corneal drying and exposure consists of frequent instillations of artificial tears, bland ointments, soft contact lenses, closure of the punctum, and in severe cases, tarsorrhaphy.

Metabolic Disorders

Numerous metabolic disorders in children, both congenital and acquired, can affect the cornea.

Corneal clouding may occur as a local manifestation of errors in metabolism. The two principal categories are mucopolysaccharidoses and mucolipidoses. Conjunctival biopsy may be of value in diagnosing the kind of storage disorder. Congenital glaucoma and interstitial keratitis can also cause corneal clouding. Corneal transplantation may improve vision, but clouding may recur in the graft.

Arcus juvenilis results from the deposition of lipids (cholesterol) in the corneal periphery. The arcus tends to appear during the early teen years and remains confined to the peripheral cornea. It usually has no effect on vision. The corneal deposits are usually permanent and do not resolve even if the blood lipid level returns to normal.

In *Fabry's disease*, patients develop characteristic corneal changes early in childhood that may be the first manifestation of this lipid storage disease. Lipid deposits in the cornea take the form of fine opacities in the epithelium, radiating from the central cornea to the periphery in a fanlike manner.

In *cystinosis* (Fanconi's syndrome), crystals of cystine are deposited in the cornea, conjunctiva, sclera, extraocular muscles, uvea, and retina. The crystals, evident by 6 to 15 months of age in the cornea, appear as needlelike, glistening dots throughout the entire thickness of the cornea.

Wilson's disease (hepatolenticular degeneration) is an autosomal recessive disorder of copper metabolism. The Kayser-Fleischer ring of the cornea is pathognomonic and may be the first sign of the disease. The ring contains copper and appears as a greenish golden annular opacity lying just inside the limbus in the deep layers of the cornea. Cataracts and retinal degeneration may coexist.

Band keratopathy, superficial deposits of calcium in the cornea, can occur secondary to other corneal disease (keratitis, alkali burns of the cornea), other ocular disease (chronic uveitis associated with Still's disease), or systemic diseases associated with increased serum calcium levels (hyperparathyroidism, vitamin D intoxication, renal failure, and sarcoidosis). Band keratopathy appears initially as a grayish white opacification of the superficial cornea at the nasal and temporal limbus. It eventually extends across the cornea in a band-shaped configuration. Holes in the degenerated area are characteristic. Treatment consists of preliminary curettage of the epithelium, followed by the application of a chelating agent such as ethylenediaminetetraacetic acid (EDTA). Improvement in vision can be dramatic, but the procedure may have to be repeated.

THE SCLERA

Blue Sclera

The normal sclera of young infants, being relatively thin compared with that of adults, is often mistaken for the true congenital anomaly of blue sclera. By the end of the first year, most infants show the normal porcelain-white color of the sclera. The anomaly of blue sclera is secondary to persistent thinning and alteration in the structure of the sclera, which allows the pigmented choroid to show through and gives the sclera a blue appearance. Blue sclera occurs in high myopia and in systemic disorders that affect connective tissue, such as osteogenesis imperfecta, Marfan's syndrome, and others.

Scleral Pigmentation

The normal sclera is white with occasional pigment spots present in varying amounts, depending on the general racial pigmentation of the person. Brown pigment may collect at the sites of exit of a main blood vessel and nerve from the sclera near the limbus, particularly in blacks, and may be mistaken for a foreign body or melanoma. The yellowish appearance of the sclera in jaundice is due to the presence of bilirubin in the overlying vascular conjunctiva. Only a minimal amount of bilirubin is found in the relatively avascular sclera.

Episcleritis

Inflammation of the episclera, or *episcleritis*, is a benign and recurrent disorder occurring in young adults. Edema and congestion of the episclera are often sectorial but may be diffuse or nodular. Ocular pain and mild uveitis are associated. The cause is usually unknown, although many patients have a family history of atopy. Episcleritis may be associated with rheumatoid and collagen diseases (5 percent), herpes zoster (7 percent), or gout (3 percent). Recovery usually occurs within 3 weeks without treatment, but topical corticosteroids can relieve pain and hasten resolution.

Scleritis

Scleritis is a more severe process than episcleritis, involving deeper and more diffuse destructive inflammation, even leading to significant thinning (27 percent of cases) and perforation of the sclera. Severe pain is the most prominent feature, and uveitis occurs in approximately 35 percent of cases. Adults in the fourth and fifth decades are most often affected, particularly those with some kind of connective tissue disorder such as adult rheumatoid arthritis or ankylosing spondylitis. Juvenile rheumatoid arthritis is more often associated with uveitis than with scleritis. Treatment with topical corticosteroids and nonsteroidal antiinflammatory drugs (NSAIDs) such as indomethacin are usually ineffective; systemic therapy generally is necessary. If long-term corticosteroid therapy is needed for recurrent or persistent scleritis, periodic examinations for cataracts and increased intraocular pressure is necessary. Surgery may be needed to reinforce the sclera if the thinning is pronounced and there is danger of perforation.

THE LACRIMAL APPARATUS

Dacryostenosis

Dacryostenosis, or congenital obstruction of the nasolacrimal duct, is manifested in newborns and infants by tearing (epiphora) and discharge. It occurs in 1 to 6 percent of newborns and is more common in firstborn children. Persistent tearing from dacryostenosis must be differentiated from infantile glaucoma. If a discharge is present, conjunctival and corneal disease must be excluded. Obstruction of the nasolacrimal duct is usually unilateral and secondary to failure of spontaneous atrophy of the thin membrane that separates the lower ostium of the duct and the inferior nasal meatus. Other causes include clogging of the duct with epithelial debris, a stricture of the bony canal, and redundancy of the nasal mucosa at the lower opening of the duct into the nose.

As a consequence of the obstruction, stagnation and infection from pyogenic bacteria, most often gram-positive, occur in the lacrimal sac (*dacryocystitis*). Dacryocystitis is accompanied by a tender swelling of the skin overlying the lacrimal sac and the adjacent eyelids. Pressure on the lacrimal sac causes reflux of pus from the punctum. Acute or chronic conjunctivitis and keratitis can occur together. The acute infection is treated with hot compresses and local or systemic antibiotics. Untreated or recurrent disease may go on to abscess formation with rupture through the skin and establishment of a draining sinus. Scarring of the lacrimal sac with obliteration of the lacrimal passages is a troublesome consequence of chronic infection.

Congenital obstruction of the nasolacrimal drainage system usually resolves spontaneously by 6 to 8 months, so during this period conservative treatment is advocated. The parents are instructed how to properly express material from the lacrimal sac by massage several times a day, and any infection is treated with topical broad-spectrum antibiotic drops (ointments are less likely to penetrate the nasolacrimal system). Topical corticosteroids are contraindicated, because there is no therapeutic rationale for their use and undiagnosed secondary ("steroid") glaucoma may result. Digital pressure over the nasolacrimal sac increases the hydrostatic pressure in the sac and causes rupture of the membranous obstruction at the bottom of the duct. When the obstruction fails to resolve by age 6 to 8 months, or if recurrent dacryocystitis intervenes and does not respond to two courses of intensive massage and topical antibacterial therapy, decompression of the lacrimal sac by nasolacrimal duct probing and irrigation is indicated. Brief, light anesthesia is recommended for this procedure. A single probing and irrigation is usually curative. If the nasolacrimal duct cannot be opened by probing, intubation of the nasolacrimal system with silicone tubing for a short period or dacryocystorhinostomy may be required to restore drainage of the tears into the nose.

Although obstruction of the nasolacrimal duct accounts for most tearing in infants, other conditions must be differentiated. Congenital mucocele is an obstruction of the upper portion of the lacrimal system. Resultant fluid accumulation causes distention of the lacrimal sac at birth. A tense blue-gray swelling is seen inferior to the medial canthal tendon. The diagnosis is aided by ultrasound. Treatment is immediate lacrimal system probing in the neonatal period. Other causes of lacrimal system outflow obstruction include canaliculitis (herpes simplex, chicken pox), punctal and canalicular agenesis, congenital fistula, trauma, craniofacial defects, and functional eyelid problems. Hypersecretion of tears without outflow obstruction is seen in infantile glaucoma, conjunctivitis, and corneal abrasions.

Dacryoadenitis

Acute *dacryoadenitis* presents clinically with pain and fullness over the lacrimal gland, edema and redness of the temporal half of the upper lid and conjunctiva, possible mucoid or purulent discharge, and orbital cellulitis. There may even be diplopia and restricted movements of the globe if the orbital lobe of the gland is involved. With eversion of the lid, the gland can be seen to be enlarged and inflamed. Frequently the cause is an associated systemic infection such as mumps, infectious mononucleosis, influenza, or an exanthem. Local causes are staphylococcal infection, trachoma, and herpes zoster. Treatment consists of appropriate systemic workup, local cultures, and cytology, followed by antibiotics (if indicated) and heat.

Trauma

Injuries to the nasolacrimal duct result from fracture of the orbit and lateral wall of the nose. Dacryocystorhinostomy will usually relieve the obstruction of the nasolacrimal duct; age is no barrier for this procedure. The canalicular system is most commonly avulsed by hooks or dog bites in children. Canalicular injury may not be recognized initially, and therefore an examination under anesthesia may be necessary to determine the extent of the injury. Primary repair of the severed canaliculus should be undertaken immediately with placement of a metal or Silastic stent in the severed canaliculus for 2 to 3 months.

Alacrima and Hypolacrima

Most newborns secrete tears in the first week of life, and within a few weeks normal rates of secretion are present. The reason we do not see newborn infants cry tears is that their lacrimal drainage system works efficiently, so tears do not spill over the cheeks. Persistent deficiency or absence of tearing (*hypolacrima* and *alacrima*) may be due to a neurogenic cause (secondary to brain damage), lacrimal gland aplasia, anhidrotic ectodermal dysplasia, or familial dysautonomia. In familial dysautonomia, decreased tearing is associated with anesthesia of the cornea that leads to corneal drying, erosion, ulceration, and scarring. Differential diagnosis can be helped by instilling methacholine (Mecholyl) (2.5 percent) or pilocarpine (0.06 to 0.125 percent). One drop repeated in 5 minutes will usually cause miosis after 30 minutes in patients with familial dysautonomia but not in normal eyes, a response consistent with parasympathetic denervation. Treatment is directed in all disorders at protecting the cornea with artificial tears, bland ointments, moisture chambers (airtight goggles), soft contact lenses, and tarsorrhaphy.

THE LENS

Congenital Anomalies

Microspherophakia is a bilateral condition of small and spherical lenses that are prone to subluxation as a result of weakened zonules. The presence of defective zonules leads to poor iris support resulting in a tremulous iris (iridodonesis). Pupillary-block glaucoma can occur secondary to anterior subluxation; this may be prevented by peripheral iridectomy. The increased curvature of the lens induces myopia. This lens anomaly may be inherited as an autosomal recessive or dominant trait, or it can occur as part of a syndrome such as congenital rubella, homocystinuria, aniridia, and Marfan's syndrome.

Lenticonus is an anterior or posterior conical protrusion of the central pole of the lens that produces a dark disc ("oil droplet") in the center of the pupil seen on ophthalmoscopy. This anomaly results in a marked disturbance of vision owing to irregular astigmatism or myopia and the frequent presence of lens opacities. Anterior lenticonus is often bilateral and may be a feature of Alport's syndrome. Posterior lenticonus is often unilateral and occurs more frequently in females than in males. Surgical removal may be necessary for useful vision.

Ectopia lentis refers to either subluxation or complete dislocation of the lens secondary to weak and absent zonular fibers. High refractive errors are usually evident (usually astigmatism in subluxation, hyperopia in dislocation). Ectopia lentis can occur in a wide variety of ocular and systemic syndromes, or it can be inherited as an isolated abnormality, usually with ectopic pupils. Superior bilateral symmetric subluxation of the lenses is found in about 75 percent of eyes with Marfan's syndrome by the fourth or fifth decade. Inferiorly subluxated lenses are the most frequent ocular complication of homocystinuria, occurring in nearly 90 percent of such patients. The ectopia is detected early in life, and almost one third of those patients eventually experience lens dislocation into the vitreous or anterior chamber. *Pupillary dilation should be avoided because it can precipitate dislocation and secondary glaucoma.* Associated ocular anomalies include congenital glaucoma, aniridia, megalocornea, and coloboma of the iris and choroid.

Cataracts

Congenital Cataracts

Congenital cataracts are usually present at birth, but they frequently are not discovered until some time during the first year of life. The terms *congenital cataract* and *infantile cataract* are, thus, synonymous. The degree of opacity varies widely from a small dot to total clouding of the lens. Although congenital cataracts are usually static, they may progress during childhood. Congenital lens opacities occur in less than 0.5 percent of live births and account for about 10 percent of blindness in preschool children. They are a common cause of amblyopia.

Congenital cataracts appear in a number of ways, depending on their laterality and density. Parents may notice decreased visual attention to environment, light sensitivity, decreased vision, or leukokoria if the cataract is dense. A wandering type of nystagmus may be noted if the cataracts are bilateral. A deviation of the eyes (strabismus) can be a clue, as can a systemic disorder. *Because early diagnosis is critical for visual rehabilitation, all infants must be checked routinely for cataracts.*

Congenital cataracts may be classified according to location of the opacity in the lens (i.e., polar, lamellar, nuclear), degree of opacity present (partial, immature and complete, mature), and cause. Partial cataracts involve only a portion of the lens (i.e., the nucleus), leaving part of the lens clear (i.e., the cortex). A partial cataract appears as a dark opacity surrounded by clear lens through which the red reflex is seen. Complete or mature cataracts may be present from birth or may result from the progression of partial cataracts. Complete opacification of the lens creates a white pupillary reflex (leukokoria).

Approximately 50 to 60 percent of congenital cataracts are idiopathic, but the remainder have diagnosable—and possibly treatable—causes, so careful ocular and systemic evaluation must be undertaken for all patients with congenital cataracts. Patients in whom a cause can be established can be categorized as shown in Table 14.1. Hereditary or familial cataracts are usually inherited as an autosomal dominant trait, and the cataract is nuclear in morphology. Autosomal recessive and X-linked heredity are rare.

Ocular disease can produce congenital or acquired cataracts. Cataracts may occur as part of a systemic disease or syndrome. For a list of the disorders and their causes refer to Table 14.1. Intrauterine infection with rubella frequently causes congenital cataracts. The cataract is noted at birth or during the first year of life and can be either nuclear or complete and either unilateral or bilateral. Microphthalmia, spherophakia, congenital glaucoma, mesodermal dysgenesis of the anterior segment, strabismus, and nystagmus are often present. Other intrauterine infections that may cause cataracts are varicella,

Table 14.1 CAUSES AND DISORDERS ASSOCIATED WITH CATARACTS IN CHILDREN

Heredity or familial secondary to ocular disease (complicated cataract)
  Congenital glaucoma, retinal detachment, retinoblastoma, retinopathy of prematurity, trauma, uveitis

Associated with ocular anomalies
  Aniridia, ectopia lentis, mesodermal dysgenesis of anterior segment, microphthalmia/microcornea, persistent hyperplastic primary vitreous, sclerocornea, coloboma, posterior lenticonus

Prematurity associated with systemic disease

Intrauterine infections
  Viral: Rubella, rubeola, smallpox, varicella, herpes simplex, herpes zoster, cytomegalic inclusion disease
  Bacterial: Syphilis
  Parasitic: Toxoplasmosis

Chromosomal aberrations: Trisomy 13,18, 21; monosomy 21 (Turner's syndrome); partial deletion 4p, 5p, 11p, 18q; ring syndrome 4, D, 21; partial duplication of 15q

Genetic and metabolic: Albright's syndrome, aminoaciduria (Lowe's syndrome), amyloidosis (primary), cholestanolosis (familial cerebrotendinous xanthomatosis), cretinism, diabetes mellitus, Fabry's disease, galactokinase deficiency, galactosemia, hepatolenticular degeneration (Wilson's disease), homocystinuria, infantile hypercalcemia, infantile hypoglycemia, infantile hypoparathyroidism, mannosidosis, Morquio's syndrome (MPS IV), pseudohypoparathyroidism, pseudo-pseudohypoparathyroidism, Refsum's disease

Dermatoses (syndermatotic cataracts): Atopic dermatitis, congenital ichthyosis, ectodermal dysplasia, Gorlin-Goltz syndrome, incontinentia pigmenti, Judassohn-Lewandowski syndrome, monilethrix, Naegeli's syndrome, Rothmund-Thomson syndrome, Schafer's syndrome, Sieman's syndrome, Werner's syndrome

Systemic syndromes: Aberfeld's (Schwartz-Jampel), Alport's, Apert's, Bonnevie-Ullrich, Cockayne's, Conradi's, craniofacial dysostosis, Ellis-van Creveld, Francois-Haustrate, Hallermann-Streiff, Hutchinson-Gilford, Lanzieri's, Laurence-Moon-Biedl, mandibulofacial dysostosis, Marfan's, Marinesco-Sjogren, Meckel's, Miller's (aniridia-Wilms' tumor), myotonic dystrophy, Nieden's, osteogenesis imperfecta, osteopetrosis, Pierre-Robin, Robert's, Rubenstein-Taybi, Sjogren's

Miscellaneous
  Drugs: Corticosteroids, vitamin D excess, chlorpromazine hydrochloride, naphthol or naphthalene, 2,4-dinitrophenol, triparanol (Mer-29), tetracycline
  Ionizing radiation

From Apt L, Gaffney WL: The eyes. In Rudolph AM, Hoffman JIE (eds). Pediatrics, 18th ed. Norwalk, CN: Appleton & Lange, 1987. Modified and reproduced with permission.

herpes simplex, cytomegalic inclusion virus, syphilis, and toxoplasmosis.

Acquired Cataracts

A host of *metabolic disorders* can produce cataracts. In galactosemia and galactokinase deficiency, cataracts are secondary to an increased level of blood galactose. In the first weeks of life the lens takes on an oil-droplet appearance, and later a nuclear or lamellar cataract develops. Some reversal of the opacities is possible if galactose is withheld from the diet early in life. Children with juvenile-onset diabetes can develop bilateral multiple anterior or posterior subcapsular snowflake dots over a network of vacuoles.

These opacities appear late in childhood or adolescence and are not usually visually significant.

Various *chromosome disorders* are associated with cataracts. Nearly all children with Down's syndrome have microscopic lens opacities (60 percent of young children and 100 percent of adolescents) that fall into four types: arcuate opacities along the equator of the nucleus (lamellar), sutural (lamellar), posterior polar, and acquired types secondary to other factors.

Drug-induced cataracts are seen in children on long-term systemic corticosteroid therapy for asthma, nephrotic syndrome, systemic lupus erythematosus, and juvenile rheumatoid arthritis. These cataracts are posterior subcapsular in type, and their development is related to dosage and duration of corticosteroid therapy. Because these cataracts may be reversible at an early stage, patients under treatment with systemic corticosteroids should be evaluated by slit-lamp examination yearly if the dosage is less than 10 mg prednisone per day, or at least every 6 months if the dosage is higher. The posterior subcapsular cataract will appear as a central black dot against the red reflex. If cataracts are diagnosed, the patient might benefit from a reduced dose of systemic corticosteroids or a schedule change in the therapeutic regimen. A patient being treated for bronchial asthma might benefit from the concomitant use of beclomethasone or cromolyn by inhalation.

The key to management of congenital cataracts is early diagnosis, early surgical removal, appropriate optical aphakia correction, and careful postoperative monitoring, especially for amblyopia. Vision rehabilitation is generally better in bilateral than in unilateral cataracts and in partial than in total cataracts, and poorer in patients with other ocular defects. If children with extensive or complete cataracts fail to receive foveal stimulation during the most sensitive 8 to 16 weeks of vision development, nystagmus usually develops in bilateral cases. Surgery, therefore, preferably should be performed before 8 weeks of age in an attempt to avoid

nystagmus and the concomitant amblyopia. The visual prognosis for a child with a unilateral congenital cataract is poorer than for one with bilateral cataracts, because even with early surgery optical correction and amblyopia prevention therapy are difficult. Spectacle correction produces a 25-percent magnification in the aphakic eye and thus prevents normal binocularity. Contact lens correction offers the best alternative to date for the development of functional acuity in the aphakic eye and some binocularity. The number of reports documenting good visual outcomes in patients who had neonatal surgery and appropriate postoperative care is increasing. The use of daily-wear soft contact lenses has made the postoperative care of infants with infantile cataracts easier and more successful. Better types of extended-wear soft contact lenses are being investigated and may become more popular and safer in the future (see Chapters 9 and 17). The use of intraocular lens implants is currently experimental in children. Other forms of treatment of childhood cataracts include prolonged dilation of the pupil with a mydriatic (not cycloplegic) and optical iridectomy. These treatments are more likely to be successful in patients with a clear lens periphery, as in hereditary zonular cataracts.

THE UVEA

Congenital Anomalies

Coloboma

The uveal tract, comprising the iris, ciliary body, and choroid, is the pigmented and vascular layer of the eye. The common defect, *coloboma*, is described above under the developmental anomalies of the globe. Anomalies include multiple pupils (polycoria), displacement of the pupil to one side of the center of the iris (corectopia), and small pupil (microcoria). Microcoria is also frequently associated with ophthalmoplegia. Unequal pupils (anisocoria) is an autosomal dominant trait present in about 25 percent of normal persons. Persistent pupillary membrane remnants are extremely common (80 percent) and may be associated with congenital cataracts.

Aniridia

Aniridia has been defined as a complete or partial absence of the iris. It is actually a misnomer. Most aniridia is bilateral. Vision is generally poor, but better visual acuity is sometimes encountered in some pedigrees. Nystagmus is probably related to macular hypoplasia. Optic nerve hypoplasia may be due to fewer neurons traveling from the hypoplastic macular area. Cataracts frequently develop. Corneal pannus is also encountered. Glaucoma often develops before adolescence and is difficult to treat medically and surgically. Associated systemic abnormalities are commonly absent.

Heterochromia Iridis

A difference in the color of the two irides (*heterochromia iridis*) may represent either hypopigmentation or hyperpigmentation of the abnormal eye compared with the normal one. When the lighter-colored eye is abnormal, Horner's syndrome, Waardenburg's syndrome, or iris atrophy, as in rubella embryopathy, may be suspected. A darker-colored abnormal iris can be due to siderosis, iris tumor, neurofibromatosis, or juvenile xanthogranuloma.

Ocular Albinism

Ocular albinism is an inborn error of metabolism caused by a disturbance in melanogenesis; it is inherited as a sex-linked or autosomal recessive trait. Like generalized oculocutaneous albinism, ocular albinism presents with striking changes in the iris, choroid, and retina. The iris is thin and devoid of pigment, which allows the red fundus reflex to be transmitted through the translucent iris. The choroid has little or no pigment exposing the choroid vasculature. Retinal pigment granules are pale and few, and the macula is hypoplastic on ophthalmoscopic examination. Patients have reduced but functional vision, nystagmus, marked photophobia, myopia, and astigmatism. Special contact lenses with an opaque iris painted on the surface are being used to reduce the light scatter in the eye in an attempt to improve vision. Skin biopsy is an accurate means of confirming the diagnosis, especially in blacks.

Tumors

Approximately 50 percent of all whites have pigment flecks on the iris surface; these flecks are not *tumors* and have no pathologic significance. More elevated and compact pigment areas on the iris are nevi, often appearing at puberty. There is no progression of these benign nevi, and they do not interfere with pupil function. Choroidal nevi are common and likewise do not impair visual function. Melanomas of the uveal tract are the most common intraocular tumors of adults, but they are rarely encountered in children.

Uveitis

Uveitis is an inflammation of the uveal tract. Children and adolescents account for only 8 percent of all patients with uveitis, but it often tends to go undiagnosed and leads to blindness. This occurs because uveitis in children is usually low grade and chronic, with few outward signs such as pain, redness, photophobia, and tearing. In fact, these patients are often seen not as a result of the signs or symptoms of uveitis but for the complications of amblyopia, band keratopathy, cataracts, or glaucoma. If uveitis is suspected, slit-lamp and dilated fundus examinations are essential.

Uveitis has been subdivided into two forms: granulomatous and nongranulomatous. In the former, the uveal tissue is believed to be actively invaded by specific organisms; the latter is considered to be an allergic response to an antigen that may have been elaborated locally or at a remote site. These distinctions are not hard and fast and they are often difficult to make. A more useful and clinically practical classification of uveitis emphasizes the site of involvement: anterior uveitis (iritis, iridocyclitis), peripheral uveitis (pars planitis, chronic cyclitis), and posterior uveitis (choroiditis, chorioretinitis).

Anterior Uveitis

Anterior uveitis in the pediatric age group is most often due to juvenile rheumatoid arthritis (JRA, Still's disease). Pauciarticular JRA with positive antinuclear factor (ANF) is associated with severe asymptomatic chronic uveitis most frequently in females, whereas pauciarticular JRA with negative ANF is associated with acute symptomatic (pain, redness, photophobia) iridocyclitis more often in males. The polyarticular form of JRA is less often associated with anterior uveitis. Iridocyclitis may predate joint disease by 2 to 10 years, and without proper therapy the incidence of serious sequelae is high and includes band keratopathy, posterior synechiae with distortion of the pupil, secondary glaucoma, and cataract. The only certain means of detecting iridocyclitis early is routine periodic slit-lamp examinations, initially in all patients with JRA, then every 3 months in patients with pauciarticular JRA and every 6 months in polyarticular JRA, until adulthood. Treatment, consisting of topical corticosteroids and mydriatic-cycloplegic agents, is effective in the majority of patients. Periocular or systemic corticosteroids and even immunosuppressive drugs may be required; however, an incapacitating vision loss can develop despite intensive therapy. Other less common causes of anterior uveitis in children are sarcoidosis, syphilis, herpes simplex and zoster, and trauma.

Peripheral Uveitis

Peripheral uveitis (pars planitis, chronic cyclitis) is a chronic nongranulomatous inflammation of the ciliary body that usually causes no symptoms except perhaps visual blurring or the awareness of floating black spots. In severe infections, vision is appreciably reduced, with macular edema, posterior subcapsular cataract, optic neuritis, visual vasculitis, or exudative retinal detachment. The causes are unknown. *Toxocara canis* has been reported occasionally to cause a similar chronic peripheral uveitis. Generally the disease is stationary or gradually improves over 5 to 10 years. Treatment with periocular or systemic steroids is given if macular edema develops. If steroids are ineffective immunosuppressive drugs or cyclocryotherapy may be tried.

Posterior Uveitis

Posterior uveitis in children is frequently caused by either toxocariasis or toxoplasmosis. Uveitis due to *T. canis* appears mainly between ages 4 and 8 years, the average age being 7.5 years. Infection is acquired by ingesting soil contaminated by *T. canis* ova deposited in dog feces, particularly puppies'. Less often a similar disease may be transmitted by cats. Ocular inflammation is usually unilateral and can take the form of a posterior pole granulomatous mass, a peripheral inflammatory mass with cyclitis, or other forms. Children come to the eye care practitioner because of strabismus, poor vision detected on vision screening, complaints of blurry vision, or leukokoria.

Diagnosing of ocular *toxocariasis* is usually based on the clinical history, ocular findings, and results of the serum enzyme-linked immunosorbent assay (ELISA) test for toxocara. Patient's stools are negative for ova and parasites, because the larva do not mature in the human gastrointestinal tract. Because ocular toxocariasis can be managed without enucleation, the distinction from retinoblastoma is most important. Ultrasonography, radiographs of the orbit for the detection of intraocular calcium, and computed tomography can be used to help make the diagnosis. Therapy for ocular toxocariasis, including corticosteroids, antihelminthics, laser photocoagulation, and vitrectomy, has had little success. The best treatment is prevention—deworming dogs and cats, better sanitation measures at children's playgrounds, and proper personal hygiene.

Toxoplasmosis is the most common proved cause of chorioretinitis. When a previously healthy mother acquires her first infection of *Toxoplasma gondii*, the fetus has about a 40 percent chance of being affected. Chorioretinitis is present in 80 percent of children with congenital toxoplasmosis and is bilateral in 85 percent of the affected group. The chorioretinitis is rarely active at the time of birth. The typical fundus lesion is seen as a healed, densely pigmented chorioretinal scar in the posterior pole, often in the macular area. In infants who have been spared the central nervous system damage of toxoplasmosis, the chorioretinitis may not become apparent until months or years later, when the child is seen because of strabismus or reduced vision from the macular scarring. About two thirds of affected individuals seen in later childhood or adulthood represent instances of relapsing recurrences of congenital infections. The acute focal satellite lesions arise within or adjacent to healed chorioretinal scars and cause a secondary inflammation of the vitreous and anterior chamber. Papillitis and papilledema may occur. The patient notes blurred vision and floaters. A recommended therapy for active chorioretinitis in children when the macula or optic nerve is threatened involves the combined use of pyrimethamine (Daraprim) and sulfadiazine.

THE RETINA

Leukokoria

Many congenital and acquired diseases of the retina can cause *leukokoria* (white pupil). The presence of leukokoria should evoke an awareness of the possibility of retinoblastoma because this malignancy is the most serious cause of a white pupil in children from the standpoint of both vision and life. Some of the more common fundus disorders that mimic retinoblastoma are discussed in this section. The differential diagnosis of leukokoria is summarized in Table 14.2. *Patients with leukokoria should be referred immediately to an ophthalmologist for diagnosis and treatment.*

Congenital Anomalies

Congenital *retinal fold* represents either a remnant of the primary vitreous or a variant of retinopathy of prematurity. It appears as a vascularized fold of retina extending from the

Table 14.2 DIFFERENTIAL DIAGNOSIS OF LEUKOKORIA

Developmental abnormalities
  Coloboma of choroid or optic nerve
  Congenital retinal detachment
  Congenital retinal fold
  High myopia
  Myelinated nerve fibers
  Norrie's syndrome
  Persistent hyperplastic primary vitreous (PHPV)
  Retinal dysplasia
  Warburg's syndrome
  X-linked retinoschisis

Neoplastic lesions
  Hamartoma and choristoma fundus (phakomatoses)
  Medulloepithelioma (diktyoma)
  Retinoblastoma

Retinal vascular anomalies
  Angiomatosis retinae
  Coats' disease
  Retrolental fibroplasia (retinopathy of prematurity)

Inflammatory conditions
  Endophthalmitis
  Toxocariasis
  Uveitis, including pars planitis

Trauma
  Massive retinal fibrosis
  Organizing vitreous hemorrhage
  Retinal detachment
  Intraocular foreign body

Other
  Cataract
  Corneal opacity

From Apt L, Gaffney WL: The eyes. In Rudolph AM, Hoffman JIE (eds). Pediatrics, 18th ed. Norwalk, CN: Appleton & Lange, 1987. Reproduced with permission.

optic disc to the equator of the lens. Congenital detachment of the retina can result. This disorder can be inherited as a recessive trait, occurring most often in one eye of full-term infants.

Myelinated nerve fibers are one of the most common developmental anomalies found on fundus examination. Myelinization fails to stop at the lamina cribrosa and appears on the retina as a glossy white patch adjacent to the optic disc. This patch follows the course of the nerve fiber layer of the retina and tapers off with feathered edges. Rarely, the myelinated nerve fibers may be extensive enough to cause leukokoria or lead to a mistaken diagnosis of papilledema. Vision is usually not affected, but relative scotomas do occur. Unilateral extensive myelinization of the nerve head and retinal fibers may be associated with ipsilateral myopia, strabismus, and amblyopia. Early detection and treatment of this set of abnormalities in infants can prevent or minimize the amblyopia.

Persistent hyperplastic primary vitreous (PHPV) is an eye abnormality caused by a failure of regression of the tunica vasculosa lentis. A white retrolental mass persists behind a lens which becomes cataractous. The contracting retrolental mass causes the ciliary processes to elongate, a characteristic feature. PHPV is almost always unilateral and presents in a microphthalmic eye. The retina is formed normally but could detach because of adherence to the retrolental mass. The natural history is one of progressive cataract formation with decreasing anterior chamber depth and resultant angle-closure glaucoma. Untreated eyes are lost because of intraocular hemorrhage, glaucoma, retinal detachment, and phthisis bulbi. In the past, vision was usually limited or absent, even when surgery was performed on the cataract and membrane. In recent years, however, the trend to doing surgery early in infants before changes in the lens and membrane have started to progress, coupled with the use of improved surgical instrumentation and techniques, has produced much better vision. For the best vision outcome, contact lenses must be fitted shortly after surgery and the power must be monitored very carefully (see Chapter 9). Diligent patching of the good eye must also be done to preserve vision in the affected eye. Since leukokoria is common in PHPV, it must be differentiated from retinoblastoma. Distinguishing features of PHPV are its oc-

currence in a microphthalmic eye (retinoblastoma is usually found in normal-sized eyes), the absence of calcium on radiographic study of the orbit, ultrasonography, computed tomography findings, and the clinical picture.

The eye findings in infants with *fetal alcohol syndrome* include tortuosity of the retinal arteries and veins, optic disc hypoplasia or atrophy, blepharophimosis, hypotelorism, ptosis, epicanthus, thickened eyebrows, and strabismus.

Coats' disease, or retinal telangiectasia, is considered a congenital anomaly of the retinal vessels that affects primarily young males and manifests itself unilaterally. The vascular abnormalities include large microaneurysms, irregularly dilated capillaries, and bizarre, sausage-shaped vessels. These telangiectatic anomalies are surrounded by retinal exudates and hemorrhages. A total exudative retinal detachment can occur with cataract, glaucoma, and phthisis bulbi. Early stages may respond well to laser photocoagulation or cryotherapy of surface vascular abnormalities. The cause is unknown, but some cases are associated with hypogammaglobulinemia.

Juvenile retinoschisis is an X chromosome–linked recessive disorder. The retina is split in the nerve fiber layer area. An elevation of the inner layer of the retinoschisis, usually in the inferotemporal quadrant, can be identified by indirect ophthalmoscopy. Retinoschisis is generally a bilateral, progressive, degenerative disorder. Vision initially may be moderately reduced but gradually decreases with age to end in the range of 20/200. Patients have bilateral cystoid macular edema with a typical appearance of radial folds that assume a spokelike configuration. In half of affected patients the macular changes are the sole pathologic finding. When this macular appearance is seen in a young male with or without reduced vision, the retinal periphery, especially inferotemporally, should be examined by indirect ophthalmoscopy. This disorder is one of the most common abnormalities responsible for unexplained vision loss in a young male patient and is easily overlooked. When retinal detachment occurs, it is treated in the customary fashion. Vitreous hemorrhages complicating the retinal detachment may require vitrectomy in addition to the retinal detachment repair.

Retinopathy of Prematurity

Retinopathy of prematurity (ROP) primarily affects infants weighing less than 1,700 grams at birth; the incidence is inversely proportional to birth weight. In the early 1950s this disease was discovered to be secondary to the toxic effects of oxygen therapy for premature infants with respiratory distress. Careful control of oxygen therapy did cause an initial decline in the incidence of the condition, but its persistence suggests that its causes are complex and must be secondary to factors in addition to high oxygen tension. Actually the incidence has increased in recent years, owing to the higher survival rate of extremely low-birth-weight infants, who happen to be at high risk for developing ROP.

The natural history of ROP begins in the temporal peripheral retina, which is the last part of the retina to vascularize. Initially a prominent white, circumferential, intraretinal vascular border is seen demarcating vascularized and nonvascularized retina. Subsequently the border enlarges and becomes elevated as a ridge. Later, arborizing vessels approach the border in brushlike fashion but do not extend beyond the border. This border represents an arteriovenous shunt and becomes pink. Fibrovascular proliferation extends posteriorly from the elevated border. Gradual resolution occurs at or before this stage in over 90 percent of patients. Patients in whom regression has occurred may still develop problems in later life, such as myopia, amblyopia, strabismus, and peripheral retinal degeneration. In the other 10 percent, a progressive cicatricial phase ensues with continued elevation of the vascular border, extension of the fibrovascular process into the vitreous, vitreous hemorrhage, peripheral retinal scarring, temporal dragging of the disc, vessels, and macula, and

partial retinal detachment. Patients with severe disease eventually show total retinal detachment, extensive fibrovascular proliferation with a retrolental white mass, and leukokoria.

A new classification system and a standardized method of recording and reporting the acute ophthalmoscopic changes seen in ROP have been developed recently by an international committee. It is now used in all ROP research and clinical investigations.

All infants weighing less than 1,700 g at birth should be screened routinely with indirect ophthalmoscopy, preferably with scleral depression after pupil dilation with 2.5-percent phenylephrine hydrochloride and 0.5- to 1.0-percent tropicamide. Infants with greater birth weights do not need routine screening unless there is a history of prolonged oxygen therapy or unusual clinical features. The optimum age for detecting ROP is 7 to 9 weeks after birth, because ROP rarely appears for the first time after 9 weeks and retinal detachment is rare before this time. The initial examination should be postponed until at least 1 month of age because the first signs of ROP do not appear before this age, earlier visualization of the fundus is difficult, and the risk of hypoxia or intracranial hemorrhage is minimal at this age. If ROP is identified the infant is reexamined at 1- or 2-week intervals until spontaneous resolution occurs. Once the peripheral retina is fully vascularized, no acute changes ensue. If cicatricial changes develop the patient must be observed indefinitely, as subsequent complications such as late retinal detachment, cataract, band keratopathy, and angle-closure glaucoma can occur. If the fundus examination is normal at 1 month of age, reexamination is indicated at age 2 to 3 months. Beyond this time, no new cases of retrolental fibroplasia have been reported and no further follow-up is necessary.

Until recently, no treatment has proved effective in progressive ROP. Vitamin E has been prescribed to reduce the severity of acute ROP, but serious side effects of high blood levels of vitamin E keep this mode of treatment experimental. A nationwide multicenter clinical trial on the use of cryotherapy to treat moderately severe cases of ROP has shown very encouraging results. Cryotherapy applied to the peripheral avascular retina (beyond the ridge) prevents formation of new vessels in the area. The results so far have indicated that twice as many eyes have improved after therapy when compared with a no-treatment group. It should be remembered that about 95 to 97 percent of infants identified with ROP never need treatment; the disease resolves spontaneously. Only a small proportion go on to develop stage 3 of the disease and require treatment.

Retinoblastoma

Retinoblastoma is a malignant tumor composed of embryonal retinal cells. It is the most common intraocular tumor in childhood, although it is rare (annual incidence, about 3.4 per million). The prevalence has apparently increased in the past three decades owing to an increase in the mutation rate. The current incidence is 1 in 20,000 live births, whereas sporadic disease occurs with a mutation frequency of 1 in 30,000 live births. Survivors transmit the defective retinoblastoma gene to their children by autosomal dominant inheritance. The tumor may be present at birth, but most are discovered before age 3 years, the average age at diagnosis being 17 months. Unusual features of this tumor include instances of spontaneous regression, multicentric origin, high incidence of secondary primary tumor, and atypical inheritance.

The heredity of retinoblastoma is complicated, but basically there are two kinds of retinoblastoma: hereditary, 40 percent of all cases, and nonhereditary, the remaining 60 percent. Hereditary retinoblastoma arises in one of three ways: inheritance from an affected parent by autosomal dominant transmission, inheritance from an unaffected gene carrier parent, or acquisition as a new germinal mutation from a normal parent.

About 10 percent of the hereditary cases of retinoblastoma have chromosomal deletion in the region of 13q14. Also, the esterase

D (ESD) gene is located at the region of 13q14. Because deletion carriers have cellular enzyme levels 50 percent of the normal value quantitation of ESD level has been used as an objective means of identifying carriers.

Hereditary familial occurrences are usually bilateral and account for 4 to 6 percent of all retinoblastomas. Usually the tumor is first diagnosed in one eye only, with the tumor appearing in the second eye later, even several years later. With reduced penetrance the probability of the tumor being transmitted by parents to a patient is 40 percent. The probability of transmission of the tumor by healthy siblings or healthy children of a patient is 70 percent. New germinal mutations produce bilateral tumors in most patients; only 10 to 15 percent of unilateral tumors are due to a germinal mutation. The mutation usually occurs at the time of egg or sperm formation, so the risk of recurrence is less than 5 percent. Nonhereditary tumors are sporadic and are mainly unilateral. There is a negligible risk among siblings of a person with unilateral retinoblastoma and descendants of a person with unilateral retinoblastoma (approximately 5 percent). The hereditary patterns would suggest that if a single instance of retinoblastoma appears in a family, each new member must be examined with mydriasis and general anesthesia at 3- to 6-month intervals in the first 2 years of life and subsequently every 3 to 6 months up to the age of 7 years. In addition, because of the frequent multicentric origin of the tumor or delayed appearance in the second eye, all treated patients must be examined periodically.

Retinoblastoma appears in the eye grossly as a pinkish white or cream-colored nodular mass. Histologically the tumor is composed of tightly packed, undifferentiated retinoblasts that may show variable degrees of differentiation toward rods and cones (rosettes and fleurettes). The blood supply is invariably inadequate, and patchy necrosis and degeneration with calcium deposition are characteristic. Because it is uncommon in children's eyes in any other condition, the demonstration of intraocular calcium on radiographic study is an important diagnostic sign.

The clinical characteristics depend on the stage of growth of the tumor at the time of its discovery. When the tumor is small and at the posterior pole of the eye, the initial sign may be strabismus secondary to impaired vision. Therefore, every young pediatric patient with strabismus should have a careful ophthalmoscopic examination. As the tumor grows, a creamy white pupillary reflex (leukokoria, cat's-eye reflex) develops, and the mass may be visualized easily. There is a tendency to seed other ocular tissues through the vitreous or subretinal fluid, which leads to secondary glaucoma, uveitis, endophthalmitis, and buphthalmos. Unusual presentations include hyphema, heterochromia, unilateral pupillary dilation, orbital cellulitis, and proptosis.

Early diagnosis is important because treatment in the early stages can be very effective and may preserve vision, and in some cases the baby's life. Several diagnostic points are worth emphasizing. Usually the eye harboring the retinoblastoma does not appear abnormal externally, is of normal size for age, and the anterior chamber is of normal depth. Transillumination of the eye reveals a solid tissue mass. The finding of calcium on high-resolution thin-section computed tomography of the orbit is characteristic of retinoblastoma and is seen in over 80 percent of tumors. A- and B-mode ultrasonography, computed tomography, and magnetic resonance imaging may be of particular help when visualization of the fundus is impaired. Optic foramen radiographs may show enlargement due to extension of the tumor along the optic nerve.

It must be emphasized that retinoblastoma is a true ocular emergency. Immediate referral to an ophthalmologist, preferably one experienced with retinoblastoma, is essential.

Retinoblastoma has a predilection for invading the optic nerve, and by extension it may reach the subarachnoid space and the brain. Intracranial extension is the most common cause of death. Local spread may also occur into the choroid, the orbit, and the lymphatics. Hematogenous metastases to bone (skull, ribs, humerus) are frequent; metastases to viscera and muscle occur less often.

The prognosis in retinoblastoma patients depends on the size and location of the tumor or tumors and the presence and degree of ocular and extraocular involvement. Prognosis has improved impressively over the past 25 years because of earlier discovery of tumors and improved methods of diagnosis and treatment. If the tumor is unilateral and small and the eye is treated promptly, the chance of survival is over 90 percent. Once the tumor has extended into the optic nerve, the cure rate decreases to about 50 percent. Survival decreases to 25 percent with extraocular extension. Overall mortality is 18 percent. Spontaneous regression occurs in only 1.8 percent of patients. Secondary primary tumors are found in 15 percent of survivors of bilateral retinoblastoma, with an average latent interval of 11 years.

Current treatment options include enucleation (primarily, especially in unilateral cases), radiotherapy (external beam from linear accelerator or local application of cobalt 60), photocoagulation, or cryotherapy.

Tapetoretinal Dystrophies

Retinitis Pigmentosa
Retinitis pigmentosa is a retinal pigmentary degenerative disorder inherited as an autosomal dominant, autosomal recessive, or sex-linked recessive trait, but only 50 percent of patients have a family pattern of inheritance. Characteristic symptoms are nyctalopia (night blindness), delayed dark adaptation, and constriction of the visual field leading to total blindness. In a well-developed disorder the appearance of the fundus is typical. The vessels are attenuated, and the disc is pale. Bone corpuscle–shaped pigment is scattered throughout the fundus adjacent to retinal blood vessels. Posterior subcapsular cataracts and cystoid macular edema occur in time. In early stages, abnormalities in the

electroretinogram (ERG) may predate visible changes in the fundus. In advanced disease the ERG is severely depressed or absent. Dark adaptation is also markedly abnormal. As a rule, incapacity does not develop until early adulthood, but signs and symptoms do appear early in childhood. When the onset occurs in childhood, the prognosis is poor and no treatment is effective. Retinitis pigmentosa may be associated with a number of systemic disorders, including Friedreich's ataxia, mucopolysaccharidoses, and syndromes such as Bassen-Kornzweig, Batten-Mayou, and others.

Pseudoretinitis Pigmentosa

A number of conditions can produce a pigmentary disturbance of the retina in the form of punctate, bone-corpuscular, or heaped-up masses of pigment. These are not true tapetoretinal dystrophies and are termed *pseudoretinitis pigmentosa,* or secondary retinitis pigmentosa. Included in this group are infections (e.g., syphilis, rubella, cytomegalic inclusion disease, influenza), obstetric trauma, radiotherapy, drugs (e.g., phenothiazines, chloroquine), trauma, and retinal vascular occlusion. Rubella retinitis requires special comment because of its frequent occurrence in congenital rubella along with microphthalmia, glaucoma, cataract, and nystagmus. It is usually bilateral and more advanced in one eye. The fundus shows a diffuse salt-and-pepper pigmentary mottling. The retinitis is inactive at birth, and little or no progression occurs. The effect on visual acuity caused by these pigmentary changes is difficult to estimate because of the ocular abnormalities that impair vision. Visual acuity seems to be unaffected in most patients, and color vision, visual field, and ERG are normal.

Leber's Congenital Amaurosis

Leber's congenital amaurosis is an infantile tapetoretinal degeneration characterized by connatal blindness (visual acuity less than 20/200), nystagmus, and a markedly reduced or absent ERG response. Inherited disease shows an autosomal recessive pattern. The fundus presentation is polymorphous and includes a normal appearance, arteriolar narrowing, optic disc pallor, bone-spicule pigmentation, local or diffuse chorioretinal atrophy, and various pigmentary changes. Associated neurologic and renal abnormalities have frequently been reported. The ERG is essential in differentiating Leber's amaurosis from blindness of central origin, especially in Leber's amaurosis with a fundus that appears normal.

Hereditary Macular Dystrophies

Macular degenerations occur in children both as primary disease and in association with a systemic disease.

Vitelliform degeneration of Best is an autosomal dominant macular dystrophy with onset at birth or in the first decade. Early, the fundus may show a well-defined, round, "egg-yolk" lesion in the macula, with good vision. Pigmentary degeneration of the macula with vision loss follows. The homogeneous appearance of the macular lesions fragments with time, and a pigmented "scrambled egg" appearance makes the lesions indistinguishable from other types of macular degenerations. No treatment is known.

Stargardt's disease is the most common form of macular degeneration in childhood. It is usually transmitted as an autosomal recessive disorder, but autosomal dominant cases have occurred. Decreased vision is usually noted between 6 and 20 years of age and may precede ophthalmoscopic changes. Loss of the normal macular reflex is followed by pigmentary mottling and occasional hemorrhages. Eventually the macula assumes a "beaten bronze" appearance with pigment clumping. Soft, amorphous flecks are scattered throughout the fundus, but the disorder may be overlooked because the peripheral lesions are overlooked. Vision decreases slowly but relentlessly and by the fourth decade is 20/200 or less. Total blindness does not occur, and the peripheral field remains fairly intact. The ERG examination and night vision are usually normal. If the retina shows yellow flecks randomly scattered in the fundus and macular atrophy is not present or occurs late, the disorder is called *fundus flavimaculatus.*

Retinal Detachment

Retinal detachment is rare in infants and is usually associated with ROP or intraocular tumors such as retinoblastoma. Older children may have had a hereditary disposition or prenatal ocular maldevelopment. Trauma, aphakia, high myopia, inferior temporal dialysis, lattice degeneration, uveitis, Coats' disease, and chorioretinitis may also be causative factors. It is important to examine the retina of any young patient after blunt injury because of the possibility of a long latency period between trauma and detachment and the inability of children to give a history of decreasing vision. A number of syndromes with juvenile retinal detachment have been reported, including Wagner's hyaloideoretinal degeneration (retinal detachment, cleft palate, flat facies) and Norrie's, Marfan's, and Ehlers-Danlos syndrome (see Chapter 18).

THE OPTIC NERVE

Congenital Anomalies

Optic nerve aplasia is a rare anomaly characterized by complete absence of the optic nerve and disc, ganglion cells, nerve fibers, and retinal blood vessels. It occurs when the mesoderm fails to be incorporated into the optic stalk, which normally takes place at the 4- to 10-mm stage. The affected eye is blind. Bilateral aplasia is more often associated with gross malformations of the globe and the brain. Unilateral aplasia is likely to occur in an otherwise healthy patient whose affected eye may have other intraocular and extraocular abnormalities.

Optic nerve hypoplasia is a reduction in the number of axons in the affected nerve. Some disorders result from a defect in the normal differentiation of the retinal ganglion cells in the 13- to 15-mm stage or a failure of their processes to reach the optic stalk by the 19-mm stage; others are due to transsynaptic degeneration of optic nerve fibers. In either instance the diagnosis presents little difficulty in the typical patient. The nerve head is small and gray, with a yellow peripapillary halo and ring of pigment (double-ring sign) corresponding to the normal size of the disc. Retinal vasculature is normal. Vision varies from normal to very poor and there is often an afferent pupillary (Marcus Gunn) defect. On radiographic study, the optic canal is smaller than normal. The diagnosis of lesser degrees of optic nerve hypoplasia can be difficult because the decrease in the size of the disc may not be obvious and vision may be only slightly reduced or unaffected. Measurement of the optic nerve head on enlarged fundus photographs can be helpful. The visual acuity level in optic nerve hypoplasia is usually stable. In unilateral disorders, serious central nervous system abnormalities are generally absent. The patient is typically seen because of strabismus and decreased vision. Functional amblyopia may be superimposed on an organic vision deficit. In bilateral disorders, particularly relatively severe ones, poor vision and ocular nystagmus are noted early in life, and associated neurologic and endocrine abnormalities are more common. Reported associated abnormalities include mental retardation and delayed development, seizures, deafness, cerebral atrophy, hemiparesis, ventricular defects, porencephalic cyst, hypopituitarism, hyperthyroidism, and diabetes insipidus. Bilateral optic nerve hypoplasia associated with agenesis of the septum pellucidum and growth hormone deficiency is known as de Morsier's syndrome, or septooptic dysplasia. Because of the high incidence of associated central nervous system abnormalities and endocrine problems, all patients with optic nerve hypoplasia (particularly if bilateral) need a complete neurologic work-up, including computed tomography or magnetic resonance imaging of the brain and long-term endocrine follow-up.

In *congenital tilting of the optic disc* the optic nerve head may be tilted at a 45-degree angle with the retinal vessels exiting from the disc in an abnormal fashion. This anomaly is notable because it can produce bitemporal visual field defects that are easily mistaken for a pituitary lesion, except that the field defect slopes across the vertical meridian in an irregular manner.

Optic nerve pits are congenital, and the stationary, dark gray holes are usually located on the temporal side of one disc. The involved optic nerve head is larger than normal. The pits are important clinically, because they may produce arcuate scotomas and macular edema with permanent loss of central vision.

Drusen (hyaline bodies) of the optic nerve head are white or yellow translucent spheres lying in front of the lamina cribrosa, especially on the nasal side of the optic disc. In young children they are inconspicuous, but within one or two decades the drusen become visible on the disc surface as shiny, refractile bodies that glow with indirect light. They may elevate the nerve head, simulating papilledema (pseudopapilledema). Ultrasonography usually is diagnostic. Fluorescein angiography is often a helpful diagnostic aid. In adulthood visual field defects may appear and progress slowly. Central visual acuity is usually unaffected. Drusen have an irregularly dominant inheritance, tend to be bilateral, and are not related to a specific refractive error. They occur predominantly in blond white children and do not occur in Asians or blacks. They have been described with retinitis pigmentosa, tuberous sclerosis, angioid streaks, and meningiomas but usually are not associated with other ocular disease.

Papilledema

Papilledema is a swelling of the optic nerve head due to multiple causes, including increased intracranial pressure. It is characterized by elevation of the optic papilla, with blurring of the disc margins, obliteration of the physiologic cup, venous congestion, loss of venous pulsations, splinter hemorrhages distributed radially around the disc margins, and edema of the adjacent retina producing an enlarged blind spot on visual field testing. Vision is rarely affected; when it is, it is usually only after the swelling has persisted for months.

Papilledema differs from papillitis (optic neuritis) by the absence of inflammatory signs (cells in the vitreous), central scotoma, and pain with movement of the eye. Both papilledema and papillitis may be confused with pseudopapilledema, in which an elevation of the disc is secondary to drusen, excessive glial tissue on the disc surface, hyperopia, and medullated retinal nerve fibers. Conditions that characteristically produce papilledema in children are brain tumors (craniopharyngioma, cerebellar medulloblastoma), head injuries, hydrocephalus, central nervous system infections (Guillain-Barré syndrome, meningitis), and pseudotumor cerebri.

Optic Neuritis

Optic neuritis is a disorder that refers to both *papillitis* (apparent on the nerve head) and *retrobulbar neuritis* (involvement of the nerve behind the globe with a normal-looking nerve head). It is characterized by profound loss of central vision, pain on movement of the eye or on retrodisplacement of the globe, central scotoma, depressed color vision, and afferent pupillary defect. In children optic neuritis is often bilateral, whereas in adults it is more frequently unilateral. Papillitis is more common in children than in adults.

Optic neuritis in children may result from inflammation in contiguous structures or from systemic infection. Optic neuritis secondary to meningoencephalitis is most common in children. The optic nerves can be involved by spread from orbital abscesses, cellulitis, and foci of infection in the teeth, tonsils, and sinuses. Optic neuritis can occur in infective diseases such as measles, chicken pox, mumps, pertussis, and poliomyelitis, as well as in infectious mononucleosis, influenza, and smallpox. Optic neuritis can also follow vaccination for viral diseases. Usually the optic neuritis appears 1 to 2 weeks after the onset of the infectious illness and resolves completely. Even with "full recovery," pallor of the disc and nerve fiber layer defects may be seen. Occasionally a significant vision loss results, with partial or complete atrophy of the nerve. Optic neuritis may also occur with various systemic diseases, ocular inflammation, drugs, or metabolic diseases. It may also be an early sign of multiple sclerosis.

Treatment of optic neuritis with corticosteroids (systemic, intraorbital) is controversial. Although steroids may hasten the return of vision in some patients, there is no proof that they change the ultimate vision prognosis.

Optic Atrophy

Optic atrophy indicates a permanent loss of function of part or all of the optic nerve. There is pallor of the nerve head due to decreased vascularity and gliosis. The optic nerve head of the normal infant is paler than that of the adult; therefore, a diagnosis of optic atrophy and blindness in the infant should be made only when one is sure of the findings. Kestenbaum's sign (a decrease in number of arterioles traversing the optic disk margin) may be a reliable indicator of optic atrophy. Normally, approximately 10 arterioles cross the margin of the disc, but Kestenbaum consistently noted fewer than seven in optic atrophy.

When optic atrophy in a child presents a difficult diagnostic problem, the investigation should include detailed family history; search for metabolic or toxic factors; accurate eye examination; radiography and computed tomography of the skull, orbits, and optic foramina; and other ancillary aids such as ultrasonography, arteriography, electroencephalogram, ERG, and visually evoked response. Many children with visual impairment exhibit self-mutilating behavior such as eye pressing. A useful clinical point is that children blind from optic nerve (i.e., optic atrophy) or cortical disease do not press their eyes whereas children blind from a retinal disorder are more likely to.

The most common cause of childhood optic atrophy is an expanding lesion of the orbit, frequently glioma of the optic nerve. This diagnosis should be suspected in a child who exhibits unilateral optic atrophy, proptosis, and radiographic evidence of an enlarged optic foramen. Optic nerve gliomas are most common in the first decade, particularly in girls. The gliomas grow slowly, do not metastasize, and usually follow a benign course with favorable survival rates. Their treatment is controversial; surgical excision, irradiation, and observation are options, depending on the specific case.

Hereditary forms of optic atrophy have a characteristic spontaneous and often sudden loss of vision of 20/200 or less with bilateral central scotomas. Thereafter vision deteriorates only slightly and is rarely lost completely. Leber's optic atrophy can develop at any age, but it usually begins in the late teens or early twenties, predominantly in males. It is usually described as an X-linked recessive condition, but there is evidence that it is not a simple or true X-linked recessive disease. True congenital optic atrophy can be transmitted as a dominant or a recessive trait. The dominant form is a relatively mild type in which the eyes appear normal at birth but decreased vision and optic atrophy progress through childhood and adolescence. Vision usually remains between 20/20 and 20/60 and rarely decreases to 20/200 or less. Some patients have night vision complaints. A blue deficiency is detected on color vision testing. Only the temporal or papillomacular part of the disc may appear atrophic. Central or paracentral scotomas are found. In the recessive form, severe bilateral vision loss and nystagmus are noted early in infancy. *The ERG is normal.* Severe color defects (achromatopsia) and restricted visual fields are common. On ophthalmoscopic examination the entire disc is atrophic and pronounced arteriolar narrowing is seen.

OCULOMOTOR NERVES

Third Cranial Nerve Palsy

Palsies of the third cranial nerve are uncommon in children. The child is seen with unilateral blepharoptosis, a larger pupil on the affected side, and an eye that is exotropic and hypotropic with poor ability to move up, down, or in. The palsy may be congenital or acquired. Episodic oculomotor palsy may be seen in children with ophthalmoplegic migraine. Pupil abnormalities are often absent in the congenital and migraine forms of third nerve palsy. Most of the acquired disorders in children are caused by increased intracranial pressure and trauma; some disorders occur after a viral infection. An isolated oculomotor palsy has limited localizing value. Associated neurologic signs are usually necessary for a topographic diagnosis. Most commonly there is selective paresis of the levator and superior rectus muscles together. Selective palsy of the superior rectus and the inferior oblique muscles (double elevator palsy) also can occur.

Fourth Cranial Nerve Palsy

Children with a *fourth cranial nerve palsy* have a head tilt to the shoulder opposite the affected eye, and the affected eye is higher than normal when the head is held straight because the main actions of the superior oblique muscle are depression and inward torsion. Most disorders are congenital in origin. The head tilt may be mistaken for torticollis and the infant may be referred to an orthopedist. Patching one eye may eliminate the head tilt. Eye muscle surgery should be performed to avoid permanent neck contraction and to promote fusion and normal development of binocular vision. The most common cause of acquired fourth nerve palsy is closed head trauma. A tumor in the region of the roof of the midbrain (e.g. pinealoma) can also cause fourth nerve palsy.

Sixth Cranial Nerve Palsy

Sixth nerve palsies are very common and are of special interest in children. They are characterized by inability to turn the eye out beyond the midline, diplopia, and head turn toward the side of the palsy. The more frequent acquired causes are purulent meningitis, in-

creased intracranial pressure, skull fractures, intracranial neoplasms (pontine glioma, posterior fossa astrocytoma, and medulloblastoma), viral infections, immunization inoculations, and idiopathic paralysis of the lateral rectus muscle, which may be recurrent. Sixth nerve palsy can have serious implications as a sign of serious intracranial disease, but if it seems to be an isolated occurrence without neurologic and systemic abnormalities, particularly if there is a history of recent febrile illness, it may be considered benign and can be observed closely without extensive neurologic testing. Either the palsy will resolve spontaneously within weeks to several months if benign, or additional neurologic or systemic disease will appear, which then calls for a detailed neurologic evaluation.

A special case of sixth nerve palsy follows middle ear infections or mastoiditis (Gradenigo's syndrome); osteitis of the petrous pyramid develops, producing diplopia, facial pain (due to fifth nerve involvement), and deafness. Sixth nerve palsy may occur transiently in a newborn due to birth trauma or other factors. The left side is more often affected. Full recovery of function within 6 weeks is the rule.

Duane's Syndrome

Duane's syndrome can be considered a form of sixth cranial nerve palsy because recent autopsy studies have shown aplasia of the sixth cranial nerve nucleus and fascicular portion of the sixth peripheral nerve, and in some cases aberrant innervation of the lateral rectus muscle by third-nerve fibers in the orbit. Abduction is limited or absent, and characteristically there is narrowing of the palpebral fissure and enophthalmos on adduction. An upshoot or downshoot of the affected eye may also occur during adduction. Electromyographic studies show anomalous innervation to the medial and lateral rectus muscles with co-contraction of both muscles on horizontal gaze. Almost all disorders are congenital, and 10 percent of those reported show a familial pattern. Usually visual acuity is normal and the eye is otherwise normal. The left eye is more frequently affected than the right, and both eyes are involved in about

20 percent of cases. The syndrome is slightly more common in females. Strabismus may or may not accompany the syndrome; esotropia is much more frequent than exotropia. Patients with no strabismus will have no head turn, but those with esotropia will turn the head in the direction of the affected eye and those with exotropia will turn the head to the opposite side to obtain fusion. Eye muscle surgery is not performed in patients with Duane's syndrome unless there is an objectionable head turn or strabismus in the primary position.

Seventh Cranial Nerve Palsy

Bell's palsy is a unilateral peripheral facial palsy of sudden onset arising from inflammation and swelling of the *seventh cranial nerve* within the facial canal of the petrous temporal bone. The cause may be viral. Lagophthalmos results, and exposure keratopathy can occur, necessitating the use of protective bland ointments, patching, soft contact lenses, or even tarsorrhaphy. Fortunately, recovery with complete return of eyelid function is usual within weeks to months.

Tic

A *tic* is a spasmodic repetitive blinking of the eyelids seen especially in children 5 to 10 years of age. It is usually psychogenic and it can be initiated voluntarily. It ceases when the child is diverted or sleeps. Rarely do refractive errors, chronic blepharitis, or conjunctivitis cause tics. Tics tend to abate with time, especially in childhood, if little attention is paid to them by doctors, teachers, and parents and if the causes of emotional tension are managed.

MOTILITY DISORDERS SECONDARY TO BRAIN STEM LESIONS

Parinaud's Syndrome

Parinaud's syndrome results directly from lesions in the vicinity of the upper midbrain (near the superior colliculi) or indirectly from conditions that elevate the pressure in the third ventricle. The characteristic signs are paralysis of upward gaze, poor convergence and accommodation, retraction nystagmus with attempted upward gaze, failure of the pupil to react to light with preservation of reaction to near objects, and lid retraction (Collier's sign). The most common causes of this syndrome include pinealoma, internal hydrocephalus, third ventricle tumor, aqueduct stenosis, trauma, encephalitis, syphilis, and congenital defect.

Skew Deviation

Skew deviation is any acquired vertical imbalance of the eyes (hypertropia) not due to extraocular muscle or nerve lesions. It indicates supranuclear or vestibuloocular damage from a lesion in the brain stem, cerebellum, or vestibular apparatus. Brain stem contusion or tumor and posterior fossa tumor or injury are the most frequent causes. The low eye is often, although not invariably, on the side of the lesion. Skew deviation may be associated with the Arnold Chiari malformation. It often is seen transiently in otherwise healthy newborns.

Ocular Motor Apraxia

Ocular motor apraxia is a defect in volitional horizontal saccades that appears in the early months of life. The affected child, usually a boy, thrusts the head laterally, thereby stimulating vestibular centers, which compensates for the defect in voluntary horizontal gaze movements as the child attempts to move the eyes to the desired point of fixation. An overshoot of the head occurs and when the desired position of the eyes is reached, the child jerks the head back, often concurrently blinking the eyes. In young infants, the thrusts are absent because of lack of head control, and this can lead to the erroneous impression that the infant is blind. In these patients the visually evoked response, which is normal, can offer an important diagnostic clue. The site of the underlying lesion is unknown. A delay in myelination of the ocular motor pathways for conjugate gaze has been suggested. The congenital form of this disorder tends to subside during the first and second decades. Affected children may be otherwise normal or may have other neurologic disorders such as hydrocephalus or brain stem or posterior fossa tumors, so a neurologic examination, including computed tomography or magnetic resonance imaging, is indicated in most patients.

Ocular Myoclonus

Ocular myoclonus, or dancing-eye syndrome, is an unusual form of nystagmus that follows encephalitis. Bilateral intermittent bursts of high-frequency, to-and-fro saccades (no slow phase) tend to be the same frequency in all affected persons. Mainly horizontal, these jerk movements persist during sleep.

Opsoclonus

Opsoclonus consists of bizarre, chaotic conjugate eye movements that occur in young patients after an acute febrile illness or in unconscious patients with encephalitis or brain stem disease. The to-and-fro oscillations are irregular and nonrhythmic horizontally and vertically. An awake person may have to close the eyes to reduce the awareness of ocular movement. Truncal ataxia may be associated. The illness usually clears spontaneously in a few weeks to months if there is no major underlying disease. Opsoclonus is a major feature of Kinsbourne's infantile myoclonic encephalopathy. This syndrome, characterized by opsoclonus, cerebellar ataxia, hypotonia, and myoclonic jerks of the face and body, is frequently associated with neuroblastoma.

NYSTAGMUS

Pendular Nystagmus

Pendular nystagmus is often referred to as ocular or sensory nystagmus because it is secondary to some binocular impairment of vision early in life (before 2 years) that pre-

vents the development of normal fixation reflexes. Loss of binocular vision between ages 2 and 6 years can lead to pendular nystagmus, but usually does not. After age 6 years binocular loss of vision does not lead to nystagmus. The nystagmus is usually horizontal and remains so on vertical gaze, but on lateral gaze converts to jerk nystagmus with the fast phase in the direction of the gaze. Causes include congenital anomalies of the optic nerve (hypoplasia, optic atrophy), bilateral failure of normal macular development (albinism, aniridia, high myopia, total color blindness), disorders of the macula as in chorioretinitis or coloboma, and congenital opacities of the cornea or lens.

Latent Nystagmus

Latent nystagmus is a special form of jerk nystagmus elicited by covering one eye. The fast component is in the direction of the occluded eye. Strabismus, frequently esotropia, may be present.

Congenital Nystagmus

Congenital nystagmus may be pendular or of the jerk variety. Usually it is pendular over a narrow range of gaze and jerky elsewhere. Congenital nystagmus is present at birth, but usually it is not detected before age 2 or 3 months, when fixation and conjugate movements develop. The nystagmus is almost always horizontal and invariably bilateral. Although hereditary disorders have been described (X-linked recessive or dominant), most congenital nystagmus is sporadic and of unknown cause. Children with isolated congenital nystagmus may have subclinical albinism or a form of albinoidism. An important characteristic of congenital nystagmus is that it remains horizontal in vertical gaze; the pendular type also converts to jerk nystagmus on lateral gaze. Nystagmus caused by an acquired brain stem lesion is often upbeating in upward gaze and downbeating on downward gaze. Frequently, especially in patients with congenital jerk nystagmus, there is a position of gaze in which the nystagmus is greatest and one in which it is least (null point). The child may develop a head turn or tilt to take advantage of the eye position with least nystagmus, for in this position the visual acuity is best. When the position of least nystagmus is small, yoked prisms (prisms with the bases in the same direction, i.e., bases left or right) can be used to move the null point to the primary position, thus eliminating the head turn. When the position of least nystagmus is in extreme gaze with a marked head turn, extraocular muscle surgery can be performed to place the null point in the primary position. Contact lenses have been of limited value in reducing the amplitude and frequency of the nystagmus; however some patients report a subjective improvement in visual acuity when using contact lenses. Congenital nystagmus is characteristically variable. It can be quite violent in association with excitement or stress, and it may be absent when the child is relaxed or sedated. Almost invariably there is some visual impairment, but near vision may be remarkably good. Perhaps this is because convergence often reduces the nystagmus amplitude and frequency.

Acquired Nystagmus

Acquired nystagmus usually is of the jerk type and secondary to lesions in the vestibular apparatus, cerebellum, brain stem, or chiasm. Peripheral vestibular disease (labyrinthine) produces horizontal and rotary nystagmus with vertigo. Vestibular nuclear lesions produce horizontal, rotary, or vertical nystagmus with the fast phase toward the diseased side. Brain stem lesions often cause vertical nystagmus. Cerebellar lesions are associated with nystagmus to the same side as the lesion. Chiasmal glioma typically is seen with monocular nystagmus and optic atrophy.

Spasmus Nutans

Spasmus nutans, an acquired disorder, consists of the clinical triad of head bobbing (or nodding), head tilt (torticollis), and nystagmus. Head nodding often precedes the nystagmus; the abnormal head position is the most variable feature of the entity. Nystagmus is more often bilateral than unilateral

and is characterized by rapid, fine, pendular, asymmetric horizontal movements (quiverlike) that vary in different directions of gaze. Nystagmus may disappear when the head is supine. Affected infants are normal. Generally the onset is between 4 and 12 months of age and the condition resolves spontaneously by 36 months. The cause and pathogenesis are unknown. Occasionally manifestations suggestive of spasmus nutans are seen in a patient who has a glioma in the region of the optic chiasm or hypothalamus. Complete eye examination and neurologic evaluation, including computed tomography or magnetic resonance imaging, are therefore advisable.

OCULAR MYOPATHY

Myasthenia Gravis

Myasthenia gravis may occur in a transient form in an infant whose mother has the disease. Paresis of the levator muscle may be the initial sign of myasthenia gravis. Ptosis that develops at any age without pain or pupillary abnormality or the appearance of an atypical ocular muscle imbalance requires exclusion of myasthenia gravis. In addition to the myopathies, the differential diagnosis of acquired ptosis in childhood includes tumors of the orbit or eyelid, neurofibromatosis, third nerve palsy, trauma, and acquired Horner's syndrome.

External Ophthalmoplegia

Chronic progressive external ophthalmoplegia is a bilateral, usually symmetric, gradual external ophthalmoplegia (pupil and accommodation are not affected) and ptosis. In 50 percent of patients there is a family history, and transmission is usually dominant. Occasionally the disorder may be congenital, but it usually begins in childhood or adolescence. Associated findings include retinitis pigmentosa (frequently involving only the posterior pole with a normal electroretinogram), spinocerebellar atrophy, cardiac arrhythmias, weak face and pharyngeal muscles, pancreatic insufficiency, and testicular atrophy. Ptosis surgery must be avoided because of the inability to close the lid.

Myotonia Congenita

Myotonia congenita or Thomsen's disease is an autosomal dominant disease that manifests itself before 5 years of age. It has been regarded as the congenital form of myotonic dystrophy. Systemic manifestations are myotonia (tonic spasm), primarily of muscles of the upper and lower extremities in association with muscle hypertrophy and weakness, and a pronounced delay in relaxation of contracted voluntary muscles. The eyelids also fail to open for a few seconds after sudden closure. Ptosis and sluggish extraocular muscles or paresis may be seen. Eye signs are infrequent.

THE PUPIL

Amaurotic Pupil

An *amaurotic pupil* has no direct response to light, no consensual response in the opposite eye, and an intact consensual response in the blind eye. This results from profound deficiency of vision in one eye due to extensive retinal or even mild optic nerve disease.

Afferent Pupillary Defect

A sensitive indicator of optic nerve dysfunction is the *afferent pupillary defect* (Marcus Gunn pupil). This pupil abnormality can be demonstrated by the swinging flashlight test: with the patient looking at a distant target, the flashlight is moved back and forth rhythmically from pupil to pupil. Both pupils constrict to direct light shone into the normal eye, but when the light moves to the affected eye, both pupils slowly dilate.

Light-Near Dissociation

Light-near dissociation of the pupillary reaction consists of a decreased or absent response to direct light with a good reaction to

a near stimulus. Causes include Parinaud's syndrome, pinealoma, hydrocephalus, diabetes mellitus, encephalitis, syphilis, and vision loss.

Fixed Dilated Pupil

Fixed dilated pupils are often due to inadvertent instillation of an atropine-like drug into the eye. Instillation of pilocarpine (1 percent) will differentiate drug-induced mydriasis (no pupil constriction) from one with neurologic cause.

Adie's Tonic Pupil

Adie's tonic pupil occurs unilaterally, usually in females, often during the teen years. Early the pupil is dilated and reacts poorly to light, both direct and consensual. The near response is slow and tonic (pupil remains constricted long after the patient has discontinued the accommodative effort). This light-near dissociation is due to an abnormality in the ciliary ganglion or short ciliary nerves (exact cause unknown). Accommodation is impaired, with blurred near vision. About 50 percent of patients recover full accommodation within 2 years. The pupil becomes smaller but retains its poor light response, with slow and tonic near response. In the Adie syndrome, the iris sphincter has undergone denervation and exhibits the phenomenon of denervation hypersensitivity to dilute cholinergic agents. One drop of pilocarpine (0.06 to 0.125 percent) or methacholine (Mecholyl) 2.5 percent instilled into both eyes and repeated after 5 minutes will usually cause more miosis of the affected eye after 30 minutes.

Horner's Pupil

Horner's pupil is part of a syndrome of ptosis (usually mild), miosis, and anhidrosis of the ipsilateral side of the face caused by the interruption of sympathetic pathways to the eye. Conjunctival hyperemia and elevation of the lower eyelid (Kearn's sign) suggest that the disorder occurred early in infancy, frequently from birth trauma. The pupil in

Horner's syndrome dilates poorly to cocaine. Pharmacologic testing with topical cocaine 4 percent and hydroxyamphetamine (Paredrine) 1 percent confirms or denies the diagnosis and helps localize the site of the lesion. Failure of the pupil to dilate after a drop of 1-percent hydroxyamphetamine is instilled indicates third-order neuron (superior cervical ganglion or postganglionic fiber) Horner's syndrome. The Paredrine test can separate third-neuron Horner's from first- (central) and second-neuron (preganglionic) Horner's, but no pharmacologic test can differentiate first- from second-neuron syndrome. A complete neurologic evaluation is indicated to rule out serious intrathoracic, cervical, or intracranial disease.

Paradoxic Constriction

Paradoxic constriction of the pupil to darkness is unique to children with retinal disease and is seen in congenital stationary night blindness of X-linked or autosomal recessive type, congenital achromatopsia, and optic nerve hypoplasia. If an infant has vision loss, nystagmus, and this pupillary sign, the cause is in the retina.

GLAUCOMA

Congenital Glaucoma

Congenital or infantile glaucoma is rare (one in 10,000 live births). Most disorders are sporadic, but genetic transmission does occur with variable penetrance. Most genetic disorders are autosomal recessive, but autosomal dominant transmission does occur. For this reason, siblings and children of patients with infantile glaucoma are at significant risk and must be checked. Most disorders (75 percent) are bilateral and are apparent at or shortly after birth. Males are affected more frequently than females (65 : 35). The cardinal symptom of infantile glaucoma is photophobia. This light sensitivity may be so extreme that infants will shield their eyes from bright light by hiding their face in a pillow. Usually there is associated blepharospasm and tear-

ing, which may lead to the mistaken diagnosis of dacryostenosis and conjunctivitis. The characteristic signs are increased intraocular pressure (usually worse in one eye if bilateral), edema and slight congestion of the conjunctiva, corneal haziness due to edema, increased diameter of the cornea (greater than 11 mm in the newborn or 12 mm in the first year of life), horizontal linear white opacities in the cornea (tears in Descemet's membrane), deep anterior chamber, and cupping and atrophy of the optic nerve. Because of the distensibility of the infant's eye in the first 3 years of life, enlargement of the globe may occur; thus, the name buphthalmos (ox eye) is sometimes given to the disease. Unilateral enlargement of the globe from high myopia (quiet eye with no corneal haze and normal intraocular pressure) and megalocornea (normal intraocular pressure) must be differentiated. In addition, any of the other causes of corneal opacity in infants must be considered.

The increase in intraocular pressure results from interference with outflow of aqueous humor from the anterior chamber angle caused by developmental anomalies in the angle structures. The anatomic defect is trabeculodysgenesis associated with anterior insertion of the iris on the scleral spur. The characteristic gonioscopic finding is either a crowded angle, sometimes with anomalous persistence of a membrane covering the trabeculum (Barkan's membrane), or thick iris processes covering angle structures. When passage of fluid out of the eye is impaired, pressure increases, distending the coats of the eye and producing the clinical picture of glaucoma.

Topical and systemic medications (miotics, epinephrine, acetazolamide, timolol maleate) are relatively ineffective in permanently lowering pressure in infantile glaucoma, so *early surgical treatment is essential*. The initial surgical procedure is usually goniotomy. Alternative operations are trabeculotomy and trabeculectomy. In these procedures, an opening is made in the trabecular meshwork to allow aqueous humor to drain from the eye. Occasionally the procedures must be done several times to obtain an adequate opening. In uncomplicated glaucoma, early surgery often is successful in controlling the intraocular pressure. Cyclocryotherapy to reduce aqueous inflow is ordinarily a last resort to control the pressure.

The visual prognosis in infantile glaucoma depends on the age at onset (the earlier the onset, the worse the prognosis), the amount of myopia induced by enlargement of the eye, the degree of corneal scarring, the extent of atrophy of the optic nerve, and the presence of lens opacification or other injury to the eye secondary to surgical trauma. Frequently the more severely involved eye becomes exotropic with time, less often esotropic, and it may be amblyopic. Usually the pressure in one eye can be controlled, and this eye can maintain satisfactory visual acuity. Early amblyopia therapy, including correction of any refractive error, is essential.

Juvenile Glaucoma

Juvenile glaucoma is a form of open-angle glaucoma that occurs early (usually after 3 years and before 20 years of age). It is seen most often in myopes and sometimes is inherited as an autosomal dominant trait with high penetrance. Because juvenile glaucoma is rare and is seen late in childhood, it can be easily overlooked or underdiagnosed until corneal and optic nerve damage are advanced.

Steroid Glaucoma

Prolonged topical or systemic corticosteroid therapy can produce severe *steroid glaucoma* that is often refractory to topical antiglaucoma therapy even after the corticosteroids are discontinued. The clinical picture may be identical to primary infantile glaucoma. All steroid-dependent children should have periodic eye examinations, not only for tonometry but also to check for posterior subcapsular cataract formation. *It is because of steroid-induced glaucoma that indiscriminate use of corticosteroids in the treatment of blepharitis or conjunctivitis should be avoided.*

THE ORBIT

Exophthalmos

The most frequent sign of disease of the orbit is *proptosis*, forward protusion of the eye caused by a retrobulbar mass. Exophthalmos is often used synonymously, but it is probably best used with reference to the condition seen in hyperthyroidism. A mass behind the eye may press on the optic nerve, producing papilledema and eventually optic atrophy. Extraocular movements may be impaired by involvement of nerves or direct interference with muscle action, which produces diplopia. Retinal striae may be visible as faint parallel lines extending temporally from the optic disc. Edema of the lids and chemosis are accompanied by variable degrees of orbital congestion. The cornea can suffer exposure damage if lid closure is inadequate. If the tumor is in the anterior half of the orbit, it may be palpated through the lids. Some orbital tumors may produce a bruit.

The type of proptosis may give a clue to the cause. Intermittent proptosis is often due to a varix or vascular tumor in the orbit. Pulsating proptosis may result from an orbital aneurysm, meningocele, or carotid-cavernous fistula. The reducibility of the proptosis can be helpful. In general, inflammatory or malignant tumor masses are not compressible and do not allow the eye to be pushed back into the orbit.

The degree of proptosis can be appreciated by viewing the eyes from above and behind by looking over the brow of the patient, but measurements with an exophthalmometer should be taken because visual estimates can be misleading. Pseudoexophthalmos can be produced by a number of conditions, including lid retraction, shallow orbits, buphthalmos, and high myopia. The average distance from the lateral orbital margin to the cornea is about 16 mm. A difference of more than 2 mm between the two eyes is considered significant. The evaluation of proptosis frequently includes radiographs of the orbits and optic foramina, orbital venography or angiography, ultrasonography, and computed tomography. A biopsy of an orbital mass may be necessary for diagnosis. The common causes of proptosis in children are listed in Table 14.3.

Inflammatory Diseases of the Orbit

Infections of the lids and orbit are potentially serious diseases that can extend to involve the eye or central nervous system and even lead to death. Two types of cellulitis are distinguished.

Preseptal Cellulitis

Preseptal (periobital) cellulitis involves the eyelids and surrounding tissue anterior to the orbital septum without involving the eye or orbital contents. The globe has full range of motion and vision is unimpaired. This type is characterized by tenderness, erythema, and edema of the lids and adjacent face, and drainage from a wound or the conjunctiva may be present. Because the inflammation is anterior to the septum, it does not pose the same risk as orbital cellulitis and generally has the same course and prognosis as cellulitis of the face and neck. The most common cause in children under 5 years is *H. influenzae* type B. Frequently there is an associated upper respiratory infection or otitis media in affected children.

Preseptal cellulitis should not be considered a benign disease. Infections caused by virulent organisms may enter the bloodstream and progress to orbital and intracranial involvement. Therefore most patients are hospitalized for treatment.

Bacteriologic studies involving the conjunctiva, nasopharynx, and blood (Gram-stained smears, cultures, antibiotic sensitivity tests) should be obtained. Radiography and computed tomography of the orbital and sinus areas are ordered if there is any indication of orbital inflammation, sinusitis, fracture, or foreign body. If a fluctuant mass is present, surgical drainage is performed and smears and cultures of the drained material are taken. If no area of fluctuation is present, percutaneous aspiration of the swollen area, with smear and culture of the aspirated material, should be considered for possible detection of the causative organism. If a causative organism cannot be found, broad-spectrum antibiotic therapy is recommended until results of bacteriologic studies are returned. At present full parenteral doses of a penicillinase-resistant penicillin such as oxacillin or nafcillin and chloramphenicol are given. Antibiotic therapy usually is given for 1 to 2 weeks. Appropriate antibiotics may

---

Table 14.3   CAUSES OF PROPTOSIS IN CHILDREN

Developmental
　Craniosynostosis
　Craniofacial dysostosis
　Mandibulofacial dysostosis
　Meningocele
　Encephalocele

Neoplastic
　Primary
　　Hemangioma
　　Lymphangioma
　　Rhabdomyosarcoma
　　Dermoid cyst
　　Glioma of optic nerve
　　Inflammatory pseudotumor
　Secondary and metastatic
　　Lymphoma
　　Leukemic infiltration
　　Neurofibroma
　　Retinoblastoma
　　Neuroblastoma
　　Ewing's sarcoma
　　Reticuloendotheliosis
　　Juvenile xanthogranuloma

Traumatic
　Orbital hemorrhage
　Fracture

Inflammatory
　Orbital cellulitis
　Mucocele

Metabolic
　Hyperthyroidism

From Apt L, Gaffney WL: The eyes. In Rudolph AM, Hoffman JIE (eds). Pediatrics, 18th ed. Norwalk, CN: Appleton & Lange, 1987. Reproduced with permission.

be given orally when there is clear clinical improvement.

Orbital Cellulitis

Orbital cellulitis is rare in young children and occurs primarily in older children. It is characterized clinically by orbital pain, ophthalmoplegia, decreased vision, proptosis, and chemosis of the conjunctiva. The usual cause is extension of infection from paranasal sinusitis, particularly the ethmoid sinuses. Other causes include expansion of processes from adjacent structures other than paranasal sinuses (facial cellulitis, local trauma, dental abscess), ocular and orbital disorders (rhabdomyosarcoma, dermoid cyst rupture), or conditions secondary to systemic disease (bacteremia, viremia). *It is imperative that orbital cellulitis be recognized promptly and treated aggressively.*

Progressive inflammation in the orbit may lead to decreased vision or blindness. Extension of the process may result in meningitis, central nervous system abscess, and death from cavernous sinus thrombosis. Treatment is carried out in the hospital. Bacteriologic studies, orbit and sinus radiographs, and orbital computed tomography, as described for preseptal cellulitis, should be obtained. If, on admission, Gram-stained smears of material gotten from the nose and throat, infected sinus, or surgical drainage of an acutely compromised orbit are *not* informative for selection of appropriate initial antibiotic therapy, broad-spectrum antibiotic therapy is given, as for preseptal cellulitis. Results of cultures and antibiotic sensitivity studies may dictate a change in the choice of antibiotics. Treatment usually is given for 2 to 3 weeks or for at least 7 to 10 days after the patient is afebrile and definite clinical improvement has been seen.

TUMORS

Capillary Hemangiomas

Capillary hemangiomas are the most common vascular anomaly of the orbit in children. They are nonheritable, benign developmental vascular tumors appearing at birth or during the first 2 months of life. Girls are affected more often, and low-birth-weight infants are predisposed. These hemangiomas occur in the orbit (usually anterior) or superiorly in the eyelids. Approximately one third have periocular cutaneous involvement in the form of a raised red lesion called a strawberry mark. In the absence of this mark, hemangiomas can be diagnosed by the presence of a dark red or bluish discoloration of the subcutaneous tissue and a change in size on crying. Orbital radiographs show an increased orbital volume without bone erosion typical of inflammatory disease and other tumors of the orbit. Computed tomography and ultrasonography may be helpful in the differential diagnosis of space-occupying lesions and in localizing the lesion.

Shortly after birth the hemangioma tends to grow for a while, usually 3 to 6 months. It then stabilizes for a year or more and undergoes spontaneous involution. Resolution is complete in 66 percent of patients by age 4 years and up to 76 percent by age 7 years. Complications are frequent and include ptosis, amblyopia, astigmatism, strabismus, anisometropia, and optic nerve compression. Therapy has been variably successful, so it is fortunate that most patients can be managed by careful observation alone. Treatment is indicated when the hemangioma seriously distorts and disfigures the lids and brow, when it occludes the palpebral fissure and obstructs vision, or when vision is threatened by optic nerve compression. Surgical excision of these tumors is difficult and is often used as a last resort. At present the preferred method of management is intralesional injections of corticosteroids if the tumor is accessible. The treatment may be repeated once or twice at 1- to 3-month intervals. Other modes of therapy to reduce tumor size include systemic steroids, low-dose superficial irradiation, photocoagulation, cryotherapy, and laser therapy.

Lymphangiomas

Lymphangiomas may occur in the lid or orbit and frequently are confused clinically with hemangioma. Differences include associated cellulitis and hemorrhage with lymphangioma, absence of spontaneous regression, and slower progression rate. Surgical excision is difficult but is the best treatment.

Rhabdomyosarcoma

Rhabdomyosarcoma is the most common malignant tumor of the orbit in children. The average age at onset is 7 to 8 years, and white males are affected most often. The tumor arises from embryonic mesenchyme, usually in the upper and inner portion of the orbit, causing a rapidly progressive downward and outward proptosis and drooping of the upper eyelid, or merely ptosis with lid mass alone. It can often masquerade as an infectious orbital cellulitis with inflammatory signs. A subconjunctival or lid mass is palpable in only 25 percent of patients, and loss of vision is uncommon at the time of presentation. There may be pain, nasal stuffiness, and frequent nosebleeds. The best diagnostic aid is a high index of suspicion whenever a rapidly progressive proptosis or lid mass is seen in a child. Diagnosis is by biopsy. Rhabdomyosarcoma is a highly malignant cancer that infiltrates the orbit deeply, often beyond the margins of attempted excision. Metastases may appear in the regional lymph nodes, lungs, or bones. Formerly the prognosis was poor, and most patients survived less than 2 years. With extremely early diagnosis and a multidisciplinary approach utilizing surgery, radiation therapy, and chemotherapy, the 3-year survival rate is now 75 percent.

General Considerations

Optometrists should be aware of malignancies that originate outside the eye area, and the pediatrician should be cognizant of ophthalmic manifestations of these outside tumors. Cancer is second only to trauma as the leading cause of death in children under 14 years of age in the U.S., and it accounts for approximately 15 percent of all deaths from disease in this population. Therefore a list of pediatric malignancies with primary and secondary eye findings is provided in Table 14.4.

FOREIGN BODIES

Conjunctival

Conjunctival foreign bodies can usually be removed easily by flushing with a stream of isotonic saline solution or by using a moistened cotton-tipped applicator. The upper eyelid should be everted and inspected if the foreign body is not readily located. Local anesthesia facilitates the examination.

Corneal

Corneal foreign bodies generally cause more pain and congestion of the eye and are potentially more serious than conjunctival foreign bodies. Fluorescein staining may help to demonstrate the foreign body. If the foreign body cannot be removed with irrigation or a moist cotton applicator, a minor office surgical procedure with a slit lamp for high magnification and stereoscopic viewing may be necessary under topical anesthesia. Broad-spectrum topical antibiotics should be used after the foreign body is removed. Patching usually is not necessary. All patients should have the cornea reexamined in 24 hours to rule out an infection of the abraded area. Metallic foreign bodies frequently leave a localized rust stain (rust ring) that must be removed.

CORNEAL ABRASION

Abrasions of the cornea result from traumatic removal of a portion of the surface epithelium. Fluorescein may be added to the eye and the extent of the corneal abrasion determined under cobalt blue light. In general, abrasions are very painful and are accompanied by marked blepharospasm, tearing, and photophobia. An initial instillation of a topical anesthetic facilitates the examination. Treatment consists of instillation of a broad-spectrum antibiotic and a short-acting cycloplegic and application of a firm pressure patch for 24 hours. Most abrasions heal completely in this time. Young children may resist patching, and it can be omitted if necessary. All patients should be reexamined in 24

Table 14.4   EYE FINDINGS ASSOCIATED WITH PEDIATRIC MALIGNANCIES

Disorder or Syndrome	Findings	Tumors
Primary intraorbital cancers		
Malignant melanoma	Blindness, strabismus, intraocular mass	Melanoma
Retinoblastoma	Strabismus, developmental glaucoma, intraocular mass, second primary cancers	Retinoblastoma
Rhabdomyosarcoma	Periorbital inflammation, strabismus, intraorbital mass	Rhabdomyosarcoma
Metastatic orbital cancers		
Leukemia	Lid edema, subcutaneous and subconjunctival nodules, intraretinal hemorrhage	Leukemia
Lymphoma	Lid edema, ecchymosis, exophthalmos	Lymphoma
Neuroblastoma	Exophthalmos, periorbital hemorrhage, periorbital infection, strabismus, ptosis, blindness	Neuroblastoma
Dermatologic disorders		
Albinism	Pale irides, photophobia	Basal cell carcinoma, squamous cell carcinoma
Ataxia-telangiectasia	Conjunctival telangiectasia, nystagmus, saccadic conjugate eye motion, mental retardation	Lymphoma
Bloom's	Facial telangiectasia, cutaneous atrophy, depigmentation, low birth weight, stunted growth	Leukemia
Chédiak-Higashi	Pale irides, photophobia, strabismus, anemia, recurrent infection	Leukemia, lymphoma
Nevus basal cell	Developmental glaucoma, cataract, hypertelorism, strabismus, nystagmus, odontogenic cysts, facial bone abnormalities, nevi	Basal cell carcinoma
von Recklinghausen's	Café-au-lait spots, neurofibromas of the lids, conjunctiva, iris, optic nerve	Schwannoma, sarcoma
Xeroderma pigmentosa	Pigmentary degeneration, telangiectasia, foci of cutaneous atrophy, keratoconjunctivitis, pterygia	Basal cell carcinoma, squamous cell carcinoma
Nonorbital cancers		
Aniridia	Developmental glaucoma, cataract, aniridia, photophobia	Nephroblastoma (Wilms' tumor)
Down's	Epicanthus, hypertelorism, myopia, cataract, strabismus, Brushfield's spots, mental retardation	Leukemia
Hemihypertrophy	Aniridia	Nephroblastoma (Wilms' tumor), adrenocortical carcinoma, hepatoma
Neuroblastoma	Opsoclonus, blindness	Neuroblastoma

hours to rule out the possibility of infection. Topical anesthetics should never be dispensed for home use; they delay epithelial healing and can cause serious toxic keratopathy.

CONTUSIONS

Contusion injuries result from blunt trauma to the globe and adnexa. They may vary in severity from ecchymosis of the eyelid (black eye) to anterior chamber hemorrhage (hyphema), iris angle recession, dislocated lens, vitreous hemorrhage, retinal detachment, or rupture of the globe. What may appear to be a minor blunt injury to the eye or adnexa may in fact be a serious intraocular injury (see Chapter 18).

Hyphema

Traumatic hyphema occurs more often in males and from a variety of objects that strike the anterior segment of the globe with enough kinetic force to rupture an iris blood vessel or a small ciliary artery or to cause a tear in the ciliary body. There is no consensus on what constitutes proper management. Traditionally the child with even a small hyphema was hospitalized and kept at total bed rest with heavy sedation and eye patches applied to both eyes. Recent studies suggest that patients with small hyphemas that occupy less than 25 percent of the anterior chamber may be treated just as well at home with limited ambulation and bed rest and a patch to cover only the injured eye if the child is cooperative. Patients with larger hyphemas generally continue to be hospitalized and treated with complete bed rest, monocular patching, and avoidance of near accommodation as by reading. Bed rest is continued for 5 to 7 days and then limited ambulation is begun. Most hyphemas fill less than one third of the anterior chamber, are absorbed within a week, and leave no serious ocular sequelae. Recurrent hemorrhages tend to develop between the third and fifth day after injury. After this time hemorrhage is less likely to recur. A recurrent hemorrhage may lead to total obscuration of the anterior chamber by clot-

ted blood, secondary glaucoma, and blood staining of the cornea. *To reduce the incidence of secondary hemorrhage some physicians use prophylactic oral aminocaproic acid (Amikar), an antifibrinolytic agent, or corticosteroids.* Glaucoma from a traumatic recession of the iris angle may not appear for months or years after injury. Possible damage to the lens and retina must be checked when the hyphema clears. Extensive bleeding may cause a "black ball" hyphema and lead to high intraocular pressure. Surgical evacuation is indicated if medical therapy (timolol, carbonic anhydrase inhibitors) fails to control the glaucoma, if corneal blood staining begins to appear, or if clot formation persists. Cataract may result from the injury or the black ball hemorrhage. Cycloplegics and topical corticosteroids may be used for pain and iridocyclitis.

LACERATIONS

Lacerations involving the eyelid margin or lacrimal passages should be treated by an ophthalmologist. Careful primary closure is required to avoid permanent notching of the eyelid margin, resulting in chronic tearing or permanent closure of the lacrimal canaliculus. Lacerations or perforating injuries of the globe are an ocular emergency. The lids and conjunctiva may be moderately swollen, the anterior chamber shallow or flat, and the pupil nonreactive; the intraocular contents may be seen presenting at the wound site. Because lid squeezing may cause expulsion of intraocular tissues, examination should be cautious and limited. The eye should be covered with a patch or shield, and immediate referral should be made to an ophthalmologist. In the emergency room, antibiotics should be given immediately.

BURNS

Chemical

Chemical burns of the conjunctiva and cornea should be treated at once by copious irrigation with water or isotonic saline solution. Acid burns are less serious than alkali burns, because the acid precipitates proteins and forms its own barrier to penetration. Alkaline agents, in contrast, have a lytic action and readily penetrate the cornea, causing rapid and severe damage. With alkali burns, irrigation must be continued while awaiting an ophthalmologic consultation. Further treatment consists of local antibiotics, cycloplegics, and corticosteroids.

Thermal

Thermal burns of the cornea with cigarette ashes, match heads, and the like usually are not serious and can be treated in the same manner as an abrasion.

Radiation

Radiation burns in the form of ultraviolet light from the sun, sun lamps, or welding arcs can produce a diffuse superficial punctate keratitis that is very painful. The keratitis follows the radiation exposure by 8 to 10 hours. Treatment consists of firm bilateral patching for 24 to 48 hours. No permanent sequelae usually develop.

BIRTH TRAUMA

Mechanical trauma to the eye and lids can occur during any delivery, but it is more common after prolonged and difficult deliveries or when instrumentation is used. Some injury to the eye or adnexa occurs in 20 to 25 percent of births; fortunately it is usually mild.

Corneal injury may result in a cloudy cornea secondary to edema. Forceps are the usual cause, producing ruptures in Descemet's membrane and allowing aqueous humor to leak into the cornea. The condition is usually monocular, and ecchymoses of the lids and subconjunctival hemorrhage may be associated. The corneal edema usually clears in 4 to 6 weeks, but later in life high myopia, marked astigmatism, or conical cornea can result in severe visual impairment with amblyopia and strabismus.

The most common ocular birth injury is *retinal hemorrhage*, which has a reported incidence of 20 to 40 percent of all births. The cause and significance of these hemorrhages are not known. Proposed fetal factors include venous congestion of the head and neck secondary to prolonged and difficult labor, sudden release of intracranial pressure with birth asphyxia, capillary fragility, impaired blood coagulability, constriction of the neck by the umbilical cord, cephalic molding, the stress of the first breath, and prematurity. Maternal predisposing factors include first birth, prolonged labor, vaginal delivery, and use of instrumentation (forceps or vacuum extraction greatly increases the occurrence of retinal hemorrhages). The hemorrhages are bilateral in half the affected infants and occur in three forms: superficial flame-shaped hemorrhages close to the optic disc; large, round hemorrhages near the optic disc; and small, round or elongated hemorrhages adjacent to the macula or optic disc. Usually the hemorrhages are absorbed in 2 to 3 weeks without sequelae. Large hemorrhages can organize into elevated scars that resemble tumors (massive retinal fibrosis). There is no apparent relationship between retinal hemorrhages and brain damage, but minor changes in the central nervous system may be detectable.

Other intraocular injuries that have been ascribed rarely to birth trauma include hyphema, vitreous hemorrhage, cataract, iridodialysis, choroidal tears, and subluxation of the lens. Minor injuries to the eyelids and conjunctiva are common. Edema, ecchymoses, hematoma, and lacerations heal without sequelae. Lagophthalmos, the inability to close the eye, occurs occasionally in newborn infants. Usually it is unilateral and may be due to injury to the facial nerve from forceps pressure. The condition usually disappears within a week. Traumatic ptosis also occurs in newborn infants and usually disappears in a few days.

BATTERED-CHILD SYNDROME

Ocular trauma may be the first sign or a prominent symptom of the *battered-child syndrome*. Approximately 40 percent of children who are physically abused show evidence in the eyes. The most common ocular finding is retinal or subhyaloid (preretinal) hemorrhages, and their discovery in a traumatized child less than 4 years old with multiple injuries, especially fractures of the long bones, and an inconsistent history is pathognomonic of battering. Other signs include periorbital swelling and ecchymoses (frequently bilateral), subconjunctival hemorrhages, hyphema, subluxation of the lens, cataract, iridodialysis, angle recession, secondary glaucoma (simulating congenital glaucoma), vitreous hemorrhage, retinal detachment, Purtscher's retinopathy (hemorrhagic retinal angiopathy usually seen with sudden compression of the thoracic cage), optic atrophy, strabismus, and psychogenic vision disorders.

Injuries resulting from whiplash are called the *shaken-baby syndrome.* Retinal and cerebral hemorrhages are present with few or no signs of external trauma. Thirty-five percent of these children suffer blindness or visual impairment.

AIDS

Acquired immunodeficiency syndrome (AIDS) in children was first reported in 1982. Acquisition of the infection was believed to have resulted from transfusions with blood infected by the human immunodeficiency virus. By April 1986, 278 cases of pediatric AIDS were reported, and by November 1988, 1,234 cases in children under 13 years of age had been reported to the Center for Disease Control, representing 1.6% of all the AIDS cases reported since 1981. Seventy-eight percent of the pediatric cases were infected perinatally. The evidence suggests both transplacental infections as well as postnatal transfer of the virus through breast milk. Nineteen percent were infected by transfusion of blood or blood products.

The incubation period in the pediatric age group is variable, and can be quite short. The average age at onset of symptoms in perinatally infected infants is 9 months. In neonates infected by early blood transfusion, symptoms begin at an average age of 14 months. There is a more rapid deterioration seen in pediatric AIDS. For children diagnosed under 1 year of age, half died within 6 months. For those diagnosed after 1 year of age, half died within 20 months.

About 20% of the pediatric AIDS cases have ocular involvement. This is in contrast to 50–73% in adult AIDS. In a recent series of 40 cases, 20% had ocular involvement, 8% had cotton-wool spots, 5% had hemorrhages, 5% had cytomegalovirus retinitis, and 8% had external infections around the eyes.

The incidence of ocular manifestation of AIDS is much lower in the pediatric than the adult population. Therefore, screening of all seropositive HIV children is unnecessary. However, eye examinations should be performed on all children with known encephalopathy or disseminated opportunistic infections, or when clinical signs or symptoms suggest ocular involvement.

BIBLIOGRAPHY

The Lids

Crawford JS: Congenital eyelid anomalies in children. J Pediatr Ophthalmol Strabismus 21:140, 1984.

Fedukowicz HB, Stenson S: External Infections of the Eye. New York, Appleton-Century-Crofts, 1985.

Perry HD, Serniuk RA: Conservative treatment of chalazia. Ophthalmology 87:218, 1980.

Robin JB, Gindi JJ, Schanzlin DJ: Blepharitis: Current concepts in classification, pathogenesis and therapy. Ocular Therapy 1:10, 1984.

Smolin G, Okumoto M: Staphylococcal blepharitis. Arch Ophthalmol 95:812, 1977.

Smolin G, Tabbara K, Whitcher J: Infectious Diseases of the Eye. Baltimore, Williams & Wilkins, 1984.

The Conjunctiva

Brooke I: Anaerobic and aerobic bacterial flora of acute conjunctivitis in children. Arch Ophthalmol 98:833, 1980.

Fedukowicz HB, Stenson S: External Infections of the Eye. New York, Appleton-Century-Crofts, 1985.

Gigliotti F, Williams WT, Hayden FG, et al: Etiology of acute conjunctivitis in children. J Pediatr 98:531, 1981.

Hobson D, Rees E, Visualingam WD: Chlamydial infections in neonates and older children. Br Med Bull 39:128, 1983.

Laga M, Plummer FA, Piot P, et al: Prophylaxis of gonococcal and chlamydial ophthalmia neonatorum: A comparison of silver nitrate and tetracycline. N Engl J Med 318:653, 1988.

Matola A: Ocular viral infections. Pediatr Infect Dis 3:358, 1984.

Stenson S, Newman R, Fedukowicz H: Conjunctivitis in the newborn: Observations on incidence, cause and prophylaxis. Ann Ophthalmol 13:329, 1981.

The Cornea

Grayson M: Diseases of the Cornea. St Louis, CV Mosby, 1984.

Laibson PR, Waring GO: Diseases of the cornea. In Harley RD (ed): Pediatric Ophthalmology. Philadelphia, WB Saunders, 1984.

Nahmias AJ, Visentine AM, Caldwell DR, Wilson LA: Eye infections with herpes simplex in neonates. Surv Ophthalmol 21:100, 1976.

Poiriers RH: Herpetic ocular infections of childhood. Arch Ophthalmol 98:704, 1980.

Waring GO: Congenital and neonatal abnormalities. In Leibowitz HM (ed): Corneal Disorders: Clinical Diagnosis and Management. Philadelphia, WB Saunders, 1984.

The Sclera

Watson P: Diseases of the sclera and episclera. In Duane TD, Jaeger EA (eds): Clinical Ophthalmology, vol 4, ch 13. New York, Harper & Row, 1979.

The Lacrimal Apparatus

Apt L, Cullen BF: Newborns do secrete tears. JAMA 189:95, 1964.

Kushner BJ: Congenital nasolacrimal system obstruction. Arch Ophthalmol 100:597, 1982.

Paul TO: Medical management of congenital nasolacrimal duct obstruction. J Pediatr Ophthalmol Strabismus 22:68, 1985.

Peterson RA, Robb RM: The natural course of congenital obstruction of the nasolacrimal duct. J Pediatr Ophthalmol 15:246, 1978.

The Lens

Beller R, Hoyt CS, Marg E, et al: Good visual function after neonatal surgery for congenital monocular cataracts. Am J Ophthalmol 91:559, 1981.

Davidorf FH (ed): Congenital cataracts. Ophthalmic Forum 3:117, 1984.

Hiles DA: Infantile cataracts. Pediatr Ann 12:556, 1983.

Maumenee IH: Classification of hereditary cataracts in children by linkage analysis. Ophthalmology 86:1554, 1979.

Nelson LB: Diagnosis and management of cataracts in infancy and childhood. Ophthalmic Surg 15:688, 1984.

Rogers GL, Tishler CL, Tsou BH, et al: Visual acuities in infants with congenital cataracts operated on prior to 6 months of age. Arch Ophthalmol 99:999, 1981.

The Uvea

Giles CL: Uveitis in childhood. In Duane TD, Jaeger EA (eds): Clinical Ophthalmology, vol 4, ch 56. Hagerstown MD, Harper & Row, 1981.

Kanski JJ, Shun-Shin GA: Systemic uveitis syndrome in childhood: An analysis of 340 cases. Ophthalmology 91:1247, 1984.

Schlaegel TF: Toxoplasmosis. In Duane TD, Jaeger EA (eds): Clinical Ophthalmology, vol 4, ch 51. Hagerstown MD, Harper & Row, 1981.

Shields JA: Ocular toxocariasis: A review. Surv Ophthalmol 28:361, 1984.

The Retina

Burns RP, Lourien EW, Cibis AB: Juvenile sex-linked retinoschisis: Clinical and genetic studies. Trans Am Acad Ophthalmol Otolaryngol 75:1011, 1971.

Chang M, McLean IW, Merritt JC: Coats' disease: A study of 62 histologically confirmed cases. J Pediatr Ophthalmol Strabismus 21:163, 1984.

Committee for the Classification of Retinopathy of Prematurity: An international classification of retinopathy of prematurity. Arch Ophthalmol 120:1130, 1984.

CRYO-ROP Cooperative Group: Multicenter trial of cryotherapy of prematurity. Arch Ophthalmol 106:471, 1988.

Ellsworth RM: Retinoblastoma. In Duane TD, Jaeger EA (eds): Clinical Ophthalmology, vol 3, ch 35. New York, Harper & Row, 1979.

Juan Verdaguer T: Juvenile retinal detachment. Am J Ophthalmol 93:145, 1982.

Payne JW: Retinopathy of prematurity. In Avery ME, Taeusch HW Jr (eds). Schaffer's Diseases of the Newborn. Philadelphia, WB Saunders, 1984.

Phelps DL, Rosenbaum AL, Isenberg SJ, et al: Tocopherol efficacy and safety for preventing retinopathy of prematurity: A randomized, controlled, double-masked trial. Pediatrics 79:489, 1987.

Pruitt RC, Schepens CL: Posterior hyperplastic primary vitreous. Am J Ophthalmol 69:535, 1970.

The Optic Nerve

Apple DJ, Robb MF, Walsh PM: Congenital anomalies of optic disc. Surv Ophthalmol 27:3, 1982.

Hayreh SS: Optic disc edema in raised intracranial pressure: V. Pathogenesis. Arch Ophthalmol 95:1553, 1977.

Kennedy C, Carroll FD: Optic neuritis in children. Arch Ophthalmol 63:747, 1960.

Miller NR: Walsh & Hoyt's Clinical Neuro-Ophthalmology. Baltimore, Williams & Wilkins, 1982.

Schwartz JF, Chutorian AM, Evans RA, et al: Optic atrophy in childhood. Pediatrics 34:670, 1964.

Skarf B, Hoyt CS: Optic nerve hypoplasia in children: Association with anomalies of the endocrine and CNS. Arch Ophthalmol 102:62, 1984.

Walton DS, Robb RM: Optic nerve hypoplasia: A report of 20 cases. Arch Ophthalmol 84:572, 1970.

Nystagmus

Albright AL, Schlabassi RJ, Slamovitis TL, et al: Spasmus nutans associated with optic gliomas in infants. J Pediatr 105:778, 1984.

Lavery MA, O'Neill JF, Chu FC, et al: Acquired nystagmus in childhood: A presenting sign of intracranial tumor. Ophthalmology 91:425, 1984.

Ocular Myopathy

Zasorin NL, Yee RD, Baloh RW: Eye movement anomalies in ophthalmoplegia, ataxia and areflexia (Fisher's syndrome). Arch Ophthalmol 103:55, 1985.

The Pupil

Pratt SG, Beyer CK, Johnson CC: The Marcus Gunn phenomenon: A review of 71 cases. Ophthalmology 91:27, 1984.

Saver C, Levinsohn M: Horner's syndrome in childhood. Neurology 26:216, 1976.

Glaucoma

Alfano JE: Steroid-induced glaucoma simulating congenital glaucoma. Am J Ophthalmol 78:501, 1974.

Costenbader FD, Kwitko ML: Congenital glaucoma. An analysis of seventy-seven consecutive eyes. J Pediatr Ophthalmol Strabismus 4:9, 1967.

Deluise VP, Anderson DR: Primary infantile glaucoma (congenital glaucoma). Surv Ophthalmol 28:1, 1983.

Goethals M, Missotten L: Intraocular pressure in children up to five years of age. J Pediatr Ophthalmol Strabismus 20:49, 1983.

Kwitko ML: Glaucoma in Infants and Children. New York, Appleton-Century-Crofts, 1973.

Robin AL, Quigley HA, Pollack IP, et al: An analysis of visual acuity, visual fields and disc cupping in childhood glaucoma. Am J Ophthalmol 88:847, 1979.

The Orbit

Macy JI, Mandelbaum SH, Minckler DS: Orbital cellulitis. Ophthalmology 87:1309, 1980.

Shapiro ED: Periorbital and orbital cellulitis. In Nelson JD (ed): Current Therapy in Pediatric Infectious Disease. Philadelphia, BC Decker, 1986.

Weiss A, Friendly D, Eglia R, et al: Bacterial periorbital and orbital cellulitis in childhood. Ophthalmology 90:195, 1980.

Tumors

Kushner BJ: Intralesional corticosteroid injection for infantile adnexal hemangioma. Am J Ophthalmol 93:496, 1982.

Abrasions, Contusions, Lacerations, Burns

Nelson LB: Management of ocular trauma. In Nelson LB (ed). Pediatric Ophthalmology, ch 16. Philadelphia, WB Saunders, 1984.

Pfister RR: Chemical injuries of the eye. Ophthalmology 90:1246, 1983.

Stanworth A: Emergencies involving the eyes. In Black JA (ed): Pediatric Emergencies, ch 14. London, Butterworths, 1979.

Wilson FM: Traumatic hyphema. Pathogenesis and treatment. Ophthalmology 87:910, 1980.

Birth Trauma

Besio R, Caballero C, Meerhoff E, Schwarz R: Neonatal retinal hemorrhages and influence of perinatal factors. Am J Ophthalmol 87:74, 1979.

Hoffman RF, Paul TO, Pentelei-Molner J: The management of corneal birth trauma. J Pediatr Ophthalmol Strabismus 18:45, 1981.

Battered Child and AIDS

Ammann AJ: Human immunodeficiency virus infections in infants and children. Adv Pediatr Infect Dis 3:91, 1988.

Amodio JB, Abramson S, Berdon WE, et al: Pediatric AIDS. Semin Roentgenol 22:66, 1987.

Dennehy PJ, Warman R, Flynn JT, et al: Ocular manifestations in pediatric patients with acquired immunodeficiency syndrome. Arch Ophthalmol 107:978, 1989.

Friendly D: Ocular manifestations of physical child abuse. Trans Am Acad Ophthalmol Otolaryngol 75:318, 1971.

Pahwa S, Kaplan M, Fikrig S, et al: Spectrum of human T-cell lymphotropic virus type III infection in children. JAMA 255:2299, 1986.

Smith SK: Child abuse and neglect: A diagnostic guide for the optometrist. J Am Optom Assoc 59:760, 1988.

General References

Apt L, Gaffney WL: The eyes. In Rudolph AM, Hoffman JIE (eds). Pediatrics, 18th ed. Norwalk, CN: Appleton & Lange, 1987.

Apt L, Urrea PT: The eye. In Gellis SS, Kagan BM (eds). Current Pediatric Therapy. Philadelphia, WB Saunders, 1990.

Bartlett JD, Jaanus SD: Clinical Ocular Pharmacology. Boston, Butterworths, 1984.

Barya M, Baum J: Ocular infections. Med Clin North Am 67:131, 1983.

PART III

Specific Conditions in Diagnosis and Management

Chapter 15

The Visually Impaired Child

Randall T. Jose

Alfred A. Rosenbloom

The earlier treatment begins for a visually impaired child, the better will be the results and the more normal will be the child's life. Children who learn at an early age to make adjustments for their visual impairments have more confidence later in life and are more skilled in using specific techniques and low-vision devices.

It is important that the low-vision optometrist understand developmental characteristics of visually impaired children. There is almost universal agreement in the literature that the motor development of the congenitally blind child is similar to that of the sighted child (37). Barraga and her colleagues have attempted to systematize the study of visual development in children with a visual impairment.

They proposed hierarchial stages of perceptual development. The normally sighted child masters skills in the following sequence:

1. Pay attention to a test object in the field of vision
2. Easily track a moving light
3. Manipulate objects to match a model (e.g., the block design subtest of the Wechsler Adult Intelligence Scale [WAIS])
4. Copy such configurations as occur in the Bender Gestalt test of visual perception
5. Match single elements to complex pictures, as in the picture completion subtest of the WAIS, which can be modified so that the test is multiple choice
6. Distinguish figure from ground (the baseline measure for this level is the Frostig Figure-Ground Test.)

7. Recognize and distinguish printed letters and words (There are specific tests for these last two levels.)
8. Read efficiently.

The visually impaired child develops in the same way as a sighted child but more slowly. The later the onset of the visual impairment, the more normal is the child's development and the less evidence there is of developmental lag (31). This is the usual sequence, but there are exceptions: for example, some children who have poor eye movements have good matching skills on visual perception tests. It should be noted that children who are unable to perform one or more of these tasks may still have normal intellectual functioning.

Visual impairments in infants usually delay development of the sequence of gross and fine motor movements, cognitive development, socialization, and communication skills. The optometrist must know the nature and extent of the impairment to treat the child effectively.

GROSS MOTOR DEVELOPMENT

Research has established that children who have severe visual impairments or are blind experience delayed mastery of some gross motor tasks, but this is not necessarily true for children with low vision (5). Visual stimulation facilitates growth, even if it is delayed (9). Frequently, infants with visual impairment develop head control when placed in a position that encourages it, such as lying over the caregiver's shoulder or sitting in someone's lap. Visually impaired children often do not develop head and related trunk and arm control in the prone position until about 10 months of age, when the near-object association begins to develop. Sighted children develop these skills at an earlier age, because they use vision to explore their environment (1). Children with visual handicaps roll over and get up on their hands and knees at the same age as sighted children do. Visually handicapped children do not, however, progress from lying to sitting or standing until

several months after their sighted age peers have done so. They have a delayed crawling stage. Their average age for walking independently is 18 to 24 months, compared with 12 to 16 months for normally sighted children. Visually handicapped children may also have an unstable gait. Parents need to be patient, understanding, and supportive of such children. Orientation and mobility services can help children use their low vision most effectively (23).

FINE MOTOR DEVELOPMENT

Infants with a visual handicap should be encouraged to locate, reach, and touch objects. Like all babies, they may explore with their mouths as well as their hands. Parents should encourage another source of tactile stimulation by letting the child walk barefoot whenever it is safe to do so. Children with severe visual handicaps are slower to develop gross and fine motor skills, because their visual feedback is limited and they find it difficult to imitate others. They do receive some auditory feedback from sounds.

COGNITIVE DEVELOPMENT

According to Piaget's theory of cognitive development, the first 2 years constitute the sensorimotor period, during which the infant's behavior progresses from simple reflexes to problem solving (37). Piaget emphasized the importance of an infant's interaction with his environment, an interaction that Stephens (35) believes depends largely on vision in the normal infant.

Severe visual impairment or blindness places many experiences and concepts beyond the child's grasp—distinguishing colors, the visual concept of three dimensions, figure-ground relationships, and size and shape (when the gestalt of an object cannot be perceived by touching its individual parts). Low vision often adversely affects cognitive development but does not usually hinder speech although in some cases language is delayed; in fact, many visually handicapped children are avid conversationalists

(30). Daugherty and Moran (7) performed case studies of 50 low-vision children and found significant delays in their cognitive, psychomotor, and academic development. It is important to note that this study dealt with group data and that individual blind and visually impaired children may demonstrate excellent cognitive and motor development.

SOCIALIZATION

By definition, "socialization involves the growing process of interacting with other people and with the demands they impose on the child" (37). Since socialization involves other people, the reaction of others to the vision handicap is significant to the socialization process. Social involvement of visually impaired children should be encouraged through the development of peer relationships in and out of school. Delays in social development are often related to lack of experience (30).

COMMUNICATION SKILLS DEVELOPMENT

An infant is introduced to extrinsic communication by his parents. Language acquisition, from babbling to the production of sentences, is a complex developmental process, which is impeded by the presence of a visual handicap. Warren (37) notes that language is involved in other areas of development, such as verbal mediation in problem solving and verbal and nonverbal aspects of interpersonal relations. Once a diagnosis of visual impairment is made, family members can describe details of the environment to the child to help compensate for the restricted visual input. The parents' consistent use of particular names for persons and objects will help build a basic vocabulary.

In general, children who are visually impaired but have no other disabilities develop language skills at the same rate as sighted children, but their vocabulary building may fall behind after 2 years or so. Some children verbalize less in infancy and spend more time in the echolalic, or repetitive, phase.

Children's songs and story books available on records or cassettes are quite helpful in expanding a child's language skills. They are available without charge from the National Library Service for the Blind and Physically Handicapped Talking Book Program.

EDUCATIONAL RESOURCES

To help teachers and other school professionals become comfortable with visually handicapped children the American Foundation for the Blind (AFB) offers *No Two Alike* (Phoenix Films, Inc.), *You Seem Like a Regular Kid to Me* (Phoenix Films, Inc.), and *A Different Way of Seeing*, a pamphlet in letter form to the classmates of a visually impaired child. The foundation has also made available *When You Have a Visually Handicapped Child in Your Classroom: Suggestions for Teachers and Other Materials*, and *Getting Help for a Disabled Child: Advice for Parents*.

Support groups such as the National Association for Parents of the Visually Impaired (NAPVI) and the International Institute of Visually Impaired, 0-7, Inc. (IIVI) can be of great help. The AFB offers a book titled *Parenting Preschoolers: Suggestions for Raising Young Blind and Visually Impaired Children*. Books such as *Get a Wiggle On* and *Can't Your Child See?* (University Park Press, Baltimore, 1977) are also excellent materials for optometrists working with visually handicapped children.

SERVICE PLANNING FOR LOW-VISION CHILDREN

Optometrists must approach low-vision children as normal children with a vision problem. Children must learn their *own* capabilities and limitations and should not be restricted by a doctor or by overprotective (or aggressive) parents. The clinician's role is to ensure that the child has access to and understands the compensatory systems and techniques available (e.g., eccentric viewing, moving the object of regard in a parallel plane) and attains a thorough understanding of her or his visual impairment.

Reliable statistics on the number of blind and visually impaired children in the United States are not available, because there is no national registry (31). In 1987, 43,000 legally blind children registered with the American Printing House for the Blind (2). This figure includes both visual and Braille readers and students attending residential schools, their local public schools, programs for multiply handicapped students, infant and preschool programs, and rehabilitation programs. That number translates to about 63 per 100,000 children from birth through 17 years of age or about 1 child in 1,400 (19).

Children made up approximately 10 percent of the patient population at The Lighthouse of Houston/University of Houston Vision Rehabilitation Clinic from 1980 to 1988. Data from the American Printing House Register of Legally Blind Pupils (1978), the 1976 U.S. National Center for Health Statistics Health Survey Interview, and the 1976 Bureau of Census Survey of Income and Education indicate that the number of visually impaired children in the U.S. school systems is about 55 per 100,000 (20). Since few school systems provide low-vision services, the authors estimate that less than 25 percent of visually handicapped students receive low-vision care.

Since 1963 there has been a steady increase in the number of multiply impaired students with visual handicaps in all types of schools. P.L. 94-142, passed in 1975, mandates that a child with a disability be given a "free and appropriate education in the least restrictive environment" (12). This is commonly interpreted to mean a public school classroom, although that may not serve the child's needs best. For some children, a residential school may offer the greatest educational opportunity. There is no universally accepted definition of visual impairment, so each local education provider or state education agency determines which children are eligible for special services. Optometrists should be familiar with the local school systems and available services. Because the federal law defines handicap in functional terms as determined by professional evaluation, op-tometrists could be instrumental in establishing specific evaluation procedures or in modifying established guidelines.

In planning services for visually impaired children, it is important for optometrists to realize that, within the population of persons who are legally blind, a small minority (usually estimated at 15 percent) are functionally or totally blind (20). The remaining legally blind persons have useful vision and need help to efficiently utilize what vision they have (2). This help may be provided in a self-contained classroom where visually impaired children are educated with other handicapped children or by an itinerant teacher program, where children receive direct educational services. The latter usually allows the child with a visual impairment to remain in a community school in a regular classroom. The teacher of the visually handicapped, however, can also work with multiply handicapped children in a self-contained classroom setting. In either case, the child is visited routinely by a specially trained teacher who provides counseling and educational materials and develops instructional plans in cooperation with the classroom teacher. In addition to receiving training from the itinerant teacher, the child may attend a resource room for several hours each day for selected subjects.

Optometrists involved with the care of visually impaired children should be familiar with the services available in the area and should visit the various children's service centers and meet the people involved. Information obtained there will prove valuable in designing a visual and learning environment for a particular child (lighting, glare, visual devices, visual and auditory noise, teacher attitudes, etc.).

A list of common ocular diseases associated with visual impairment is seen in Table 15.1 (36). Faye reports that from 1979 to 1983 the leading cause of visual impairment in persons aged 19 years and younger was optic atrophy, followed by cataracts, albinism, and myopia (8). Jose et al. report that in 1985 to 1987 the most prevalent causes of visual impairment in school-aged children were cata-

Table 15.1 COMMON CAUSES OF VISUAL IMPAIRMENT IN AMERICAN CHILDREN AND ADOLESCENTS

Congenital
  Cataracts
  Coloboma
  Corneal dystrophy
  Functional amblyopia
  Glaucoma
  Keratoconus
  Toxoplasmosis

Adventitious (acquired)
  Brain tumor
  Infection
  Trauma
  Uveitis

Hereditary
  Achromatopsia
  Albinism
  Aniridia
  Cataracts
  Juvenile macular degeneration
  Leber's optic atrophy
  Marfan's syndrome
  Retinitis pigmentosa
  Retinoblastoma

Vascular
  Diabetic retinopathy
  Coats' disease
  Retinopathy of prematurity
  Sickle cell retinopathy

(From Stern ET: Helping the person with low vision. Am J Nurs 80:1789, 1980.)

racts or aphakia, albinism, and optic atrophy (18). Some children's visual impairment results from accidental head injuries, child abuse, or gunshot wounds. Multiply impaired children with mental retardation, motor deficits, hearing loss, or medical problems (cardiovascular) may need vision care (see Chapter 16).

Specific pathologic entities, genetic and acquired, are discussed in greater detail in Chapters 5 and 16. It is important to understand these pathologic conditions and to explain them to children, parents, and teachers, who must know the functional limitations of the child's vision and what specific medical or surgical techniques may improve or maintain vision.

LOW-VISION ASSESSMENT

The purpose of a low-vision assessment is to determine the child's potential to function visually and to provide optical devices or environmental modifications to enhance visual performance. Some of the more common *functional* effects are listed.

1. *Reduced visual acuity* can range from loss of sight to a sensation of letters being dim. This dimness can be from a light-loss problem, as with cataracts, or from a contrast sensitivity problem.
2. *Fluctuating vision* can be due to actual physiologic changes (as in diabetes) or to changes in fixation. This is not typically a problem with young children, but the optometrist should still evaluate the quality of fixation and the consistency of eccentric viewing. Lighting changes for very photophobic children may also result in this subjective complaint.
3. *Metamorphopsia* is described by the majority of patients as, "I can see OK, but things just look funny." Even young children can notice distortion on an Amsler grid.
4. *Photophobia* can be difficult to identify. Most children complain of problems with brightness or glare. They do not know what a normal response is in moving from a dim to a bright setting. The optometrist must differentiate between a normal and an abnormal response.
5. Teachers and parents usually discover a *color vision deficiency.* Even patients 14 to 16 years minimize the effects of a color deficiency having learned good color naming skills to compensate for the physiologic loss (see Chapter 19).
6. *Visual field limitations* often go unnoticed by the patient and by teachers and parents. Major field defects make it difficult for children to perform a number of educa-

tion-related tasks, ranging from reading to mobility.

7. *Night blindness* is usually easy to identify from the history. It is important to confirm this functional loss so that appropriate mobility services can be provided.

8. *Oscillopsia* is a fairly rare condition. A child's report that the world is moving or jumping around may not be reliable. The optometrist should make sure that the child is not reporting problems related to endpoint nystagmus, anxiety, stress, or another cause.

9. *Illumination requirements.* Some children need additional lighting to maximize their available vision. A carefully recorded history can alert the optometrist to this problem area, but a definitive diagnosis is usually made in the clinical examination and training sequences.

These are some important functional vision deficits a child can have as a result of a particular ocular disease trauma or anomaly. The optometrist should understand the functional implications of the visual impairment to better manage the child's vision habilitation program.

REFERRAL CONSIDERATIONS

Because most congenital visual problems express themselves in the first few years of life, the pediatric optometrist or ophthalmologist is likely to make the initial diagnosis in children 2 to 5 years of age. Children often are not referred for low-vision or specialty care when their visual acuity is better than 20/70, a popular cut-off point for the definition of visual impairment, formerly known as partial sight. When the visual acuity is the sole criterion for screening, children with 20/50 acuity are frequently recorded as having no vision problem and are not referred for vision care. They are therefore "on record" as having no visual deficiencies. Many of these children do have progressive problems, such as visual field losses, color defects, or binocular problems that can interfere with the child's edu-

cation and require optometric intervention. The parents are generally the first to notice their child's functional problems. When some of these children are identified later as "having a problem," they are given *large-print* reading materials. Handing out large-print materials is a common substitute for individualized comprehensive low-vision care. It works to some extent, but it further delays proper identification of—and good optometric intervention for—the child's real problems. Appropriate optical devices allow the child to read nonenlarged materials such as textbooks and magazines and also facilitate distance vision, such as the use of a telescope for viewing the chalkboard.

Unfortunately, many children with low vision are not identified until significant delays in development (see Chapter 1) or education (see Chapters 21 and 22) are noted. Early optometric intervention is very important.

VISION SCREENING FOR VISUALLY IMPAIRED CHILDREN

The literature of infant vision care increasingly emphasizes the importance of early identification and intervention for vision anomalies (15). Langley and Dubose (21) cited the following problems inherent in conducting vision screening assessments of visually impaired children. They note that many children fear the testing situation, fail to understand the tests, lose interest, are easily distracted, and give unreliable and inconsistent responses. They proposed special techniques for functional vision screening of partially sighted children with possible visual impairment.

Goldie et al. (11) describe a comprehensive federally funded program (under P.L. 94-142) in Oakland County, Michigan for visually impaired children. The successful program involves low-vision screening, comprehensive low-vision evaluation, prescribing of low-vision devices, training, and aftercare. A discussion of contemporary vision screening is presented in Chapter 20.

OPTOMETRIC EXAMINATION OF THE VISUALLY IMPAIRED CHILD

The objectives of an optometric examination are to (1) provide an accurate description of the child's ability to function visually and (2) facilitate the prescription of optical or nonoptical systems to enhance the present level of visual functioning.

Consequently, the optometrist must obtain as much information as possible about the child's visual functioning. A functional assessment by teachers, before the clinical appointment, provides a more comprehensive history and complements the description of the child furnished by the parents. Appendix 2 is a sample low-vision intake form to be completed prior to examination by the optometrist or ophthalmologist.

Bishop presents an organized approach to low-vision evaluation by suggesting protocols for three broad categories of patients: "normal" visually impaired school-aged children, "normal" visually impaired preschoolers, and multiply handicapped/visually impaired children. With these protocols she identified appropriate diagnostic tests for selected visual abilities that can assist parents or classroom teachers in planning intervention and stimulation activities. This information also establishes eligibility for special services and for educational program decisions based on individual needs (4).

Case History

Case histories, including the teacher's report, if available, in conjunction with information from the child's parent or guardian are valuable. Parents and teachers should be encouraged to attend the examination, as their reactions can be as important to the case management as the child's responses. The optometrist should also consider the attitudes of parents and teachers in evaluation and management. The more the teacher and parent are encouraged to participate in the evaluation, the better the chances for coordinated educational planning. The parent or teacher involved in the examination, especially of a multiply handicapped child, can be helpful in eliciting or interpreting responses to a particular test. Optometrists should not make educational recommendations (e.g., the need for Braille, large print, mobility training, etc.) that affect educational services *without* consulting the child's teacher and parents. Collaboration is the most important key to the success of a low-vision examination and to the subsequent treatment plan.

A good case history covers specific items related to general and ocular health, family history, previous low-vision care, present educational programs, mobility skills, lighting needs, and the presence of other special sensory or communication disorders and their effects on developmental milestones (see Appendices 1 and 2).

When taking a case history the optometrist should face the child and should watch and listen to the child's nonverbal responses when a parent answers the questions. If the child can answer, the optometrist should ask for an explanation of the visual impairment. It is very important for the child to have a thorough understanding of the visual impairment.

Acuity

Typically, children can answer questions about letters, pictures, or numbers. The examination outlined here assumes these skills are present. Different optotypes will provide slight variations in acuity. These variations should be considered when taking measurements for reports, especially reports used to determine what educational services are needed. *The optometrist must be sure to know the eligibility requirements for services.* A child can be denied services if a higher level of acuity is measured when symbols are presented at 5 feet than when letters are presented at 10 feet. The distance at which the child is tested can affect the final data, even though, theoretically, a 10-foot acuity should be equivalent to that at 20 feet, because in the latter case the letters are twice as large. Differences in acuity may be due not to visual function but rather to factors such as attention span, figure-ground problems, lighting changes, number and arrangement of optotypes, and accuracy of test distances.

A test distance of 10 feet is best for all acuity measurements in children over 5 years of age. A 5-foot test distance is better for children aged 2 to 5 years, as it affords fewer visual distractions. If acuity has not previously been recorded and there appears to be a severe acuity problem, the appropriate first test is the Designs for Vision number chart. The 700-foot number of the Designs for Vision chart will allow the child with an acuity of 20/7000 to respond successfully (2/700). Once the acuity has been established as 20/400 or better, more accurate and repeatable measurements can be made utilizing Bailey-Lovie charts, Lighthouse Distance charts, or Snellen wall charts. The clinician must *watch* the child during the test procedure to be sure responses are reliable and to detect eccentric viewing or unusual head and eye postures.

If the child is hesitant about responding to numbers, symbol cards may be used. The most popular ones are the Lighthouse Symbol Cards (apple, house, umbrella) and the Efron Distant Symbol Cards (shoe, circle, cup). The Efron cards are easier for children aged 2 to 5 to identify. If problems exist, however, either of these sets can be used for matching to obtain acuity measurements. The combination of number cards, symbol cards, and matching techniques allows the optometrist to obtain an acuity measurement for almost any verbal child who is not severely mentally retarded. Several preferential-looking cards (Vistech, Bailey-Hall Mr. Smile Cards, STYCAR protocol) can be used to estimate acuity of nonverbal children.

Visual acuity measurement provides two important pieces of information. First, it provides a baseline measurement from which magnification needs and improvements in performance can be measured. Second, it allows the optometrist to discuss with parents and teachers what the child can be expected to see. This information helps optometrists, parents, and teachers to provide individualized services for the child. It is important for teachers and parents to know whether a child really can't see to perform a task (homework), fatigues easily, or doesn't want to cooperate.

At near point, symbol charts are more comfortable for children; but letters, words, numbers, or matchings can be used, depending on the child's abilities. It is best to let the child hold the material at a comfortable distance. Most children have already learned that they can see smaller print by holding the material close. *The distance at which they read the chart is as important (if not more so) than the size of the optotypes read.* A child may read text print easily at 5 cm. This is a 20 D accommodative demand and may result in a short attention span while reading. The addition of a plus lens to reduce the accommodative demand will not improve acuity, but parents and teachers should be told that it may substantially improve the child's "reading" ability and may even reduce behavior problems. Because of crowding, contrast, and contour interaction, there is a significant difference between letter or number acuities and reading acuities. Typically, the child needs a single letter acuity two lines better than the letter size of the reading material (38). If the reading material is 1.6 M, then the single-letter acuity should be 1.0 M (1.6 M, 1.2 M, 1.0 M).

There are many advantages for the visually impaired children in the use of a smaller, regular text print rather than large print. If the child is working with large print, the optometrist should find out whether it is appropriate to prescribe for regular print. (This can mean the difference between prescribing a 2× or a 4× system.) Children who learn to use standard-sized print with standard lenses or optical devices will have more opportunities to read.

Distance and near point acuities should be about the same when similar optotypes are used (e.g. 10/100 and 4 M at 40 cm or 10/50 and 1 M at 20 cm). If not, the optometrist must try to find the psychological, clinical, or physiologic reasons for any significant discrepancy. Some children hold material much closer than necessary. They read 1 M at 10 cm but when persuaded can also read at 25 cm. This preference for reading up close may be due to a habitual posture, resulting in restriction of the field or is a method to reduce nystagmus or an attempt to achieve easier visual prehension.

For the multiply handicapped or nonverbal child, the report may have to read "identifies or responds to a 1 inch–high object at 10 inches," as normal optotypes cannot be used for testing. This gives the teacher or parent an idea of the *size and distance* objects should be placed for the child's optimal visual function. (A 1-inch object at 10 inches is equivalent to a 2-inch object at 20 inches or a $\frac{1}{2}$-inch object at 5 inches.) Such test objects should be presented against a plain, solid-colored background.

The optometrist should observe any unusual head or eye postures. Is there a null point (specific position of gaze) at which the nystagmus is reduced? A child may turn his head to the far right to view a chart in front of him. This may be a way of placing the eyes into a left field of gaze to reduce nystagmus (null point), or it could mean that the best vision is in the temporal peripheral field of the left eye. There are no absolute rules for a low-vision child. If an unusual behavior is observed, the cause should be sought. The optometrist must make sure there is no restriction of eye movements, describe the type of nystagmus present, and check pupillary reflexes and the retinal reflex. Unusual postures should be recorded. A careful and complete examination of the internal eye should be performed.

Refraction

Good refraction is important for younger visually impaired patients. A child may never have been refracted correctly because of lack of services or an inability to respond to normal refractive procedures. When refracting a child it is vital *always to start from scratch.* A comfortable trial frame and an interesting target at 10 feet should be used. Retinoscopy is still the best technique for determining a

refractive state. *The phoropter should be avoided.* If there is not a clear retinoscopic reflex at the normal work distance, the optometrist must try to obtain a reflex at a shorter distance. This is called radical retinoscopy. The procedure may require a 20-cm work distance (and a 5 D compensating lens) to obtain a clear reflex. At least one baseline cycloplegic retinoscopy/subjective, if appropriate, is recommended.

Other objective instruments used to measure refractive state include the keratometer, keratoscope, ophthalmoscope, ultrasound, and automated refractometer. All available methods are used to determine an appropriate and accurate refractive correction. The better the acuity obtained with conventional refraction, the less magnification will be required to improve visual function. Also, a magnified image can be of better quality if the refractive state is accurately corrected.

Even if no reliable results are obtained with objective techniques of measuring the refractive state, a subjective evaluation can often be performed successfully. Special children's trial frames are available. A new distance acuity reading is taken to establish an *immediate* baseline measurement. The child may have become fatigued since the first acuity measurement, or he may have become more relaxed and will give better responses. The child is asked which lens makes the picture or number look better or worse. Because these children have poor acuity, it may be difficult for them, initially, to grasp the concepts of *clearer* or *better.* The optometrist should use terminology that the child understands. Typically, the child will respond to differences. Dioptric power changes may be increased until a just noticeable difference is achieved.

Once refraction is determined subjectively, distance acuity should be measured again to note the improvement in acuity. The young patient will have learned the chart, will feel more comfortable, and will respond better. He or she also will have adapted to the lighting or may have learned to view better eccentrically during the course of the refraction procedure. Perception is not solely a function of a sharp retinal image. Therefore, *the habitual distant acuity is always rechecked before new lenses are prescribed.*

Binocular Assessment

The optometrist must determine whether the child can function binocularly (simultaneous perception) or monocularly, or if she or he is potentially biocular (uses the two eyes independently). Biocular vision is present infrequently in visually impaired children. In the review of clinic records of The Lighthouse of Houston/University of Houston Vision Rehabilitation Clinic and the Chicago Lighthouse Low-Vision Service, less than 10 percent of the total population demonstrated some binocular vision skills—alignment, gross stereopsis, red-lens fusion, or Worth Dot fusion.

The most reliable tests for binocularity are the cover test and monocular acuities. If the vision is 10/40 to 10/60 at distance (2 M to 2.5 M at 40 cm near point acuity) in the better eye, with no more than two lines difference in the poorer eye, there is a good chance for prescribing a binocular correction. Typically, 3× magnification for microscopes (+12 D) is the limit of binocularity. Telemicroscopes can be designed binocularly up to 6×, but the practical limit is probably 4×. The authors do not recommend binocular prescriptions of bioptic telescopes for distance use.

In cases where optimum acuity exists but there is no indication of binocular vision (or simultaneous perception), the optometrist should explore the possibility of biocularity. Biocularity is present when the child can use either eye independently while suppressing the other. This condition provides opportunities to prescribe for one eye for near and the other eye for distance. A conventional prescription may be used for mobility in one lens, and the other may contain a full-field (or reversed) telescope. The same reading lens in each eye for alternate viewing may also be prescribed. *No prescribing option should go unexplored, no matter how unconventional it may seem.*

When a child is definitely monocular, a decision must be made about patching the weaker eye.

Retinal rivalry can exist even if acuity in the poorer eye is 20/800 and in the better eye 20/100. The poorer eye should be occluded with the low-vision device before the better eye, to check acuity *and performance.* In some cases, the child needs to touch the lids to stop the interference of the poorer eye. Significantly improved localization and tracking skills may be realized by patching the poorer eye.

Visual Fields

The purpose of visual field evaluation is to determine the extent of peripheral or central field losses. A precise measurement may not be necessary. The optometrist needs to know whether the field losses are significant enough to affect the child's performance or to interfere with the effectiveness of a specific low-vision device. In some cases, the type of field loss dictates the particular prescription (reversed telescopes, prisms, etc.). The optometrist needs information about the peripheral fields and the macular area.

All young patients who can respond should be tested with the Amsler grid. A child with a central scotoma who views an Amsler grid and then reports absence of the fixation spot has not learned to use eccentric fixation. A scotoma to the right of fixation will cause reading problems because the print will "pop out" of the scotomatous area. The Amsler grid can be very helpful in establishing the type of fixation under these conditions (17). With a younger or nonverbal child, it is fairly difficult to ascertain this information from the Amsler grid test.

Peripheral fields are usually evaluated with a modified tangent screen test. Ninety percent of children with peripheral field losses demonstrate field losses on a tangent screen (12). If scotomata are found, more complete perimetry is performed.

The Lighthouse of Houston/University of Houston Clinic uses the tangent screen as the routine field test for younger patients. When conditions with probable peripheral field losses are examined (e.g., retinitis pigmentosa, diabetes, optic atrophy), the Humphrey field screener (or comparable test) is utilized. An arc perimeter is still the most reliable instrument for obtaining responses from children. Initially, 8 to 10 meridians are evaluated on the arc perimeter. This gives sufficient information about the presence of peripheral field losses that may interfere with mobility. For 15- to 18-year-olds who want to drive, more comprehensive peripheral fields are required to determine eligibility.

With visually impaired children, the optometrist may wish to increase the response reliability by using larger test targets and moving them more slowly. The optometrist should always watch the child's eyes for fixational changes; should use larger targets or crosses as fixation targets (22); and, of course, should try to make a game of the test.

For younger children, an arc perimeter is used, and little finger puppets pop up above the arc. By watching the child's saccadic movement when the puppet pops up in the periphery, the optometrist can infer the presence of peripheral vision in that area. Pointing at the puppet or shining a light helps the game (Fig. 15.1). Nonverbal children may have objects brought from the periphery while they attend to a blinking light. They can point at the object (usually a favorite toy or clinical object that attracts their attention) when it comes into view from behind. There is the "blow out the light" game, which children love. A penlight is the target; the child blows on the light and it goes off. A flickering red light is a good stimulus to use as a confrontation target for severely retarded or severely visually and physically impaired children. This confrontation test provides the clinician with a gross description of the child's visual fields. Whether a loss of peripheral field is cortical (awareness loss) or retinal (physiologic dysfunction) is irrelevant at this stage. The optometrist reports that there does not appear to be any visual function in the periphery and indicates that planning for educational tasks or activities should take this into consideration. The teacher is advised to present objects in the child's central field if a response is expected.

Applying this clinical information to the educational setting is important. A child with

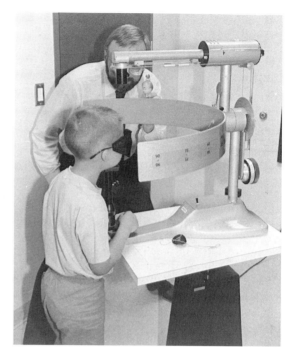

Figure 15.1 A flickering red light can be used for confrontation testing of the visual field of young or mentally slow children. For greater accuracy, the child can be asked to stand within a perimeter, staring at a central target, and to report when a puppet pops up.

a severe peripheral field loss will be given mobility or vision efficiency training. *One field test does not yield a permanent diagnosis.* Only after the clinical tests indicate an area of loss, which finding is supported by the evaluations of teachers and parents, should the loss be considered permanent. Clinicians who work with many visually impaired children will find the information from the teacher and parent as valuable as the clinical tests, especially in field evaluations.

Illumination

The need for special sun filters or lighting for younger children (including nonverbal ones) is usually determined by the history and by the child's performance as evaluated by a mobility instructor or educator. Older children can more easily report their reaction to the introduction of sun filters, filters for contrast at near point, or illumination or contrast control devices such as typoscopes, hooded lamps, and visors. Brightness sensitivity testing is also valuable.

Magnification Assessment

The optometrist must determine whether magnification is required, and if so, how much.

For distance vision, the initial magnification is found by dividing the denominator of the distance acuity by the denominator of the acuity needed for the task. If a child has 10/60 acuity with best correction and wants to see the chalkboard at school (which requires a 10/30 acuity) then a 2× telescope should be evaluated. (Or the child could move closer to the board by half the usual distance.) In this case, a full-field 2.2× telescope can be used in a Halberg clip over the child's regular glasses to obtain an acuity of 10/25, indicating the potential benefit of telescopes.

At near point, the child reads 2-M print (18 pt) at 20 cm. The reading material in the class is 1 M (9 pt). To achieve 1 M, the material must be moved to half the distance in order to double the size (or at 10 cm the child should be able to see 1-M letters instead of 2-M letters at 20 cm). A 10-cm viewing distance requires a +10-D lens, or 10 D of accommodation. If the child holds the material at 10 cm and reads 1-M letters, a tentative prescription is noted. Accommodative demand, however, must be considered. As an initial approach, it is wise to leave the visually impaired child with 4 or 5 D of accommodative reserve. This can be modified later with reading performance tests and the use of loaned devices in class. Again, full-field microscopes are best for initial evaluations and training regimens.

The optometrist should choose what she or he considers the most suitable device for near and far vision and should train the child in its use. If the child is unable to localize through a 2.2× spectacle full-field telescopic system, then telescopic corrections should not be considered until further training is provided. The child must be able to use a device before it is released as a prescribed or loaned device.

Perceptual Testing

In some cases, perceptual testing is an important part of the evaluation. Visually impaired persons can have learning disorders, hand-eye coordination is often poor, and gross motor skills can be deficient. Intervention can reduce the effects of visual perceptual deficits and improve the child's learning skills, and for others training visual perceptual skills will lead to more successful use of optical prescriptions.

All the information from the examination must now be analyzed and converted into a prescription for the child. The therapeutic regimen must be consistent with the child's behavior, the parents' expectations and support, the teacher's perception of the child's needs, educational demands, available finances, cooperation of administrators in the school, and most important, the child's desire to improve visual functioning. In completing the evaluation, the optometrist should also address the concepts of control and predictability.

Examination of Nonverbal Children

Some modifications must be made to the examination protocol for nonverbal children such as mentally retarded ones and infants. These children usually have motor impairments (e.g., cerebral palsy) and have hearing as well as vision problems and require special testing. The optometrist must help answer this question: Is the child's inability to perform a particular task or activity related to his inability to see that task or is it a cortical problem in which the child cannot grasp the concept of that task or activity?

The answer is very important to the teacher. For example, a teacher can attempt, unsuccessfully, to teach color coding to a child who is color vision deficient or mentally unable to differentiate colors. If a clini-

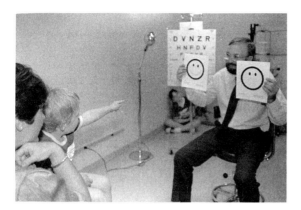

Figure 15.2 The Bailey-Hall Mr. Smile Cards can be used to estimate a child's contrast sensitivity and acuity level.

cian can determine this color deficiency early (new Pease-Allen Preferential Looking tests allow this), the teacher can emphasize activities that will benefit the child, such as simple color matching tasks or elimination of confusing backgrounds. Once the optometric evaluation is completed, the information must be incorporated into the child's educational programming. This is particularly true for the child involved in a vision stimulation curriculum.

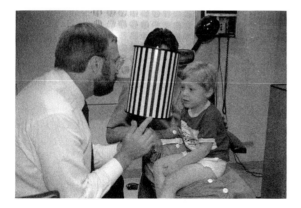

Figure 15.3 In the hands of a trained examiner the Optokinetic Nystagmus Drum provides an approximate measure of visual acuity and an indication of normal or reduced vision.

The principal difference in working with nonverbal children is that objective tests must be used. The acuity can be obtained from presentation of compelling targets (Fig. 15.2), or the OKN drum can provide an approximate value. The clinician must remember that to a teacher, a size and distance measurement is more meaningful for designing appropriate programming than an acuity number (e.g., 2-inch block at 8 inches is better than 20/400).

All children, no matter what their age or ability, enjoy the reward for good behavior of exploring the treasure chest for a special toy!

TREATMENT OPTIONS

Typically, visually impaired children need to perform educationally related tasks; read smaller print (or go from Braille to print); learn Braille and print letters simultaneously; and see the chalkboard, movies, and television. They may need devices to reduce glare in order to participate in school recreation.

Parents' questions to the optometrist often involve how much the child really sees and what may be hoped for: "Is there anything or anyone *in the world* that can help my child? What about this new treatment in South America?" A difficult situation arises when the parent is angry because the school system will not provide *blind* services for a child with low vision. Equally troublesome for the optometrist is the situation in which it is appropriate (or even mandated by law) for the school to provide special services for a low-vision child but it does not do so. Parents may have to consider educational placement in a residential program. This requires that parents who know the child's functional visual capabilities be supportive and understanding. Knowledge of the child's acuities, fields, binocularity, contrast, illumination, work distances, etc., can be of great value in planning an individualized learning program. Knowledge of a child's vision problems must lead to actions using appropriate devices to develop visual efficiency. An optical system should not be prescribed if acceptable environmental modifications have resolved the problem. For the multiply impaired, nonverbal child with a severe visual handicap, a program of vision stimulation may be recommended as a treatment option.

VISION STIMULATION OF THE VISUALLY IMPAIRED CHILD WHO IS SEVERELY HANDICAPPED*

Children who have severe and profound handicaps including visual impairments do not generally learn about their environments in an incidental or self-initiated manner. In order to interact with and learn from their environments (including people and objects) they must be stimulated by parents, teachers, brothers, and sisters. Those working with severely impaired children with visual impairments must learn how to motivate the children to interact with their environments. These children must be helped to match visual events with events causing or resulting from changes in their body position or movements with events involving other people and objects. If the visual impairments are severe, these children may have difficulty understanding the consequences of visual events or their own movements on changes in the environment. Indeed, these children may not understand of what objects and people the environment is composed, and therefore, how actions alter their environment. Sophisticated instrumentation and procedures are not necessary to help children "make the match"; with simple procedures and objects, caretakers can encourage children to become visually aware of themselves and of objects and people.

Flashlight Activities

A flashlight can be very important for enhancing children's awareness of self, objects, and people external to the self. For some chil-

dren, however, seeing the light of a flashlight may be an unpleasant experience; for others, it may become an object for self-stimulation to the extent that the purpose of the flashlight as an instrument for visual regard becomes nonfunctional. Such penlight activities as the following serve to develop "tracking" skills and enable a child to relate to an external object visually, kinesthetically, and proprioceptively.

1. The penlight is placed in the child's hand and moved slowly and smoothly in various quadrants of gaze. Turning the head in conjunction with the movement of the flashlight is also encouraged. This activity helps develop eye movement skills and position in space.
2. Two flashlights close together are flashed alternately as the examiner observes the child's eyes. Then they are moved apart and positioned in different quadrants of gaze to teach fixational movements.
3. The optometrist guides the child's head with his or her own while using the light to outline various geometric shapes (circle, square, triangle). This provides visual and kinesthetic feedback on various geometric shapes.
4. A developmentally able child can be encouraged to go toward a light source in a darkened room by pairing the light with a positive reinforcer such as food or a hug. After the child masters the exercise with one light, lights can be placed in various positions in a room, enabling the child to understand the geometry of space involving fixed and stable points of reference.

Other activities might use a light box (e.g. American Printing House for the Blind materials) or closed-circuit TV as a visual tool, to teach a child to follow a moving dot on the screen. Additional activities might involve real objects and people (e.g., pieces of cheese on contrasting backgrounds, balloons, watching pets move). It is also useful to point out what is available in the child's home (e.g., indicating when a drawer is open or asking a child to tell when there is an egg yolk in a bowl). If there is sufficient acuity, these activ-

---

* The editors thank Drs. Anne Corn and Paul Freeman for their valuable help in preparing this section.

ities may be as useful as those with the flashlight or more so.

Formal Instructional Programs

Teachers of visually handicapped children first review any clinical information available from an optometrist, ophthalmologist, or other professional who can provide information on students' visual acuity, visual fields, and contrast sensitivity. Then, the teacher performs a functional vision assessment, to determine in what ways the child is able to use vision to perform a variety of school- and home-based tasks, under what environmental conditions the child's vision seems to be enhanced or hindered, how the child functions with prescribed optical devices, and to gain other information about how the child's vision may affect cognitive and social development. The teacher also determines whether a low-vision clinical evaluation is recommended (if none was performed previously). Also when children have very low levels of visual functioning, the teacher of the visually handicapped may determine if vision can be elicited through a variety of techniques which may not be available in a clinical setting.

Although there is still controversy about whether children with low visual acuity use their vision spontaneously, research seems to show that, with a structured series of activities, children with low vision can increase their visual efficiency (3). In addition, those with low vision can be taught to use their available vision more efficiently by utilizing optical devices, nonoptical devices, and environmental modifications or techniques. Through a comprehensive program of vision stimulation, visual efficiency training, and utilization of vision, a child with low vision can learn such skills as how to alter environmental cues to make an object appear more observable, change body position to take greater advantage of available environmental cues, and learn to make visual judgments based on outlines of images or on images with low, medium, or high levels of complexity of internal information (6).

Using the information from a functional vision assessment, the teacher of the visually handicapped will be able to develop an instructional program for the use of available vision, make a recommendation for a low-vision clinical evaluation, determine a medium for reading (print, Braille), and make recommendations about the use of vision for learning to classroom teachers, parents, and other significant persons in the child's environment. The teacher may discuss the assessment findings with children who are old enough and able to understand, in order to help them utilize their vision most efficiently. The teacher may also determine when the use of vision is not the most desirable or preferred method of approaching a task. For one task, a visual approach may be the most efficient, but for another, a combination of auditory and visual input is beneficial; for still another task, a tactual approach may be more efficient or more cosmetically acceptable. The teacher of the visually handicapped is also a professional to whom children and their parents may ask questions regarding social, vocational, and personal situations in which low vision is a factor in the child's success. Counseling in such areas is well within the scope of the roles of the teacher. It is important, however, that the teacher know when to refer the child back to the optometrist or ophthalmologist, to a psychologist, or to another professional whose expertise is needed.

A teacher who recommends a low-vision clinical evaluation will forward a copy of the functional report. This report should be most helpful to the optometrist, who is trying to provide additional information to the child and the school.

It is essential that a positive working relationship be established between clinicians and members of the school's educational team. Often, the clinician functions as a member of a multidisciplinary special education team whose input is utilized for educational decision making (e.g., which reading medium to use or how lighting may be altered to enhance visual efficiency in the classroom).

SUMMARY OF PRINCIPLES AND TECHNIQUES FOR EXAMINING A VISUALLY IMPAIRED CHILD

The examination and management of visually impaired children should conform to their special needs and requirements. Although details may vary, the pediatric low-vision evaluation must include the case history, evaluation of ocular health status, and visual performance at all working distances, prescribing of low-vision devices, adaptive training and counseling in their use, communication and coordination with other health providers and team professionals, and planning for progress evaluations and ongoing care.

The observations of parents, physicians, and teachers become especially important when testing infants and preliterate children, and they should be included in the case history. Gross visual response testing, electrodiagnostic testing (i.e., VER), ocular motility and binocularity functions, and determination of refractive state are important diagnostic procedures (29, 30). (For details and recommended procedures, see Faye and Jose) (8, 19).

Literate children may be tested subjectively from approximately $3\frac{1}{2}$ years on (8). Important elements of the evaluation include the following:

Case history with regard to individual differences and purposes (goals) of the low-vision evaluation

Ocular health status (internal and external)

Assessment of vision, including visual acuities at distance and for reading

Oculomotor evaluation (eye movements; fixation and fusion; binocular vision skills; gross and fine motor performance)

Contrast sensitivity function

Color vision discrimination

Visual fields

Sensitivity to light

Refraction methods, objective and subjective

Binocular vision, including accommodative abilities

Reading performance (print size and working distance; proper use of optical device; ability to sustain fusion and amplitude of accommodation over time; facility, speed, and comprehension in reading)

PRESCRIBING

Peer image is a major factor in children's refusal to use optical devices, especially after second grade. In the third grade, educational demands change (e.g., smaller text print) and optical intervention usually is needed. Optometrists should avoid prescribing devices that other children will ridicule. Cosmesis of the prescription must have high priority in the final design and mounting system. Other than the concern for appearance, the optometrist follows the same rules for determining an appropriate prescription by seeking answers to the following questions:

1. What magnification is needed for comfortable, sustained performance?
2. What field of view through the optical system is needed?
3. What work distance is required to function safely and comfortably?
4. Is mobility required?

Other considerations for final lens design are:

1. Stability of the eye condition
2. Refractive anomalies that need to be incorporated into the prescription
3. The child's (or parent's) concern for cosmesis
4. Travel time involved for after-care
5. Cost
6. Is more than one low-vision device appropriate?

With the above questions, the optometrist will identify functional optical parameters of magnification, working distance, field of view, mobility requirements and then determine which type of optical system to prescribe. For instance, viewing the chalkboard is a distance task that may require the use of a telescope. If the child must look under the telescope to write, a hand-held or a bioptic design may be more appropriate. If the child has trouble following the teacher's board writing through a bioptic (small field), a full-field system (spectacle or clip-on) can provide a larger field. A hand-held system may afford the larger field of vision needed. (Note that, the closer the ocular element of the telescope is to the eye, the larger is the field of view.) If possible, the child should use the telescope without spectacles. This reduces the vertex distance significantly and affords a larger field of view. A hand-held telescope may provide the needed larger field of view. The full-field system, however, will still preclude mobility. If the child needs to read (4× magnification) and can hold the material close to the eye (6 cm), then a microscope is the device of choice, as it provides a large field. If mobility is required, the microscope design can be changed to a half-eye (if no distance prescription is needed) or an executive-type bifocal (if a distance prescription is needed). If the required reading is from an CRT screen at 20 cm working distance, then a 4× telescope with a +5 cap (20 cm work distance) is the system of choice. These systems give adequate or better magnification. If the field of view is too small, then the clinician could consider a clip-on 4× telescope, which is larger and more cumbersome but allows a larger field of view. Also, a hand-held telescope will allow for a larger field (as the ocular lens is placed close to the eye), and it requires fewer head movements. Large-print software or a closed-circuit television (CCTV) are other options to consider.

Low-vision devices can be categorized as follows:

Telescopes

Hand-held
Clip-on
Bioptics or behind-the-lens telescopes
Full-field spectacle
Binoculars

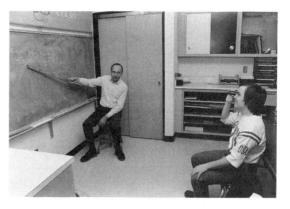

Figure 15.4 A 6× hand-held focusable telescope is useful for spotting small details at a distance, as in reading the chalkboard. (Courtesy of Chris Cowan, Austin TX)

Contact lens telescope
IOL telescope

Telescopes are used for distance tasks, beyond arm's length. The largest fields are achieved with field binoculars, intermediate

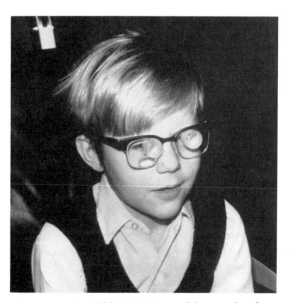

Figure 15.5 A child with Stargardt's macular disease uses a 2.5× bioptic telescope (corrected vision to 20/30+) to "spot" the chalkboard. A +10.00 high-add bifocal on the right eye enables him to read all sizes of textbook print.

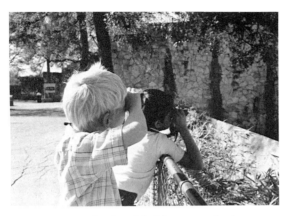

Figure 15.6 An 8× hand-held monocular focusable telescope enables these visually impaired boys to watch animals at the zoo. (Courtesy of Chris Cowan, Austin TX)

fields with hand-held monocular telescopes, and smaller fields with bioptic systems. Bioptic telescopes allow mobility, as do some flip-up systems. Powers up to 6× are practical in bioptics, 10× in monoculars, and up to 20× in binoculars. The appearance of these systems is a major hindrance to their acceptance by young adults. This should be discussed with patients before they are prescribed. The new, behind-the-lens design may obviate some of the aesthetic objections.

Telemicroscopes

Spectacle reading telescope
Surgical telescope
Bioptic focusable telescope
Clip-on focusable telescope
Nonfocusable telescope with reading caps
Hand-held telescope used for short-term tasks
Binoculars with reading cap

Telemicroscopes are used for intermediate distance tasks (20 cm to 1 m), such as reading music. Typically, the telemicroscope has a small field of view; the longer the working distance, the smaller the field compared to a similar microscope. The telemicroscope

allows for mobility, if it is not mounted on center. To provide the large field of the full-field system and still allow for mobility, a clip-on telescope system is used. Magnification beyond 6× at a distance of 30 cm to 1 m is not useful in telemicroscope form.

Microscopes

Single-vision (aspheric, full-field)
Doublet
Executive bifocal
Ultex bifocal
Round segs
Franklin bifocal
Fresnel bifocal
Ary loupe (others)
Contact lens
Myopic bifocal
Half-eye

Microscopes are used for tasks within a short distance (2 to 20 cm). They provide the largest field of view for comparable magnification. Field size decreases in half-eye form, and even more in bifocals. The functional significance of a small field for such tasks as reading or identifying objects at near distance may be less important for a person with low vision and good fixation skills than for one without good fixation skills. A full-field design precludes mobility, whereas a bifocal allows adequate mobility and a smaller functional field. The Ary loupe allows a larger field and flips up for mobility. The half eye is a good compromise between mobility and field if no significant refractive state exists. Low-power +5 add bifocals of round seg design can still interfere with a child's mobility. Magnification is available in powers of 1× (+4 add) to 20× (+80 D add). Binocular corrections with a half-eye are practical up to 3× (+12 D add with 14 base-in prism).

Magnifiers

Hand-held
Stand magnifier
Mirror magnifier
Illuminated magnifier
Bar magnifier

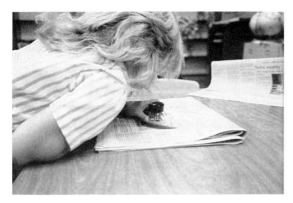

Figure 15.7 An 8× Agfa loupe enables this girl with 20/200 acuity to read newsprint. (Courtesy of Chris Cowan, Austin TX)

Magnifiers afford a compromise between the work distance of a telemicroscope and the field of view of a microscope. Their disadvantage is that they do not allow both hands to be free for reading. This is not always a requirement for proficient reading, however. Magnifiers are cosmetically acceptable to children and provide an adequate working distance. The optometrist must remember, however, that the distance from the eye is an important determinant of the functional field of view.

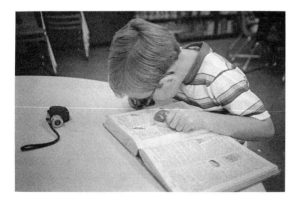

Figure 15.8 This student has ocular albinism and 20/180 acuity. The 6× hand-held monocular telescope is used to read words on the chalkboard while the 5× planoconvex magnifier enlarges dictionary print so that he may participate in mainstream classroom instruction. (Courtesy of Chris Cowan, Austin TX)

The patient will usually find a compromise in work distance that is comfortable and provides a reasonable field of view. Mobility is not a problem, since magnifiers are not attached to spectacles. Pocket magnifiers are portable but their small field of view may be limiting to some readers. Stand magnifiers may not fit in pockets or school bags and are often left at home, but if this option is desirable, it may be worthwhile for the child to have one to leave at school.

Magnification up to 7× (+28 D) is available in stand magnifiers and up to 20× (+80 D) in hand-held magnifiers. Some of the stand systems are illuminated. (Halogen lighting is particularly good for contrast.) Above +28 D, the lens design is either a pocket magnifier or a high-power stand magnifier. Each has a very small field of view, which requires the child to hold the material very close to the eyes. The optometrist must keep in mind that aphakic and older patients typically use a bifocal to compensate for their lack of accommodation, so they may obtain optimum magnification from a stand magnifier (23). Stand magnifiers may also be useful to persons who have difficulty holding a magnifier steady or who lose their place on the line of print.

The closed circuit television is used in some school systems as a cure-all for children in the visually handicapped program and for compliance with P.L. 94-142. (Federal regulations require school systems to provide appropriate devices for learning.) CCTV does provide younger children easy access to printed material, but it presents a long-term problem. Children who use only CCTV may find later, in high school and college classes, that a more portable system is needed. Also, using CCTV gives no experience in localizing tracking, or scanning. The combination of CCTV and an appropriate optical device provides an optimum and competitive learning environment for the child.*

---

* For source lists of modern optical and nonoptical devices, the reader should write the Low Vision Section, American Optometric Association, 243 N. Lindbergh Blvd., St Louis, MO 63141.

Educational Considerations of Prescribing

High plus lenses require a short working distance from eye to object. The child may need to increase his head movements when eye movements alone do not allow for reading at short focal distances along the line of print in a text. Some children find that working at short distances is very fatiguing. They may prefer a hand-held lens that must be moved, but allows for varied working distances (with smaller fields at greater distances). Hand-held lenses also allow the child to read and examine objects above or below eye level: bulletin boards, sewing machine needles, objects in positions where the head cannot comfortably be placed (as in reading card catalogues). Students may require several lens designs for various educational purposes (5).

ADAPTIVE TRAINING AND AFTER CARE

Children who can benefit from a low-vision device should be trained in its proper use. This is very important! Working distance, field of vision, and spatial distortions require them to learn new motor patterns involving head, hand, and eye coordination. Optometrists must not dispense a low-vision device until the child has demonstrated proficiency in its use. There are a number of factors to consider: working distance, field of view, level and type of illumination, and use of auxiliary supports, such as reading stands, which hold the material and facilitate smooth lateral movements of the print at a fixed distance and in a plane parallel and frontal to the face.

Successful training must follow a regular sequence of teaching the required motor skills. Training involves repeated demonstrations, explanations, and supervision. Jose describes the key elements in the training regimen (17). Children should begin with low magnification, large print, good contrast, widely spaced letters, short words, optimum illumination, and a typoscope or reading guide if necessary. The optometrist gradually

introduces higher magnification, smaller print, more closely spaced and longer words, careful control of illumination, and increased movement. The fundamental principle of the procedure is to adjust the environment and the task so that children can perform tasks successfully. As they learn to function, more normal visual conditions can be used. They are trained gradually to use lenses of magnification appropriate to the type and complexity of daily tasks he or she will encounter. In this regard it is important to remember that the fast-paced classroom may present a different environment than that in the office (e.g., uncontrolled lighting).

The training should be appropriate to the recommended devices. Telescopic lenses for distance vision require both an explanation and a demonstration of the inherent limitations of field of view and parallax displacement of objects. Children should be taught to use fewer eye movements and more head movements in viewing an object and in judging its distance and position from other objects. They must be made aware of the limitations of microscopic lenses or high plus reading corrections. Adaptive training must be provided to teach the child to cope with limitations in depth of focus, working distance, and field of view. When eccentric viewing is present, the head must be turned into a position that facilitates maximum use of peripheral retina. One responsibility of teachers of visually handicapped persons is, in cooperation with the optometrist, to teach the use of prescribed optical devices.

When testing, the optometrist must be sure that the test cards for near point acuity do not have words that are too difficult or unfamiliar. Single letters or numbers may be more appropriate. A familiar school book is a good testing tool. Primary print textbooks that require less ocular accommodation frequently enable the optometrist to use less magnification to achieve the desired level of near vision.

It is often desirable to provide children with "loaner" low-vision devices to use at home or school. The determination of which device or devices is most effective should be made only after the child has completed one or more periods of supervised adaptive training during which parents, social workers, and teachers, as well as the optometrist, have an opportunity to evaluate the effectiveness of the low-vision device.

A follow-up examination is essential within 3 to 6 months after completion of the initial low-vision service and then at intervals of 6 months to 1 year. Proper dispensing of the low-vision device is essential. This includes adjustment of the device to the patient's head, the verification of performance with the device, and instructing the child in its use. Not only must the device be comfortable for extended wear, but the visual axis of the optical system must be properly aligned to minimize aberrations. (See Chapter 8 for a complete discussion of spectacles for children.)

The optometrist should advise the school authorities about the nature of the child's visual impairment and the corrective measures taken. The report should clearly and completely explain the type of low-vision device(s) prescribed, its purpose and conditions of use, and lighting considerations and the child's placement in the classroom. Finally, it is important to emphasize the need to work closely with social service workers, psychologists, educators, and others who help the child to accept and adapt to his new visual role. It is vital to supply requested information about eligibility for services and to ease decision making on educational matters. For example, measures of visual field may alert teachers to specific approaches to reading instruction.*

Young adults who want to drive even though they have low vision are a special problem. Driving is an important issue to the patient, and it makes parents anxious. Many times a teenager can be coaxed to use a bioptic in the classroom as a training measure preparatory to driving. State vehicle licensure laws must be checked before a young patient is offered the hope of driving. Typically, a corrected acuity of 20/120 or better through the carrier lens with an improvement to 20/40 or better through the telescope is needed. Also, 140-degree fields are required in order to obtain a license. The Lighthouse of Houston/University of Houston clinic recommends that the first week of behind-the-wheel driver training be conducted without the bioptic, so that the student can become used to the mechanics of the automobile. The bioptic is then introduced to enhance the margin of safety for driving. The clinic requires that the prospective driver wear the bioptic for 3 months before applying for a driver's license. The patient is encouraged to first wear the bioptic while riding as a passenger in a car and while riding a bicycle. Most important, it is desirable for the patient to "go public" with the device. If not, it is likely the patient will get the driver's license and let the bioptic sit unused on the seat beside him instead of using it while driving.

A teenager and his parents should also be apprised of issues surrounding such a prescription, and they should be encouraged to discuss the psychologic and social ramifications and consequences of becoming a "handicapped" driver. Such a discussion is not meant as a deterrent; rather, it is a way to provide a meaningful discussion of the issues and responsibilities of optometrist, parents, and teenager.

Prescribing for younger children is usually not complicated. Young children adapt easily and learn quickly. Prescription devices that can be loaned for a few weeks are excellent for these situations. Normally, in a year or two, the student will ask parents or teachers about those "special glasses" the doctor showed them at the clinic. Every child grows up with individual goals and needs and matures at his or her own pace.

---

* (For a discussion of national standards and guidelines designed to serve as a resource for parents, educators, and administrators in identifying, assessing, and program planning for the unique needs of visually impaired students, see: Hazelkamp J, Huebner, KM (ed): Program Planning and Evaluation for Blind and Visually Impaired Students: National Guidelines for Educational Excellence. New York, American Foundation for the Blind, 1989.)

SUMMARY

Working with visually impaired children is rewarding. Early intervention is the key to successful growth and development. The low-vision optometrist must concentrate on delivering services to visually impaired children in the infancy to 8 years age group. If the impact of a visual impairment can be reduced at an early age, the barriers to learning will be minimized. The longer it takes to provide an optimal visual medium for learning, the farther behind the child will fall. In addition, bad habits will be formed, and resistance to school and learning may become a part of the child's psychological makeup. Prescribing an optical system does not always avoid or alleviate these problems, but it certainly helps in the process of motivating the child to achieve academic and social potential and excellence.

The transition between the supported environment of education and the sudden independence of the working world has been a weak link in the educational and vocational system. Suddenly, no one is there to help with the next step. Educational and vocational organizations are aware of this weakness and are developing programs to facilitate the transition. The low-vision optometrist can help by discussing vocational goals with high school (or even younger) students and beginning to address these goals through vocationally related prescriptions.

Assuming "visual responsibilities" takes on great importance at this time. The student who knows how best to use optical devices and how to modify the environment to enhance visual functioning will be better able to adapt and to solve new visual problem situations on the job and off.

This model of care is based on a delivery system developed under a grant by the Texas Education Agency, Project DOVES. The program provides appropriate vision care to visually impaired children. Modifications to this model may be necessary to suit the resources and needs of a particular area (11), but the concept of an interdisciplinary approach to vision care for the visually impaired student is mandatory (18).

A low-vision optometrist can take a proactive role in providing services to children by helping school administrations and rehabilitation personnel to understand the importance of cost benefits of low-vision care. Optical devices are no longer a luxury; they are an integral part of a child's educational program. Without optical devices, students are relegated to more dependent, and thus, more restrictive educational environments. Ultimately, without the visual independence such devices afford, young adults will be limited in their vocational and lifestyle choices (6).

Future research must address devices for specific tasks, such as viewing the chalkboard in adverse visual environments. It would also be desirable to have a multipurpose mobility aid, but this research is still in the beginning stages. Active research is in progress to develop new devices (34) and to address the important cosmetic concerns in the design of bioptics and other devices for writing, reading, seeing computer printouts, and related tasks. It is hoped that this research will make the benefits of the devices far outweigh their limitations. More students will be helped at earlier ages, thus substantially reducing the handicapping effects of their visual impairment. More visually impaired children will attain their growth potential and become substantive contributors and leaders in society, a goal that is worthy of optometrists' very best efforts.

APPENDIX 1

Sample Form

LOW VISION INTAKE FORM: VISUALLY IMPAIRED CHILD

DATE _____

NAME _____ SEX _____ AGE _____

ADDRESS _____

PARENT/PRIMARY CARETAKER _____

PHONE (H) _____ (O) _____

REFERRED BY _____ REPORT TO _____

REASON FOR REFERRAL _____
_____

VISUAL HISTORY (Onset; Dx; description; surgery; treatment; etc.) _____
_____
_____
_____
_____

CURRENT OPTOMETRIST _____ OPHTHALMOLOGIST _____

FAMILY VISUAL HISTORY: _____
_____

DEVELOPMENTAL HISTORY (Pregnancy/birth complications; health; medications; motor functions; disabilities; auditory/speech development; etc.) _____
_____
_____
_____
_____

EXPECTATIONS FOR LOW VISION EVALUATION _____
_____

FUNCTIONAL VISUAL ASSESSMENT AVAILABLE Yes _____ (Please attach) No _____

SCHOOL _____ STANDARD Rx _____

PUBLIC _____ PRIVATE _____ _____

EDUCATIONAL PLACEMENT _____ OPTICAL/LOW VISION DEVICE _____

APPENDIX 1 (*continued*)

ACADEMIC GRADE LEVEL __ GRADES __

READING LEVEL _____

SPECIAL EDUCATIONAL PROGRAM ____

RELATED EDUCATIONAL SERVICES ____

_____

SCHOOL RELATED VISION NEEDS

HOW DOES THE CHILD WORK WITH:

CHALKBOARD _____

COMPUTER ACCESS _____

TEXTS & WORKBOOKS _____

PRINT SIZE _____

CURRENT READING MODE (large; regular; Braille) _____

OTHER VISION NEEDS _____

_____

RELATED SERVICES (occupational; physical; speech; counseling/remedial) ____

_____

_____

Distance _____ Near _____

NON-OPTICAL DEVICES _____

_____

NEAR VISION (Toys; print; food) _____

_____

_____

MID-RANGE VISION (TV; play objects; faces; colors)_____

_____

_____

DISTANCE (play activities; sports; movies; street signs, etc) _____

_____

_____

ORIENTATION (gait; posture) _____

_____

ENVIRONMENTAL (seating; lighting) __

_____

ASSESSMENT (appearance; mood; orientation; intellectual functioning; gross and fine motor movements; attitude; motivation; social/emotional)

_____

_____

_____

OTHER: _____

_____

APPENDIX 2

Example of Eye Report Form

EXAMPLE OF EYE REPORT FORM
Educationally Oriented Vision Report
(To be completed by the eye specialist)

Date:	Month	Day	Year	Student's name:	Last	First	Middle

The following information would be helpful in determining educational programming based on the needs of the student. We would appreciate your completing this form in addition to the "Eye Report for Children with Visual Problems."

1. What is the cause of visual impairment?

2. Is any special treatment required? If so, what is the general nature of the treatment?

3. Is the visual impairment likely to get worse, better, or stay the same?

4. What symptoms would indicate a need for reexamination?

5. Should any restrictions be placed on the student's activities?

6. Should the student wear glasses or contact lenses? If so, under what circumstances?

7. If it was not possible to do a visual acuity measure, what is your opinion regarding what the student sees?

8. Are the student's focusing ability, tracking, and eye muscle balance adequate? If not, please describe:

9. If the student's visual field was not testable, what is your opinion regarding this student's field of vision?

10. Please describe the object size and distances that are optimal for the student:

APPENDIX 2 (*continued*)

11. What lighting conditions would be optimal for the student's visual functioning?

_____

12. Do you have any additional specific recommendations concerning this student's use of vision in learning situations?

_____

13. When should this student be examined again?

_____

Please return this form to:

_____

Reprinted from *Program Guidelines for Visually Impaired Individuals* (rev. ed.: Sacramento, CA: California State Department of Education, 1987).

REFERENCES

1. Adelson E, Fraiberg S: Gross motor development in infants blind from birth: Child Dev 45:114, 1974.

2. American Printing House for the Blind: Reaching Out Since 1858: One Hundred Nineteenth Annual Report of the American Printing House for the Blind for the Year Ended June 30, 1987. Louisville, KY, 1988.

3. Barraga N, Collins M: Development of efficiency in visual functioning: Rationale for a comprehensive program. J Visual Impairment Blindness 73:121, 1979.

4. Bishop V: Making choices in functional vision evaluations: "Noodles, needles, and haystacks." J Visual Impairment Blindness 82:94, 1988.

5. Corn A: Low vision and visual efficiency. In Scholl G (ed): Foundation of Education for Blind and Visually Handicapped Children and Youth, ch 6. New York, American Foundation for the Blind, 1986.

6. Corn A, Ryser G: Access to print for students with low vision. J Visual Impairment Blindness 83:340, 1989.

7. Daugherty K, Moran M: Neuropsychological, learning and developmental characteristics of the low vision child. J Visual Impairment Blindness 9:398, 1982.

8. Faye E, Padula W, Padula J, et al: The low-vision child. In Faye E (ed): Clinical Low Vision, ch 18. Boston, Little, Brown, 438, 1984.

9. Fraiberg S: Parallel and divergent patterns in blind and sighted infants. Psychoanal Study Child 23:264, 1968.

10. Furth HS, Wachs H: Thinking Goes to School. New York, Oxford University Press, 1974.

11. Goldie D, Gormezano S, Raznik P: Comprehensive low vision services for visually impaired children: A function of special education. J Visual Impairment Blindness 80:844, 1986.

12. Harrington DO: The Visual Fields. St Louis, CV Mosby, 1981.

13. Hazekamp J: The team approach to advocacy. In Schell G (ed): Foundation of Education for Blind and Visually Handicapped Children and Youth. New York, American Foundation for the Blind, 275, 1986.

14. Hofstetter H, Wolter R: Unmet vision care needs. J Vision Rehab 3:1985.

15. Hyvarinen L: Vision and Eye Screening in Finland: An Overview. Helsinki Finland, Institute of Occupational Health, 1988.

16. Jose RT (ed): Understanding Low Vision. New York, American Foundation for the Blind, 1983.

17. Jose R, Ferraro J: A functional interpretation of the visual fields of the low vision patient. J Am Optom Assoc 54:885, 1983.

18. Jose R, Labossiere S, Small M: Project D.O.V.E.S. J Vision Rehab 1:5, 1987.

19. Jose R, Smith AJ, Shane K: Evaluating and stimulating vision in the multiply impaired. J Visual Impairment Blindness 74:2, 1980.

20. Kirschner C: Data on Blindness and Visual Impairment in the United States. New York, American Foundation for the Blind, 82, 1985.

21. Langley B, Dubose R: Functional Vision Screening for Severely Handicapped Children. New Outlook Blind 70:346, 1976.

22. Mehr E, Freid A: Low Vision Care. Chicago IL, Professional Press, 1975.

23. Mills R: In Welsh R, Blasch B (eds): Additional handicaps. In: Foundation of Orientation and Mobility. New York, American Foundation for the Blind, 429, 1980.

24. Miner LE: Speech improvement for visually handicapped children. New Outlook Blind 57:160, 1963.

25. O'Brien R: Alive-Aware-A-Person. Montgomery County Public Schools, Rockville, MD, 1976.

26. Pease P, Allen J: Preferential color vision test. Houston, TX, University of Houston College of Optometry, 1988.

27. Rosenbloom A: Principles and examination techniques for the care of the partially sighted child. Part IV in Manual on the Partially Seeing Child. St Louis, American Optometric Association, 55, 1961.

28. Rosenbloom A: The partially seeing child. In Hirsch M, Wick R (eds): Vision of Children: An Optometric Symposium, ch. 10. Philadelphia, Chilton, 251, 1963.

29. Rosenbloom A: Low vision. In Peyman G, Sanders D, Goldberg M (eds): Principles and Practice of Ophthalmology, vol 1. Philadelphia, WB Saunders, 241, 1980.

30. Scholl G: Visual impairments. In Scholl G (ed): The School Psychologist and the Exceptional Child, ch 10. Reston VA, The Council on Exceptional Children, 210, 1985.

31. Scholl G: Growth and development. In Scholl G (ed): Foundations of Education for Blind and Visually Handicapped Children and Youth, ch 4. New York, American Foundation for the Blind, 93, 1986.

32. Spitzberg L, Keuther C, Jose R: The new writing magnifier. J Vision Rehab 1:23, 1987.

33. Spitzberg L, Jose R, Kuether, C: The behind the lens telescope—A new concept in bioptics. Am J Optom 66:616, 1989.

34. Stabinsky A: Project STRIDES—Program for Multiply Impaired. Available through Region IV Education Service Center, Houstin, TX, 1988.

35. Stephens B: Cognitive Processes in the Visually Impaired. Education of the Visually Handicapped 4, 106, 1972.

36. Stern EJ: Helping the person with low vision. Am J Nurs 80:1789, 1980.

37. Warren D: Blindness and Early Childhood Development. New York, American Foundation for the Blind, 32, 1984.

38. Watson G, Jose R: A training sequence for low vision patients. J Am Optom Assoc 47:1407, 1976.

Chapter 16

Assessment and Management of the Exceptional Child

Mitchell Scheiman

Many textbooks devoted entirely to the subject of mentally and multiply handicapped (MMH) children contain detailed information about various handicapping disorders. What is not readily available, however, is a presentation that stresses the special needs of different MMH children for optometric assessment and management of vision disorders. The objective of this chapter is to present information that will be most useful to primary care optometrists who encounter MMH children in practice.

Several issues make the topic of MMH children very important for optometry. First, unless a practice is limited to adult patients, the likelihood of encountering MMH children is great. The incidence figures discussed later in this chapter indicate that a significant percentage of children have mental or multiple handicaps. In addition, a large percentage of children with handicapping conditions also may have one or more vision anomalies, such as refractive errors, strabismus, amblyopia, nystagmus, accommodative disorders, visual perceptual anomalies, and ocular pathology. Therefore, not only are there many children with MMH, but a majority of these children have functional vision problems or ocular pathology that may need the optometrist's attention.

Another important issue is the current trend in society toward deinstitutionalization of this population as a result of governmental programs and pressure (21, 115). More and more MMH children are being mainstreamed into regular educational settings and are living at home. As a result, today a primary care optometrist is more likely to encounter these children than ever before.

Finally, the infant vision research that has accumulated in recent years clearly suggests the importance of early identification and intervention for vision anomalies (6, 35, 110). Prompt identification and treatment of any disorder is critical, particularly when a child is faced with multiple problems that might affect development and health.

When these four factors are considered, it becomes evident that if optometrists are to fulfill their role as a primary care profession, they must become knowledgeable about the special needs of these special people, who have such a high incidence of vision disorders. The specific objectives of this chapter are as follows:

Provide a brief but adequate description of the most prevalent conditions.

Provide incidence and prevalence data for the various conditions.

Provide data about the prevalence of vision disorders in each condition.

Recommend and describe modifications of assessment techniques that may make them more effective for gathering data from MMH children.

Recommend and describe modifications in treatment that may be necessary to most effectively manage vision problems in MMH children.

Stress the importance of an interdisciplinary approach to managing the vision problems of MMH children.

Stress the importance of the role of providing guidance and advice to parents of MMH children and to professionals who work with these children.

COMMON MENTALLY/MULTIPLY HANDICAPPING CONDITIONS IN CHILDREN

The most common handicapping conditions an optometrist is likely to encounter are mental retardation, cerebral palsy, Down's syndrome, spina bifida (myelomeningocele),

hearing impairment, and low-birth-weight syndrome.

Mental Retardation

Description and Incidence

Mental retardation is a condition found in many disorders with known and unknown causes (109). Because it is a complication associated with all of the handicapping conditions to be described, it represents the most common childhood problem of exceptionality that the optometrist is likely to encounter in practice. It is, therefore, important to begin any discussion of mentally or multiply handicapping conditions with the subject of mental retardation.

The definition of mental retardation according to the American Academy of Mental Deficiency (AAMD) includes three specific components (88): (1) a significantly subaverage general level of functioning (2 SD below the norm, that is, less than 70), normal IQ is considered to be above 70) and (2) a concurrent deficit in adaptive behavior, and (3) both of which are manifest during the developmental period between birth and age 21 years.

To be classified as mentally retarded a person must have an IQ below 70 and must display poor adaptive functioning. Depending on the demands placed on a child and his or her ability to adapt, the child may be classified at one point as mentally retarded and several years later as normal. The reported incidence of mental retardation may, therefore, vary depending on age level. The number of children classified as retarded rises during the school years and decreases toward age 15 to 19, when scholastic demands are no longer an issue in determining functional adequacy. It is estimated that 30 to 70 percent of young adults with IQs in the 55 to 69 range make adequate vocational and social adjustment to community life (109). By definition, therefore, they are not considered retarded.

Based on a low IQ level alone, the prevalence of mental retardation has been estimated at approximately 2.5 percent of the general population, but recent studies that also carefully consider adaptive functioning suggest a prevalence closer to 1 percent of children under 18 years of age (88).

Etiology

There are numerous potential causes of mental retardation (Table 16.1). Mental retardation is also associated with all of the other syndromes and conditions discussed in this chapter. In the majority of cases, particularly when the retardation is in the mild to moderate range, the cause is unknown (11).

Classification

Two systems of classification are currently in general use. One is more popular with educators of mentally retarded children and the other is generally used by health care professionals. Which terminology is used depends on which type of professional the optometrist communicates with. In the following description, the primary terminology used is the educational classification and the medical system is shown in parentheses.

Educable Mentally Retarded (Mildly Mentally Retarded) This category includes 90 percent of children who are classified as retarded. Most need special class placement, and some can achieve fourth- to sixth-grade reading levels. Those who are well adjusted may be able to function independently as adults. Approximately two thirds are employed, and 80 percent are married (88). The IQ as measured with the Wechsler Scales is between 55 and 69.

Trainable Mentally Retarded (Moderately Mentally Retarded) Children in this group usually function in classes that emphasize self-care skills and perhaps some academic skills. They are capable of learning concepts equivalent to about third-grade level. Those who are well-adjusted may be able to function semi-independently in supervised living and sheltered workshop settings. They can generally write their name and learn enough arithmetic to do their own basic shopping as adults. Their IQs fall between 40 and 54 on the Wechsler Scales.

Severely Retarded (Severe) Children in this category can learn minimal self-care skills and simple conversation. They need extensive supervision from parents or relatives and

Table 16.1 POSSIBLE CAUSES OF MENTAL RETARDATION

Condition or Associated Event	Examples
Metabolic Disorders	Tay-Sachs Disease
Chromosomal Abnormalities	Down's Syndrome
Mother Exposed to Teratogens during Pregnancy	Chemicals, Alcohol, Radiation
Infection during Pregnancy	Rubella Cytomegalovirus
Fetal Malnutrition	Mother with High Blood Pressure, Kidney Disease
Events Associated with Birth Process	Prematurity, Hypoxia, Trauma from Forceps
Events Occurring in Postnatal Period	Meningitis, Automobile Accidents, Child Abuse, Near Drowning, Lead Poisoning, Parental Psychiatric Disorders

are often institutionalized. IQ is between 25 and 39.

Profoundly Retarded (Profound) The IQ is less than 25, and the children need total supervision. Very minimal self-care skills are possible. Some may be toilet trained. Language development is limited. Such persons need permanent nursing care.

It is important to be aware that severely and profoundly retarded persons make up only 5 percent of the retarded population. Optometrists are most likely, therefore, to encounter only mildly or moderately retarded patients.

Vision Problems in Mentally Retarded Children

Table 16.2 is a compilation of some of the studies that have reported on the prevalence of vision problems in mentally retarded children (60, 62, 64, 71, 111, 114). It is apparent from this table that the prevalence of refractive conditions, strabismus, nystagmus, and optic atrophy is considerably higher in this population than in children with normal intelligence.

Although few studies have attempted to relate the prevalence of vision anomalies to the degree of retardation, a study by Tuppurainen (111) reported that more than 75 percent of moderately to profoundly retarded children have vision disorders, whereas only 36 percent of mildly retarded ones do.

Other Problems Associated with Mental Retardation

Approximately 85 percent of mentally retarded children have at least one additional handicap, which may be a problem with ambulation and speech, emotional difficulties, a vision or hearing disorder, dental disease, obesity, anemia, heart disease, or diabetes.

Cerebral Palsy

Description and Incidence

Cerebral palsy does not describe a single disease. Rather, it is a group of signs and symptoms that may be associated with many

different diseases. The term *cerebral palsy* refers to any disorder of movement and posture that results from a nonprogressive abnormality or injury of the brain (50). A critical aspect of the definition of cerebral palsy is that the injury occurs during the early stages of development and before the child's brain has fully matured. Most authorities suggest that this period encompasses approximately the first three years of life (51, 112). Any injury to the brain during fetal, perinatal, and early development can lead to cerebral palsy. It is important to remember that with cerebral palsy the difficulty lies in the *brain's* ability to control the muscles and nerves rather than with the muscles and nerves directly.

The incidence of cerebral palsy is about 1.5 to 2 per 1000 live births (51); the actual prevalence is higher than this because of postnatal causes. Approximately 700,000 persons in the United States have cerebral palsy (14). Each year an estimated 10,000 babies are born with cerebral palsy or acquire it early in life, and it is considered to be the most widespread lifetime disability.

Etiology

Virtually any disease that can affect brain development can lead to cerebral palsy. The causal factors are generally divided into prenatal, natal, and postnatal categories. Prenatal causes include maternal stroke, intrauterine infection, exposure to radiation, ingestion of teratogenic drugs, abruptio placentae, and fetal malformations. Perinatal factors include complications of labor and delivery, prematurity, low birth weight, and apnea. Finally, the most common postnatal causes are early childhood disorders such as meningitis, lead poisoning, head trauma, and drowning (47, 82). The most recent studies have suggested that the cause of cerebral palsy is prenatal about 50 percent of the time, perinatal in 33 percent of cases, and postnatal in about 17 percent (54).

In spite of extensive investigation of the causes of cerebral palsy researchers report that the cause is unknown approximately 50 to 75 percent of the time (78, 79).

Table 16.2 PREVALENCE OF VISION ANOMALIES IN MENTALLY RETARDED CHILDREN

Study (Ref.)	No. of Subjects	Hyperopia	Myopia	Astigmatism	Anisometropia	Strabismus	Nystagmus	Cataract	Optic Atrophy
Kolb (62)	96	20 (21%)	8 (8%)	20 (21%)	—	16 (17%)	11 (11%)	7 (7%)	—
Kirschen (60)	93	45 (48%)	25 (27%)	—	—	20 (22%)	18 (19%)	—	—
Lennerstrand (64)	26	8 (30%)	10 (38%)	9 (35%)	—	13 (50%)	8 (31%)	—	11 (42%)
Manley (71)	25	12 (48%)	3 (10%)	—	—	—	—	—	—
Tuppurainen (119)	149	— 42%	—	31 (21%)	15 (10%)	37 (25%)	16 (10%)	3 (2%)	8 (5%)
Wiesinger (114)	75	38 (51%)	22 (29%)	—	—	38 (51%)	11 (15%)	7 (9%)	11 (15%)

Classification of Cerebral Palsy

Classification of cerebral palsy is based on motor signs and symptoms. Although as many as seven types of cerebral palsy have been identified (76), there are three principal subtypes of cerebral palsy that are important to remember: spastic (pyramidal), athetoid (extrapyramidal), and mixed. Which particular type of cerebral palsy occurs as a result of any injury depends on the timing of the event, the location of the damage, and the causal factor.

Spastic (Pyramidal) Cerebral Palsy   When the injury is located in the motor cortex or the pyramidal tract, spasticity occurs. This is the most common form of cerebral palsy, accounting for 60 percent of all cerebral palsy, and results in muscle stiffness. Harryman (50) compares the muscle tone in spasticity to the movement that occurs when a pocket knife is closed. As the extremity is moved, resistance initially is strong, but it gives way suddenly.

The final damage depends on the location of the injury in the motor cortex or pyramidal tract. Spastic cerebral palsy can be subclassified as paraplegia (involvement of legs only), diplegia (involvement of trunk and all four extremities, generally legs more than arms), hemiplegia (involvement of one side of the body only), and quadriplegia (involvement of arms, legs, head, and trunk). The most common form of spastic cerebral palsy is hemiplegia, which occurs about 60 percent of the time.

Athetoid (Extrapyramidal) Cerebral Palsy   Approximately 20 percent of all cerebral palsy is caused by injury to the basal ganglia and is referred to as dyskinesia. The basal ganglia are the part of the nervous system that regulates movement. Extrapyramidal cerebral palsy can be subclassified as choreoathetosis—abrupt, involuntary movements of the extremities—and asthetosis—slow, writhing movements, particularly of the wrists and fingers. In the former, the affected person has difficulty maintaining balance rather than controlling movement.

Mixed   Twenty percent of persons with cerebral palsy have a combination of the two types described above, although one type tends to predominate.

Vision Problems and Cerebral Palsy

A very high incidence of vision problems in cerebral palsy children has consistently been reported (3, 12, 24, 25, 28, 31, 46, 53, 65, 66–68, 95, 97, 98, 100, 104). Table 16.3 displays the various studies and their respective results. Reported vision disorders include strabismus (15 to 60 percent), amblyopia (6 to 16 percent), significant refractive error (19 to 69 percent), nystagmus (2 to 9 percent), and optic atrophy (2 to 17 percent). A recent study by Scheiman (104) was the first to report on a group of cerebral palsy children with normal intelligence. All previous reports had studied cerebral palsy populations that included persons of normal intelligence and mentally retarded ones. Scheiman hypothesized that the high incidence of vision problems found in previous reports would be present only in the most severely affected cerebral palsy children. His study, however, revealed that even in cerebral palsy children with normal intelligence the incidence of vision anomalies is high. He found 69 percent had strabismus, 4 percent had clinically significant heterophorias, 30 percent had accommodative anomalies, and 64 percent had significant refractive error.

Duckman also studied a group of cerebral palsy children with normal intelligence and found that 100% of his sample were unable to pass standard accommodative facility testing (25, 28). The presence of visual perceptual anomalies has also been investigated. Using the Bender Gestalt test, Patel and Bharucha (81) found a greater incidence of visual motor problems in cerebral palsy children than in a control group. Duckman (25) administered the Piaget Test of right-left concepts, the Winterhaven Copy Forms, and the Motor Free Visual Perception Test to 25 cerebral palsy children and found that 78 percent had visual perceptual dysfunction.

There has been only one longitudinal study of vision in cerebral palsy. Lo Casio

Table 16.3　PREVALENCE OF VISION ANOMALIES IN CEREBRAL PALSY CHILDREN

Study (Ref.)	No. of Subjects	Hyperopia (%)	Myopia (%)	Astigmatism (%)	Combined Refractive Error (%)	Esotropia (%)	Exotropia (%)	Amblyopia (%)	Nystagmus (%)	Optic Atrophy (%)
Scheiman (96)	73	22	15	28	64	32	37	32	18	4
Altman (2)	64	33	16	21	69	30	14	6	5	14
Breakey (12)	100	—	—	—	—	40	8	—	2	3
Fantl (31)	417	27	23	—	—	—	—	—	—	—
Guibor (46)	147	—	—	—	—	52	9	25	9	2
Lossef (68)	88	—	—	—	67	17	17	—	7	17
Seaber (100)	232	—	—	—	—	28	23	—	3	5
Schrire (98)	73	3	11	5	19	11	4	16	4	4
Schachat (95)	98	—	—	—	54	22	21	—	—	—
Lo Casio (66)	124	—	—	—	61	23	21	—	—	—
Douglas (24)	168	—	—	—	—	13	6	—	2	8

(67) followed the progress of 34 children with cerebral palsy over an 11-year period. Initially the sample had a high incidence of vision anomalies: 72 percent had significant refractive errors, 68 percent had strabismus, 9 percent nystagmus, and 9 percent optic atrophy. His final data analysis indicated that, left untreated, the strabismus remained relatively stable. In regard to refractive state, the athetoid children became less myopic and astigmatic, whereas all types of refractive anomalies of those in the spastic category deteriorated.

The literature, therefore, clearly indicates a very high incidence of vision problems in cerebral palsy children, both the mentally retarded ones and those with normal intelligence. The high incidence appears to be associated with all categories of cerebral palsy.

Other Problems Associated with Cerebral Palsy

In addition to vision anomalies, cerebral palsy children often have other disabilities of which optometrists must be aware in order to make appropriate modifications in assessment and management techniques—mental retardation, auditory and language disorders, epilepsy, behavioral and emotional disorders. Approximately 60 to 70 percent of cerebral palsy children are mentally retarded. The incidence and degree of retardation are related to the type of cerebral palsy. The lowest incidence of retardation is in the spastic subclass, while a large percentage of the mixed category are generally retarded. Although mental retardation is fairly common in cerebral palsy, only 50 percent of patients are severely to profoundly retarded; 35 percent are moderately retarded, and 15 percent are mildly retarded (89).

Optometrists generally encounter cerebral palsy children who have normal intelligence or are only mildly to moderately retarded. These children tend to live at home and may be in special education programs or mainstreamed. Severely to profoundly retarded cerebral palsy children are more likely to be institutionalized. Optometrists

who are not consultants for an institution are less likely to encounter such children.

The type of cerebral palsy associated with kernicterus (in which bilirubin deposited in the basal ganglia damages the extrapyramidal tracts) is often associated with hearing loss. Robinson estimates (89) that 20 percent of cerebral palsy children have hearing and language deficits.

Another problem associated with cerebral palsy is epilepsy. Spastic types of cerebral palsy are most often associated with epilepsy, but approximately 35 percent of all children with cerebral palsy develop seizures at some time in their lives (50).

Finally, psychosocial problems of adjustment to permanent disability are common, particularly in cerebral palsy children with normal intelligence during adolescence (34).

Down's Syndrome

Description and Incidence

Also referred to as trisomy 21, Down's syndrome results from a chromosomal abnormality in which there is an extra chromosome 21 or an extra part of it in each body cell. Instead of the normal 46 chromosomes, persons with Down's syndrome have 47. This abnormality causes the physical and developmental features of Down's syndrome—mental retardation, congenital heart disease, short stature, speckling of the iris (Brushfield's spots), upward slanted eyes, epicanthal folds, small oral cavity and protruding tongue, wide gap between first and second toes, and short, broad hands with a single palmar crease (simian crease).

The most significant of these defects is the mental handicap, which can be mild or severe. Most Down's syndrome children are moderately retarded. One of the very important concepts about Down's syndrome for optometrists is the prognosis for development and quality of life. Until the past 2 decades, Down's syndrome children generally were raised in adverse environments such as institutions (102). Little was expected of them, so they were taught little and, therefore, achieved little.

Recently, however, the positive effects of home rearing (106) and early education programs (69) have revealed greater potential and variability among Down's syndrome children than had been previously anticipated. A recent study by Sharav et al (102) suggested that, just as the level of maternal education is one of the determining factors in the development of normal children, it is also an important factor in the development of Down's syndrome children. Sharav concluded that "the intellectual functioning of the child with Down's syndrome is not a global one that produces a uniform level of mental retardation. It appears that the trisomy 21 may produce an effect of subtracting a constant amount of intellectual potential from what would have been expected if the child had not had Down's syndrome." A recent editorial in the Australian Pediatric Journal expressed an even more optimistic viewpoint. ". . . The majority of Down's syndrome children provided with effective early education can be expected to acquire a wide repertoire of skills within, or close to, the normal range for their age by the end of the preschool period" (19).

The importance of this information is that the same environmental influences that determine whether a normal child fulfills his or her potential are important for Down's syndrome children. Thus, just as we stress the importance of vision in the development and school-related activities of normal children, we must emphasize the role that vision may play in the lives of mentally retarded children.

The incidence of Down's syndrome is generally considered to be approximately 1 in 600 to 800 live births. A very important finding, however, is that the incidence increases significantly with the age of the mother. A recent study by Heuther et al (52), for instance, found a reported rate of approximately 0.5 per 1000 at age 20, 1 per 1000 at 30, 3 per 1000 at 35, 10 per 1000 at 40, 36 per 1000 at 45, and 250 per 1000 for women older than 49.

Vision Problems Associated with Down's Syndrome

The appearance of children with Down's syndrome is so characteristic that these children tend to resemble each other more than they resemble their relatives (70). Part of this characteristic appearance is due to the ocular features of Down's syndrome children. This includes short and oblique palpebral fissures and prominent epicanthal folds (70). The outer canthus is higher than the inner canthus, and the palpebral aperture is 3 to 5 mm shorter horizontally than in normal eyes.

Table 16.4 summarizes some of the studies that have reported the prevalence of vision problems in Down's syndrome children. It is evident that the visual system is significantly affected in Down's syndrome. In addition to the high prevalence of functional vision problems such as refractive anomaly and strabismus, Down's syndrome children also are likely to have blepharitis, keratoconus, and Brushfield's spots.

In Cullen and Butler's study (22) of Down's patients, 5.5 percent had keratoconus. They described acute keratoconus in five of the eight patients with the condition. In these instances the patients experienced an acute episode in which Descemet's membrane ruptured. The clinical picture was one of sudden cloudiness and ecstasia of the cornea associated with pain, redness, and lacrimation.

Brushfield's spots were first described by Wolfin in 1902 and later associated with Down's syndrome by Brushfield (13). They are white to yellow, slightly raised, discrete pinhead-sized areas in the iris periphery. Generally they form an even, concentric ring, but they may also occupy only a portion of the iris periphery or may be scattered irregularly in the middle and peripheral zones of the iris (83). They tend to be more common in blue and hazel eyes than in brown ones. In Jaeger's sample, Brushfield's spots were found in 95 percent of subjects with blue eyes but in only 17 percent of those with brown eyes. The cause of this anomaly is unknown, and Brushfield's spots have no known functional significance (56).

Table 16.4 PREVALENCE OF VISION ANOMALIES IN DOWN'S SYNDROME CHILDREN

Study (Ref.)	No. of Subjects	Hyperopia	Myopia	Astigmatism	Strabismus	Nystagmus	Cataract	Keratoconus	Brushfield Spots	Blepharitis
Cullen (22)	143	—	—	—	46 (32%)	7 (5%)	22 (15%)	8 (6%)	—	3 (2%)
Fanning (30)	24	13 (54%)	2 (8%)	—	7 (29%)	1 (4%)	—	—	—	—
Gardiner (39)	62	9 (15%)	31 (50%)	23 (37%)	—	—	—	—	—	—
Jaeger (56)	75	14 (19%)	23 (31%)	—	31 (41%)	8 (11%)	27 (37%)	2 (3%)	44 (59%)	—
Lyle (70)	44	5 (11%)	14 (32%)	—	16 (36%)	7 (15%)	12 (27%)	2 (5%)	27 (62%)	18 (41%)
Pesch (83)	41	15 (37%)	10 (24%)	6 (15%)	23 (56%)	14 (34%)	1 (2%)	—	19 (46%)	10 (24%)
Shapiro (101)	53	—	—	—	23 (43%)	5 (9%)	7 (13%)	5 (9%)	43 (81%)	25 (47%)
Total	442	25%	33%	29%	38%	11%	19%	6%	62%	20%

Other Problems Associated with Down's Syndrome

Other serious health problems that are often associated with Down's syndrome include congenital heart disease and duodenal atresia, or blockage of the small intestine. These anomalies can usually be treated successfully by medical and surgical means. After such treatment is completed there is essentially no difference in health status between normal children and those with Down's syndrome.

Myelomeningocele (Spina Bifida)

Description and Incidence

Myelomeningocele is considered to be a congenital malformation or developmental defect of the nervous system. Specifically, during the latter part of the first month of gestation, the spinal cord and vertebrae around it do not form properly and the posterior portion of the neural tube fails to close, usually in the lumbosacral region.

There are three types of open spine defects: spina bifida occulta, meningocele, and spina bifida cystica (myelomeningocele) (63). Spina bifida occulta is a mild malformation present in about 10 percent of children, usually in the lumbar region. The backs of the vertebrae fail to form, but there are no abnormalities in the membranes or spinal cord. Generally there is nothing more than a hairy dimple on the skin of the lower back, and it is usually an isolated insignificant finding with little functional consequence.

With meningocele, the spinal cord itself does not pouch out but the membranes (meninges) surrounding it do distend. In spite of this distension of the membranes, neither motor nor sensory defects in the legs nor incontinence is usually present in this form of spine defect. Laurence reported on a 10-year longitudinal study of 39 patients with meningocele and found that all 39 survived (63). Only six were even slightly or moderately incapacitated, having a bad gait or partial paralysis. In 6 of the 39 hydrocephalus developed but it resolved spontaneously.

Myelomeningocele (Fig. 16.1) is the most serious open spine disorder. Both the meninges and the spinal cord or nerve rootlets protrude through the abnormal opening in the spine. The nerves to the lower limbs and internal organs, particularly the bladder and kidneys, may be cut off, causing paralysis and lack of function. Various abnormalities of the skeletal system such as clubfoot and dislocated hips and anomalies of the heart and bowel may be present. In addition, hydrocephalus caused by obstruction of the normal flow of cerebrospinal fluid is a very common complicating factor. Often hydrocephalus first develops after surgical repair of the myelomeningocele. Mental retardation is

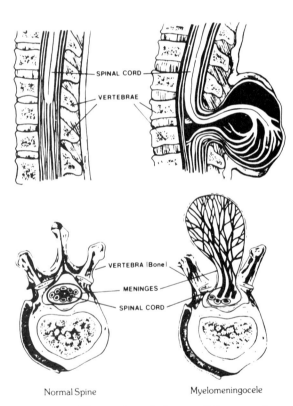

Figure 16.1 Illustration of abnormalities associated with myelomenigocele. (From Wolraich ML: Myelomeningocele. In Blackman JA: Medical Aspects of Developmental Disabilities in Children Birth Through Three. Reprinted with permission of Aspen Publishers, Inc., 1983.)

commonly associated with the hydrocephalus. In myelomeningocele the most frequent cause of obstruction is the Arnold-Chiari malformation, which is due to aberrant development of the lower brain stem and cerebellum.

Untreated hydrocephalus can produce brain damage and retardation. The standard treatment for hydrocephalus is surgical diversion of the cerebrospinal fluid (CSF) from the cerebral ventricle to the peritoneum or the right atrium. This is referred to as a shunt. Figure 16.2 illustrates how a shunt functions. A tube is inserted into the ventricles with a one-way valve that drains the cerebrospinal fluid out of the brain. This is generally connected to a tube that is threaded just under the skin down into the cavity of the abdomen. There are complications associated with shunts, including infection, obstruction, and the need for reoperation. Even with prompt treatment approximately 60 percent of children with hydrocephalus have significant intellectual and motor problems (103).

Laurence reported on 368 children with myelomeningocele who were followed over a 10-year period (63). Approximately 50 per-

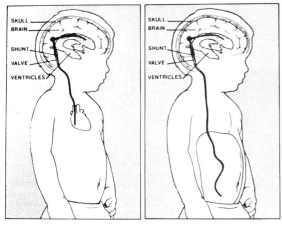

SKULL
BRAIN
SHUNT
VALVE
VENTRICLES

SKULL
BRAIN
SHUNT
VALVE
VENTRICLES

Ventriculo-Peritoneal (VP) Shunt   Ventriculo-Atrial (VA) Shunt

Figure 16.2 Illustration of how a shunt functions in hydrocephalus. (From Wolraich ML: Myelomeningocele. In Blackman JA: Medical Aspects of Developmental Disabilities in Children Birth Through Three. Reprinted with permission of Aspen Publishers, Inc., 1983.)

cent did not survive the full 10 years. The most common causes of death were intracranial infection and hydrocephalus. Shurtleff (103) reported on 112 patients with myelomeningocele and found that 90 percent survived for at least 10 years.

For the children who survive, an important issue is the quality of life. Although myelomeningocele itself is a nonprogressive disease, associated secondary disorders can worsen and have a significant effect on the child's lifestyle. Musculoskeletal deformities and complications can have very detrimental effects on a child's mobility and self-care potential (55). In addition, learning self-care and mobility skills also depends very much upon intellectual capacity.

Myelomeningocele or spina bifida cystica is one of the most common developmental anomalies of the nervous system, with an incidence of 0.4 to 4 per 1000 (115).

Vision Problems in Spina Bifida Cystica

The most common vision anomaly associated with myelomeningocele is strabismus. Studies by various authors have found that approximately 30 to 55 percent of children with myelomeningocele and hydrocephalus have strabismus (17, 33, 41, 43, 49, 90, 105). Rothstein and France both reported (33, 90) that approximately 70 percent of the strabismus was esotropia and 30 percent exotropia. Unusually high incidences of A pattern esotropia and exotropia have been found by one author (33). While A and V patterns may be found in 15 to 25 percent of typical samples of strabismus patients, France found that over 60 percent of his sample of children with myelomeningocele had an A pattern.

Several studies have tried to determine whether the strabismus is associated with the myelomeningocele or the hydrocephalus. Rothstein (90) reported on 52 patients with myelomeningocele and hydrocephalus, 44 percent of whom had strabismus. In a group of 15 children with myelomeningocele and no hydrocephalus, no strabismus was found. Stanworth et al (105) found the same trend, reporting that strabismus was found in 52 percent of those who had hydrocephalus but in only 12 percent of those who did not. Thus, hydrocephalus rather than the myelomeningocele appears to be the cause of the high rate of strabismus in this population.

According to Harcourt (49) the causes of strabismus associated with hydrocephalus can be divided into two broad categories. The first category includes hydrocephalus unrelated to shunting procedures. The strabismus in such cases, usually noncomitant and convergent, is caused by elevated intracranial pressure or stretching and angulation of the brain stem and cranial nerves. Meningitis and encephalitis may occur by direct infection through the site of the myelomeningocele and can lead to strabismus. Finally, the strabismus may be secondary to poor visual acuity due to optic atrophy following papilledema or chiasmal compression (49).

The second category or causes of strabismus associated with hydrocephalus includes those that are directly related to the shunting procedure. After a shunting procedure is completed, development of strabismus has significant implications. If a valve becomes infected, leading to meningitis, various patterns of noncomitant strabismus may result. If a valve is blocked there may be a dramatic rise in intracranial pressure, producing a rapidly progressive alternating, noncomitant esotropia due to pressure on the sixth nerves.

Hearing Impairment

Description and Incidence
There are several methods of classifying hearing loss (8): by location of the damage, age at onset, or degree of loss. Three types of damage can occur: conductive, sensorineural, and mixed. Damage to the external or middle ear causes conductive hearing loss, whereas malfunction of the cochlea or auditory nerve results in sensorineural loss. Mixed type is a combination of the two. Hearing impairment can be congenital or acquired. Finally, one can classify hearing deficits by the severity of the loss.

The two major categories of hearing impairment are deafness and partial hearing. Deafness is generally defined as hearing loss so severe at birth and in the prelanguage period that it precludes the normal development of speech (73). Partial hearing refers to persons who had normal hearing in the prelanguage period but lost their hearing later. Less severe forms of hearing loss include mild, moderate, and severe impairment.

Hearing loss occurs in approximately 0.5 percent of the population. Of these individuals, 40 percent have a mild loss, 20 percent a moderate loss, 20 percent a severe loss, and 20 percent a profound loss (8). Profound loss or deafness occurs in about 1 in 1000 children, 65 percent of whom are born deaf.

For about 50 percent of children with hearing loss the cause is unknown. For the other 50 percent there are several possible etiological factors. Mild to moderate conductive hearing loss may be caused by chronic otitis media or middle ear infections. Approximately 50 percent of severe sensorineural losses are caused by genetically inherited conditions. Others are acquired, intrauterine infection being a significant cause. Viruses such as rubella, toxoplasmosis, herpes virus, and cytomegalovirus can lead to hearing loss.

In the perinatal period, anoxia can damage the auditory nerve, resulting in deafness. In newborns, damage to the basal ganglia as a result of build-up of bilirubin (kernicterus) is associated with sensorineural loss. Finally, bacterial meningitis and head trauma that leads to skull fracture and intracranial hemorrhage may cause a hearing problem.

Vision Problems Associated with Deafness
The literature on the vision characteristics of deaf children suggests that they have a higher incidence of vision problems than normal children do. Previous studies have revealed an incidence of 38 to 76 percent of visual anomalies among deaf children (42, 44, 77, 85, 118) (Table 16.5).

Mohindra (77) reported on a sample of 77 deaf children and examined six general areas: visual acuity, refractive status, binocularity, color vision, ocular pathology, and visual perceptual skills. She found that 76 percent

Table 16.5 PREVALENCE OF VISION ANOMALIES IN DEAF CHILDREN

Study (Ref.)	No. of Subjects	Hyperopia	Myopia	Astigmatism	Strabismus	Amblyopia	Heterophoria Accommodative	Cataract	Other Pathology	Visual Discrimination Form Perception
Mohindra (77)	77	30%	7%	14%	9%	5%	10%	—	14%	26%
Pollard (85)	511	8%	13%	1%	5%	2%	2%	1%	4%	—
Greene (44)	156	25%	7%	9%	12%	—	46%	4%	21%	—
Gottlieb (42)	81	—	—	—	31%	—	—	—	37%	—

of the children had a problem in one of the six areas. One third of the sample had a significant degree of hyperopia; strabismus was present in 9 percent; whereas a significant heterophoria was a problem in 10 percent. In 14 percent of the sample, external or internal pathology was detected. An important finding from her study was the high percentage of visual perceptual problems. Twenty-six percent had problems in form reproduction, 42 percent in spatial organization, and 50 percent in visual memory.

Greene (44) also found a much higher prevalence of all visual anomalies except myopia. He found hyperopia in 25 percent of his sample, approximately four times the expected rate. The most common problem detected was nonstrabismic binocular and accommodative anomalies. Forty-six percent of his sample had such problems; accommodative insufficiency was the most prevalent.

A different approach was taken by Woodruff in a recent study of vision in deaf children. He assessed the differential effects of various causes of deafness on the prevalence of vision anomalies (118). In his sample of 460 patients the cause of deafness was unknown in 51.1 percent of cases; the common causes were rubella (20.6 percent), meningitis (7.6 percent), inherited deafness (7.4 percent), Rh incompatibility (4.8 percent), and neonatal sepsis (3.9 percent). The results demonstrated that congenital rubella has the most devastating effect on the visual system. It was the only underlying cause that resulted in blindness. Eight children with congenital rubella had unilateral cataracts. Congenital rubella cases accounted for 28 percent of all the strabismus and 30 percent of the amblyopia, despite the fact that they constitute only 20.6 percent of the sample. The congenital rubella group also had a high rate of astigmatism greater than 40%. Woodruff speculated that this could be related to the higher prevalence of microphthalmia among children with this disease.

The sample of children whose strabismus resulted from Rh incompatibility had the highest rate of myopia in the group. Woodruff suggested that a history of Rh incompatibility

should, therefore, be considered a risk factor for the occurrence of myopia, and that appropriate advice be given to parents. Children with a history of neonatal sepsis also presented with a different profile of visual anomalies. This particular group appears to be at risk mainly for astigmatic anisometropia and hyperopia. A history of deafness caused by neonatal sepsis, therefore, suggests the need for early vision care.

Although the children with inherited deafness had fewer vision problems than other groups, they still demonstrated prevalence rates high enough to warrant early vision examination.

It is readily apparent that although deaf children need to depend more on the visual system as a source of information for learning than normal children do, they have a very high incidence of vision anomalies. The detection and treatment of these conditions must be a prime concern of optometrists.

Low-Birth-Weight Syndrome

Description and Incidence

Developmental follow-up studies of children have demonstrated that low-birth-weight infants are at risk for both mental and physical disabilities (86). With recent advances in neonatal intensive care, more children with a history of low birth weight are surviving, so optometrists are likely to encounter them in practice.

The typical birth weight for a full-term baby is $5\frac{1}{2}$ to $8\frac{1}{2}$ pounds (2500 to 3800 g). Anything under 2500 g is considered low birth weight (10). The entire classification is listed in Table 16.6.

Low birth weight is usually associated with prematurity, intrauterine growth retardation (IUGR), or both (10). Babies with a gestational age of less than 37 weeks are considered premature regardless of weight. Prematurity is associated with factors such as maternal trauma, multiple or teen-age pregnancies, poor prenatal care, and drug and alcohol abuse.

In IUGR, the infant's birth weight falls

Table 16.6 LOW-BIRTH-WEIGHT CLASSIFICATION

Classification	Birth Weight (g)
Normal Birth Weight	2500–3800
Low Birth Weight	2500–1500
Very Low Birth Weight	1500–1000
Extremely Low Birth Weight	<1000

below the tenth percentile for a given gestational age (7). For example, a baby born at 34 weeks weighing 2250 g has appropriate weight for gestational age, but one born at term weighing 2250 g is considered to have low birth weight (Fig. 16.3).

Some of the more common causes of low birth weight secondary to IUGR include alcohol abuse during the pregnancy, maternal malnutrition, viral disease such as cytomegalovirus, and rubella. Maternal alcohol abuse

is considered to be the primary predisposing factor in today's society; the infant may be born with a constellation of signs referred to as fetal alcohol syndrome (FAS) (57).

Clarren and Smith (16) reported on a study of 245 subjects with FAS and described the principal features of the syndrome. They established three main categories: central nervous system dysfunction, growth deficiency, a characteristic cluster of facial abnormalities and variable major and minor malformations.

The most important central nervous system problems are microcephaly and mental retardation. More than 80 percent of affected patients fall more than 2 SD below the mean on intelligence tests and are thus categorized as mentally retarded. This is without doubt the most serious defect associated with FAS. Other central nervous system features are irritability in infancy and hyperactivity in later childhood (16).

Most infants with FAS are growth deficient at birth for both length and weight.

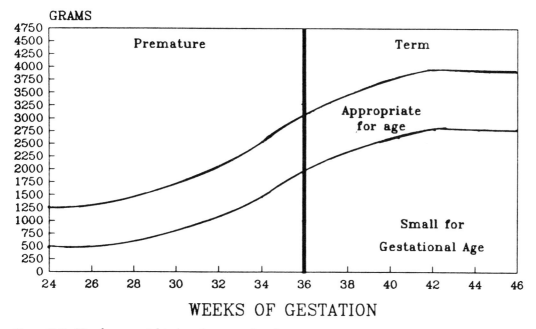

Figure 16.3 Newborn weight chart by gestational age.

They do not demonstrate postnatal catch-up growth and generally remain more than 2 SD below the means for length and weight.

In addition to being mentally retarded and small, 80 percent of these children usually have distinctive facial characteristics: short palpebral fissures (the horizontal measurement), hypoplastic philtrum (medium groove on upper lip), and thinned upper vermilion (Fig. 16.4). The nose is frequently short with a low bridge. The facial characteristics of FAS children are considered to be as distinctive as those of Down's syndrome. The incidence of FAS is approximately 3 to 6 per 1000 (16, 32). About 50 to 75 percent of children born to women who are chronic alcohol abusers may be affected with FAS.

For optometrists, the important issue is that a significant percentage of low-birth-weight infants develop complications that may lead to mental retardation or physical handicaps. Both the evaluation and management of their vision problems must be modified.

Vision Anomalies and Low-Birth-Weight Syndrome

The visual status of children with FAS has been studied extensively. Clarren (16) has reported that myopia, strabismus, and

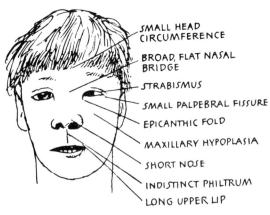

Figure 16.4 Typical facial characteristics of FAS children. (From Stromland K: Ocular abnormalities in the fetal alcohol syndrome. Acta Ophthalmol [Suppl] (Copenh) 63, 1985.)

ptosis are more common in FAS. Garber (37, 38) found a very high prevalence of astigmatism in a population of 30 children with FAS. Astigmatism of greater than 2 D in at least one eye occurred in 42.1 percent of FAS children. Corneal curvature of 46.00 D or more occurred in 90.6 percent of those studied. Garber suggested that the steep corneal curvature is due to the small eye size, which also explains the short palpebral fissure that is characteristic of FAS. Because of its very high prevalence, he recommended that steep corneal curvature should be considered another characteristic of FAS. Thus, keratometry could be applied as a screening device in the detection of FAS (37). Significant refractive anomalies were also reported by Miller et al (74). All nine children in her sample had significant refractive anomalies. Four of the nine had a high degree of myopia.

Strabismus, most often esotropia, is a common abnormality in FAS. Miller et al (74) reported that 55 percent had strabismus, while Stromland found (107) 43 percent.

Other characteristics that have been reported are telecanthus (increased distance between the medial canthi) (3, 74, 75, 107, 108), short palpebral fissures, and ptosis. Miller et al (74) showed that the most frequent external eye changes consist of short horizontal palpebral fissures and ptosis. Ptosis has been reported in approximately 20 percent of FAS children (107).

A wide range of anterior segment abnormalities has also been found: corneal opacities, anterior chamber angle abnormalities, and iris defects (75, 107, 108). A characteristic anterior segment finding is Peter's anomaly. The principal features of this condition are a central corneal opacity accompanied by adhesions between the iris collarette and the leukoma. The condition is generally bilateral. Histopathologically, there is an absence of endothelium and Descemet's membrane under the area of the leukoma (75). Seven of the eight FAS children reported by Miller et al demonstrated Peter's anomaly (75).

Fundus changes have also been found. Miller et al reported optic nerve hypoplasia in two of nine cases (74). Stromland found that the most frequent intraocular anomalies in FAS children occur in the fundus (107). The most common anomaly found in his sample was optic nerve hypoplasia, which was present in 48 percent of the children. Other retinal changes included retinal vessel tortuosity, earlier than normal branching of the vessels, and a greater than normal number of small unspecified vessels (108).

Of low-birth-weight syndrome with causes other than FAS, Desmond et al (23) report, "Visual impairments are the most frequently encountered problem of the very small infant." Vision problems include transient myopia of prematurity, retinopathy of prematurity, myopia secondary to retinopathy of prematurity, and strabismus. Transient myopia varying from 1 to 10 D may occur in preterm infants with a change toward emmetropia during the first year of life. At preschool age, visual perceptual problems may become evident, particularly in children who have other motor and behavior problems.

In a study of 111 children with very low birth weight, Keith and Kitchen found strabismus in 19 percent, significant refractive anomalies in 17 percent, and retinopathy of prematurity in 10 percent (58). In 20 of the 21 children with strabismus, esotropia was present.

Vision Problems Associated with Handicapping Conditions: Summary

It is clear that there are a variety of vision problems which one must be aware of for the various conditions. Table 16.7 is a summary of this information. For example, once the diagnosis of spina bifida is elicited, it is important to determine whether hydrocephalus has been a problem and if so, whether a shunt procedure was performed. If there is a history of a shunt, the optometrist would be concerned about signs or symptoms that might suggest elevated intracranial pressure. Recent changes in binocular vision, a noncomitant strabismus, esotropia greater at distance than at near point, and papilledema are some of the conditions that should be considered during the examination of such a child.

Other Issues

Conditions such as cerebral palsy, spina bifida, and other problems in which there are physical impairments may necessitate modifications in testing due to postural problems, paraplegia, diplegia, hemiplegia, or quadriplegia. An important issue to discuss with parents or other professionals involved with these children is proper positioning of the child for the evaluation. It has been sug-

Table 16.7 HANDICAPPING CONDITIONS AND THEIR MOST COMMONLY ASSOCIATED OCULAR ANOMALIES

Condition	Most Common Ocular Anomalies
Mental Retardation	Refractive Error, Strabismus
Cerebral Palsy	Refractive Error, Strabismus, Amblyopia
Down's Syndrome	Refractive Error, Strabismus, Cataracts, Blepharitis, Keratoconus, Brushfield Spots
Deafness	Refractive Error, Strabismus
Myelomeningocele	Strabismus (Esotropia > Exotropia)
Low Birth Weight	Retinopathy of Prematurity, Myopia, Strabismus
Fetal Alcohol Syndrome	Steep Corneal Curvature, Astigmatism, Telecanthus, Short Palpebral Fissure (Horizontal), Ptosis, Anterior Segment Abnormalities

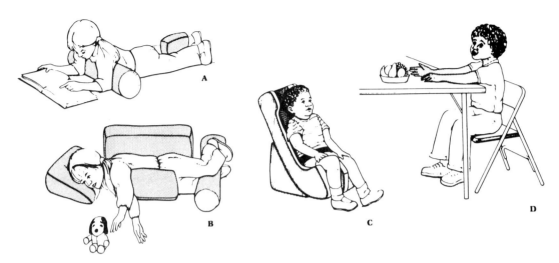

Figure 16.5 Examples of adaptive positioning for MMH children. [From Coley, Ida Lou, and Procter, Susan: Self-maintenance activities. In Clark, Pat Nuse, and Allen, Anne Stevens: Occupational therapy for children, ed. 2, St. Louis, 1989, The C. V. Mosby Co. (in press).]

gested that inappropriate responses to testing procedures may be due not to a visual disorder but to a motor defect and improper positioning (1, 4). It is, therefore, vital to ensure that the child is positioned properly before beginning the assessment. The objective of positioning a child with developmental disabilities may require adapted or specially designed equipment in order to achieve better posture and performance (Fig. 16.5).

Occupational therapists believe that a child who is positioned properly is more comfortable and performs better (61). There is no one best position for maximizing function (20). Finding the best functional position for a particular child usually requires consultation with an occupational therapist. Often the parents or guardian will have this information with them at the time of the examination. If a case history questionnaire is sent out in advance and positioning is an issue, the optometrist can call and consult the occupational therapist involved with the child.

Hearing loss, of course, requires modification of communication techniques during an examination. McConnell (73) suggests that a child with impaired hearing listens with the eyes as well as the ears, so it is important to

face such children at all times and to talk slowly. In addition, this need for face-to-face contact suggests that the use of a phoropter may be inappropriate. The ability of an optometrist to communicate through hand signing would be helpful but is generally not absolutely necessary. Invariably the parent or professional who accompanies the child will assist in the communication process.

Some MMH children often use one or more types of medication. Woodruff (117) has reported that 25 percent of a population of mentally retarded children were on medication. Of the various drugs being used, eight produced side effects on the visual system (Table 16.8).

EVALUATION

One of the key differences in examining MMH children is the need to rely on observational skills. Generally, the lower the child's developmental level and more severe the impairment, the greater the dependence of the optometrist on the process of observation to seek answers and solutions. Curtis and Donlon (99), in a recent textbook devoted to the observational evaluation of MMH chil-

Table 16.8 DRUGS COMMONLY USED BY MMH CHILDREN AND THEIR SIDE EFFECTS

Brand Name	Generic Drug Name	Condition for Which Prescribed	Side Effect
Primidone	Myosoline	Epilepsy	Diplopia, Nystagmus
Phenobarbital	Phenylethylmalonylurea	Epilepsy	Photosensitivity
Dilantin	Diphenylhydantoin	Epilepsy	Nystagmus
Largactil	Chlorpromazine	Hyperactivity	Miosis, Photosensitivity, Reduced Accommodative Ability
Valium	Diazepam	Hyperactivity	Blurred Vision, Diplopia
Benadryl	Diphenhydramine HCl	Aggressive Behavior	Blurred Vision
Mellaril	Thioridazine	Aggressive Behavior	Blurred Vision
Lanoxin	Digoxin	Congenital Heart Problems	Blurred Vision, Yellow Vision

dren, state, "Observation is the major source of information about the severely multihandicapped child." They have developed a very sophisticated and structured observational evaluation routine for this population. Specific details of this approach are beyond the scope of this chapter, but any optometrist currently examining MMH children or planning to do so in the future would benefit significantly by referring to this reference. Before beginning the evaluation it is helpful to have the parents fill out a questionnaire and provide detailed information about the child's condition and medical history (see Appendix).

The importance of gathering information about visual acuity is well recognized. Because it can be time consuming and somewhat stressful, it is not the ideal first technique for the evaluation. Beginning the examination process with something nonthreatening like playing with blocks, handheld toys, or a puzzle is an appropriate strategy. Although the child may perceive it as a game, the optometrist can use it as an opportunity to observe the child's visual behavior. Some information can be gathered about head posture, nystagmus, strabismus, motil-

ity, perceptual skills, handedness, and how the child interacts visually with the task at hand. Once the child is more relaxed, the optometrist can begin to gather the specific information necessary.

After this initial period of "play," several general principles should be followed throughout the assessment. Most were discussed at length in Chapter 7. Some factors are so critical to success, however, that a brief discussion relative to MMH children is appropriate. The key modifications in examination technique include the following:

Technique

1. Select procedures appropriate for the developmental age, regardless of the chronologic age of the child. In Chapter 7, Rouse and Ryan discussed both visual acuity and binocular testing relative to age. An important question that must be addressed is whether some of the newer techniques, such as forced-choice and operant preferential looking, are also effective with developmentally delayed and multiply handicapped children. Although these procedures were originally designed for

normal infants and preverbal children, several researchers have already demonstrated that they are also effective in special population groups (9, 26, 29, 64, 72, 97).

Once developmental age has been established the optometrist can select an appropriate assessment procedure from the acuity procedures discussed in Chapter 7. The procedure of choice is often forced choice or operant preferential looking. When using operant preferential looking it is important to select the most effective reinforcer possible. A very effective reinforcer with the MMH population is food, specifically Cheerios (97). An important consideration with MMH children is the use of home training to prepare the child for a specific assessment technique. For instance, with preferential looking, the parent can practice the procedure with the child during the week prior to the evaluation.

An important new development in the infant research literature has been the introduction of behavioral assessment techniques for the evaluation of stereopsis. Ciner et al (15) recently reported that for children under age $2\frac{1}{2}$ years, operant preferential looking with Cheerios for reinforcement was significantly more effective than other stereopsis tests. Using this technique they were able to measure stereopsis in 90 percent of children under age 30 months.

Preferential looking tests that use hand-held, portable cards are now readily available to optometrists, and stereopsis tests using such cards will be available soon. These procedures should form the basis of the optometric examination of MMH children.

2. The ability to work quickly is absolutely essential. It is important to decide which information is most important and to organize the evaluation to gather that data first.
3. It is important to be flexible and to quickly switch to another procedure if the initial approach is unsuccessful.
4. The traditional chair and stand, with all its

instrumentation, is not very useful for MMH children. A phoropter simply cannot be used. Instead lens racks should be used for refraction techniques and prism bars for binocular testing.
5. Two, or even three, short examinations may be preferable to one prolonged evaluation, owing to the short attention span of many of these children.
6. Traditional subjective testing techniques used for older children and adults have little value; however, newly developed behavioral assessment techniques, such as preferential looking, are valuable, even though they are subjective.
7. Because of the difficulty associated with proper fixation during traditional static skiametry, refraction using a cycloplegic may be necessary. Care, however, is necessary when selecting a cycloplegic agent. There have been reports of psychotic reactions in some MMH children (59). With these children it is best to be particularly cautious about dose, keeping the concentration and number of eye drops to a minimum (80). Either 0.5 percent cyclopentalate or 1.0 percent tropicamide is preferable to 1 percent cyclopentalate. Another possibility is a combination drop (Cyclomydril) that contains 0.2 percent cyclopentalate and 1 percent phenylephrine. This drug permits better evaluation of the fundus because it contains phenylephrine, yet in combination both cyclopentalate and phenylephrine are both less concentrated than the two separate drops (80). Chapter 18 contains a more complete discussion of these issues.

Although some investigators advocate near retinoscopy to evaluate refractive status in young children (80), no studies have demonstrated the reliability and validity of this technique in infants and MMH children.

A very promising new development in the area of refraction of MMH children is photorefraction. The procedure is ideal for infants and young children because it is nonthreatening. Most children enjoy being photographed. Duckman (29) reports positive results using photorefraction to assess the refractive status of MMH children, and it may soon be the technique of choice for them.

8. Because of problems in posture and mobility it is often possible to complete only certain aspects of the ocular health evaluation by utilizing hand-held, portable equipment. Instruments such as the Kowa hand-held slit lamp, a monocular indirect ophthalmoscope, and the Keeler Pulsair noncontact tonometer are invaluable for the examination of MMH children.

9. Assessment of visual perceptual skills is as important in MMH children as in normal ones. Such an evaluation is usually recommended when a child is not performing up to potential in school. The objective of visual perceptual testing is to determine whether a problem in this area may be interfering with school performance.

Some differences must be taken into consideration with MMH children. Tests should be selected by developmental rather than chronologic age, and the child's performance should be compared to the norm for developmental age peers rather than chronologic peers, in order to determine whether there is a significant lag. Finally, if a motor problem is present, visual motor integration tests such as the Developmental Test of Visual Motor Integration (Beery), and the Test of Visual Analysis Skills (Rosner) cannot be utilized.

As long as these procedures are taken into consideration, the visual-perceptual battery suggested in Chapter 7 is applicable to MMH children.

MANAGEMENT

The keys to effective management of MMH children are:

1. A realization that the potential of these children cannot be known until after corrective procedures are instituted.
2. A commitment to do everything possible to maximize the child's visual capabilities.

3. Understanding the information needs of the parents and of professionals who refer these children for examination.

The critical question that needs to be addressed is whether correction of refractive anomaly or the use of vision therapy has any positive impact on the performance of MMH children. Certainly, in the case of children who have a physical or hearing disability and normal intelligence, there should be no question that conventional optometric intervention for a vision problem should be as useful and important as for normal children. The sequential considerations discussed in Chapter 13 and the specific suggestions about vision therapy in Chapter 14 are applicable to these children.

Questions about whether to treat or not generally arise when managing a child with mental retardation alone or in combination with other disabilities. Several studies have been designed to answer this specific question. Bader and Woodruff (5) investigated whether spectacle correction produces behavioral changes in mentally retarded patients. Two hundred eighty-seven patients were divided into control and experimental groups. The control group was subdivided into a placebo group, a group that did not need any glasses, and a group for whom new glasses were delayed for 2 months. They found that significantly more patients in the new-glasses (experimental) group showed improved ability to identify objects or people; to have eye-to-eye contact; improved performance in sports, such as catching, kicking, and throwing a ball; improved posture while eating, and in fine motor control such as, reaching and grasping for objects, stacking blocks, stringing beads, and cutting paper.

Overall, almost 60 percent of the experimental group were judged to have benefited from glasses as compared to only about 20 percent of the placebo group. The authors concluded that spectacle correction can enhance development and achievement of mentally retarded children and that it may be possible to enhance preschool and school performance in reading, writing, and other abilities necessary for academic success.

When prescribing eyeglasses for MMH children most conventional rules apply (refer to Chapter 6), although bifocals may not be appropriate in certain situations. For example, children with physical problems that affect head posture cannot always use bifocals properly. If the child needs additional plus, overcorrection can be tried for desk work at school.

VISION THERAPY

Several authors (27, 36, 40) have suggested that vision therapy is also a viable option for MMH children, including those with mental retardation. Duckman (27) reported on a group of nine cerebral palsy children, five of whom were also mentally retarded. An individualized program of vision therapy was prescribed for each child, aimed at remedying specific problems. Eliminating strabismus, which was present in most of the children, was not considered realistic. Rather, the objectives of the therapy were to improve skills in the areas of fixation, ocular motility, accommodation, binocularity (if strabismus was not present), spatial organization, visual memory, hand-eye coordination, and form perception. His results indicated significant improvement in ocular motility in all subjects, and six of the nine (including two of the five mentally retarded children) showed improved accommodative facility and flexibility. Eight of the nine subjects showed significant changes in the perceptual areas.

Another study assessing the effects of therapy on ocular motility in 10 cerebral palsy children was reported by Gauthier and Hofferer (40). An important aspect of this research was that the authors used a photoelectric eye movement recording system to assess ocular motility before and after therapy. This objective assessment approach eliminated observer bias. The ten subjects, aged 8 to 13 years, received therapy 1 hour per week for 6 to 10 weeks. Measurements were made of smooth pursuit maximum velocity, saccadic delay and precision, and maximum velocity of the saccades before and after therapy. The results demonstrated that 6 to 10 weeks of training significantly improved oculomotor performance in all areas measured.

Specific issues that must be kept in mind when prescribing vision therapy for the MMH population are the mode of therapy (individual or multiple training) and the specific therapy procedures.

Most office vision therapy is done in a group setting in which one therapist may have the responsibility of working with two or more patients at a time. MMH children may be easily distracted, have short attention spans, and have other special needs that necessitate individual therapy sessions in which one therapist works with one child (36). The specific considerations and therapy techniques are similar to those recommended in Chapters 13 and 14 and other texts (45, 87), although modifications may be necessary to deal with communication problems, and physical disabilities.

Communication with Parents and Professionals

One of the most important aspects of managing MMH children is communicating the findings and recommendations to parents and others involved in the child's care. More important than a detailed technical account and report of the examination is attention to several key questions:

What does the child see?
What is the visual acuity?
Will glasses help?
Is vision therapy appropriate?
How does the child use vision to interact with the environment?
How can the child's environment be modified to take into consideration the visual problems, including areas such as feeding, mobility, and educational issues.

SUMMARY

Although the care of MMH children is a complex undertaking that must address problems of children with many different conditions, a high prevalence of vision anomalies is an almost universal characteristic. These children have a great need for optometric care. With the new testing procedures described in other chapters in this text, optometrists are now able to assess visual acuity, stereopsis, refraction, and eye health in infants and preverbal children. The same techniques are applicable to MMH children and permit optometrists to gather considerably more information than they could in the past. Hopefully, the availability of these new assessment procedures will eliminate the tendency of practitioners to label children as too difficult or too unresponsive to test.

Research clearly indicates an optimistic outlook for many MMH children if they receive early intervention. It is critical for optometrists to become involved as part of the team of professionals providing such early care, to ensure that these children attain the highest possible visual function.

APPENDIX

PEDIATRIC SERVICE PARENT QUESTIONNAIRE
THE EYE INSTITUTE OF
PENNSYLVANIA COLLEGE OF OPTOMETRY

Child's full name _____ Nickname _____

Birthdate ____/____/____ Current age _____ Today's date ____/____/____

Parent's name(s) _____ Occupation _____

Is child presently attending: _____ Day care, _____ Nursery school

If yes: Name of school _____ Hours attending _____

My child is here today because:

_____ Eye drifts in

_____ Eye drifts out

_____ Squint alot

_____ Eyes don't focus

_____ Bumps into things

_____ Red eyes

_____ Routine checkup

_____ Vision problems in family

_____ Second opinion

_____ Recheck examination

_____ Other _____

_____

_____

My child is: _____ Natural; _____ Adopted; _____ Foster; _____ Other

FAMILY VISION HISTORY

Does anyone in the family have:

Relationship to child

_____ Nearsightedness

_____ Farsightedness

_____ Astigmatism

_____ Amblyopia (lazy eye)

_____

_____

_____

_____

APPENDIX (*continued*)

_____ Strabismus (eye turn)   _____
_____ Blindness   _____
_____ Eye disease   _____
_____ Other   _____

Has child received any previous eye care?

	Approximate date	By whom
_____ Glasses		
_____ Patching		
_____ Medication		
_____ Surgery		
_____ Therapy		

PREGNANCY (if known)

How long was pregnancy? _____ less than 7 months
_____ between 7 and 8 months
_____ between 8 and 9 months
_____ over 9 months

Please check which of the following occurred during pregnancy:

_____ Excessive vomiting   _____ Smoking
_____ Excessive staining/blood loss   _____ Use of alcohol
_____ Infection(s)   _____ Use of drugs
_____ Toxemia   _____ Regular obstetrical care
_____ Operation(s)   _____ Little medical care
_____ Other illnesses   _____ Poor nutrition
_____ Prescribed medications   _____ Poor hygiene
_____ X-rays during pregnancy
_____ Other _____

DELIVERY

Was labor: _____ Induced _____ Spontaneous
_____ Forceps: _____ High _____ Mid _____ Low
Duration of labor: _____ hours
Type of delivery: _____ Normal _____ Breach _____ Caesarean

Complications (check those that apply)

_____ Cord around neck
_____ Cord presented first
_____ Hemorrhage
_____ Infant injured during delivery
_____ Other (specify) _____

APPENDIX (*continued*)

POST DELIVERY PERIOD (while in hospital)

_____ Birth weight
_____ Apgar score (if known)
_____ Total number of days baby was in hospital after delivery
_____ Jaundice
_____ Incubator care/Need for oxygen   _____ number of days
_____ Infections
_____ Sucking problems
_____ Breathing difficulty
_____ Swallowing difficulty
_____ Birth defects

If the child has been diagnosed as multiply impaired or mentally retarded please answer the following questions.

In previous testing what diagnosis was established: _____
_____
_____
_____

Does the child respond to speech, signing, visual stimuli? _____
_____
_____
_____

How does the child express emotions such as anger, fear, pleasure, unhappiness? _____
_____
_____
_____

Are the child's favorite objects smooth, shiny, etc? _____
_____
_____

Is the child interested in playing with other children, Adults? _____
_____
_____

What is the current educational setting? _____
_____
_____

Describe the child's "self help skills" such as dressing, grooming, toileting, eating and mobility. _____
_____
_____
_____
_____

Describe any unusual behavior we should be aware of: _____
_____
_____
_____

APPENDIX (*continued*)

INFANCY–TODDLER PERIOD

Were any of the following present—to a significant degree?

_____ Did not enjoy cuddling
_____ Was not calmed by being held and/or stroked
_____ Colic
_____ Excessive restlessness
_____ Diminished sleep because of restlessness and easy arousal
_____ Frequent headbanging
_____ Constantly into everything
_____ Excessive number of accidents compared to other children

GENERAL HEALTH/DEVELOPMENTAL HISTORY

Check those items that pertain to your child:

_____ Asthma, eczema or allergies
_____ Presently taking any medications
_____ Previous injuries or accidents
_____ Significant or frequent illnesses
_____ Medical condition and/or surgery
_____ History of epilepsy
_____ Previous neurological evaluation
_____ Diagnosed as developmentally delayed (including Cerebral Palsy, Down's Syndrome, Mental Retardation, etc.)

Is child's development normal in:

Average

Sitting	_____ Yes	_____ No	(5–8 months)
Crawling	_____ Yes	_____ No	(5–8 months)
Walking	_____ Yes	_____ No	(11–15 months)
Speech	_____ Yes	_____ No	(Single words—12–22 months)
Emotional	_____ Yes	_____ No	

What was the date of your child's last medical exam? _____

Name of pediatrician _____

Is there any additional information you would like us to know about your child?
_____
_____
_____

REFERENCES

1. Allen J, Fraser K: Evaluation of visual capacity in visually impaired and multi-handicapped children. Rehabil Optom 1:5, 1983.

2. Altman B: Fetal alcohol syndrome. J Pediatr Ophthalmol 13:255, 1976.

3. Altman HE, Hiat RL, Deweese MW: Ocular findings in cerebral palsy. South Med J 59:1015, 1966.

4. Appel SA, Steciw M, Graboyes M, et al: Managing the child with special needs. J Vis Rehab 3:2, 1985.

5. Bader D, Woodruff ME: The effects of corrective lenses on various behaviors of mentally retarded persons. Am J Optom Physiol Opt 57:447, 1980.

6. Banks MS, Aslin RN, Letson RD: Sensitive period for the development of human binocular vision. Science 190:675, 1975.

7. Batshaw ML, Perret YM: Born too small, born too soon. In Batshaw ML, Perret YM (eds): Children with Handicaps: A Medical Primer. Brookes, Baltimore, 1981.

8. Batshaw ML, Perret YM: Children with Handicaps: A Medical Primer, ch 18. Brookes, Baltimore, 1981.

9. Birch E, Hale L, Stager D, et al: Operant acuity and developmentally delayed children with low vision. J Pediatr Ophthalmol Strabismus 24:64, 1987.

10. Blackman JA: Low birth weight. In Blackman JA (ed): Medical Aspects of Developmental Disabilities in Children Birth Through Three. Rockville, MD, Aspen Publishers, 143, 1983.

11. Blackman JA: Mental retardation. In Blackman JA (ed): Medical Aspects of Developmental Disabilities in Children Birth through Three. Rockville, MD, Aspen Publishers, 147, 1983.

12. Breakey AS: Ocular findings in cerebral palsy. Arch Ophthalmol 53:852, 1955.

13. Brushfield T: Mongolism. Br J Child Dis 21:240, 1924.

14. Cerebral palsy—Facts and figures. New York, United Palsy Association, 1982.

15. Ciner E, Scheiman M, Schanel-Klitsch E, et al: Stereopsis testing in 18–35 month old children using operant preferential looking. Optom Vis Sci 66:782, 1989.

16. Clarren SK, Smith DW: The fetal alcohol syndrome. New Engl J Med 298:1063, 1978.

17. Clements DB, Kausal K: A study of the ocular complications of hydrocephalus and meningomyelocele. Trans Ophthalmol Soc UK 40:383, 1970.

18. Clunies-Ross GG: Accelerating the development of Down's syndrome infants and young children. J Spec Ed 13:169, 1979.

19. Clunies-Ross GG: The development of children with Down's syndrome: Lessons from the past and implications for the future. Aust Pediatr J 22:167, 1986.

20. Coley IL, Procter SA: Self maintenance activities. In Clark PN, Stevens-Allen A (eds): Occupational Therapy for Children. St Louis, CV Mosby, 219, 1985.

21. Courtney GR, Watson PD: Suggested criteria for vision classification on the AAMD adaptive behavior scale. J Am Optom Assoc 47:469, 1976.

22. Cullen JF, Butler HG: Mongolism (Down's syndrome) and keratoconus. Br J Opthalmol 47:321, 1963.

23. Desmond MM, Wilson GS, Alt EJ, et al: The very low birth weight infant after discharge from intensive care: Anticipatory health care and developmental course. Curr Probl Pediatr 10:1, 1980.

24. Douglas AA: The eyes and vision in infantile cerebral palsy. Trans Ophthalmol Soc UK 80:311, 1960.

25. Duckman R: The incidence of anomalies in a population of cerebral palsied children. J Am Optom Assoc 50:1013, 1979.

26. Duckman R, Sclenow A: The use of forced choice preferential looking for measurement of visual acuity in a population of neurologically impaired children. Am J Optom Physiol Opt 60:817, 1983.

27. Duckman RH: The effectiveness of visual training on a population of cerebral palsied children. J Am Optom Assoc 51:607, 1980.

28. Duckman R: Accommodation in cerebral palsy: Function and remediation. J Am Optom Assoc 4:281, 1984.

29. Duckman R, Meyer B: Use of photoretinos-

copy as a screening technique in the assessment of anisometropia and significant refractive error in infants/toddlers/children and special populations. Am J Optom Physiol Opt 64:604, 1987.

30. Fanning GS: Vision in children with Down's syndrome. Aust J Optom 54:74, 1971.

31. Fantl EW, Perlstein MA: Refractive errors in cerebral palsy. Their relationship to the causes of brain damage. Am J Ophthalmol 63:857, 1967.

32. Finnegan LP: The effects of narcotics and alcohol on pregnancy and the newborn. Ann NY Acad Sci 362:136, 1981.

33. France TD: Strabismus in hydrocephalus. Am Orthop J 25:101, 1975.

34. Freeman RD: Psychiatric problems in adolescents with cerebral palsy. Dev Med Child Neurol 12:64, 1970.

35. Freeman RD, Mitchell DE, Millodot M: A neural effect of partial deprivation in humans. Science 175:1384, 1972.

36. Friedenberg HL: A discussion of physical and perceptual environment in visual training of mentally retarded children. J Am Optom Assoc 34:535, 1963.

37. Garber JM: Corneal curvature in the fetal alcohol syndrome: Preliminary report. J Am Optom Assoc 53:641, 1982.

38. Garber JM: Steep corneal curvature: A fetal alcohol syndrome landmark. J Am Optom Assoc 55:595, 1984.

39. Gardiner PA: Visual defects in cases of Down's syndrome and in other mentally handicapped children. Br J Ophthalmol 51:469, 1967.

40. Gauthier GM, Hofferer JM: Visual motor rehabilitation with cerebral palsy. Int Rehabil Med 5:118, 1983.

41. Goddard UK: Ocular changes in hydrocephalus. Br Orthop J 22:72, 1965.

42. Gottlieb DD, Allen WA: Incidence of visual disorders in a selected population of hearing impaired students. J Am Optom Assoc 56:292, 1985.

43. Graham MV: Squint in meningomyelocele: Incidence and etiology. Ophthalmol Dig 10:20, 1974.

44. Greene HA: Vision and the deaf school child. Rev Optom 114:39, 1977.

45. Griffin JR: Binocular Anomalies: Procedures for Vision Therapy. Chicago, Professional Press, 1982.

46. Guibor GP: Some eye defects seen in cerebral palsy with some statistics. Am J Phys Med 32:342, 1953.

47. Hagberg B, Hagberg G, Olow I: The changing panorama of cerebral palsy in Sweden. IV. Epidemiological trends 1959–78. Acta Paediatr Scand 73:433, 1984.

48. Hammer HM, Noble BA, Harcourt RB, et al: Ophthalmic findings in very low birth weight children. Trans Ophthalmol Soc UK 104:329, 1985.

49. Harcourt RB: Ophthalmic complications of meningomyelocele and hydrocephalus in children. Br J Ophthalmol 52:670, 1968.

50. Harryman S: Cerebral palsy. In Batshaw ML, Perret YM (eds): Children with Handicaps: A Medical Primer. Baltimore, Brookes, 1981.

51. Healy A: Cerebral palsy. In Blackman JA (ed): Medical Aspects of Developmental Disabilities in Children Birth Through Three. Rockville, MD, Aspen Publishers, 1983.

52. Heuther CA, Gummere GR, Hook EB, et al: Down's Syndrome: Percentage reporting on birth certificates and single year maternal age risk rates for Ohio 1970–80: Comparison with Upstate New York data. Am J Public Health 71:1367, 1981.

53. Hiles DA: Results of strabismus therapy in cerebral palsied children. Am Orthop J 25:46, 1975.

54. Holm VA: The causes of cerebral palsy: A contemporary perspective. JAMA 247:1473, 1982.

55. Huttenlocher PR: Defects of closure of the neural tube. In Behrman RE, Vaughan VC (eds): Nelson Textbook of Pediatrics. Philadelphia, WB Saunders, 103, 1987.

56. Jaeger EA: Ocular findings in Down's syndrome. Trans Am Ophthalmol Soc 80:808, 1980.

57. Jones KL, Smith DW, Ulleland CN: Pattern

of malformation in offspring of chronic alcoholic mothers. Lancet 1:1267, 1973.

58. Keith CG, Kitchen WH: Ocular morbidity in infants of very low birthweight. Br J Ophthalmol 67:302, 1983.

59. Kennerdell JS, Wucher FD: Cyclopentalate associated with two cases of grand mal seizure. Arch Ophthalmol 87:634, 1972.

60. Kirschen M: A study of visual performance of mentally retarded children. Am J Optom Arch Am Acad Optom 31:282, 1954.

61. Knutson-Lough L: Positioning and handling. In Blackman JA (ed): Medical Aspects of Developmental Disabilities in Children Birth to Three. Rockville, MD, Aspen Publishers, 203, 1983.

62. Kolb EH: Examining the mentally retarded. Am J Optom Arch Am Acad Optom 39:660, 1962.

63. Laurence KM: The natural history of spina bifida cystica. Arch Dis Child 39:41, 1964.

64. Lennerstrand G, Axelsson A, Andersson G: Visual acuity testing with preferential looking in mental retardation. Acta Ophthalmol (Copenh) 61:624, 1983.

65. Levy NS, Cassin B, Newman M: Strabismus in children with cerebral palsy. J Pediatr Ophthalmol 13:72, 1976.

66. Lo Cascio GP: A study of vision in cerebral palsy. Am J Optom Physiol Opt 54:332, 1977.

67. Lo Cascio GP: Longitudinal study of vision in cerebral palsy. Am J Optom Physiol Opt 61:689, 1984.

68. Losseff S: Ocular findings in cerebral palsy. Am J Ophthalmol 54:1114, 1962.

69. Ludlow J, Allen L: The effect of early intervention and preschool stimulus on the development of Down's syndrome child. J Ment Defic Res 23:29, 1979.

70. Lyle WM, Woodruff ME, Zuccaro VS: A review of the literature on Down's syndrome and an optometrical survey of 44 patients with the syndrome. Am J Optom Physiol Opt 49:715, 1972.

71. Manley JN, Schuldt WJ: The refractive state of the eye and mental retardation. Am J Optom Arch Am Acad Optom 47:236, 1970.

72. Mayer DL, Fulton AB, Sossen Ol: Preferential looking acuity of pediatric patients with developmental disabilities. Behav Brain Res 10:189, 1983.

73. McConnell F: Children with hearing disabilities. In Dunn L (ed): Exceptional Children in the Schools: Special Education in Transition. New York, Holt, Rinehart & Winston, 351, 1973.

74. Miller M, Israel J, Cuttone J: Fetal alcohol syndrome. J Pediatr Ophthalmol Strabismus 18:6, 1981.

75. Miller M, Epstein R, Sugar J: Anterior segment anomalies associated with the fetal alcohol syndrome. J Pediatr Ophthalmol Strabismus 21:8, 1984.

76. Minear WL: A classification of cerebral palsy. Pediatrics 18:841, 1956.

77. Mohindra I: Vision profile of deaf children. Am J Optom Physiol Opt 53:412, 1976.

78. National Institutes of Health Report on Causes of Mental Retardation and Cerebral Palsy. Pediatrics 76:457, 1985.

79. Nelson KB, Ellenberg JH: Antecedents of cerebral palsy. New Engl J Med 315:81, 1986.

80. Palmer EA: How safe are ocular drugs in pediatrics? Ophthalmology 93:1038, 1986.

81. Patel S, Bharucha EP: The bender gestalt test as a measure of perceptual and visuomotor defects in cerebral palsied children. Dev Med Child Neurol 14:156, 1972.

82. Perlstein MA: Cerebral palsy: Incidence, etiology, pathogenesis. Arch Pediatr 79:289, 1962.

83. Pesch RS, Nagy DK, Caden B: A survey of the visual and developmental abilities of the Down's syndrome child. J Am Optom Assoc 49:1031, 1978.

84. Pieterse M: Recent developments and future trends in the early education of the handicapped. Recent Dev Spec Educ Disabl 10:11, 1979.

85. Pollard G, Neumaier R: Vision characteristics of deaf students. Am J Optom Physiol Opt 51:839, 1974.

86. Resnick MB, Eyler FD, Nelson RM, et al: Developmental intervention for low birth

weight infants: Improved early developmental outcome. Pediatrics 80:68, 1987.

87. Richman J, Cron M: The Bernell Guide to Vision Therapy. South Bend, IN, Bernell, 1987.

88. Roberts KB, Vining EPG: Development and retardation. In Roberts KB (ed): Manual of Clinical Problems in Pediatrics. Boston, Little, Brown, 74, 1985.

89. Robinson RO: The frequency of other handicaps in children with cerebral palsy. Dev Med Child Neurol 15:305, 1973.

90. Rothstein TB, Romano PE, Shoch D: Meningomyelocele. Am J Ophthalmol 77:690, 1974.

91. Rouse MW, London R: Development and perception. In Barresi BJ (ed): Ocular Assessment: The Manual of Diagnosis for Office Practice. Boston, Butterworth, 173, 1984.

92. Rutstein RP, Wesson MD, Gottlieb S, et al: Clinical comparison of the visual parameters in infants with intrauterine growth retardation vs infants with normal birth weight. Am J Optom Physiol Opt 63:697, 1986.

93. Rynders JE, Peuschel SM: History of Down syndrome. In Peuschel SM, Rynders JE (eds): Down Syndrome: Advances in Biomedicine and the Behavioral Sciences. Cambridge MA, Academic Guild Publishers, 1982.

94. Rynders JE, Spiker D, Horrobin JM: Underestimating the educability of Down's syndrome children: Examinations of methodological problems in recent literature. Am J Ment Defic 82:440, 1978.

95. Schachat WS, Wallace HM, Palmer M, et al: Ophthalmologic findings in children with cerebral palsy. Pediatrics 19:623, 1957.

96. Scheiman M: Optometric findings in children with cerebral palsy. Am J Optom Physiol Opt 61:321, 1984.

97. Scheiman M, Ciner E, Gallaway M: A comparative study of operant preferential looking and the Broken Wheel Cards in a population of developmentally delayed children. Poster Program. Am Acad Optom Annual Meeting, Atlanta, 1985.

98. Schire L: An ophthalmological survey of a series of cerebral palsy cases. South Afr Med J 30:405, 1956.

99. Scott-Curtis W, Donlon ET: Observational evaluation of severely multi-handicapped children. Swets North America, 1985.

100. Seaber JH, Chandler AC: A five year study of patients with cerebral palsy and strabismus. In Moore S, Mein J, Stockbridge L (eds): Orthoptics: Past, Present, Future, New York, Stratton Intercontinental Medical Book, 271, 1976.

101. Shapiro MB, France TD: The ocular features of Down's syndrome. Am J Ophthalmol 99:659, 1985.

102. Sharav T, Collins R, Shlomo L: Effect of maternal education on prognosis of development in children with Down syndrome. Pediatrics 76:387, 1985.

103. Shurtleff DB: Myelodysplasia: Management and treatment. In Gluck L (ed): Current Problems in Pediatrics. Chicago, Year Book, 7, 1980.

104. Smith VH: Strabismus in cerebral palsy. Br Orthop J 22:84, 1965.

105. Stanworth A: Squint in hydrocephalus: An analysis of cases. In: Strabismus '69. St Louis, CV Mosby, 73, 1970.

106. Steadman D, Eichom D: A comparison of the growth and development of institutionalized and home reared mongoloids during infancy and early childhood. Am J Ment Defic 69:391, 1964.

107. Stromland K: Ocular abnormalities in the fetal alcohol syndrome. Acta Ophthalmol [Suppl] (Copenh) 63:7, 1985.

108. Stromland K: Ocular involvement in the fetal alcohol syndrome. Surv Ophthalmol 31:277, 1987.

109. Taft LT: Mental retardation. In Behrman RE, Vaughan VC (eds): Nelson Textbook of Pediatrics. Philadelphia, WB Saunders, 103, 1987.

110. Thomas J, Mohindra I, Held R: Strabismic amblyopia in infants. Am J Optom Physiol Opt 56:197, 1979.

111. Tuppurainen K: Ocular findings among mentally retarded children in Finland. Acta Ophthalmol (Copenh) 61:634, 1983.

112. Vining EPG: Cerebral palsy. In Roberts KB (ed): Manual of Clinical Problems in Pediatrics. Boston, Little, Brown, 1985.

113. Warshowsky J: A vision screening of a Down's syndrome population. J Am Optom Assoc 52:605, 1981.

114. Wiesinger H: Ocular findings in mentally retarded children. J Pediatr Ophthalmol 1:37, 1964.

115. Wolraich ML: Hydrocephalus. In Blackman JA (ed): Medical Aspects of Developmental Disabilities in Children Birth Through Three. University of Iowa, 137, 1983.

116. Wolraich ML, Siperstein GN: Assessing professionals' prognostic impressions of mental retardation. Ment Retard 21:8, 1983.

117. Woodruff ME: Prevalence of visual and ocular anomalies in 168 non-institutionalized mentally retarded children. Can J Public Health 68:225, 1977.

118. Woodruff ME: Differential effects of various causes of deafness on the eyes, refractive errors, and vision of children. Am J Optom Physiol Opt 63:668, 1986.

Chapter 17

The Management of the Aphakic Neonate

Emilio C. Campos

Jay M. Enoch

In the last decade or so significant advances have been made in understanding the maturation of the human visual system and events that can compromise it. Sensory deprivation amblyopia is one of the most frequently encountered causes of pathologic maturation of the visual system. As a consequence, visual function may be severely damaged and only very early treatment can normalize vision, or, more often, at least improve the existing situation. Cataracts in neonates are by far the most common cause of sensory deprivation amblyopia. Both congenital and traumatic cataracts can be present in this age group. Some feel that the term congenital is no longer appropriate. In fact, some children are destined at birth to develop cataracts that become clinically detectable in the first weeks, months, or even years of life. Therefore, one should speak of developmental cataracts (13).

As far as sensory deprivation amblyopia is concerned, the effects of developmental and traumatic cataracts are identical in patients *of the same age*. So the timing of surgery and the rehabilitation of patients with both conditions are discussed together here. There are two major differences between them:

1. The posterior segment of an injured eye in which a traumatic cataract develops is usually normal. Eyes with developmental

This research has been supported in part by the National Eye Institute Research Grant EY 03674 (to JME), National Institutes of Health, Bethesda, MD and by a grant of the Ministero della Pubblica Istruzione (to ECC).

cataracts often exhibit additional malformations such as microphthalmia, persistent hyaloid artery, and persistent hyperplastic vitreous (PHPV). As a consequence, visual prognosis after uncomplicated surgical intervention may be poorer for developmental cataracts.

2. Surgical problems are different for developmental and traumatic cataracts. Trauma may be accompanied by penetrating corneal injuries, vitreous loss, or secondary glaucoma, so surgery for traumatic cataracts may be difficult. This aspect is not discussed here because it departs from the topic of the rehabilitation of the aphakic neonate.

SURGERY AND ITS TIMING

It is not our aim to discuss in detail each of the surgical procedures that is used when operating on neonates with congenital cataract. No magic approaches are available at this time. Each technique can have pitfalls. The old concept of multiple discission in these babies has been abandoned, because considerable time elapses between diagnosis and the end of treatment. Preference is given to procedures that attempt to solve the problem in one surgical session. Classic techniques of discissions combined with aspiration-irrigation with a two-way needle can still be effective (35). Although the technique is not very traumatizing, the results often are not definitive. Today, mechanical instruments for suction-infusion are used widely. Phakoaspiration is employed as well, although infantile cataracts usually do not require it because of their softness and the absence of a hard nucleus. The best results have been obtained when the instrument is introduced via the pars plana (36), but there is evidence that using this approach during the first year of life may be dangerous. Complications include risk of infection, uveal reaction, and retinal lesions. For this reason, most surgeons prefer a limbal approach (57, 66), but it is quite obvious that this approach does not eliminate all of the problems associated with the area behind the iris. Campos uses the limbal approach with an infusion suction machine introduced in the anterior chamber through a 3-mm keratotomy.

Obviously, all of these procedures are extracapsular. Often after surgery, the posterior capsule thickens and a secondary cataract develops. Many surgeons suggest a posterior central capsulectomy. An aperture is formed on the optical axis of the eye. This procedure, although effective, may be risky, as it is easy to rupture the anterior vitreous membrane and find vitreous in the anterior chamber. Practically speaking, Campos feels this to be a risk worth taking. In his experience, even patients with posterior capsulectomy occasionally develop Elschnig's pearls, resulting in a nonfunctional or partially functional visual pathway. The absence of a good retinoscopic reflex is a good indication that this kind of problem is developing. If we are unable to perform reliable retinoscopy, it is likely that the patient is unable to see through the openings that were made previously. The association of posterior capsulectomy with anterior vitrectomy also has been suggested (57). It is advantageous, particularly if posterior lens opacities are present.

In a recently published series by C. Hoyt and Nickel (42), it appears that the use of phakoemulsification may result in cystoid macular edema. Indeed, this problem should be studied further.

In conclusion, the least traumatizing technique should be used. Depending on the surgeon's experience and the reliability of instruments at hand, discission, aspiration-irrigation, or phakoemulsification can be used. Finally, patients must be monitored closely after surgery because secondary cataracts are likely to develop. If intraocular lenses (IOLs) are implanted or epikeratophakia is performed, surgery is certainly more complicated. Separate from this issue, we oppose using IOLs in neonates; the reasons are discussed below.

The timing of surgery for congenital cataracts is crucial because of its influence on the development of the visual system. This topic was recently considered also by Gelbart et al. (33).

At least three functions should be considered: visual acuity, the fixation reflex, and binocular vision (7). Of course, one can never overlook concerns about patient welfare.

Visual Acuity

Apparently, visual acuity develops in two stages. From birth to 6 months of age or shortly thereafter, visual acuity increases from about 20/800 to 20/20 (2, 6, 14, 37, 55). This reflects a variety of factors, including anatomic development of the fovea and central retina (39, 51), maturation of the neural system, and visual experience. From 6 months to roughly 6 or 7 years, visual acuity is still in a plastic phase. If vision is interrupted for any reason and the cause of such a visual decrease is not eliminated promptly, vision will remain poor and amblyopia will develop. After roughly 7 years of age, it is no longer necessary to quickly eliminate a vision-decreasing defect. Thus, if optimal vision is to develop, surgery must be conducted as early as possible, preferably not later than 2 or 3 months of age.

If both eyes require treatment, surgery is performed on them separately, within a few days' time, to avoid the risk of bilateral infections. The correcting contact lens may be fitted on the eye that has already been operated on during an examination under anesthesia prior to surgery for the second eye. Meanwhile, bilateral patching is prescribed after the first surgery until optical corrections can be made. This is done in order to prevent an imbalance in image size and quality from causing anisometropic amblyopia and disrupting binocular vision (66) (see Prevention and Treatment of Amblyopia for details).

Until recently, many professionals believed that patients with congenital cataract caused by maternal rubella during pregnancy who exhibit viremia should not undergo surgery immediately. It was claimed that they are at high risk of developing endophthalmitis after surgery, but a report on a large series of patients (65) showed that this risk no longer exists. It is sufficient to isolate the patient so that the disease is not transmitted to other children.

The Fixation Reflex

The capability of making small, corrective movements to fixate a target develops during the first 2 years of life. If, for any reason, bilateral vision is poor during this period, the fixation reflex does not develop properly and pendular nystagmus results. This has been termed sensory nystagmus. Interestingly, this nystagmus generally does not develop before the fifth or sixth month of age. It will develop even if the reduction of visual acuity occurs after the eighth or ninth month and through the second year. The presence of pendular nystagmus adds another causal factor to the preexisting amblyopia (8). In fact, the moving images on the retina are themselves the cause of amblyopia. Generally, it is very difficult to eliminate such nystagmus once it is well-established. Sensory nystagmus develops only if visual acuity is poor bilaterally.

Binocular Vision

Binocular vision matures at a different time than visual acuity; that time has not yet been well defined. There is evidence that some cooperation between the two eyes is present as early as the third or fourth month of life (5, 28, 29, 58), but this development can be interrupted by various causes (e.g., poor vision in one eye). If such interruption takes place before the sixth or seventh year of life, treatment has to begin immediately, because once binocular vision is interrupted effectively, it may be lost forever. This is important for unilateral congenital cataract patients, who, as noted above, do not develop nystagmus but lose ocular alignment. In these cases, surgery should be performed even earlier than for bilateral cataracts. Preferably, surgery should be performed by the second or the third month of life. In these cases of sensory deprivation amblyopia caused by monocular cataract, strabismic amblyopia may occur subsequently, resulting in the loss of ocular alignment and the development of sensory strabismus.

In conclusion, timing of surgery for congenital cataract is crucial, particularly if vision in the two eyes, or in the one affected eye, is very low. It is impossible to obtain good functional results if surgery is delayed (as it has been in the past) until the second year of life or later.

On the other hand, some congenital cataracts are not very dense and visual acuity is sufficient to allow the patient to live a reasonably normal life. In these cases, surgery should not be done at an early age but should be deferred until age 7 or 8 years. In fact, if surgery is performed earlier in this group of patients, strabismus may be precipitated simply because the interval necessary to fit the patient with a visual correction after surgery may be long enough to interrupt binocularity. It is sometimes better to trade a modest amount of visual acuity for binocular vision.

When speaking of surgery, we think it is important to comment on the introduction of IOL's into the eyes of patients who are operated on for congenital cataracts (4, 41). We feel that because such a procedure is still very dangerous and unpredictable it should be restricted to adult patients. There are various unknown elements inherent with this procedure: (1) Follow-up studies are not long enough to justify introducing into a child a foreign body that is to remain there for the rest of a lifetime; (2) additional correction is still necessary; (3) introducing a fixed optical device in a growing eye is dangerous; (4) the procedure increases the possibility of secondary infection in these patients (i.e., they are more likely to react adversely to this type of surgery than do adult patients). Probably the ideal approach is to use contact lenses and to implant an IOL once the patient is an adult. Epikeratophakia (55) has been suggested for correcting the high refractive error of aphakic neonates. This method, although promising, needs further evaluation.

OPTICAL CORRECTION AND MENSURATION

The optical correction of this group of patients is largely dependent on the fact that one is dealing with a growing, developing eye. Soft contact lenses, which are designed for eyes with adult measurements, do not fit infants' eyes (20, 23). At birth most infants' eyes are about 16 mm long, and they grow to about 25 mm in adulthood. Often, at birth a cataractous eye is somewhat smaller than a normal eye, generally by about 1 mm. This proves to be an advantage, because it reduces by a small factor the image size discrepancy after unilateral cataract surgery. Much of the literature on the mensuration of infant eyes is not useful. Measured corneal curvatures tend to be only slightly steeper than those of adult eyes, perhaps by 1 to 3 D. Thus, the large optical power difference between infants' and adults' eyes is largely centered in the eye lens component. This means that after cataract surgery hyperopic refraction measured at the cornea is extremely high and requires special optical elements. Generally, if the eye is smaller the corneal diameter also is smaller, so it becomes important to routinely measure the cornea of these eyes with calipers as a means of assessing growth. If there is a unilateral cataract, it is common for both that eye and its corneal diameter to be slightly smaller.

In order to correct these infants' refraction, it is useful to determine ocular mensuration data at the time of surgery or examination under anesthesia (EUA). The diameter of the cornea is measured not only to gauge growth but also to aid in fitting the contact lens. The base curve of the prescribed contact lens can be derived from a measurement of corneal curvature. It is possible to obtain this just prior to surgery in the operating suite by using a keratometer, although this is sometimes difficult, particularly with an anesthetized child. A far more sensitive and successful approach in our hands is to use a precision set of hard contact lenses of known curvature as templates and the usual fluorescein techniques to determine the best-fitting lens. This also allows us to assess the corneal astigmatism, because astigmia produces an elliptical fluorescein pattern. Generally, if an eye is to have surgery performed on it after obtaining mensuration data during EUA, one determines the best-fitting contact lens (template) first on the more normal eye. This provides an initial estimate of the corneal curvature for the eye that will have surgery and serves to minimize contact with and to protect the corneal epithelium of the eye to be operated upon prior to surgery (16, 17, 20, 22, 45, 46).

It is useful to obtain A-mode ultrasound data at the same time for eye length estimates (6, 20, 22, 45, 48). Infants' eye lenses are less dense, so acoustic velocity is somewhat higher than in adults (although cataractous lens changes can alter acoustic velocity). Eye length in the aphakic eye can also be estimated by retinoscopy after the cataract is removed. The corneal curvature, in diopters, plus the refractive correction at zero vertex distance represents the total power needed to focus an object at infinity on the retina. The focal length of the eye in meters, from the corneal apex to the retinal surface, is simply 1.336 (the index of refraction of the aqueous and vitreous humors) divided by the sum of the refractive correction at zero vertex distance and the corneal curvature, both in diopters.

A third estimate of ocular length can be obtained from microspherometry measurements of scleral curvature (which will be described later) (21, 22). Each technique has its weaknesses. The axis of the eye is difficult to define by A-scan. If the length of the eye is to be used to define scleral radius, the A-scan provides no adequate correction for the corneal vault. Alignment relative to the fovea or to the point of fixation is a problem in retinoscopy. The microspherometer is limited to measuring scleral curvature at the front of the eye, which is exactly what one wants for fitting the scleral portion of a soft contact lens, but this value may not provide accurate information on total ocular length.

To fit a hard contact lens, one needs a

to define the base curve, the diameter of the lens, and the power. To keep the lens lightweight, as small a lenticular element as possible is used, because the power of the correcting lens is extremely high. A contact lens with a diameter as large as practical is used in order to increase the bearing area to maintain lens centration and to counter the weight of the high plus prescription.

Our experience suggests that soft lenses are far more comfortable for the child, though hard lenses are probably easier to fit. (We obtain our soft lenses from the Flexlens Corporation, 114 Industrial Park Place, Rio Rancho, NM 87124 [JME] and the Hydron Corporation, London, England [ECC]). It should be remembered that soft lenses are actually scleral lenses, so not only the corneal portion of the lens must be specified but also the scleral portion. For the infant eye, the manufacturer needs the scleral radius or some estimate of eye length, the diameter of the cornea, and the vault (or sagittal height) of the cornea above the scleral plane. Using the familiar sagittal equation, and knowing the corneal radius (based on the K reading, or central cornea curvature determination, using hard contact lens templates) and the corneal diameter, one may assume the presence of a spherical cornea:

$$S = \frac{d_1^2}{8r_c}$$

where S = sagittal height, d_1 = corneal diameter, and r_c is the radius of curvature of the cornea (may vary with meridian).

A more practical technique is to use a small microspherometer made from modified iris forceps. The blades are flattened and blunted at the tips. The two blades are separated by a small metal block that contains a screw mount supporting a small centrally located clear optical flat. The two blades of the forceps are separated by a fine screw adjustment to provide a fine caliper measurement of the diameter of the cornea. The optical flat is lowered to just touch the cornea, which has had a drop of fluorescein placed on it. Using a blue light, one can observe just contact of the optical flat on the cornea. To determine the sagittal height one measures the height of the optical flat above the base of the blades of the forceps.

Another simple technique is to add a second measurement to the one just described (i.e., the same measurement is repeated with the blades arbitrarily separated about 12.5 or 13.0 mm). The sagitta thus determined, the original measurement can be used to compute scleral radius from the following equation:

$$r_s = \frac{d_2^2 - d_1^2}{8(s_2 - s_1)}$$

where r_s is the radius of curvature of the sclera in the meridian measured, d is the separation of the caliper blades for each of the two measurements, and s is the corresponding measurement of sagitta. Data for each of the several measurements must be determined routinely in order to record growth and to provide estimates for new contact lens fittings. To summarize, the following measurements are needed: corneal curvature and diameter, refraction, length of eye and/or scleral radius and sagittal vault of the cornea above the sclera.

In neonates, the conjunctival cul de sac is poorly developed and the palpebral fissure is small. Maximum lens diameter is 13.5 mm. By the end of the first year, lenses of up to about 14.5 mm overall diameter can be fitted.

A pair of spectacles with plastic lenses for wear when contact lenses cannot be worn are prescribed in order to maintain acuity at all times. Vertex distance is rarely more than 10 mm, and it may be 8 or 9 mm. Strap-type bands about the head are used to secure the spectacles to the eyes of very young children.

At birth, we overcorrect the unilateral or bilateral aphakic infant by about 3 D. That is, the infant's world is largely centered at the near point. This add is gradually reduced, so that by 1 year of age it is reduced to about 1 to 1.5 D. At age 2 years, the distance correction is prescribed in the aphakic spectacle correction, and an add is provided in the form of a bifocal. The same principle will be followed in the contact lens correction.

It is interesting that it is often easy to measure refraction of an aphakic infant's eye by means of a retinoscope with a lens such as a +20 D trial lens, varying, not the power of the lens, but the vertex distance (18). Effective plus power increases as the lens is moved from the eye. The vertex distance can readily be measured after locating the point of retinoscopic reflex reversal. By simply using a Distometer vertex distance measuring wheel, one can quickly determine the power of the lens at either the spectacle or contact lens plane. At these powers, which generally range +20 and +30 D in neonates, an error of 1 mm in measurement can be equivalent to 0.75 to 1.25 D. Care must be used in all measurements. Alignment with the perceived optical axis (corneal reflex) is also critical!

ANISEIKONIA

There can be no possibility of binocular function if unilateral aphakia is present in the infant unless the resultant aniseikonia is corrected. The actual correction in each eye can be computed. For initial visual correction of most infants, particularly if the aphakic eye is smaller than the more normal eye, it is probably sufficient to use an inverted Galilean telescope in front of the aphakic eye with added plus power in the contact lens (19, 25, 26, 34).

The table on page 426 shows the resultant magnification values and the required negative powers in the spectacle lens plane when one increases the power of the contact lens by +7 D at vertex distance = 0 mm in the aphakic contact lens in order to create a reverse Galilean telescope. For more complete discussion of the nature of these corrections, see Enoch and Hamer (24). One concern is that in a micro eye, the ideal goal may not be equal size images. While generally we seek equal size images, this approach has not been proven. Other bases of corrections are no better defined.

It is important to check the actual resultant correction after the contact lens–spectacle combination or the spectacle correction has been given to the child. Proper lens adjustments or corrections prior to assessing visual resolution and other visual functions, should be made. As noted, plus seven diopters are added to the contact lens prescription placed on the aphakic eye. A minus lens is placed in the spectacle plane. The power and magnification are functions of the vertex distance as shown in the following table:

Vertex Distance (mm)	In Spectacle Plane (D)	Size Reduction (%)
7	−7.36	4.9
8	−7.42	5.7
9	−7.47	6.3
10	−7.53	7.0
11	−7.58	7.7

Checking the overrefraction is a quick process in these patients, particularly if there is an add in the contact lens and the spectacle lens. The actual add in each is simply the reversal position for the retinoscopic reflex. So, to determine whether the power in the contact lens is correct, if an inverted telescope was prescribed, the spectacle correction is removed and the retinoscopic reversal point is determined. If a +7 D plus element of the telescope (inverted) was prescribed over the Rx in the contact lens plane, the retinoscopic reversal point should be 14.3 cm from the corneal apex. With a +3 D add in the spectacle overcorrection, reversal position should be 33 cm from the spectacle (in the spectacle prescription alone or in the combined spectacle/contact lens). If these results are not found, the desired powers were not achieved. The correction can be altered to achieve the proper correction.

A key to fitting contact lenses to a neonate is to transfer all lens handling to the parent *as soon as possible.* One approach is to fit the mother with a soft lens or a hard lens first, to let her learn to manipulate the lens on her own eye during the period required to obtain lenses for the child. The mother learns to overcome her fear of the lenses and to know that she will not hurt the child. This approach is taken whether the mother needs lenses or not. Once she is familiar with lens technique, they may be discontinued.

One of the major problems of fitting soft contact lenses to an infant is the sometimes rapid and nonlinear development of the corneal vault. Dimensions may change rapidly, altering an otherwise perfect fit. An excellent fit may have been obtained, but within a few weeks the central corneal epithelium can be denuded by an area of central corneal touch causing the child discomfort and resulting in his rubbing the eye. The contact lens fit can be evaluated quickly and easily using large-molecule fluorescein. In such a case, one must increase the corneal vault above the scleral flange, which serves as a base for the corneal portion of the soft lens. An increase of 0.05 mm or 0.10 mm of vault height should be tried.

As with hard contact lenses, the high plus central portion of the soft lens drags the lens down unless the largest scleral flange that is practical is used. The lenses sometimes crack between the more rigid heavy plus central element and the thinner supporting soft contact lens component. Some practitioners use high–water content contact lenses, others use extended wear lenses (limited time period before removal and cleanup), and some, a dual material (Saturn lenses). Extended wear without periodic removal and cleaning is not recommended.

VISUAL FUNCTION TESTING

It is natural to assume that a child with cataracts has seen very little in his or her lifetime. This is not always so if the cataract does not fill the eye lens and pupillary aperture.

As soon as the visual correction is available, it becomes desirable to obtain baseline estimates of visual performance, which include determination of fixation capability, even rudimentary estimates of hand-eye coordination, and general estimates of visual awareness. Measurement of visual resolution is attempted, even though visual resolution or visual acuity is not the principal organizing feature of the visual experience. As indicated earlier, visual acuity does not reach fine dimensions until the child is about 6 months old and has had more visual experience. Thus, it is not clear which visual functions are crucial to the initial development of vision, and visual acuity is only one estimate of visual capability. However, at present it is the best clinical tool available (7).

Currently, there are three generally accepted approaches to the estimation of visual resolution in infants (9). Clinicians prefer to use the term "visual acuity," and often use similar notation for the different measurements, although this may not be technically correct. The three techniques are optokinetic nystagmus (OKN), preferential looking, and visually evoked response. Each has its strengths and weaknesses.

Optokinetic Nystagmus (See Chapter 4)

There is some question as to whether measured OKN response in the neonate is the same as in an older child or adult, because it is not clear that following eye movements are present in many infants at birth (56, 62). There is some suggestion that following movements do not develop until later in life, yet by observing the saccades in the direction of the movement of the OKN strips, one can also estimate visual capability. Also in the newborn, nasal eye movements tend to be better organized than temporal eye movements, and sometimes this becomes the more sensitive measurement. It is also unclear what part of the optokinetic response is organized at the cortical level (8); certainly there are subcortical components to this response (55, 68).

The apparatus for eliciting an OKN response is most often available and most commonly used by clinicians. Because aphakic children do not have accommodative capability their vision must be corrected for a specific test distance, so it is desirable to have several different line or bar frequencies available for testing at the distance for which the child's vision is corrected.

We prefer to take the striped display off the drum and hold it horizontally in front of the child and to move it back and forth by hand. This provides a more complete visual environment and a larger field. In our experience, it is rare that a neonate attends to any object placed more than 4 feet from the eye. Often an assistant uses a hand puppet or other distraction, moving it up and around the OKN display to help direct the child's interest in the general area of the display pattern.

Preferential Looking

Preferential looking is a relatively new technique that was first reported by Fantz, Ordy, and Udelf (27) and more recently was developed as a clinical test in a series of laboratories, including those of Davida Teller and Velma Dobson at the University of Washington (14, 15, 52), Anne Fulton at the Children's Hospital in Boston (38, 53), Philip Salapatek at Minnesota (61), Richard Held at MIT (37, 38), and Martin Banks at the University of California School of Optometry, Berkeley (2). The technique requires the observer to judge at which of two discs or squares the child looked. One is seen as unpatterned and appears similar to the background to the patient. The second is a patterned grating with a specific line frequency. The rationale is that the child would look at the grating if he or she sees it because it is intrinsically more interesting than an otherwise uniform field. This is generally true, but the test is fatiguing for the child. A child of 5 or 6 months of age needs a reward as an incentive to continue the task. Often many trials are needed. One determines the limiting size grating chosen or preferred just above chance. Generally, line frequency is varied in steps of two, that is, octave variation, and a psychophysical function is determined. The technique takes time and therefore presents problems for broad clinical application. Test areas may cover several degrees, and the locus of fixation is not well defined. Again one must be concerned about proper focus in the aphakic eye.

Visually Evoked Response

Two types of stimuli exist, namely flashes and patterns. Essentially, the technique examines variations in the electroencephalogram (EEG) following the presentation of a visual stimulus. On the basis of the angle subtended by the stimuli at the eye, it is possible to extrapolate a measurement of equivalent visual acuity or resolution (60). This may be a questionable procedure; in fact, the presence of a VER signal indicates only that the visual system is working up to the point where the electrodes are placed. This does not mean that the patient has a visual acuity corresponding to the resolution obtained with the VER. In fact, visual acuity is a complicated and integrated psychophysical function. Therefore, it is more reliable to state that a given patient has a VER compatible with (not necessarily corresponding to) a given visual acuity or resolution (9). VER requires fairly expensive equipment, which is not available to all clinicians. Recordings can easily be performed with a child awake and not anesthetized, but care must be taken when applying the electrodes. In the case of neonates, a stimulator can be positioned conveniently so that the baby can remain in its crib.

In order to make a reliable measurement of the patterned VER that provides useful information about the baby's operational visual resolution, it is crucial to correct the baby's refractive state for the testing distance. In fact, the VER is strongly influenced by blur, so any assessment that is done without lenses appropriate for the test distance in an aphakic infant is useless. Since ambient electrical signals can produce spurious results, an operator must have a fair amount of experience before routinely using this method.

All three visual resolution measuring techniques have a place in the assessment of visual function of aphakic babies. It is useful to use more than one test and to obtain multiple estimates, so that if one or another of the techniques does not work well on a given occasion, alternative data are available. Once baseline data are obtained after the initial correction, regular determinations are made to monitor progress.

There is another very quick method for assessing visual resolution. It is useful only for clinical purposes and is obviously gross. It can be applied only to babies with monola-

teral congenital cataracts and subsequent surgical aphakia and secondary esotropia (9). In these patients, the aphakic eye is deviated. As a consequence, it is amblyopic. Once the point is reached where visual acuity is almost the same in both eyes, the patient will be able to maintain fixation and eventually even begin to alternate. This is a gross estimate, but it provides useful information on the development of vision in the aphakic eye.

PREVENTION AND TREATMENT OF AMBLYOPIA

Once the optical correction of these babies has been assessed, there are only limited means of improving visual function in bilateral aphakia. In order to prevent imbalance between the two eyes in patients with bilateral cataracts, bilateral occlusion is used after surgery of the first eye pending surgery of the second eye. This procedure has been advocated by von Noorden (66). While this procedure has not yet been subjected to controlled clinical trials, the argument makes good sense and should help in the development of binocular cooperation and aid in preventing subsequent strabismus.

Treatment is mandatory for monolateral aphakia. As stated above, in these cases it is necessary to sequentially treat stimulus deprivation amblyopia, anisometropic or aniseikonic amblyopia, and strabismic amblyopia. Occlusion is still the most effective treatment for the aphakic eye; however, the patching schedule for these patients should be carefully evaluated because of the high risk of patching the sound eye during its development. The risk of creating an occlusion amblyopia in the good fixing eye may be very great for infants during their first year of life.

We prefer to do our best for the neonate's aphakic eye *while minimally hampering functional development* of the fixing eye. Therefore, parents are asked to make a detailed daily waking and sleeping schedule. Occlusion of the fixing eye is scheduled so that it receives at least 50 percent of visual exposure during the baby's waking hours. This amount of exposure is necessary to allow the eye to develop fully. Obviously, the schedule must be changed regularly and good cooperation of the parents, particularly the mother, is required.

When the fixing eye is exposed, the amblyopic aphakic deviated eye is occluded. Patients who have monolateral congenital cataract and subsequent aphakia almost always develop a secondary esotropia and also develop all the sensory sequelae typical of strabismus. When vision is dominated by the fixing eye, exposure of the aphakic eye encourages the development of suppression or anomalous retinal correspondence (ARC), making the restoration of binocularity more difficult (1, 10).

When the eikonic correction is in place, binocular function is encouraged during some portion of each day. In general, each eye is patched for one third of each day. This allows the child to experience binocular vision for the remaining third of the day (assuming conditions allowing binocularity are provided).

The patching schedule can be modified after the first year of life. At this stage, more general patching of the fixing eye is less harmful than it would have been before. The new schedule is 2 days' occlusion of the fixing eye and one day of the deviated eye. Ideally, a point would be reached at which alternation takes place; in reality full alternation is rarely achieved. Therefore, treatment of amblyopia must be anticipated as a relatively long-term time commitment. In fact, whatever level of acuity is reached at age 2 or 3 years must be maintained until the child reaches 10 or 12 years. Whatever visual acuity the child has achieved may be lost if the treatment is interrupted. Depending on the situation of the patient, prescribed cycles of occlusion are like those for more usual strabismus patients.

From the point of view of visual resolution, these babies are followed closely, particularly during initial patching. Ideally, check-up visits are recommended every 10 days. Only after the first year of life is it possible to schedule them on a monthly basis. The objective is to avoid the risk of sensory deprivation amblyopia in the fixing, or more normal, eye.

The contact lens correction is evaluated and changed as eyeball growth requires. The patency of the opening of the visual pathway created by surgery should be checked periodically. After the second year of life, bifocals should be prescribed in order to provide both distance and near-point vision for the child. A slab-off prism also will probably be needed.

TREATMENT OF SECONDARY STRABISMUS

As stated above, children with monolateral aphakia almost invariably develop secondary strabismus, which exhibits the same features as primary congenital esotropia, namely ocular deviation, suppression and/or ARC, and amblyopia (1). On the other hand, motor fusion apparently is not disturbed, as it is in congenital esotropia. In the latter condition normal motor fusion never develops. Patients with secondary strabismus due to monolateral aphakia are able to regain a certain amount of binocularity if their eyes are kept or made straight. It is worthwhile to consider a period of nonsurgical treatment to align the eyes before resorting to a surgical procedure. This can be achieved by incorporating prisms in the baby's glasses. If one prescribes an exact correction for the angle of deviation, often after a short while the patient will revert to the original deviation. In other words, the patient compensates for the prismatic correction. It is likely that this phenomenon is an expression of the presence of deeply rooted sensorimotor sequelae bound to ARC. This is commonly seen in primary congenital esotropia. Therefore, it is possible to prescribe a prismatic overcorrection of the angle of deviation, creating an artificial condition of exo-deviation. The prisms added to the spectacle lenses should be worn by the patient as much as possible during the day. During the time when prisms are not worn, it is better to patch the fixing or the deviated eye (depending on the status of the amblyopia), to avoid strengthening the suppression and ARC that are already present.

After 1 month of wearing this type of prismatic correction, some patients were able to keep their eyes straight even without prisms. These patients rarely achieve a high level of binocularity, because they often have limited or very gross stereopsis. It is better to follow the procedure outlined above than to recommend further surgery for these patients. They may already have undergone several surgical procedures. Obviously, surgery must be considered if other measures fail.

SUMMARY

Finally, ophthalmic practitioners should attempt to treat these types of cases, because vision will not develop properly without treatment. It is the complexity of the total program and the need for practitioners with different skills that has prevented success in the past.

Until recently, relatively delayed surgery of congenital cataracts was the rule, and obviously this did not provide good functional results (30, 64). It is now advocated that surgery be performed early. With early treatment of bilateral cataracts it is possible to achieve 20/30 to 20/40 acuity (8, 57, 59). Although our results are not as spectacular as those reported by others in the literature (3, 32), we think it is worthwhile to try to treat patients with unilateral cataracts (11, 31, 40, 42, 43). In the latter condition, we never achieved a lasting normal acuity better than 20/28 to 20/1000, but this is still better than a nearly blind eye.

REFERENCES

1. Bagolini B: Diagnostic et possibilité de traitment de l'état sensoriel du strabisme avec des instruments peu dissociants (test du verre strié et barre de filtres). Ann Ocular (Paris) 194:236, 1961.

2. Banks MS, Salapatek P: Infant pattern vision: A new approach based on the contrast sensitivity function. J Exp Child Psychol 31:1, 1981.

3. Beller R, Hoyt CS, Marg E, et al: Good visual function after neonatal surgery for congenital monocular cataracts. Am J Ophthalmol 91:559, 1981.

4. Ben Ezra D, Paez JH: Congenital cataract and intraocular lenses. Am J Ophthalmol 96:311, 1981.

5. Birch EE, Gwiazda J, Held R: Stereoacuity development for crossed and uncrossed disparities in human infants. Vision Res 22:507, 1982.

6. Blomdahl S: Ultrasonic measurements of the eye in the newborn infant. Acta Ophthalmol (Copenh) 57:1048, 1979.

7. Bronson GW: The postnatal growth of visual capacity. Child Dev 45:873, 1974.

8. Campos EC: Optical correction in monolateral and bilateral aphakia due to congenital cataracts. In Francois J, et al (eds): Cataract Surgery and Visual Rehabilitation. Milan, Libreria Scientifica già Ghedini, 361, 1982.

9. Campos EC: Some thoughts on visual function testing in newborn babies. In Francois J, Maione M (eds): Pediatric Ophthalmology. Chichester, J Wiley & Sons, 333, 1982.

10. Campos EC, Enoch JM, Rabinowicz IM: Prismatic therapy associated with an attempt towards restoration of visual functions in monolateral aphakia due to congenital cataract. Proc Third Meeting, Int Strabismologic Assoc, May 10–12, Kyoto, 1978. In Reinecke RD (eds): Strabismus. New York, Grune & Stratton, 319, 1978.

11. Catalano RA, Simon JW, Jenkins PL, et al: Preferential looking as a guide for amblyopia therapy in monocular infantile cataracts. J Pediatr Ophthalmol Strabismus 24:56, 1987.

12. Cohen RL: Strabismus in the aphakic patient. Ophthalmology 86:2101, 1979.

13. Crawford JS, Morin JD: The Eye in Childhood. New York, Grune & Stratton, 1983.

14. Dobson V, Teller DY: Visual acuity in human infants: A review and comparison of behavioral and electrophysiological studies. Vision Res 18:1469, 1978.

15. Dobson V, Teller DY, Lee CP, et al: A behavioral method for efficient screening of visual acuity in young infants: I. Preliminary laboratory development. Invest Ophthalmol Vis Sci 17:1142, 1978.

16. Enoch JM: The fitting of hydrophylic (soft) contact lenses to infants and young children: I. Mensuration data on aphakic eyes of children born with congenital cataracts. Contact Lens Med Bull 5:36, 1972.

17. Enoch JM: The fitting of hydrophylic (soft) contact lenses to infants and young children: II. Fitting techniques and initial results on aphakic children. Contact Lens Med Bull 5:41, 1972.

18. Enoch JM: A rapid, accurate technique for retinoscopy of the aphakic infant or child in the operating room. Am J Ophthalmol 78:335, 1974.

19. Enoch JM: Use of inverted telescopic corrections incorporating soft contact lenses in the (partial) correction of aniseikonia in cases of unilateral aphakia. Adv Ophthalmol 32:54, 1976.

20. Enoch JM: Fitting parameters which need to be considered when designing soft contact lenses for the neonate. Contact Intraocular Lens Med 5:31, 1979.

21. Enoch JM: Techniques for evaluating scleral curvature and corneal vault. Contact Lens J 8:19, 1979.

22. Enoch JM, Binder PS, Bourne WM: The need to measure added parameters in order to properly specify hydrogel lenses in the treatment of corneal pathology. Contact Intraocular Lens Med J 7:331, 1981.

23. Enoch JM, Campos EC: Helping the aphakic neonate to see. Int Ophthalmol 8:237, 1985.

24. Enoch JM, Hamer RD: Image size correction of the unilateral aphakic infant. An invited paper presented at the joint meetings of the International Society of Genetic Eye Disease and the International Society of Pediatric Ophthalmology, Oct 28, San Francisco, 1982. Ophthalmic Paediatr Genet 2:153, 1983.

25. Enoch JM, Rabinowicz IM: Early surgery and visual correction of an infant born with unilateral eye lens opacity. Doc Ophthalmol 41:371, 1976.

26. Enoch JM, Rabinowicz IM, Campos EC: Post surgical contact lens correction of infants with sensory deprivation amblyopia associated with unilateral congenital cataract. Proc Int Med Contact Lens Symp May 9–10, Kyoto, 1978. J Jpn Contact Lens Soc 21:95, 1979.

27. Fantz RL, Ordy JM, Udelf MS: Maturation of pattern vision in infants during the first six months. J Comp Physiol Psychol 55:907, 1962.

28. Fox R: Stereopsis in animals and human infants: A review of behavioral investigations. In Aslin RN, Alberts JR, Petersen MR (eds): Development of Perception, Psychobiological Perspective, vol 2. The Visual System. New York, Academic Press, 1981.

29. Fox R, Aslin RN, Shea SL, et al: Stereopsis in human infants. Science 207:323, 1980.

30. Francois J: Later results of congenital cataract surgery. Ophthalmology 86:1586, 1979.

31. Frey T, Friendly D, Wyatt D: Reevaluation of monocular cataracts in children. Am J Ophthalmol 76:381, 1973.

32. Fulton AB, Manning KA, Dobson V: A behavioral method for efficient screening of visual acuity in young infants. II. Clinical application. Invest Ophthalmol Vis Sci 17:1151, 1978.

33. Gelbart SS, Hoyt CS, Jastrebski G, et al: Long-term visual results in bilateral congenital cataracts. Am J Ophthalmol 93:615, 1982.

34. Gernet H: Augenseitige Optik und kombinierte Haftschalenkorrektur der einseitigen Aphakie. Adv Ophthalmol 32:67, 1976.

35. Girard LJ: Aspiration-irrigation of congenital and traumatic cataracts. Arch Ophthalmol 77:387, 1967.

36. Girard LJ: Pars plana lensectomy by ultrasonic fragmentation: Results of a retrospective study. Ophthalmology 12:317, 1981.

37. Gwiazda J, Brill S, Mohindra I, et al: Infant visual acuity and its meridional variation. Vision Res 18:1557, 1978.

38. Gwiazda J, Wolfe JM, Brill S, et al: Quick assessment of preferential looking acuity in infants. Am J Optom Physiol Opt 57:420, 1980.

39. Harayama K, Ameniya T, Nishimura H: Development of the eyeball during fetal life. J Pediatr Ophthalmol Strabismus 18:37, 1981.

40. Helveston EM, Saunders RA, Ellis FD: Unilateral cataracts in children. Ophthalmic Surg 11:102, 1980.

41. Hiles DA: Intraocular lens implants in children. New York, Grune & Stratton, 1980.

42. Hoyt CS, Nickel B: Apakic cystoid macular edema occurrence in infants and children after transpupillary lensectomy and anterior vitrectomy. Arch Ophthalmol 100:746, 1982.

43. Jacobson SG, Mohindra I, Held R: Development of visual acuity in infants with congenital cataracts. Br J Ophthalmol 65:727, 1981.

44. Kupfer C: Treatment of amblyopia ex anopsia in adults: A preliminary report of seven cases. Am J Ophthalmol 43:918, 1957.

45. Larsen JS: The sagittal growth of the eye: I. Ultrasonic measurement of the depth of the anterior chamber from birth to puberty. Acta Ophthalmol (Copenh) 49:239, 1971.

46. Larsen JS: The sagittal growth of the eye: II. Ultrasonic measurement of the axial diameter of the lens and the anterior segment from birth to puberty. Acta Ophthalmol (Copenh) 49:427, 1971.

47. Larsen JS: The sagittal growth of the eye: III. Ultrasonic measurement of the posterior segment (axial length of the vitreous) from birth to puberty. Acta Ophthalmol (Copenh) 49:441, 1971.

48. Larsen JS: The sagittal growth of the eye: IV. Ultrasonic measurement of the axial length of the eye from birth to puberty. Acta Ophthalmol (Copenh) 49:873, 1971.

49. Lewis TL, Maurer D, Brent HP: Optokinetic nystagmus in children treated for bilateral cataracts. In Groner R, McConkie GW, Menz C (eds): Eye Movements and Human Information Processing. Amsterdam, North Holland, 1985.

50. Lewis TL, Maurer D, Brent HP: Effects on perceptual development of visual deprivation during infancy. Br J Ophthalmol 70:214, 1986.

51. Mann I: The Development of the Human Eye. British Medical Association, London, 1964.

52. Maurer D, Lewis TL, Brent HP: The effects of deprivation on human visual development: Studies of children treated for cataracts. In Morrison FJ, Lord CE, Keating DP (eds): Applied Developmental Psychology, vol. 3. New York, Academic Press, in press.

53. Mayer DL, Dobson V: Visual acuity development in infants and young children as assessed by operant preferential looking. Vision Res 22:1141, 1982.

54. Mayer DL, Fulton AB, Hansen RM: Preferential looking acuity in pediatric patients obtained with a staircase procedure. Invest Ophthalmol Vis Sci 23:538, 1982.

55. Morgan KS, Asbell PA, May JG, et al: Pediatric epikeratophakia. In Reinecke RD (ed): Strabismus II. Orlando, Grune & Stratton, 937, 1984.

56. Naegle JR, Held R: The postnatal development of monocular optokinetic nystagmus in infants. Vision Res 22:341, 1962.

57. Parks MM: Visual results in aphakic children. Am J Ophthalmol 94:441, 1982.

58. Petrig R, Julesz B, Kropfl W, et al: The development of stereopsis and cortical binocularity in infants: Electrophysiological evidence. Science 213:1402, 1981.

59. Pratt-Johnson JA, Tillson G: Visual results after removal of congenital cataracts before the age of one year. Can J Ophthalmol 16:19, 1981.

60. Ryan SJ, Maumenee AE: Unilateral congenital cataracts and their management. Ophthalmic Surg 8:35, 1977.

61. Salapatek P, Banks MS: Infant sensory assessment: Vision. In Minifie FD, Lloyd LL (eds): Communicative and cognitive abilities: Early behavioral assessment. Baltimore, University Park Press, 1978.

62. Schor C: The development of OKN in human infants. Am J Optom Physiol Optics 58:80, 1981.

63. Sokol S: Patterned elicited ERG's and VECP's in amblyopia and infant vision. In Armington JC, Krauskopf J, Wooten BR (eds): Visual Psychophysics and Psychology. New York, Academic Press, 1978.

64. Taylor D: Amblyopia in bilateral infantile and juvenile cataract. Relationship to timing of treatment. Trans Ophthalmol Soc UK 99:170, 1979.

65. von Noorden GK, Ryan SJ, Maumenee AE: Management of congenital cataracts. Trans Am Acad Ophthalmol Otolaryngol 74:352, 1970.

66. von Noorden GK: Monolateral congenital cataracts. When and if advisable to remove. In Francois J, et al (eds): Cataract Surgery and Visual Rehabilitation. Milano, Libreria Scientifica giá Ghedini, 1982.

67. von Noorden GK: Burian-von Noorden's Binocular Vision and Ocular Motility: Theory and Management of Strabismus. St Louis, CV Mosby, 1985.

68. Yee RD, Baloh RW, Honrubia V, et al: Pathophysiology of optokinetic nystagmus. In Honrubia V, Brazier MAB (eds): Nystagmus and Vertigo: Clinical Approaches to the Patient with Dizziness. New York, Academic Press, 251, 1982.

Chapter 18

Ocular Trauma and Emergencies

Leland W. Carr

Lesley L. Walls

There are few areas of clinical optometry more challenging than proper management of ocular trauma. The difficulty of examination, the need for accuracy in diagnosis, and the necessity of appropriate measures for management characterize every case. When the patient happens to be a child, the examination tends to be even more difficult to perform, and the margin for error is smaller. These cases are always trying for patient, parent, and practitioner, but successful optometric management of the child's injured eye is a most rewarding experience.

Children are most susceptible to traumatic damage of the eye and visual system (9). They engage repeatedly in active, hazardous play, and often manifest complete disregard for their own safety and that of their playmates.

Managing a child's traumatized eye differs from managing an adult's primarily because the examination is usually much more difficult. Also there is always the risk of amblyopia when either the injury or the treatment abolishes a sharp retinal image for a protracted period. Amblyopia is a real risk for any child who is injured before the age of 6 or 7 years (4), and especially for a child younger than 6 months, the critical period for visual development (2, 22).

It is important to know the most common forms of ocular and visual trauma for those under 12 years of age, to help establish indices of suspicion and so avoid missing some forms of ocular damage.

It has been suggested that the most common eye injury for both adults and children is probably a nonperforating corneal injury (17)

434

and that the commonest intraocular complication of ocular trauma during childhood is hyphema (9).

In their excellent article on eye injuries in childhood, Drs. Grin, Nelson, and Jeffers describe the breakdown of pediatric trauma cases seen at the Wills Eye Hospital between January 1983 and December 1985 (7). They found that the majority of patients (50 percent) had nonperforating injuries of the globe, including hyphema, iridodialysis, traumatic cataract, vitreous hemorrhage, and retinal detachment. The proportion of penetrating injuries to the globe was 34.5 percent, and of extraocular injuries, 14.5 percent, including lid lacerations and foreign bodies involving the lid. Two percent had intraorbital injuries and one percent had orbital wall fractures.

Our experience at W. W. Hastings Indian Hospital suggests that thermal, chemical, and radiation burns of the lids, cornea, and conjunctiva are also quite common in children. During 1987 we examined children with the following *primary* findings or sequela associated with ocular trauma:

Corneal or conjunctival abrasions (40 percent)
Benign ecchymosis (29 percent)
Hyphema (8 percent)
Acute traumatic cataracts (5 percent)
Corneal or conjunctival lacerations (3 percent)
Orbital fractures (3 percent)
Ultraviolet blepharokeratoconjunctivitis (3 percent)
Thermal ocular burns (3 percent)
Significant lid laceration (2 percent)
Chemical spills involving the eyes (2 percent)
Anterior chamber foreign bodies (1 percent)

Other findings of primary significance included vitreoretinal foreign bodies, choroidal rupture, and two cases of retrobulbar orbital foreign body.

Each of these injuries represents a significant threat to vision. Contaminated cornea can lead to ulceration and scarring, or eventually to endophthalmitis. Hyphema indicates damage to the iris, the angle tissues, or the ciliary body. Corneal blood staining and secondary glaucoma are always possible consequences when an anterior chamber fills with blood, and patients with angle recession are at risk throughout life of developing glaucoma. Burns can produce disfigurement and functional loss through scarring of lids, conjunctiva, cornea, and trabecular meshwork.

Every injured eye warrants a thorough examination of *all* structures from the adnexal epidermis to the retina, optic nerve, the visual cortex, and integration centers of the brain. The only way to avoid catastrophic mistakes in trauma management is to *always assume the worst has happened until you can absolutely rule it out.* Clearly, if the examiner does not look for it, it will not be found. If the examination is terminated when the first deviation from normal is discovered, other findings detectable by further examination will be missed.

What follows is a basic work-up applicable to eye trauma for patients of all ages. It is an orderly approach to data collection that stresses evaluation of the entire eye and visual system in *every* case. This is particularly important in pediatrics, owing to the difficulty of obtaining an adequate history and examination.

BASIC COMPONENTS OF TRAUMA EVALUATION

Firmly Establish the Accident History

Knowing exactly what happened helps to establish the proper indices of suspicion and to guide the examination. What, when, where, why, and how are the key questions in a thorough history. The history can never be too specific but it can easily be too general. If the initial history indicates that a true ophthalmic emergency exists, then immediate action is required and takes precedence over completing the history.

Measure Visual Acuity

This is a medicolegal absolute and an essential diagnostic, prognostic, and dynamic clinical variable. It is the best corrected visual acuity that is important. Pinholes, retinoscopes, trial lenses, and phoropters are important tools for this component of trauma evaluation.

It is necessary to question patients and parents about preexisting poor visual acuity and to consider the possibility of longstanding amblyopia in cases of depressed acuity with best correction in place.

Visual acuity should be recorded for the right eye, the left eye, and both eyes viewing together. Ideally this would be Snellen letters, numbers, rotating E's, Landolt C's, or a similar instrument at 20 feet, but it is often necessary to resort to near point flashcards, finger counting, Cheerios tests, or similar well-accepted pediatric acuity testing techniques. As a minimum it is necessary to describe the eye's fixational ability as central or eccentric and steady or unsteady.

Firmly Establish Events Since the Accident

The optometrist must establish exactly what has happened to the eye since the time of injury, and whether the patient has seen other doctors. If so, what have they been told about their injury? It is important to determine whether medications were prescribed or instilled into the eye and whether anything was removed from the eye. There is little to be gained from repeating expensive radiologic, hematologic, serologic, or microbiologic studies if the information has already been obtained, and is easily accessible.

Similarly, there is no point in duplicating prescriptions the patient may already have, or in continuing ineffective treatments. There may be times when patients have been given inappropriate prescriptions and it is necessary to take the drugs away in order to avoid complicating the trauma.

Diagnostically, it is necessary to evaluate the potential impact of previously adminis-

tered drugs, including mydriatics, cycloplegics, corticosteroids, analgesics, beta-blockers, and anesthetics. It is good to remember that more fixed, dilated pupils result from atropine-like substances than from true third nerve palsies (6)! Has the patient (or another doctor) put any medication into the injured eye?

Assess for Ocular Perforation

The next step is to examine for an intact globe and to be certain there are no perforations in the cornea or sclera. The examiner must look for signs of perforation or rupture.

Many times it is necessary to utilize topical anesthetics and cycloplegics to obtain the cooperation required for this assessment. Children are particularly likely to require sedation, facial nerve block, or general anesthesia. Specific recommendations are discussed later in the section on drug utilization.

The eye must be evaluated systematically for evidence of extrusion to the exterior of intraocular tissue. Uveal tissue will appear dark gray to brownish black; vitreous appears thick, gelatinous, and mucoid; and aqueous is indistinguishable from tears by gross inspection.

An extremely useful tool for evaluating a possible site of perforation involves painting the wound with sodium fluorescein (Seidel's Test) (9). Following installation of a drop of tropical anesthetic, and with the lids held firmly apart, a moistened strip is laid flat across the suspected site of perforation. The strip is then drawn away and the wound is evaluated with cobalt blue illumination. The area will appear dark purple-blue unless the aqueous or vitreous is leaking through the wound, in which case the alkaline intraocular fluid causes the fluorescein to glow bright green and flow currents may be detectable with magnification.

Intraocular pressure is an important indicator of globe integrity. Although traumatic injury to the iris and ciliary body often result in transient lowering of intraocular pressure by 4 to 5 mm Hg, all pressures below 5 to 8 mm Hg should be considered suspicious for an ocular perforation. Pressure below 4 mm Hg is very often associated with ocular penetration (13).

Other indicators of a violated globe include anomalies detectable within the eye: vitreous hemorrhages, unilaterally deep anterior chamber, displaced and distorted pupil ("pointing pupil"), wavelike patterns in the vitreous fibrils, and more obvious signs such as large chorioretinal breaks.

It is always advisable that an eye with a known or suspected penetration undergo radiologic evaluation to rule out retained intraocular or intraorbital foreign bodies.

Neurologic Evaluation

Significant trauma to the orbital region is at times associated with neurologic injury, and it is necessary, and relatively simple, to rapidly screen for intracranial and intraorbital neurologic involvement.

Assessment of pupils, lid position, ocular motility, corneal and facial sensitivity, and visual fields are essential to determine cranial nerve integrity (CN# 2, 3, 4, 5, 6, 7) and to evaluate neurologic health in the frontal, temporal, parietal, and occipital lobes, midbrain, cerebellum, and brain stem.

Pupils must be assessed for equality, shape, direct and consensual responsiveness to bright light stimulation, afferent defects (Marcus-Gunn sign on swinging flashlight test), and constriction upon convergence to near point.

A finding of "PERRLA" (*p*upils *e*qual, *r*ound, *r*esponsive to *l*ight and *a*ccommodation) implies bilaterally intact optic nerves and intact peripheral fiber bundles for both oculomotor (third cranial) nerves. PERRLA also indicates intact midbrain pupillary centers and normal sympathetic innervation reaching the pupillary dilator muscle.

The third cranial nerve can be further evaluated through examination for acquired ptosis, diplopia, or limitations of gaze. While chemotic swelling, edema, and hemorrhage into the lid tissues are common with ocular trauma and usually result in some degree of transient mechanical ptosis, this can be con-

sidered benign *unless* the ptosis is progressive or fails to resolve as ecchymosis and swelling subside.

Head, neck, and thoracic trauma have also been associated with subtle ptosis in cases of Horner's syndrome produced by damage to the sympathetic pathway to Mueller's muscle in the lid (3). Other signs of sympathoparesis include anisocoria, with the involved pupil showing faulty dilation in dim illumination and (rarely) anhydrosis with impaired sweating on the same side of the face.

Ocular motility is an important neurologic test in all trauma cases. An eye that can be moved up and out, down and out, up and in, and in toward the nose, has normal third nerve innervation. If it can be abducted from the nose without limitation, the sixth cranial nerve is functioning. If it can be directed down and in, sufficient fourth nerve signals are reaching the superior oblique muscle (Fig. 18.1).

If binocular pursuits (horizontal gaze) can be shown to be intact, with no evidence of unilateral paresis or nystagmus, then the medial longitudinal fasciculus with the midbrain and brainstem is likely intact. Voluntary saccades into gaze-right and gaze-left positions are indicators of intact frontal lobe function. Vertical gaze is considered to depend on normal function in the upper midbrain (14) and is therefore an indicator of neurologic intactness of that region.

The fifth cranial nerve functions in sensory input from the cornea and paraorbital skin. A thin wisp teased from the tip of a cotton-tipped applicator makes an excellent tool to objectively and subjectively elicit evi-

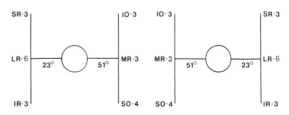

Figure 18.1 Diagram of ocular motility illustrating the primary positions for testing function of cranial nerves and extraocular muscles.

dence of sensitivity to touch. Touching the cotton wisp to a normal cornea produces an obvious blink reflex and a report of a foreign body sensation. When dragged lightly over the forehead and lower lid, it tests the sensitivity of the supraorbital and infraorbital divisions, respectively, of the ophthalmic division of the fifth cranial nerve.

Normal, complete, firm closure of the lids requires adequate input via the seventh cranial nerve to the orbicularis oculi muscle.

Intact visual fields are evidence of normal function of the visual pathway from the retina, through the optic nerves, chiasm, optic tracts, radiations, and the visual cortex. Modified confrontation fields can be performed quickly on responsive children. One excellent technique uses two red-tipped wands or two red-capped medicine bottles to run a *redness* and *brightness* comparison with test objects positioned at equal distances from fixation on either side of the vertical meridian, then on either side of the horizontal meridian. This is performed with the child fixating the examiner's nose or face. Thus, the redness and brightness are compared and contrasted for the two superior field quadrants, then the two inferior field quadrants, then the two temporal field quadrants, and finally the two nasal field quadrants. This test is remarkably accurate in screening for hemianopic and quadranopic field depressions.

With less responsive patients the visual field can be grossly assessed by introducing interesting objects, such as a flashing penlight or a small plastic toy (more colorful toys being more effective) from the periphery into the four field quadrants and observing for fixational eye movements as evidence of target detection. Some children respond very well to automated perimetry, apparently finding the task similar to a video game.

The overall responsiveness, alertness, and demeanor of the patient should be assessed for signs of neurologic injury. It has been observed that many pediatric patients with traumatic hyphema appear quite lethargic and dazed in spite of normal neurologic function (18). The exact reason remains obscure, but this phenomenon may involve the oculovagal reflex and fifth nerve stimulation in the cornea and iris.

Any patient who manifests signs of neurologic dysfunction should be referred immediately to a pediatric neurologist, trauma center, emergency room, or from another proper facility, staffed with physicians familiar with the management of pediatric head trauma. It is essential to withhold mydriatic and cycloplegic agents until the patient has been examined by the physician. Pupil function provides valuable diagnostic clues, and progressive impairment of constriction is a signal that intracranial pressure may be rising in association with subdural hematoma or from another cause of increased intracranial pressure.

Assess for Evidence of Broken Bones

Fractures in the orbital region are often accompanied by ecchymosis (black eye), mild to severe lid swelling, mild to severe enophthalmos (or more rarely, exophthalmos), and in some cases, localized skin anesthesia detectable by the cotton wisp or pinprick test. The latter results from bone-induced trauma to the supraorbital or infraorbital branches of the ophthalmic division of the fifth cranial nerve.

Defects in the orbital area are sometimes palpable by the fingertips as movable bone fragments or irregular notches. Audible clicking or cracking may be noted by the patient or by the examiner during this procedure.

Orbital emphysema (crepitus), from pockets of air from fractured paranasal sinuses may be palpable within the orbital tissues. Patients commonly describe a sensation of snap-crackle-popping associated with manipulation of these tissue air pockets.

Classic orbital floor fractures are associated with restrictions in ocular motility accompanied by diplopia. Entrapment of the inferior rectus or oblique muscle or their fascial sheaths within the fracture site typically limits upward and downward gaze. These patients are unable to look up or down without diplopia. With actual herniation into the maxillary sinus (hanging drop), the volume of intraorbital tissue is reduced and the globe becomes recessed into the orbit.

It is necessary to stress that orbital fracture diagnosis ultimately depends on radiologic studies. Orbital x-rays, tomograms, and perhaps even computed tomography may be required to confirm or refute a suspected orbital fracture. We recently examined a patient with head trauma sustained in an auto accident who showed mild ecchymosis (tattooing) where his spectacle frame was driven into his face. In addition the patient had a small inferior subconjunctival hemorrhage, full ocular motility without diplopia, and no enophthalmos on exophthalmometry, but x-ray evaluation demonstrated a total of six orbital bone fractures (including blowout fracture of the orbital floor).

The important point about orbital fractures is that they may be accompanied by much more significant damage to the eye, including globe rupture, retinal detachment, vitreous hemorrhage, hyphema, angle recession, and lens dislocation. These must all be ruled out in every case.

Goals of orbital fracture management include preservation of the eye and vision, avoidance of diplopia, and correction of significant cosmetic disfigurement. Many times these patients do not require surgery. By itself, orbital fracture is not an ocular emergency, but it is accepted practice to use antibiotic prophylaxis to prevent orbital cellulitis in cases where sinus fracture is either strongly suspected or documented. Adequate prophylaxis consists of broad-spectrum systemic antibiotics for 2 to 4 weeks after the orbital fracture (18).

Assess the External Tissues

The next step in the trauma work-up is thorough evaluation of the external tissues to check for significant lacerations, need for stitches, evidence of wound contamination, indications for systemic antibiotics, need for rabies prophylaxis, need for tetanus inoculations, and any signs that may suggest damage to the globe or orbit.

With children it is often necessary to use topical anesthetic drops to obtain even minimal cooperation during external examination. Sedatives, local nerve block, or general anesthesia may be required in certain instances. Regardless of the circumstance, the clinician must do whatever is necessary to thoroughly examine the child. The clinician should utilize gentle manipulation of the external tissues with fingertips and cotton-tipped applicators, using bright light and a magnifying device—slit-lamp, jeweler's loupe, headborne magnifier, direct ophthalmoscope. Lacerations and punctures must be evaluated for depth, contamination, and presence of intraocular or intraorbital tissue, including orbital fat.

An attempt should *always* be made to evert the upper and lower lids. The tarsus may show evidence of through-and-through laceration or puncture. It is common to find some residual foreign body trapped behind a lid, and removal of debris is essential for proper healing of an injured cornea or conjunctiva.

The recent case of a young girl seen in our clinic with "corneal abrasion secondary to ocular trauma," provides a valuable lesson. A 7-year-old child complained to her mother of eye pain after playing on a wooden clothesline pole. A large central corneal abrasion was detected by the examiner. The eye was cyclopleged, prophylaxed with antibacterial ointment, and pressure-patched. Several follow-up examinations showed the wound to be worsening, becoming more edematous, infiltrated, and widely abraded. When the girl was referred for further evaluation, we everted the upper lid and discovered a small wood splinter actively reabrading the eye every time the patch was removed! Once the foreign body was gone, the eye healed completely within 48 hours.

The U.S. Public Health Service offers the following guidelines for tetanus prophylaxis; they are very applicable to lid and conjunctival lacerations or puncture wounds (23).

For Clean, Minor Wounds Tetanus toxoid injection is recommended for all patients except those with a history of at least three previous toxoid injections who have had a booster within the preceding 10-year period.

For All Other Wounds   Tetanus toxoid or tetanus immune globulin (human) is recommended in every case except for patients who have had three or more previous injections and at least one booster within the previous 5-year period.

Topical antibiotic therapy is acceptable for managing virtually every case of lid or adnexal injury in which there is violation or loss of significant epidermis. In all cases of an open wound between the brow and maxillary ridge it is advisable to utilize ophthalmic preparations, in anticipation that some of the medication will likely end up in the eye through one mechanism or another. Common sense and medicolegal consideration indicate that drugs entering the eye should be designed for ophthalmic application.

Systemic antibiotics are indicated in cases with significant necrotic or contaminated tissue and when surgical repair and closure will be delayed more than a few hours. External wounds associated with animal bites should be managed with systemic antibiotics and proper local wound treatment.

Assess the Cornea and Conjunctiva

The cornea and conjunctiva need to be examined carefully with magnification and bright light then reexamined immediately with fluorescein dye to highlight defects. The cornea and conjunctiva must be examined for intactness, abrasions, lacerations, foreign bodies, edema, and cellular infiltrates. These findings offer clear evidence of tissue injury.

The corneal endothelium should be examined carefully with the biomicroscope in search of keratic precipitates or pigment cells, evidence of anterior uveitis and iris trauma, respectively.

Assess the Anterior Chamber

The anterior chamber requires thorough evaluation for blood, cells, flare, and pigment. Hyphema is a common finding in pediatric ocular trauma and is evidence of significant damage to the iris, iris root, angle, or ciliary body. Red blood cells in the aqueous are evidence of microhyphema (and of less severe damage). Heavy pigment cell effusion into the aqueous suggests the iris has been thrust against the crystalline lens, potentially injuring the angle or lens and leading to secondary glaucoma or cataract.

White blood cells enter the aqueous when iris or ciliary body vessels are inflamed. This iridocyclitis is commonly associated with blunt trauma to the eye and usually resolves rapidly without sequelae. Significant iridocyclitis, however, should be treated with appropriate cycloplegic/mydriatics and topical corticosteroids to avoid permanent damage to the cornea, trabeculum, iris, ciliary body, crystalline lens, and vitreous (16).

Flare is a proteinaceous plasma component from anterior uveal inflammation that signifies vessel wall damage. The presence of flare implies rather longstanding inflammation (21).

The only way to accurately diagnose cells and flare in the anterior chamber is with a high-quality slit lamp, oblique bright illumination setting, and moderate magnification (to enable detection of small cells without limiting the depth of focus, which would occur with high magnification).

Assess the Retina, Vitreous, and Choroid

Finally, in *all* cases of ocular trauma the eye should be dilated and examined by both direct and indirect ophthalmoscopy. The vitreous should be examined for blood, inflammatory cells, and pigment epithelial cells (Shafer's sign, "tobacco dust"). In some cases of operculated retinal break the rounded piece of grayish retina may be detected easily, floating within the vitreous. An annular floater (Weiss' ring) is evidence of posterior vitreous detachment and an indication that the patient must be monitored carefully for evidence of retinal break.

The retina should be examined carefully for tears, holes, breaks, detachments, hemorrhages, and edema. Key diagnostic signs of retinal detachment include elevation with undulation and loss of underlying choroidal detail due to obscuration by elevated semi-transparent retina. Holes and tears appear red as a result of increased visibility of the choroidal microcirculation.

The choroid should be examined for evidence of exudation, detachment, hemorrhage, and rupture.

Any serious problem in the posterior segment of the eye is an indication for emergency consultation with a retinal specialist.

To summarize, the management of ocular trauma involves thorough examination of each eye, from adnexa to retina and from pupils and motility to cortical perception. The optometrist should always assume the patient has a severe injury until it is positively ruled out and should be quick to refer and consult on these cases. A clinician should only handle the case when his knowledge and experience gives him a "feeling of comfort" in doing so.

EXAMINATION AND EQUIPMENT

Restraint

Examining a child is essentially identical to examining an adult, except that innovation and creative thinking may be needed to conduct a successful pediatric examination.

Most children can be evaluated with a conventional biomicroscope, although it is often necessary to have the child stand or kneel on a chair to obtain proper head positioning. Small children can be held against the head rest while seated on the parent's lap. A direct ophthalmoscope, or head-borne magnification loupe and transilluminator light source are reasonable substitutes when biomicroscopy is not possible.

Both direct and binocular indirect ophthalmoscopy should be performed on all injured eyes. At times the examiner must become a contortionist, but in most cases the fundus between the vortex vessels can be viewed if adequate dilation has been achieved. Children can be held with the head facing over the parent's shoulder. In some cases it may be necessary to position the child face up on the parent's lap with the legs straddling the parent's abdomen. If necessary, the child's arms can be extended alongside the head and held firmly against the ears in order to hold the head immobile.

Swaddling

A very young or immature child can be difficult to examine, but a complete examination is essential to ascertain the status of an injured eye. Therefore, the clinician must utilize whatever it takes in the way of restraint in order to complete the examination. When physical means are insufficient, systemic sedatives and even general anesthesia may be considered.

A very young child or infant may be adequately restrained by simple swaddling with a blanket or sheet (Fig. 18.2). The properly

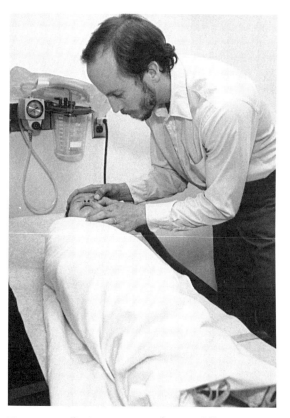

Figure 18.2 Patient restraint by swaddling.

swaddled child is unable to move the arms and body, which makes it easier for the examiner to concentrate on controlling the head and neck.

It is vital to involve the parent actively in controlling a child for examination. When swaddling is appropriate, the best person to control the body of the child is a calm, committed parent. For larger children (up to about age 4 or 5) a papoose board may be utilized (Fig. 18.3). When older and larger children cannot be controlled for examination, consideration must be given to systemic sedation or general anesthesia.

It is impossible to immobilize a patient completely with either swaddling or a papoose board. Older children who realize that the parent is involved and that the examination will take place often become cooperative enough to tolerate the examination without

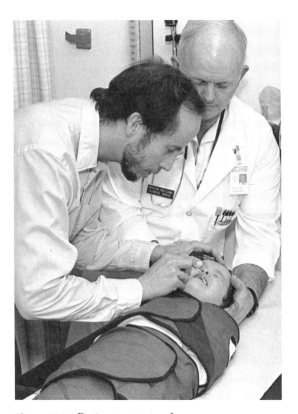

Figure 18.3 Patient restrained on a papoose board.

systemic medication. Regardless, it must be kept in mind that a complete examination is the responsibility of the doctor and that, therefore, proper utilization of restraint is always acceptable when indicated.

Systemic Medication for Examination

When there is no other way to reasonably obtain control of a child for proper examination, systemic medication must be considered. In such a case the patient should usually be taken to a hospital emergency room where consultation with an emergency department physician, ophthalmologist, and/or anesthesiologist can be obtained.

There are several ways to utilize systemic medications in order to completely examine the eye. The following are in rather common use.

A lytic cocktail administered by mouth is often sufficient. This is a combination of oral preparations of pain relievers and tranquilizers to achieve a state of sleepiness, which makes the child very amenable to examination without resistance. The only significant limitations are persuading the child to drink the solution and then waiting 30 to 60 minutes for the desired effect.

Another method of obtaining more rapid onset of the same desired sleepiness is by intramuscular or intravenous injection of tranquilizers and pain relievers. This may be indicated for the child who refuses to swallow an oral preparation or when the clinician desires more rapid drug action.

The last consideration is the administration of general anesthesia. This is performed only in a controlled environment by an anesthesiologist, because the patient loses spontaneous respiration and must have vital signs monitored. General anesthesia should never be utilized unless absolutely necessary, as it carries a small but significant risk of death.

Drugs in Diagnosis and Management of Pediatric Trauma

Diagnostic agents, including topical anesthetics and mydriatics, are essential for successful evaluation of the traumatized eye. Effective management often requires the use of therapeutic drugs, including topical and systemic antibiotics, cycloplegics, and intraocular antihypertensive drugs.

Exact compliance with a drug regimen is difficult when a child is uncooperative or if the parent is timid or overzealous. It is essential that all medications be dispensed with complete instructions given both orally and in written form on the label. All systemic drugs must be carefully adjusted to the patient's weight, development, and age. Topical drugs can usually be prescribed in accordance with adult regimens, though a few extra precautions are in order (see below).

Atropine, scopolamine, and to a lesser extent homatropine, have been associated with peripheral nervous system side effects (8, 10). Central nervous system side effects have also been associated with use of these drugs in children, and scopolamine and cyclopentolate appear to be most likely to produce dose-related toxicity (8).

Low–birth weight infants' eyes may be dilated with 1 drop of 0.5-percent tropicamide, followed by a second drop in 5 minutes. A child 8 pounds or heavier may be given a drop of 1-percent tropicamide followed in 5 minutes by a drop of 2.5-percent phenylephrine. If cycloplegic refraction is also indicated, a single drop of 0.5-percent cyclopentolate is added to this regimen (1-percent cyclopentolate is used if the child is over 12 to 15 pounds or is darkly pigmented).

When prolonged mydriasis or cycloplegia is required for a pediatric patient, 1-percent atropine sulfate in ointment or solution form is recommended. One to three instillations daily generally provide excellent pupil and ciliary muscle relaxation. Exact dosage is determined by degree of inflammation and degree of iris sphincter or ciliary muscle spasm.

Among topical antimicrobials chloramphenicol, neomycin, and sulfacetamide have been linked to aplastic anemia, allergic hypersensitivity, and Stevens-Johnson syndrome, respectively (5, 8, 15). However toxic reactions can be produced by virtually any medication if used by a patient with hypersensitivity tendencies, so all drugs must be used judiciously and with adequate precautions.

Both polysporin and gentamicin ophthalmic preparations work very well for delivering antibacterial medication to children. Frequency of instillation depends on the severity of infection, but generally three to four daily doses of a half inch of ointment placed into the cul-de-sac and spread across the lid margins provide adequate coverage.

Topical steroids and steroid–antibiotic combinations must be used cautiously in children and adults. Increased susceptibility to infection, enhanced viral replication, elevation of intraocular pressure, and inducement of posterior subcapsular cataract are well-documented risks associated with the use of topical steroids. When the structural integrity of the eye is threatened by severe inflammation the benefits outweigh the risks and judicious steroid therapy is justified.

With regard to corticosteroids (and steroid combination drugs) the best approach in general is to withhold them unless they are clearly indicated for preservation of ocular integrity. When neovascularization, scarring, or significant cell and flare make corticosteroid therapy essential, it should be given to children. When steroids are indicated, they should be used aggressively from the outset and tapered off as rapidly as resolution of inflammation permits. In general, four applications per day is considered aggressive topical corticosteroid therapy, although severe inflammation may warrant more frequent instillations. The medication *must* be withdrawn gradually to avoid rebound inflammation. The goal is to limit topical corticosteroid therapy to 2 weeks or less, if possible, in every case (21).

It is wise to consult a physician familiar with pediatric medicine and pharmacy when prescribing systemic medications for children. Erythromycin, ampicillin, methacillin, and cephradine are the systemic antibiotics used most frequently for children. Tetracycline is contraindicated in children, as it has been associated with discoloration of developing teeth (8).

MANAGEMENT

Corneal Trauma

Corneal Lacerations

Corneal lacerations must be identified with biomicroscopy and studied with fluorescein painting of the wound and tonometry. The clinician must assume intraocular penetration has occurred until it is proven otherwise. It is usually necessary to provide analgesics, to instill an anesthetic drug, and to dilate or cycloplege these eyes to obtain cooperation for thorough examination. In cases of ocular penetration it is best to avoid ointments, which may produce a plug of intraocular debris capable of damaging the endothelium, meshwork, or crystalline lens. The examiner must avoid squeezing the eye, which may lead to herniation of intraocular tissue through the wound. When a perforation is detected, a single eye pad is applied and taped in place to keep the lid closed firmly but gently over the injured eye, then a protective shield is taped over the eye pad. Immediate referral is indicated in these cases, because prophylaxis against endophthalmitis and wound closure with cyanoacrylate or sutures is probably necessary. All violated globes should be evaluated with x-ray or CT to rule out retained foreign bodies.

Corneal Foreign Bodies

Children manage to get just about anything from their environment into their eyes. Fortunately, most corneal foreign bodies remain superficial and are easily removed with a stream of preserved saline solution, a moist cotton-tipped applicator (although care must be taken to avoid abrading the cornea), a 25-gauge needle or foreign body spud.

Multiple superficial corneal foreign bodies are common in explosive or gust-type injuries. At times these cases are best referred to an ophthalmologist for alcohol or ether denuding of the entire epithelium followed by flushing and lifting of debris.

Routine corneal foreign bodies located anterior to Bowman's membrane can be lifted off with a golf-club spud or needle, though it is absolutely essential to have the patient fully cooperative to keep the eye absolutely steady during these procedures. General anesthesia is therefore often necessary with very young, rambunctious, frightened, or otherwise uncooperative children.

Instillation of two drops of ophthetic into both eyes is satisfactory for topical anesthesia. Most patients tend to perceive better anesthesia when drops are placed in both eyes. Then cycloplegia can be attained with 1 drop of 5-percent homatropine. After waiting a couple of minutes, the cornea is approached tangentially with a spud or needle. The needle is held bevel side up, so that the bevel remains directed away from the globe. The foreign body is lifted off gently and any residual rust ring debris is removed with an Alger brush. In many cases rust removal is simplified by waiting 24 to 48 hours, to allow the debris to be softened by corneal inflammatory processes and an antibiotic ointment.

Although it is not essential that 100 percent of residual rust be removed, it is advisable to remove as much as can be retrieved without damaging the cornea further. Retained rust can produce significant inflammation, gross scarring, and corneal tattooing.

Following removal of a foreign body rust ring, the lower cul-de-sac is filled with an appropriate ophthalmic antibiotic ointment, such as gentamicin, then two eye pads are applied to provide a firm pressure patch to immobilize the lids. This enhances the opportunity for epithelial healing. Systemic analgesics (but not topical anesthetics!) are prescribed as necessary. Patients are always reexamined within 24 hours to evaluate healing, rule out wound infection, and look for signs of iridocyclitis. When incomplete healing so indicates, the antibiotic and pressure patching regimen can be repeated.

Corneal Ulcers

Corneal ulcer is always an ophthalmic emergency in a child. Swab cultures, corneal scrapings, and antibiotic sensitivity studies are indicated. Appropriate antibiotics must be instilled regularly and aggressively. Hospitalization is often appropriate, to ensure compliance with medication regimens.

Anterior Segment

Hyphema

Blood in the anterior chamber is a relatively common finding in childhood ocular trauma and is always significant. Fully 25 percent of these patients can be expected to develop some vision loss as a complication of the anterior chamber injury or from associated injury to the posterior segment (26).

Complications, including corneal blood staining and glaucoma, become especially likely in cases of second bleeds (rebleeding). Around 25 percent of hyphema patients can be expected to have secondary bleeds within 5 days of the initial injury, probably as a result of clot contraction and fibrinolysis (18). Because these injuries are often associated with vision loss, an ophthalmologist should be consulted.

Clinical evaluation includes measurement of visual acuity, neurologic evaluation (do not be afraid of constricting the pupil during pupil testing, or of moving the eye during motility procedures), and intraocular pressure evaluation. It is essential to rule out rupture or penetration of the globe.

Hyphema may be a sign of injury to the posterior segment of the eye. Although dilation with hyphema remains controversial, the need to evaluate the retina and optic nerve head, and the likelihood of significant traumatic iritis, make atropine mydriasis and cycloplegia the procedure of choice whenever possible. Not only is the pupil opened for ophthalmoscopy, but the risk of both peripheral anterior and posterior synechiae is reduced. At the same time the atropine limits pupillary and ciliary muscle pull and tug on iris root tears and angle recessions. Atropine instillation reduces muscle trauma to already damaged iris vessels, so it is recommended that most patients with hyphema of 60 percent or less be dilated.

Gonioscopy should be part of the evaluation of hyphema patients to assess damage to the angle and to determine the likelihood of secondary glaucoma arising subsequently. However, it is probably best to delay gonioscopy until the hyphema has resolved and thus avoid inciting a second bleed from vessels that are not yet fully healed.

Aspirin and prostaglandin inhibitors (ibuprofen, indomethacin, etc.) should be withheld in hyphema, and only analgesics that do not affect normal blood clotting should be administered.

Proper hyphema management involves minimizing activity, elevating the head, reducing inflammation, slowing the processes of clot breakdown, preventing glaucoma, and preventing corneal blood staining. With pediatric patients this usually involves hospitalization to enforce compliance. These patients require daily evaluation of intraocular pressure and corneal transparency.

Traumatic Iritis

Mild to severe inflammation of the iris and ciliary body are common following virtually any type of trauma to the cornea or globe. The eyes may not demonstrate the classic ciliary flush of hyperemia surrounding the limbus, but patients often complain of orbital ache, blurred vision, tearing, and sensitivity to light.

Examination may reveal signs of accommodative spasm or infacility. There may be pupillary miosis or traumatic mydriasis in patients with traumatic iritis. Therefore, the small-pupil sign is not extremely useful in diagnosis; indeed, all diagnosis depends on excellent biomicroscopic examination of the anterior chamber, aqueous, and corneal endothelium.

Mild cases of traumatic iritis often benefit from mydriasis and cycloplegia and analgesics. More severe cases warrant the addition of topical corticosteroids, except when penetration or rupture is possible. The examiner must keep in mind the fact that corticosteroids increase the risk of infection and can delay healing, and must use them with great care.

Crystalline Lens Trauma

Both blunt and penetrating ocular trauma can be associated with damage to the crystalline lens, its zonular attachments, or its protective capsule. Every case of ocular trauma warrants careful biomicroscopy of the lens.

The clinician must examine for signs of lens malpositioning, including subluxation and dislocation. Findings such as irregular anterior chamber depth, tremulous iris, and visible lens edges or zonules seen upon dilation suggest lens disruption.

A lens that is dislocated into the anterior chamber requires emergency surgical intervention to avoid reverse pupillary block glaucoma and to minimize damage to the corneal endothelium (18). For similar reasons, a lens incarcerated in the pupil should be referred for surgical evaluation as an ophthalmic emergency.

When a crystalline lens dislocates into the vitreous it may persist for many years as a benign vitreous "floater," but the clinician should consider consultation with a vitreoretinal specialist in these cases. It is best to allow the surgeon to decide whether the lens must be surgically removed.

Certain systemic conditions predispose patients to lens subluxation from relatively minor ocular trauma—Marfan's syndrome, syphilis, Marchesani's syndrome, and homocystinuria (12).

Traumatic cataract is a common complication of blunt and penetrating ocular trauma. Both contusion forces from shock waves (blunt) and laceration of the capsule (penetrating) can produce localized, or more often generalized, lens intumesence and clouding (19). Traumatic cataract often arises within days after injury but may require weeks or months to become apparent. Cases of apparently mild blunt trauma may lead to formation of posterior subcapsular plaques around 6 months after the accident. A lacerated or ruptured lens capsule may spill lens cortex into the aqueous, leading to particulate or hypersensitivity glaucoma. Lens proteins in the eye warrant immediate referral for surgical intervention.

Posterior Segment Injuries

It should be assumed that ocular trauma has produced retinal breaks and detachment in every case until proper fundus examination proves otherwise. Sharp objects and high-velocity foreign bodies can easily penetrate to the vitreous and beyond. Concussive shock wave injury to vitreous, retina, and choroid is also common with ocular trauma.

Dilation with direct and indirect ophthalmoscopy, and biomicroscopy with and without auxiliary lenses (Hruby, Volk 90 D conoid, mirrored contact fundus lens) should be performed on all patients in order to carefully evaluate the vitreous. Hemorrhages, ripples, clefts, and detachments seen in the vitreous should always be considered significant. Traumatic posterior vitreous detachment must be followed at very regular intervals for the first 6 months following injury. Generally, posttraumatic retinal breaks, atrophic holes, and detachments become much more apparent within this 6-month period if they are going to occur.

Retinal edema may arise in the peripheral fundus or posterior pole and is a common sequela of direct trauma to the globe. Retinal edema has also been associated with contre-coup-type trauma from blows to the back of the head. Retinal edema typically occurs within 24 hours of the injury and appears as whitish geographic splotches of cloudy discoloration seen against the red-orange fundus.

Retinal edema will usually resorb over several days to weeks, but it can lead to permanent vision loss through formation of retinal cysts, holes, or pigmentary degenerations affecting the retinal pigment epithelium and photoreceptors.

Severe jolts to the globe can actually rupture the choriocapillaris, the remaining choroidal layers, or even the retina. Typically an acute choroidal rupture appears as a large, deep, fundus hemorrhage with feathery bleed extension up under the retinal pigment epithelium and into the sensory retina. These breaks may lead to subretinal neovascular nets and disciform degeneration months to years after the trauma (1).

Traumatic retinal breaks and detachments may occur in an eye that is predisposed to such problems because of peripheral retinal degeneration (lattice) or thinning (myopia). They are often late sequelae of the trauma, arising weeks to months after the injury. Eighty percent of traumatic retinal detachments arise within 2 years after the injury (20), and patients with severe ocular trauma must be followed at regular intervals, especially during the critical first 6 months.

Ophthalmoscopic evidence of retinal break and detachment includes free-floating opercula, vitreous bleeds, red fundus lesions with elevated borders or "lips" which elevate upon scleral indentation, semitransparent elevations, and loss of visible underlying choroidal detail. A large retinal detachment often contains folds and undulates with eye movements. Retinal detachments always create visual field depressions.

Consultation with a vitreoretinal specialist is indicated in every case of significant injury to the posterior segment of the eye. This is especially true with pediatric trauma because examination often necessitates general anesthesia and because posterior injury to the eye can be so devastating.

SUMMARY

Trauma to the eye of an infant or child is extremely common and can be a very trying experience for patient, family, and clinician. In each case, an adequate history and examination must be obtained to provide an accurate and complete diagnosis. Proper management can be provided only in the setting of a proper diagnosis. The clinician must be prepared to be innovative in the utilization of skills and to obtain appropriate consultation when indicated in order to adequately diagnose and manage ocular trauma in children.

REFERENCES

1. Bell FC, Stenstrom WJ: Atlas of the Peripheral Retina. Philadelphia, WB Saunders, 64, 1983.

2. Bellor R, Hoyt CS, Marg E, et al: Good Visual Function after Neonatal Surgery for Congenital Monocular Cataracts. Am J Ophthalmol 91:559, 1981.

3. Burde RM: Clinician's guide to the pupil. In Burde RM, Karp JS (eds): Clinical Neuroophthalmology: The Afferent Visual System. Boston, Little, Brown, 152, 1977.

4. Burian HM, vonNoorden GK: Binocular Vision and Ocular Motility (Theory and Management of Strabismus). St Louis, CV Mosby, 221, 1980.

5. Chang FW: Anti-infective drugs. In Bartlett JD, Jaanus SD (eds): Clinical Ocular Pharmacology. Boston, Butterworths, 202, 1984.

6. Gray L: The pupil evaluation. In Terry J (ed): Ocular Disease. Stoneham, Butterworths, 301, 1984.

7. Grin TR, Nelson LB, Jeffers JB: Eye Injuries in Childhood. Pediatrics 80:13, 1987.

8. Havener WH: Ocular Pharmacology. St Louis, CV Mosby, 1983.

9. Helveston EM, Ellis FD: Pediatric Ophthalmology Practice. St Louis, CV Mosby, 1984.

10. Jaanus SD: Drugs affecting the autonomic nervous system. In Bartlett JD, Jaanus SD (eds): Clinical Ocular Pharmacology. Boston, Butterworths, 106, 1984.

11. Jaanus SD: Dyes. In Bartlett JD, Jaanus SD (eds): Clinical Ocular Pharmacology. Boston, Butterworths, 11:315, 1984.

12. Jarrett WH: Dislocation of the lens. In Fraunfelder F, Roy FH (eds): Current Ocular Therapy, 2nd ed. Philadelphia, WB Saunders, 435, 1985.

13. Keeney AH: Prevention of ocular injuries. In Boruchoff SA (ed): Practical Management of Ocular Injuries. Boston, Little, Brown, 8, 1974.

14. Leigh RJ, Zee D: The Neurology of Eyemovements. Philadelphia, FA Davis, 95, 1983.

15. O'Connor Davies PH: The Actions and Uses

of Ophthalmic Drugs. Boston, Butterworths, 342, 1981.

16. O'Connor GR: Conticosteroids and immuno-suppressives reviewed. In Srinivasan BD (ed): Ocular Therapeutics. New York, Masson, 69, 1980.

17. Pashby RC, Chisholm L: Trauma. In Crawford JS, Morin JD (eds): The Eye in Childhood. New York, Grune & Stratton, 353, 1983.

18. Paton D, Goldberg MF: Management of Ocular Injuries. Philadelphia, WB Saunders, 290, 1976.

19. Roper-Hall MJ: Traumatic cataract. In Freeman HM (ed): Ocular Trauma. New York, Appleton-Century-Crofts, 151, 1979.

20. Schepens CL: Retinal Detachment and Allied Diseases. Philadelphia, WB Saunders, 71, 1983.

21. Smith RE, Nozik RM: Uveitis: A Clinical Approach to Diagnosis and Management. Baltimore, Williams & Wilkins, 49, 1983.

22. Taylor D, Clive M: Cataracts in infancy. In Wybar K, Taylor D (eds): Pediatric Ophthalmology: Current Aspects. New York, Marcel Dekker, 154, 1983.

23. U.S. Public Health Service, Advisory Committee on Immunization Practices: Morbidity and Mortality Weekly Report Supplement, vol 21, no 25. Atlanta, Center for Disease Control, June 24, 1972.

Chapter 19

Color Vision

Gunilla Haegerström-Portnoy

WHY TEST THE COLOR VISION OF CHILDREN?

The main reasons for testing color vision in children are:

1. To identify congenital color vision defects at an early age because so much modern school material—used for both reading and mathematics—is color coded. Several authors have emphasized the importance of early identification of color defects to spare children from being labeled uncooperative or stupid because they consistently pick up the wrong-colored material (63).

2. To identify and determine the severity of acquired color vision defects (such as those associated with hereditary retinal degenerations) both for the purpose of diagnosis and to make functional recommendations regarding the child's capabilities. Changes in color vision can precede alteration in other vision functions such as acuity and visual fields and can thus serve as early warning signals to the presence of disease.

DISCRIMINATING COLOR

Three separate types of cone receptors are known to exist in the normal human retina. Each contains a different photopigment. The spectral sensitivity of each of the photopigments is known, and each photopigment absorbs electromagnetic radiation over the majority of the visible spectrum (400 to 700 nm). A person who had any single photopigment alone would be totally color blind. Color vision results from the comparison of the signals from the three cone types. Signals from each cone type are directed into one of three separate neural channels immediately following absorption of light by the photoreceptors. The signals from the cones containing the middle and long wavelength–sensitive pigments (MWS and LWS, respectively) are added to form a luminosity channel that signals whiteness or blackness but is devoid of information about color. The signals from these same receptors are also subtracted to form a color channel that signals redness or greenness. A second color channel subtracts the short wavelength–sensitive (SWS) cone signals from some combination of MWS and LWS cone signals to provide information about blueness and yellowness. The SWS receptors feed only into color channels and do not contribute substantially to luminosity or visual acuity, so standard acuity or visual field testing cannot detect abnormalities of these receptors. This becomes an important point, because the SWS receptors and/or their pathways are affected very early in most retinal diseases, but such defects do not affect visual acuity or luminosity.

COLOR VISION AT BIRTH

The foveas of young infants are extremely immature in terms of receptor density and the length of the outer segments (1, 32). Even at 15 months of age, the outer segments are only half the length of adult outer segments. Cone packing density also increases rapidly after birth but may not be adultlike even at 45 months of age. The increase in cone packing density is caused by reduction of the foveal area and thinning and elongation of individual foveal cones (82). Even as this anatomic development is taking place, the functional presence of all receptor types has been established in the first few months after birth.

By 4 to 8 weeks of age, infants have been convincingly demonstrated to have functioning rods (59, 81). By 8 to 10 weeks of age, infants have been shown to have at least two functional classes of cones (29, 69). Earlier studies suggested that infants under 3 months of age were tritanopic (lacking SWS

cones) (e.g. Pulos, et al, [60]), but more recent studies have demonstrated the presence of functioning SWS cones and at least one of their neural pathways by 4 to 6 weeks of age using the technique of steady-state visual evoked potentials (79), and behavioral tritan pair discriminations (70). (Tritan pairs are colors that produce identical stimulation of LWS and MWS receptors but very different SWS cone stimulation.)

Even though all the receptor classes appear to be present at an early age, infants sometimes fail to make chromatic discriminations (29, 69). This could be due to insensitivity of the receptors or to immaturity of postreceptoral processing. One-month-olds had difficulty performing a Rayleigh discrimination task even when the field size was 8 degrees, whereas 3-month-olds had no trouble as long as the field size was at least 3 degrees; these studies conclude that the failure of the youngest infants to discriminate is more likely to be due to immaturity of neural processing than to absence of MWS or LWS receptors. Recent studies (22) suggest that the vision of 3-week-old infants is heavily dominated by rods, even at light levels that in adults (who have much more sensitive cones) are cone dominated. Very young infants operate as if they were wearing dark glasses. By 7 weeks, the cones have gained enough sensitivity to allow consistent chromatic discrimination. A conservative summary of these studies would state that rudimentary trichromatic color discrimination is present at 2 months of age (at low photopic light levels), and possibly earlier.

COLOR PREFERENCE IN INFANTS

Studies have shown that adults prefer chromatic to achromatic stimuli and prefer primary colors that are highly saturated (vivid). In a sample of 156,250 adults Helson and Lansford (31) showed that adults rate blues and greens highest, yellows lowest, and reds intermediate in terms of subjective pleasantness. Bornstein (18) studied the color preference of 4½-month-old infants and found that they displayed a pattern of preference similar to adults' except that reds were preferred over blues. Adams (6) observed fixation preferences in three groups of infants, newborns, 1-month-olds, and 3-month-olds (60 subjects in all). At each age including newborns, the infants preferred to look at colored stimuli instead of gray ones of similar (photopic) brightness. Newborns and 1-month-olds did not show a significant preference among the colored stimuli, but the 3-month-olds did. Unlike the adults, they preferred reds and yellows to blues and greens. Recent reports (12) suggest that the results of studies such as this will depend heavily on the light levels (and retinal eccentricity) used for the stimuli.

COLOR VISION DEFECTS

Color vision defects are commonly broadly classified into acquired and congenital defects (the latter being those that are inherited, remain constant with age, are not accompanied by disease, and affect both eyes equally). Color vision defects are classified as acquired if accompanied or caused by some ocular or systemic disorder. In acquired defects, the two eyes may not be affected to the same extent and the defect may change over time for worse or better.

The category of congenital defects includes the X-linked recessive red-green defects, which occur in 8 to 10 percent of the male population in the U.S. (and less than 0.5 percent of the female population), the very rare autosomal dominant tritan or (blue-yellow) defects (frequency estimated between 0.0015 and 0.007 percent), and the group of disorders called achromatopsias, which occur in about 0.003 percent of the population or less.

Congenital Red-Green Defects

The more common red-green defects are classified as anomalous trichromacy and dichromacy by the loss of chromatic discrimination when color matching on the Nagel anomaloscope (the Rayleigh match). These categories are then further classified into pro-

tan (red weak vision) and deutan (green weak vision). Each condition involves an anomaly of the photopigment in the cone receptors.

Anomalous Trichromacy

Anomalous trichromacy affects 6 to 7 percent of the male population. These men have three photopigments but the absorption spectrum peak of one of the two longer wavelength-sensitive photopigments is shifted on the wavelength axis closer to the other one than in persons with normal color vision. Since color vision results from the comparison of signals from each of the three photopigments (present in each of three types of cones), anomalous trichromats show reduced color discrimination because the wavelength peaks of the absorption spectra of the photopigments are closer to each other. The closer the two long wavelength sensitive peaks are, the more severe the defect is and the more compromised is the color discrimination.

Simple protanomalous trichromacy can be found in 1 to 2 percent of the male population. They need more red in the match on the anomaloscope. Their matching range (the range of red-green ratios that are accepted as a match) is fairly narrow but usually broader than that of normal persons. Their matching range does *not* include the normal match point. The presumed physiological basis is the peak of the absorption spectrum of the LWS photopigment shifted closer to the spectrum for the MWS photopigment. Because of this shift, reds appear dim and protanomalous observers show an anomalous luminosity function.

Extreme protanomalous trichromacy can be found among about 1 percent of the male population. It is considered to be a separate genetic entity. Affected men also need more red in the Nagel match. They show a very wide matching range, which includes the normal match but not the extreme pure red or pure green. The presumed physiological basis is the peak of the absorption spectrum of the LWS photopigment shifted even closer to the absorption spectrum of the MWS pigment. Reds appear quite dim to these observers, and they have a severely abnormal luminosity function.

Simple deuteranomalous trichromacy affects 4 to 5 percent of the male population, being the most common variety of congenital red-green disorder. Affected persons need more green in the match; they show a fairly narrow matching range, which does *not* include the normal match. The presumed physiological basis is the peak of the absorption spectrum of the MWS photopigment shifted toward the spectrum of the LWS pigment. The intensity of yellow setting on the Nagel anomaloscope is the same as that for "color normals," and the luminosity function is normal.

Extreme deuteranomalous trichromacy (a separate genetic entity) can be found in 1 percent of the male population. Affected persons need more green in the Nagel match and also show a wide matching range, which includes the normal match but not the extreme pure red or pure green. The presumed physiological basis is the peak of the absorption spectrum of the MWS photopigment shifted even closer to the spectrum for the LWS pigment. Luminosity function is normal, so the yellow intensity setting remains as for normals.

Dichromacy

About 2 percent of the male population exhibit dichromacy. Protanopia occurs in about 1 percent of males. Protanopes can match pure red with yellow and pure green with yellow. The presumed physiological basis is that only MWS photopigment is present. Presumably this pigment is also present in the receptors that normally would have LWS pigment, as the visual acuity of these observers is normal, which requires that the normal complement of cone receptors be present.

Deuteranopia occurs in about 1 percent of males. Affected men can also match pure red with yellow and pure green with yellow. The presumed physiological basis is that only LWS photopigment is present. In the Nagel anomaloscope, persons with both kinds of dichromacy match all mixtures of the red and green primaries, including the primaries themselves (540 nm and 670 nm) to the yellow (589-nm) primary. Protanopia is distinguished from deuteranopia only by the characteristic brightness settings of the yellow half of the field for matches with the red primary. Long wavelengths (reds) appear very dim to protan observers and they turn down the yellow intensity (to 3 or 4 on the scale) when matching to pure red. A patient with deuteranopia, on the other hand, gives the same setting of yellow as normal persons for all mixtures of red and green (around 15 on the Nagel I).

"Rules" of Inheritance

Since the genes controlling these color vision defects are carried on the X chromosome, certain "rules" about the inheritance pattern can be stated:

1. Color–defective fathers cannot pass the defect on to their sons.
2. All daughters of color–defective fathers are carriers (at least).
3. For a woman to be color defective, both her father *and* her maternal grandfather must have a color vision defect.
4. Sons of a color defective woman always have a color vision defect and all daughters will be carriers.

Congenital Blue-Yellow (Tritan) Defects

Congenital tritan defects are very rare and are not detectable by standard "book tests," which mostly test for red-green defects. Tritan observers make a normal match on the Nagel anomaloscope. Special tests such as special color matches (violet to green, for example, which can be matched by a tritanope) or measures of spectral sensitivity are needed for diagnosis. Since tritan defects most frequently accompany disease, it is important to rule out an acquired cause. Krill, Smith, and Pokorny (42) suggested that in order to be diagnosed with tritanopia, the patient and all family members must have normal visual acuity and normal visual fields and the optic nerves must appear normal ophthalmoscopically. These criteria are designed to eliminate autosomal dominant optic atrophy as the cause of the tritan defect.

Achromatopsias

Achromatopsias are congenital disorders that either abolish color discrimination ability (complete achromatopsia) or severely reduce it (incomplete achromatopsia). The loss of color discrimination is accompanied by reduced visual acuity, nystagmus, photophobia, and extinguished photopic electro-retinogram (ERG). The rod system is presumed to be normal even though some persons with achromatopsia have been reported to have reduced scotopic ERGs as well (39, 54). Cone and cone-rod degenerations must be ruled out for any patient who presents with the above mentioned symptoms. Complete and incomplete forms are indistinguishable from each other on standard clinical tests.

Complete Achromatopsia

Complete achromatopsia, or typical rod monochromacy, is an autosomal recessive condition with an incidence of 0.003 percent (80). It occurs with equal frequency in males and females and most often occurs in families with no history of the disorder. The most noticeable signs in infancy are nystagmus and photophobia. Any infant with those characteristics should have an ERG examination to establish the diagnosis and to have appropriate light protection measures instituted immediately. Visual acuity is usually around 20/200 at the optimal low-light level and deteriorates at higher levels. In our sample of 21 achromats, the average visual acuity was 20/160 (range, 20/100 to 20/300). The achromats report that if they keep their eyes open outdoors in bright light, their vision "washes out," that is, all objects disappear or the contrast of objects is sharply reduced. This loss of vision causes them to squint or blink to reduce the light exposure. Exposure to bright light is not painful, but it reduces their ability

to see. (The mother of one child with rod monochromatism reported that the only time her son would open his eyes as a small child driving in the car was when they drove through a tunnel!) These children also prefer to play outside at dusk or at night. Appropriate dark lenses (or preferably red ones) should be prescribed in infancy to allow maximal vision function in daylight. High refractive states and strabismus often accompany these disorders. The refractive states should be corrected even though frequently no objectively measurable improvement in acuity takes place.

Incomplete Achromatopsia

Incomplete autosomal recessive achromatopsia is a condition of reduced acuity, nystagmus, photophobia, and reduced or absent photopic ERG and signs of residual cone function on special color matching tests or on measures of spectral sensitivity. Several different kinds have been reported. Unless special color vision tests are used, incomplete and complete forms cannot be distinguished. There appears to be a tremendous variation in the extent of expression of residual cone function. Unfortunately, no one simple test of color vision separates the apparently complete forms from the incomplete ones. Persons with both kinds respond similarly on the Sloan achromatopsia test, the Farnsworth Panel D-15 (scotopic error axis between the deutan and the tritan axis), and the Nagel anomaloscope. On the anomaloscope, an achromat matches both red and green to yellow but with a characteristic steep slope relating intensity of the yellow standard to the red-green mixture. The larger field used for the Rayleigh match in the Pickford-Nicholson anomaloscope may allow identification of persons with incomplete achromatopsia who will not accept matches over the whole range of red to green ratios. Incomplete achromats with substantial residual cone function should *not* be given red filters for light control, as they effectively render them monochromatic and deprive them of what little color discrimination they have.

Blue Cone Monochromacy

X-linked recessive (blue cone) monochromacy is yet another kind of achromatopsia (9, 16, 17, 68). The clinical findings are similar to those in autosomal recessive achromatopsia; the acuity may be slightly better (but not necessarily). A family history of affected males usually suggests the diagnosis. These individuals are dichromats at intermediate light levels; they have SWS (blue) cones and rods, which provide them with some color discrimination when both receptor types are active. At high light levels, when the rods are saturated, they are again monochromats. This disorder can be distinguished clinically from autosomal recessive achromatopsia with the Berson test (see below). Red filters should not be given to these patients, as they destroy their color discrimination. Some limited personal experience with X-linked achromatopsia (which is very rare) suggests that magenta filters (which transmit red and blue) may reduce the photophobia and subjectively improve vision.

Acquired Defects

Congenital defects are primarily of the red-green variety, whereas the most common acquired defects affect blue-yellow discrimination. Köllner's rule (38) that disorders of the retina give rise to blue-yellow defects but disorders of the optic nerve cause red-green defects holds for many diseases, but there are striking exceptions. Even in retinal diseases that initially give rise to blue-yellow defects, with progression of the disease and loss of visual acuity, red-green color vision defects are overlaid. It is possible to have significant blue-yellow defects with normal visual acuity, because the SWS cones do not contribute to acuity, but it is extremely rare to have significant red-green errors and normal visual acuity, as the same receptors responsible for red-green discrimination also underlie visual acuity. Excellent descriptions of color vision defects associated with disease can be found in Pokorny et al (58) and in Krill's *Hereditary*

Retinal and Choroidal Disorders, vol. II (39). A few specific examples are mentioned here.

Albinism

Color vision is grossly normal in most persons with albinism. The Rayleigh match may be shifted toward red, and the matching range may be enlarged (41, 52).

Juvenile Hereditary Retinoschisis

Blue-yellow color defects are frequently reported in this disorder (30, 32), but normal color vision (21) and red-green errors (56) have also been reported.

Congenital Glaucoma

Many studies have confirmed, contrary to expectations from Köllner's rule, that glaucoma of any cause most commonly produces an acquired blue-yellow color vision defect. Francois et al (26) found clear-cut tritan axes on the Farnsworth D-15 test in a significant proportion of patients with congenital glaucoma. Reduced color discrimination without a specific axis is also frequently reported.

Congenital Cataract

Because congenital cataract (unlike senile cataract) is not usually associated with yellowing of the lens, no particular color vision defect is expected.

Diabetes

Diabetes leads primarily to blue-yellow color vision defects, which antedate any ophthalmoscopically visible fundus changes. For example, Adams and Zisman (5) showed that young juvenile diabetic patients showed losses of blue cone sensitivity even while acuity remained normal and the fundus showed no signs of diabetic retinopathy.

Retinitis Pigmentosa

Variable color vision results have been reported in association with retinitis pigmentosa, probably depending on foveal involvement. Blue-yellow errors primarily are reported in the early stages (11). Massof et al (46) reported a negative correlation (r =

−0.73) between the logarithm of the score on the FM 100 Hue test and the percentage of the normal visual field remaining.

Juvenile Macular Degeneration

Juvenile macular degeneration (autosomal recessive, Stargardt's disease) is a progressive disease that results in central achromatopsia. Even though it is a retinal disease, it produces classic red-green vision defects, which become more severe with time, become overlaid with blue-yellow errors as well, and later become acquired achromatopsia (27, 51, 53, 77).

Vitelliform Dystrophy

Persons with vitelliform dystrophy (Best's disease) show normal color vision in the early stages, but both blue-yellow and red-green defects have been reported in the more advanced cases (13, 40, 47).

Optic Nerve Disorders

Virtually all primary hereditary optic atrophies produce severe red-green defects and severe loss of visual acuity (Smith et al 1977), except autosomal dominant optic atrophy, which mostly gives blue-yellow errors (41–43). This disorder shows dominant inheritance; slight to moderate visual acuity loss; temporal pallor of the optic disk; blue-yellow color vision defect (with red-green errors when visual acuity drops), and field abnormalities (central or cecocentral scotomas).

TECHNIQUES FOR TESTING COLOR VISION

Testing Principles

A complete color vision assessment should include a sensitive screening test capable of detecting even the mildest color defects, a test capable of grading the severity of the defect, and a test that can identify the type of defect (protan, deutan, tritan, scotopic, or mixed). Most screening tests are not capable of grading the severity or classifying the type of defect accurately, and those that grade and classify usually are not appropriate for screening. So, at least two separate tests are needed for the assessment.

The majority of color vision screening tests make use of the pseudoisochromatic design principle. A symbol made up of colored dots is placed in a background of dots of a different color. The colors are chosen such that color defective observers perform differently than those with normal color vision. Several different types of pseudoisochromatic plates are available. The most common is the vanishing type, in which a color defective observer does not see any symbol because the colors of the symbol and the background fall on a confusion line. The plates of the American Optical Hardy-Rand-Rittler (AO H-R-R) test are of this design, as are several plates of the Ishihara test (24-plate edition; Kanehara Shuppan Co., Ltd., Tokyo, 1969).

The second type is designed to diagnose the type of defect. Two symbols are printed with different colors on a common background. Plate No. 13 of the AO H-R-R test is of this design, where one of the symbols should be visible to a person with protanopia and the other is theoretically visible to one with deuteranopia. Ishihara plates No. 16 and 17 (24-plate edition) are also of this design. These plates do not always function as expected (57).

Plate No. 3 of the Ishihara test (24-plate edition) is an example of a third type of plate designed to reduce the frustration for color defective observers, who are never able to see anything on most screening tests. In the transformation type of design, both normal and color defective observers see a symbol, but different ones. Four different colors are used and the colors are selected so that part of what normal persons see as background becomes part of the symbol for those with a color vision defect. The fourth type of plate contains a hidden symbol that only a color defective observer can see. Plates No. 14 and 15 of the Ishihara test (24-plate edition) are examples.

The list of pseudoisochromatic (PIC)

Table 19.1   PSEUDOISOCHROMATIC PLATE TESTS

Ishihara Tests for Color Blindness
American Optical Color Vision Test (AOC)
American Optical Hardy-Rand-Rittler Plates (AO
   H-R-R)
Dvorine Pseudoisochromatic Plates
Velhagen Plates
Tokyo Medical Plates
Okuma
F2 Plate
PACT
Bostrom-Kugelberg
Guy's Test for Children
Standard Pseudoisochromatic Test (Ichikawa)

"book tests" is very long. The reader is referred to Pokorny and associates and to Birch (15, 57, 58) for complete descriptions of all tests that are used and have been used in the past. Table 19.1 lists the most common PIC tests. In this chapter, only a select few tests are discussed, either because they are the most commonly available in the U.S., work best with children, or were designed especially for use with children (which does not always imply that they work particularly well), or there is some other special reason for their mention.

Color Vision Tests

The Ishihara Tests for Color Blindness

The Ishihara test is one of the most commonly used screening tests for red-green color vision defects. (The term color blindness is a misnomer; the vast majority of observers with changes in their color vision should be called color defective, not color blind; only achromatopsia is truly color blindness, and affected persons also have severely reduced visual acuity, nystagmus, and photophobia). Several different editions of the Ishihara test are available with different numbers of plates. The majority of the plates consist of colored dots forming numbers set on backgrounds of different colors. Some of the plates contain paths designed to be traced

by observers who do not know numbers. The first plate is a demonstration plate which should be correctly identified before proceeding with the test. The plates are of different designs, as discussed above, and it is theoretically possible to classify the defects as protan or deutan.

The Ishihara test has been shown in adults to have high screening efficiency. It correctly identifies all color defective observers (64), but the performance of the test in classifying the type of defect is more variable (23, 55). The numbers are in script form, which makes them difficult for young observers to interpret, even children who know their numbers. This test does *not* assess blue-yellow color defects. The plates with trails have been used to assess preschool children by Verriest et al (72, 73, 75–77) and by Cox (24). Both groups came to the same conclusion: the trails are *not* valid in the preschool group (before age 6). Various children shortened the paths, made up their own paths, or did not understand the instructions.

American Optical Hardy-Rand-Rittler Test

The plates of the AO H-R-R test (now out of print) consist of small colored spots on a grey background which form the shapes of circles, triangles, or crosses. There are four demonstration plates, including one with no figure. (A common problem with screening plates is that color defective observers never see anything and therefore get very frustrated by the task; in this test not seeing anything is demonstrated as one acceptable response.) The screening plates use desaturated colors and the diagnostic plates use colors of increasing saturation to grade the severity of the defect. Both blue-yellow and red-green defects are detectable with this test.

Verriest and coworkers (72, 73, 75, 76, 78) reported that the AO H-R-R test was successfully given to 88 percent of the youngest children in their group (3.8 years on average) and given successfully to 100 percent of the older children (up to age 6 years). They presented the test in reverse order, so that the most saturated plates with the biggest color differences were presented first (omitting the demonstration plates). They also used a matching technique, providing circles, triangles, and crosses for children who could not name these symbols. Many of the youngest children missed the first two plates of the test (presented last), which caused them to be classified erroneously as having a very mild red-green defect.

Zisman and Adams (83) used the test in 41 preschool children (ages 2.5 to 4 years) but were able to get responses from only 50 percent of this age group. The failure rate for those responding was 15 percent, considerably higher than would be expected. The method of assessment was not discussed. It is likely that the majority of those who failed to answer were among the youngest children, and the discrepancy between the studies is probably caused by the slightly older children tested in Verriest's study.

Hill et al (36) also used the AO H-R-R test on 440 boys between the ages of 3 and 11 years. The performance of the AO H-R-R was compared to color matching on the Pickford-Nicholson anomaloscope. All but one of the children were able to perform the matching task on the anomaloscope. Sixty children with normal color vision failed the AO H-R-R test, whereas six color defective boys passed, generating abysmal sensitivity and specificity numbers. Unfortunately the authors do not specify whether the majority of the failure were among those in the youngest age groups. No symbols were provided for matching and the test was not given in reverse order. The performance of the AO H-R-R was equivalent to the results on the Ishihara in this sample. The results of these studies suggest that the test should not be used until at least age 3½ or 4 years unless a modified presentation is used and the results of the first two screening plates are ignored.

F2 Plate: Standard and Forced-Choice Versions

The original version of the F2 plate was designed by Farnsworth for screening. It consists of two interlocking squares, one blue, one green on a purple background. Adams et al (2) have published a description of the Munsell colors used for making the test. They also showed that the F2 plate performs comparably to the AO H-R-R, when given to children in grade 4 and older. They suggested that the F2 plate is a good screening test for both red-green and blue-yellow errors for all school children except kindergarteners and first graders, for whom the interlocking squares were too confusing.

A variation of the F2 test was recently described by Pease and Allen (50) and named PACT (Pease-Allen Color Test). A solid square composed of two shades of blue (for the red-green screening plate) is embedded in a rectangular background composed of two shades of purple. The solid square, 5 cm on a side, is placed near one end of the 30 × 10-cm plate to allow the technique of preferential looking to be used. A second plate contains a square composed of green hues for detecting tritan defects. The test also consists of a demonstration plate and a blank plate with only the background dots.

The PACT was found to show a high coefficient of agreement with the Nagel anomaloscope in an adult population. In a group of children between ages 3 and 6 years, it performed well for detection of red-green defects and produced more reasonable failure rates than the original version of the F2 plate and the AO H-R-R, which were also given to the children. The authors also state that this version can be used successfully with infants and older developmentally delayed nonverbal children. No blue-yellow color defects were found in this study. The green square in the F2 plate (used for detecting blue-yellow defects) is considerably more visible than the blue square (used for red-green defects) and a person who fails to see the green square has a more severe tritan defect than the one with a red-green defect who fails to see the blue square. The PACT is supposed to become commercially available in 1990 from Wolfe Medical Publications, Ltd, Brooke House, 2-16 Torrington Place, London, WC1E7LT, England.

I have made another version of the F2 plate on 4-inch Plexiglas plates, one plate with the background dots only, one plate with the background and an outline of the blue square (like the original), and a third plate with the background and the green square. The test is used in a forced-choice paradigm and has been used successfully to test a series of developmentally delayed children with a variety of disorders. Normal children should be able to perform this task when presented in a forced-choice format by 2 years of age.

The Guy's Hospital Test for Children

The Guy's test of color vision for children uses pseudoisochromatic principles. The only reason I bring it up is to discourage its use. The task is to match letters (provided with the test) to the letters seen on the plates. The idea of a matching task is a good one, but unfortunately, this test contains design flaws that make it very confusing to adults and completely unreliable in children.

Verriest and coworkers (72, 73, 75–77) used the test in 100 preschool and kindergarten children ranging in age from 3 years to 6 years. They report, "Our results for the whole Guy's test were catastrophic, owing to the designer's bad choice of colors and digits." Hill et al (36) used Guy's test on their sample of 440 boys ranging in age from 3 to 11 years and validated the results by their performance on the Pickford-Nicholson anomaloscope. The Guy's test correctly failed 26 of the 28 color defective boys, but it also incorrectly failed 180(!) of the normal boys. The combined results of these studies strongly suggest that this test should not be used at all.

Arrangement Tests

A list of commonly used arrangement tests can be found in Table 19.2.

Farnsworth Dichotomous Test for Color Blindness (Panel D15)

The Farnsworth D15 test was designed to detect observers who have *severe* color defects that are likely to be of practical significance in daily life. The test measures red-green and blue-yellow discrimination loss and is capable of detecting monochromacy. It

Table 19.2 ARRANGEMENT TESTS

Farnsworth Dichotomous Test for Color Blindness (Panel D15) (saturated and desaturated versions) (4, 44, 45)
FM 100 Hue
Roth 28 Hue
The Lanthony New Color Test
Sahlgren Saturation Test

is frequently used to assess acquired and congenital defects. The test is very reliable for screening and qualitative classification and has high validity in adults (34). The majority of persons with simple anomalous trichromacy pass the test, but those with more severe defects fail and are classified appropriately.

The D15 test is difficult for very young children, and the results are *not* normal in the vast majority. This test is not recommended for young children. Even much older children have difficulty performing the task required for the D15 test—sorting into a progressive color order. Adams et al (3) administered the D15 test to 389 children between the ages of 3 and 10 and showed that the error rate declined dramatically with age and that the children tended to make errors in the second half of the test. Test order was reversed and again the last few caps accounted for most of the errors, pointing to factors such as lack of concentration and fatigue as the cause of the errors instead of reduced blue sensitivity, as was originally suggested by Sassoon (61). The task of serialization is generally too difficult for young children, and this test should not be used until around age 9 or 10. Desaturated versions of the test (4, 44) are used primarily to detect acquired color vision defects. Adams' version (not commercially available) is two chroma steps less desaturated than Lanthony's version, which is commercially available. Lanthony's version will rapidly cause accumulation of very large error scores when the defects become more severe. These tests should not be used for children under 10 years of age.

City University Color Vision Test

The City University Color Vision test uses Munsell colors from the Farnsworth Panel D15. It was designed to screen moderate and severe color vision defects and to differentiate deutan, protan, and tritan defects. Each of the 11 plates of the test contains five colored disks—a central test color and four companion colors. The task of the observer is to indicate which of the four comparison colors looks most like the central test color. The test identifies and correctly classifies dichromats but not anomalous trichromats who either pass the test or fail but are frequently incorrectly classified (36, 74). Zisman and Adams (83) used the City University test in a group of preschool children (aged 2.5 to 4) and a large group of elementary school children. All but two of the preschool children were able to perform the task. The failure rate, however, was over 7 percent, considerably higher than expected, because persons with mildly defective color vision normally pass and only those with moderate and severe defects fail. In the elementary school group, 3.5 percent of the boys showed red-green errors. This percentage is close to that expected if all persons with dichromacy and extreme anomaly fail the test.

Farnsworth-Munsell 100 Hue

The Farnsworth-Munsell 100 Hue is an excellent test of color discrimination or "color acuity" that is commonly used to detect both congenital and acquired defects. The test consists of four boxes of caps to be sorted into color order. The task of sorting into color order when the differences between caps is very small is much too difficult for children, and the test should not be used with them. Even older children may become bored with the task, with subsequent loss of accuracy (57).

Other Kinds of Tests

A list of other kinds of tests can be found in Table 19.3.

Table 19.3 OTHER KINDS OF TESTS

The Fletcher-Hamblin Simplified Colour Vision Test
The Berson Test and the Berkeley Version
Portnoy Plates
The Sloan Achromatopsia Test
The Holmgren Wool Test
The City University Test
Titmus Pediatric Color-Perception Test
Anomaloscopes
   Nagel
   Pickford-Nicholson
Lantern tests

Titmus Pediatric Color Perception Test

Pokorny et al (57) state that based on validity data, neither the Titmus Color Perception Test nor the Titmus Pediatric Color Perception Test is a suitable screening test because both tests incorrectly classify normal vision as color defective. Alexander (8) used the Titmus Pediatric Color Perception Test on 38 *adults*, many of whom were known to have color vision defects, and compared the results to those obtained with the Ishihara, the Dvorine (another PIC test), and the Farnsworth Panel D15 test. He found that the Titmus test tended to overrate the severity of the color defect even in adults but suggested that it could be used if scoring was modified. No children were tested in this study.

The Fletcher-Hamblin Simplified Color Vision Test

This is a commercially available test designed for use with children. The test consists of three plates, each with many 1-cm colored plastic squares. Units 1 and 3 are used for detection of red-green errors, whereas Unit 2 is used to detect tritan errors. Units 1 and 2 contain 16 plastic squares; plate 3 consists of five squares, one a model color. The task on units one and two is to identify which of the 16 colored squares are different from the others. The task on the third unit is to pick one of the four colored squares that most closely matches the model color. Moderate to severe defects can be detected with these plates (25). Unlike most other color vision tests this one is designed to be illuminated with ordinary tungsten light. The colored chips are quite small and are not appropriate for low-vision patients.

The Portnoy Plates

I designed this new test specifically for use with children, particularly children with low vision. On each 4 × 4-inch plate, four disks of color (1 inch in diameter) are mounted on a black background. Plexiglass is placed over the colored disks to allow touching without soiling the color samples. Three of the four disks are identical in color; the fourth is different. The colors are selected from the set of Munsell colors that are used in the Farnsworth D15 test. In addition, a set of plates uses desaturated versions of the same hues with the chroma 2 steps less saturated than the standard D15 (4). The pairs of colors lie along a protan confusion axis on one plate, along a deutan axis on another plate, and on a tritan confusion axis on the third plate. Table 19.4 lists the Munsell notation for each of the plates (Munsell papers are available from the Munsell Color Corporation, 2441 N Calvert St., Baltimore, MD 21218).

The plates are presented one at a time under appropriate illumination (Illuminant C). A demonstration plate (from the Berson test) is presented first to verify that the patient understands the task, which is simply to indicate which disk is different. If the child does not know the word different, a few minutes of training usually is sufficient to learn this concept. To minimize the effects of guessing, each plate is presented 6 times; between each presentation the plate is randomly rotated. Three or fewer correct responses is considered failing. Only patients with severe color defects are expected to fail the standard version of the test, and patients with moderate defects are likely to fail only the desaturated version. Patients with only mild color vision defects pass both versions of the test. The test has not yet been validated against the regular versions of the D15, but it has been used successfully in children as young as 2.5 years and in multihandi-

capped children of all ages. The test has also been used to assess color vision in a series of patients with Usher's syndrome (congenital deafness and retinitis pigmentosa) ranging in age from 5 years to adult. Because the task is so simple, very few instructions are needed, which makes it useful in situations where communication is difficult.

The Berson Test and the Berkeley Version

The Berson test, or the test for blue cone monochromacy, was designed by Berson et al (14) to discriminate between autosomal recessive complete rod monochromacy and sex-linked blue cone monochromacy. These two conditions usually present with very similar clinical findings, reduced visual acuity, nystagmus, and absent or severely reduced photopic ERG.

In the original version of the test, plates are presented which contain four arrows, three green and one violet. The arrows are

Table 19.4 MUNSELL PAPERS USED FOR BERSON TEST AND PORTNOY PLATES

	One Disk	Three Disks
Berson Test		
(All papers are glossy)		
Demo plate 1	N-7	5.0 BG 4/8
Demo plate 2	5.0 BG 6/8	5.0 BG 4/8
Test plate 1	PB 4/9	5.0 BG 4/8
Test plate 2	PB 4/10	5.0 BG 4/8
Test plate 3	PB 4/11	5.0 BG 4/8
Test plate 4	PB 4/12	5.0 BG 4/8
Portnoy Plates		
(All papers are matte)		
Standard D-15		
Standard Protan	5.0 BG 5/4	2.5 R 5/4
Standard Deuteran	10.0 G 5/4	5.0 RP 5/4
Standard Tritan	5.0 GY 5/4	5.0 P 5/4
Desaturated D-15		
Desaturated Protan	5.0 BG 5/2	2.5 R 5/2
Desaturated Deutan	10.0 G 5/2	5.0 RP 5/2
Desaturated Tritan	5.0 GY 5/2	5.0 P 5/2

made of Munsell papers and are selected to be scotopically equivalent, that is indistinguishable to someone who only has rods. Four different test plates are used. The chroma (saturation) of the violet arrow varies from plate to plate to take into account variations in lens and macular pigment between observers. Each plate is presented six times and three correct responses or fewer is considered failing that plate. Failing any one of the four plates is considered failing the test (14). The Berkeley version of the Berson test uses the same colors as the original test, but it uses disks (1 inch in diameter) instead of arrows. Table 19.4 lists the Munsell papers used for the test. The demonstration plates for the Berson test are also used for the Portnoy test.

A person with rod monochromacy cannot correctly identify the different arrow or disk, whereas one with blue cone monochromacy has no problem identifying the violet disk as both a different color and brighter than the three green disks. Berson et al (14) reported that the test correctly identified five cases of blue cone monochromacy while seven persons with rod monochromacy failed the test. All 20 of our patients with rod monochromacy have failed the test whereas two with blue cone monochromacy passed. The youngest observer tested successfully was 2.5 years old.

Optokinetic Techniques

An optokinetic technique for nonclinical screening of color vision of infants has been developed by Anstis and Cavanaugh (10, 20). The stimulus consisted of two oppositely drifting red-green gratings presented on a computer-controlled TV screen. To normal eyes the pattern was seen to move to the left, and to color–defective eyes it appeared to move to the right. By either observing the eyes of infants or measuring their eye movements with photoelectric sensors, in principle an estimate can be made about the normalcy of the infant's color vision. This technique reliably detects protan observers but not those with deutan errors. The technique is used primarily for research pur-

poses, as it is rarely essential to determine whether infants have congenital red-green color defects.

Anomaloscopes

Anomaloscope testing is the most accurate way of screening and classifying red-green color vision defects. Unfortunately, the Nagel anomaloscope, which uses a Rayleigh match, has a telescope viewing tube that small children find difficult to use as it requires careful alignment of the eye. The examiner and the child cannot see the stimulus display simultaneously, which makes it difficult to explain the task and to verify that the child understands. An experienced examiner should be able to use the Nagel anomaloscope with elementary school children, particularly if a forced-choice procedure is used. The examiner should vary the red-green ratio and ask about the match in such a way that the answer is yes or no. Hill et al (36) used the Pickford-Nicholson anomaloscope in their sample of 440 children who ranged in age from 3 to 11 years. All but the youngest one of the children were able to perform the task, which in this anomaloscope involves a direct view of the matching fields, which makes the explanation of the task much easier. Only experienced examiners should use anomaloscopes.

Testing Conditions

Color vision testing should always be performed under conditions of illumination for which the test was designed. For the vast majority of color vision tests, this means daylight (northern sky light in the northern hemisphere). The most commonly used source of illumination in the U.S. is Illuminant C provided by a Macbeth Easel Lamp; illuminant D_{65} is used commonly in England. A standard incandescent 200-watt bulb can also be used if Wratten 78AA filters are worn by the person being tested. In general, incandescent sources should not be used, because some persons who otherwise would fail color vision tests will pass when the test is illuminated by the reddish incandescent light (35).

In addition, the axes on some arrangement tests may change under inappropriate illumination, causing erroneous classification of the defect. High-quality fluorescent lamps specifically designed for color comparison work (e.g., GE Chroma 70; Verd-A-Ray Criticolor Fluorescent) may be used instead of illuminant C, but ordinary fluorescent tubes usually are not appropriate for color vision testing.

The level of illumination should be at least 100 lux and preferably more. In general, color discrimination deteriorates with reduced light levels, and several studies have reported changes in error scores with changes in level of illumination (35, 71).

Testing should routinely be done monocularly to allow for detection of acquired defects. If only one eye is affected, the defect will be missed under binocular testing, as the more sensitive normal eye will exclusively determine the results.

Recommended Test Batteries for Different Age Groups

On the basis of review of the literature and personal experience, the following tests are recommended for use with different age groups:

Infants and toddlers (up to $2\frac{1}{2}$ years)
>Preferential looking techniques (PACT)
Red-green OKN

It is rare to test the color vision of young infants and toddlers in a clinical setting, but if the need arises, the two tests mentioned above have been used for this population.

Preschoolers ($2\frac{1}{2}$ to 5 years)
>Forced-choice F2 plate; PACT
Portnoy color vision plates
Modified AO H-R-R (not for youngest group; show examples of symbols and start at the back of the test; omit demonstration plates; ignore results of first two least saturated screening plates)
Berson test

Children in this age group should have no trouble performing the tasks required for this set of tests; identifying where the pattern is (right or left by pointing or verbalizing) on the F2 plate; pointing to the "different" disk on the Portnoy plates and the Berson test; and matching symbols on the AO H-R-R, provided examples of all the symbols are present at the time of testing.

Kindergarten and grades 1 to 3 (5 to 8 years)
>F2 plate or PACT
Ishihara
AO H-R-R
City University test
Anomaloscope (modified administration; ask the child "does it match now?" as the red-green ratio is changed)
Berson test

Children of this age group should be able to name numbers (on the Ishihara), but some may not name two-digit numbers correctly. The Ishihara and the AO H-R-R can be used for screening for mild defects, whereas on the City University test only those with moderate to severe defects that are likely to cause problems in daily life fail. The anomaloscope is the instrument of choice, but it is rarely available. The Berson test should be used for children with low vision who are suspected of having achromacy of one form or another or who have a progressive cone dystrophy that can lead to acquired achromatopsia.

Over age 8 or 9 use adult battery (some tests with caution)
>Pseudoisochromatic plates for red-green screening:
Ishihara
Pseudoisochromatic plates for red-green and blue-yellow grading:
AO H-R-R
Arrangement tests—color confusion principle:
D15 and desaturated D15 (mainly for older kids and adults)
Anomaloscope
Blue cone sensitivity (requires specialized equipment)
Berson test for blue cone monochromacy

This adult battery is capable of detecting, classifying, and quantifying both congenital and acquired color vision defects.

Can Color Vision Defects be Corrected or Cured?

In the case of congenital defects, the answer is clear. Color vision defects cannot be cured. The only time that a color vision defect may disappear is if the defect is acquired and the ocular or systemic cause is removed. Colored filters may help those with a congenital red-green color vision defect to make certain color discriminations both by noting changes in brightness of the viewed object with and without the filter and by altering the chromaticity of the object when viewed through the filter. For example, a red object appears lighter when viewed through a red filter whereas a green object becomes darker. Magenta filters (such as Wratten No. 32) may be more helpful than red ones. The X-chrome lens (a "red" contact lens fitted for one eye only) is actually magenta, so it transmits considerably in the blue end of the spectrum. Requesting a red soft contact lens from a laboratory in the U.S. usually produces a magenta lens. Requesting a tinted red plastic spectacle lens usually has the same result, as the standard commercial red dyes allow transmission of significant amounts of blue light. Standard red lenses should not be used for achromats but rather special lenses such as Corning CPF 550 or Younger Optics PLS 550.

Children who have color vision defects confuse certain colors but not others. It is possible to select colors for school materials that cannot possibly be confused. Protanopic persons confuse yellow-greens, yellows, oranges, and reds; reds and dark browns, blues, and purples; blue-greens, whites, and purples; light greens and light browns. Deuteranopes also confuse yellow-greens, yellows, oranges, and reds. In addition, they confuse reds, oranges, and light browns; blue-greens, whites, and purples; light greens, magentas, and purple-reds. In general, the less saturated (the paler or more washed out) the color is or the darker the color (such as colors found on socks), the more difficult it is for a color–defective child. Primary colors are less likely to be confused, even though dichromats can confuse primary colors as well. The size of

the object also has an effect; the larger the objects, the less likely that they will be confused. For example, the color of two small spots on the wall may be indistinguishable from across the room, but quite different when viewed up close, when the angular subtense of the objects has increased. Classic dichromats may become anomalous trichromats when field sizes of 8 degrees or greater are used (48, 65). In addition, the higher the luminance, the better the color discrimination performance.

REFERENCES

1. Abramov I, Gordon J, Hendrickson A, et al: The retina of the newborn human infant. Science 217:265, 1982.
2. Adams AJ, Bailey JE, Harwood L: Color vision screening: A comparison of the AO H-R-R and the Farnsworth F-2 tests. Am J Optom Physiol Opt 61:1, 1984.
3. Adams AJ, Balliet R, McAdams M: Color vision: Blue deficiencies in children? Invest Ophthalmol 14:620, 1975.
4. Adams AJ, Rodic R: Use of desaturated and saturated versions of the D-15 test in glaucoma and glaucoma-suspect patients. In Verriest G (ed): Doc Ophthalmol Proc Series, 33:419, 1982.
5. Adams AJ, Zisman F: Color vision in juvenile diabetics. Invest Ophthalmol Vis Sci (Suppl) 19:169, 1980.
6. Adams RJ: An evaluation of color preference in early infancy. Infant Behav Dev 10:143, 1987.
7. Alexander KR: Color vision testing in young children: a review. Am J Optom Physiol Opt 52:337, 1975.
8. Alexander KR: The Titmus Pediatric Color Perception Test as a color vision screener: A comparative study. Am J Optom Physiol Opt 52:338, 1975.
9. Alpern M, Lee GB, Spivey BE: π_1 Cone monochromatism. Arch Ophthalmol 74:334, 1965.
10. Anstis S, Cavanaugh P, Maurer D, et al: Optokinetic technique for measuring infants' response to color. Appl Opt 26:1510, 1987.
11. Aspinall P, Adams A, Hayreh SS: Primary reti-

nal pigmentary degeneration. II. Functional changes. IRCS International Research Communication System (73-3) 24-14-2, 1973.

12. Banks MS, Bennett PJ: Optical and photoreceptor immaturities limit the spatial and chromatic vision of human neonates. J Opt Soc Am 5:2059, 1988.

13. Benson WE, Kolker AE, Enoch JM, et al: Best's vitelliform macular dystrophy. Am J Ophthalmol 79:794, 1975.

14. Berson EL, Sandberg MA, Rosner B, et al: Color plates to help identify patients with blue cone monochromatism. J Opt Soc Am [A] 95:741, 1983.

15. Birch J: Practical guide for colour-vision examination: Report of the standardization committee of the international group on colour-vision deficiencies. Ophthalmol Physiol Opt 5:265, 1985.

16. Blackwell HR, Blackwell OM: Blue monocone monochromacy: A new color vision defect. J Opt Soc Am 47:338, 1957.

17. Blackwell HR, Blackwell OM: Rod and cone receptor mechanisms in typical and atypical congenital achromatopsia. Vision Res 1:62, 1961.

18. Bornstein MH: Qualities of color vision in infancy. J Exp Child Psych 19:401, 1975.

19. Bornstein MH: Human infant color vision and color perception. Infant Behav Dev 8:109, 1985.

20. Cavanaugh P, Anstis S, Mather G: Screening for color blindness using optokinetic nystagmus. Invest Ophthalmol Vis Sci 25:463, 1984.

21. Carr RE, Siegel IM: The vitreo-tapeto-retinal degenerations. Arch Ophthalmol 84:436, 1970.

22. Clavadetscher JE, Brown AM, Ankrum C, et al: Spectral sensitivity and chromatic discrimination in 3 and 7 week old human infants. J Opt Soc Am 5:2093, 1988.

23. Crone RA: Quantitative diagnosis of defective color vision. A comparative evaluation of the Ishihara test, the Farnsworth dichotomous test, and the Hardy-Rand-Rittler polychromatic plates. Am J Ophthalmol 51:298, 1961.

24. Cox BJ: Validity of a preschool colour vision test. Can J Optom 33:22, 1971.

25. Fletcher R: Children's tests—Further applications. In Verriest G (ed): Colour Vision Deficiencies VI. Doc Ophthalmol Proc Series 33:195, 1982.

26. Francois J, Verriest G, de Rouck A: Les fonctions visuelles dans le glaucome congenital. Ann Oculist (Paris) 189:81, 1957.

27. Francois J, Verriest G, de Rouck A: Heredo-degenerescence maculaire juvenile avec atteinte predominante de la vision photopique. Ann Oculist (Paris) 195:1137, 1962.

28. Frey R: Welche pseudo-isochromatische Tafeln sind fur die Praxis am besten geeignet? Vergleichende Untersuchungen uber die Verwendbarkeit des Tafeln von Bostrom-Kugelberg, Hardy-Rand-Rittler, Ishihara, Rabkin und Stilling. Graefes Arch Ophthalmol 165:20, 1958.

29. Hamer RD, Alexander KR, Teller DY: Rayleigh discriminations in young human infants. Vision Res 22:575, 1982.

30. Harris GS, Yeung J: Maculopathy of sex-linked juvenile retinoschisis. Can J Ophthalmol 11:1, 1976.

31. Helson H, Lansford T: The role of spectral energy of source and background color in the pleasantness of object colors. Appl Optics 9:1513, 1970.

32. Helve J: Colour vision in X-chromosomal juvenile retinoschisis. Mod Probl Ophthalmol 11:122, 1972.

33. Hendrickson AE, Yuodelis C: The morphological development of the human fovea. Ophthalmology 91:603, 1984.

34. Higgins KE, Moskowitz-Cook A, Knoblauch K: Color vision testing: An alternative "source" of illuminant C. Mod Probl Ophthalmol 19:113, 1978.

35. Higgins KE, Knoblauch K: Validity of Pinckers' 100-hue version of the panel D-15. Am J Optom Physiol Opt 54:165, 1977.

36. Hill AR, Heron G, Lloyd M, et al: An evaluation of some colour vision tests for children. In Verriest G (ed): Colour Vision Deficiencies. VI. Doc Ophthalmol Proc Series 33:183, 1982.

37. Knoblauch K, Saunders F, Kusuda M, et al: Age and illuminance effects in the Farnsworth-Munsell 100 Hue test. Appl Optics 26:1441, 1987.

38. Kollner H: Die Storungen des Farbensinnes, Ihre Klinische Bedeutung und Ihre Diagnose. Berlin, Karger, 1912.

39. Krill AE: Congenital color vision defects. In Krill AE, Archer DB (eds): Krill's Hereditary Retinal and Choroidal Diseases, vol. II. Clinical Characteristics. Hagerstown, MD, Harper & Row, 355, 1977.

40. Krill AE, Deutman AF: The various categories of juvenile macular degeneration. Trans Am Ophthalmol Soc 70:220, 1972.

41. Krill AE, Fishman GA: Acquired color vision defects. Trans Am Acad Ophthalmol Otolaryngol 75:1095, 1971.

42. Krill AE, Smith VC, Pokorny J: Similarities between congenital tritan defects and dominant optic nerve atrophy: Coincidence or identity? J Opt Soc Am 60:1132, 1970.

43. Krill AE, Smith VC, Pokorny J: Further studies supporting the identity of congenital tritanopia and hereditary dominant optic atrophy. Invest Ophthalmol Vis Sci 10:457, 1971.

44. Lanthony P: Le Test Panel D-15 Desature Selon Farnsworth-Munsell. Luneau, Paris, 1974.

45. Lanthony P: The desaturated D-15. Doc Ophthalmol 19:122, 1978.

46. Massof RW, Finkelstein D, Starr SJ, et al: Bilateral symmetry of vision disorders in typical retinitis pigmentosa. Invest Ophthalmol Vis Sci 18:263, 1979.

47. Miller SA: Multifocal Best's vitelliform dystrophy. Arch Ophthalmol 95:984, 1977.

48. Nagy AL, Boynton RM: Large field color naming of dichromats with rods bleached. J Opt Soc Am [A] 69:1259, 1979.

49. Packer O, Hartmann E, Teller DY: Infant color vision: The effect of test field size on Rayleigh discriminations. Vision Res 24:1247, 1984.

50. Pease P, Allen J: A New Test for Screening Color Vision: Concurrent Validity and Utility. Am J Optom Physiol Opt 65:729, 1988.

51. Perdriel G, Lanthony P, Chevaleraud J: Pathologie du sense chromatique. Diagnostic practique. Interet clinique et application socioprofessionelles. Bull Soc Ophthalmol Fr (rapport annuel, numero special) 1, 1975.

52. Pickford RW: Colour vision of three albinos. Nature 181:361, 1958.

53. Pinckers A: La maladie de Stargardt. Ann Oculist (Paris) 204:1331, 1971.

54. Pinckers A: Achromatopsie congenitale. Ann Oculist (Paris) 205:821, 1972.

55. Pinckers A, Lakowski R: The Pickford-Nicholson anomaloscope for testing and measuring colour sensitivity and colour blindness and other tests and experiments. Br J Physiol Opt 17:131, 1960.

56. Pinckers A, Nabbe B, Bogaardet P: Le test 15-hue desature de Lanthony. Ann Oculist (Paris) 209:731, 1976.

57. Pokorny J, Collins B, Howett G, et al: Procedures for testing color vision. Report of working group 41. Washington DC, Committee on Vision, Assembly of Behavioral and Social Sciences, National Academy Press, 1981.

58. Pokorny J, Smith VC, Verriest G, et al: Congenital and acquired color vision defects. Current Ophthalmology Monographs. New York, Grune & Stratton, 1979.

59. Powers MK, Schneck M, Teller DY: Spectral sensitivity of human infants at absolute visual threshold. Vision Res 21:1005, 1981.

60. Pulos E, Teller DY, Buck SL: Infant color vision: A search for shortwavelength-sensitive mechanisms by means of chromatic adaptation. Vision Res 20:485, 1980.

61. Sassoon HF: Blue vision in children. Clin Pediatr (Phila) 12:351, 1973.

62. Sassoon HF, Wise JB: Diagnosis of colour-vision defects in very young children. Lancet No. 7643, Feb 21:1970.

63. Sloan LL: Testing for deficient color perception in children. Int Ophthalmol Clin 3:697, 1963.

64. Sloan LL, Habel A: Tests for color deficiency based on the pseudoisochromatic principle. Arch Ophthalmol 55:229, 1956.

65. Smith VC, Pokorny J: Large-field trichromacy in protanopes and deuteranopes. J Opt Soc Am 67:213, 1977.

66. Smith VC, Pokorny J, Ernest JT: Primary hereditary optic atrophies. In Krill AE, Archer DB (eds): Krill's Hereditary Retinal and Choroidal Diseases, vol II. Clinical Characteristics. Hagerstown, MD, Harper & Row, 1977.

67. Spivey B: The X-linked recessive inheritance

of atypical monochromatism. Arch Ophthalmol 74:327, 1965.

68. Spivey B, Pearlman JT, Burian HM: Electroretinographic findings (including flicker) in carriers of congenital X-linked achromatopsia. Doc Ophthalmol 18:367, 1964.

69. Teller DY, Peeples DR, Sekel M: Discrimination of chromatic from white light by two-month-old human infants. Vision Res 18:41, 1978.

70. Varner D, Cook J, Schneck M, et al: Tritan discriminations by 1 and 2 month-old human infants. Vision Res 25:821, 1985.

71. Verriest G: Further studies on acquired deficiency of color discrimination. J Opt Soc Am 53:185, 1963.

72. Verriest G: Colour vision tests in children, part I. Attiv Fond G Ronchi XXXVI:83, 1981.

73. Verriest G: Colour vision tests in children, part V. Attiv Fond G Ronchi XXXVI:111, 1981.

74. Verriest G, Caluwaerts MR: An evaluation of three new colour vision tests. Mod Probl Ophthalmol 19:131, 1978.

75. Verriest G, De Coninck MR, Uvijls A: Colour vision tests in children, part IV. Attiv Fond G Ronchi XXXVI:106, 1981.

76. Verriest G, Gandibleux MF, Pierart P: Colour vision tests in children, part III. Attiv Fond G Ronchi XXXVI:100, 1981.

77. Verriest G, Uvijls A: Spectral increment thresholds on a white background in different age groups of normal subjects and in acquired ocular diseases. Doc Ophthalmol 43:217, 1977.

78. Verriest G, Uvijls A, Malfroidt A: Colour vision tests in children, part II. Attiv Fond G Ronchi XXXVI:91, 1981.

79. Volbrecht V, Werner J: Isolation of short-wavelength-sensitive cone photoreceptors in 4–6 week-old human infants. Vision Res 27:469, 1987.

80. Waardenburg PJ: Achromatopsia congenita. In Waardenburg PJ, Franceschetti A, Klein DD (eds): Genetics and Ophthalmology, vol II. Assen, Netherlands, Royal Van Gorcum, 1695, 1963.

81. Werner JS: Development of scotopic sensitivity and the absorption spectrum of the human ocular media. J Opt Soc Am 72:247, 1982.

82. Yuodelis C, Hendrickson A: A qualitative and quantitative analysis of the human fovea during development. Vision Res 26:847, 1986.

83. Zisman F, Adams A: Screening functional color vision anomalies: A comparison of the City University and AO-HRR tests on children. In Verriest G (ed): Color Vision Deficiencies VIII. Doc Ophthalmol Proc Series 46:145, 1987.

Chapter 20

Vision Screening

Paulette P. Schmidt

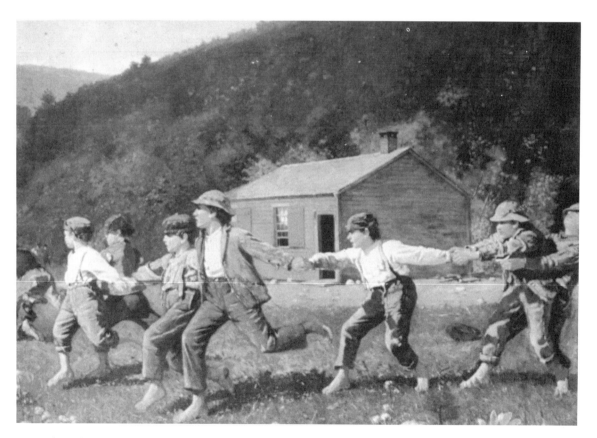

Snap the Whip by Winslow Homer. Courtesy of The Butler Institute of American Art, Youngstown, Ohio.

Jean Jacques Rousseau, in his novel *Emile* (1762), laid down in sequential fashion the arguments for the formal education of children and through that education the goal of independence and intellectual freedom for each individual. It was not until the turn of this century in America, however, that education became mandatory. With required schooling came our first opportunities for a look at the collective characteristics of children.

Early detection of vision problems is a public health goal made increasingly more important by our expanded knowledge of the critical and sensitive periods of human visual development. Increasingly this goal is more realistic not only by the fact that large numbers of children are brought together in educational settings but also by our ability to quantitatively assess the vision of infants and young children with new testing procedures.

In the introduction to this text Drs. Rosenbloom and Morgan pointed out that critical and sensitive periods in the development of the human visual system have been documented in the research literature (10, 22, 36, 86). Because developmental anomalies can be corrected most easily early in life, a system for early detection of vision problems or potential vision problems is the ideal toward which every vision health care system should be directed.

Although reasonable professionals would agree that early examination of the visual system is the most certain way to detect vision problems, universal vision examination of all children is unlikely to be mandatory in our society for years to come. In the absence of such examinations, vision screening programs have been used. A number of national organizations have employed vision screening procedures (Table 20.1).

The recent literature demonstrates a resurgence of interest in vision screening among educators, physicians, optometrists, orthoptists, and psychologists (3, 26, 27, 32, 37, 61, 76). This chapter considers the rationale for vision screening, familiarizes the reader with the historic development and wide array of vision screening techniques, and explores the limitations and comparative effectiveness of vision screening procedures.

HISTORY

Until the advent of mandatory education we did not have collective access to general populations of children to study the vision of the developing human. Early investigators began to study visual characteristics with a wide array of school-based vision screening techniques (20, 21, 50, 54, 59, 64, 78, 81–85, 89) (Table 20.2). It was not until Blum, Peters, and Bettman undertook what is commonly referred to as the Orinda Study, however, that an organized interdisciplinary analysis of procedures and devices was conducted to compare the effectiveness of those vision screening methods with that of clinical examination (13) (Table 20.3). Results from this study long served as a significant foundation for our understanding of the incidence and prevalence of vision problems in school-aged children, the rates of change in visual characteristics with age, the goal of screening programs, the criteria for referral, and the comparisons of effectiveness of a wide array of vision screening methods. Data on preschool populations are more limited and perhaps invalid.

The National Society to Prevent Blindness (NSPB) is the private organization that has made the largest single contribution to preschool screening since the 1950s, using volunteers from such organizations as Delta Gamma, the Junior League, and Parent Teacher Association to carry out the screening programs (26, 33, 34, 62). The NSPB has also served as a central agency for the compilation of vision screening data from independent societies and service groups. Ehrlich and associates indicate the prevalence rates reported by the NSPB as 0.43 percent for strabismus and 0.61 percent for amblyopia (26). Prevalence rates reported by Simons and Reinecke are 2 percent for amblyopia, 4 percent for strabismus (combined rate at least 5 percent) (69, 79). Ehrlich, Reinecke, and Simons go on to suggest that these latter rates are a conservative estimate of the prevalence

Table 20.1 VISION SCREENING PROCEDURES AND REFERRAL CRITERIA OF NATIONAL ORGANIZATIONS

Procedure	Referral Criteria
American Optometric Association	
Retinoscopy	
Myopia	−0.75 DS with acuity loss
Hyperopia	+2.00 DS
Astigmatism	±1.00 DC
Anisometropia	±1.00 DS
Cover test	
Strabismus	Any manifest strabismus
Esophoria	8Δ at distance and near fixation
Exophoria	10Δ at distance fixation
	12Δ at near fixation
Hyperphoria	2Δ at distance and near fixation
Visual acuity	Less than 5 years: Snellen acuity 20/50 or less
	5 years and older: Snellen acuity 20/40 or less
Color test	Failure of any standard color vision test
Ophthalmoscopy and external inspection	Signs of congenital organic, or infectious eye disease; traumatic injury; absence of or abnormal retinal light reflexes; or fundus abnormalities
National Association of Vision Program Consultants	
Level I screening:	
External eye inspection and history	Redness, crusts adherent to the eyelids, sties, watery eyes, discharge, head tilt, eye misalignment
	Rubbing eyes, frowning, or squinting
Distance acuity test	Visual acuity 20/40 or less in one or both eyes after retesting
Snellen E at 20 feet	
Level II screening (done by certified technicians): includes all of Level I plus:	
Eye inspection—congenital, infectious, developmental anomalies	Nystagmus; coloboma; cloudy cornea; tearing; unequal pupil size; heterochromia; possible inflammation of the globe, conjunctiva, and lids
Eye alignment:	
Cover test at near and distance fixation	Suspected intermittent and manifest tropias
Corneal reflection test	
National Society to Prevent Blindness	
Eye history and external inspection	Eye deviations or incoordination on directed gaze
	Possible eye infection such as watery eyes or discharges, history of recurrent sties, crusts on lids or lashes, reddened conjunctiva or eyelids
	Dizziness, nausea, or headaches following close work
	Positive observations during visual acuity testing such as thrusting the head forward or tilting it, watery eyes, frowning, scowling, or squinting

Table 20.1 *(Continued)*

Procedure	Referral Criteria
Distance visual acuity test—Snellen Tumbling E at 20 feet: 3- and 4-year-olds isolated symbols 5- and 6-year-olds	Visual acuity in one or both eyes after retesting at a later date: 3-year-olds: 20/50 or less in either or both eyes 4-, 5-, and 6-year-olds: 20/40 or less in either or both eyes and/or An interocular acuity difference of 1 line on isolated symbols and of 2 lines on linear presentation

(Other tests are optional but not recommended: cover test, corneal refraction test, stereopsis tests, plus lens test.)

Procedure	Referral Criteria
Volunteers for Vision External eye inspection	Severe conjunctivitis, sties, crusty accumulations on lids or lashes, apparent malalignment, apparent injury
Test for sight and vision: Miniature toy identification Picture cards held 16 feet away Child must name object or selected toy object that matches the picture he sees	Failure to identify 3 or 4 objects of an unspecified number of presented ones
Eye movement control: Follows penlight and converges	Any eye movements that are restricted in any given direction, jerky and erratic, or uncoordinated where one eye does not follow as well as the other
Muscle imbalance: Cover test at near and distance fixation	Movement of the covered eye in, out, up, or down
Spatial orientation test: The child walks along a track 9 feet long and 7 inches wide. An object is placed 3 feet to the side of the midpoint of the track. The child must stop at the point where the object is seen in his peripheral field while fixating at the other end of the track.	Failure to stay within the confines of the track or to adequately orient to the peripheral object

of amblyopia and strabismus. The exceptionally low prevalence rates in 3- and 4-year-olds reported by the NSPB, they concluded, were the result of the ineffectiveness of the screening methodology. See Table 20.1 for the procedure advocated by the NSPB.

To date, school screening is mandatory in 24 states and optional in two; 24 states make no provision for vision screening.* Only two states are reported to have specific preschool vision screening laws. Even with rapidly completed visual acuity screening methods,

---

* Miller SC (American Optometric Association): Personal communication.

Table 20.2 EARLY VISION-SCREENING STUDIES

Year	Name of Study	References	Screening Procedure	Comments
1944	Andover Study N = 797 Ages 12–19 years	81	Visual symptoms inquiry & MVK*	Fewer than 50% of those who failed MVK failed symptoms inquiry.
1947	Columbus Study N = 188 Ages 6–17 years	78	Teacher observation, Snellen E chart, MVK*, & Telebinocular	Concluded teacher observation is unreliable. Telebinocular has excessive overreferral rate, MVK has excessive underreferral rate, and Snellen acuity is most reliable single method.
1952	St. Louis N = 1215 Ages 6 & 11 years	20, 21	Snellen acuity & instruments	Ingenious instruments do not reliably measure visual function; Snellen acuity best.
1952	Toronto N = 1200 Ages 5–13 years	59	Snellen acuity, instruments, Maddox Rod, cover, test, & others	Snellen acuity is adequate screener: E's for kindergarten, numbers for grade 1, letters for grades 2 to 8
1952	Shrewsbury N = 1575 Ages 6–18 years	89	Assess MVK*	One third of those referrals were overreferrals.
1955	Danbury N = 4662 Ages 5–18 years	54	Assess MVK* with retest; optometrists & ophthalmologists consulted	Few overreferrals; 50% of those wearing glasses failed; 20% of those not wearing glasses failed.
1955	New York	64, 84, 85	Ortho-Rater, Vision Tester, & MVK*	New York school vision test performs as well but no better than MVK.*
1956	North Carolina N = 213 Age 7, 11, & 14 years	50	Telebinocular	Minimum tests necessary for vision screening include distance & near acuity, lateral phoria, and fusion test.
1959	Orinda N = 1163 Ages 7–12 years	13	Compared MCT† and other procedures; optometrists and ophthalmologists consulted	MCT† more effective than other procedures; 97.2% of those screened with MCT were correctly identified.

* MVK is the Massachusetts Vision Kit or Test; see page 477.
† MCT is the Modified Clinical Technique; see page 477.

Table 20.3 THE ACCURACY OF VISION SCREENING TECHNIQUES

Study	Correct Referrals[a]			Incorrect Referrals[d]		
	Referrals[b] (%)	Nonreferrals[c] (%)	Total (%)	Overreferrals[e] (%)	Underreferrals[f] (%)	Total (%)
St. Louis (20, 21): n[g] = 1215 people						
Clinical criteria*	31.0	69.0	100.0	0.0	0.0	0.0
Instruments						
MVK[h]	17.3	57.3	74.6	15.7	9.7	25.4
Ortho-Rater	24.5	38.5	63.0	30.5	6.5	37.0
Sight-Screener	23.5	42.0	65.5	27.0	7.5	34.5
Telebinocular	20.5	40.1	60.6	32.9	6.5	39.4
Snellen letter acuity						
High standards†	12.7	66.7	79.4	6.3	14.3	20.6
Low standards‡	5.8	72.0	77.8	1.0	21.2	22.2
Orinda (13): n = 1163 people						
Clinical criteria*	17.9	82.1	100.0	0.0	0.0	0.0
MCT[i]	17.2	80.0	97.2	2.0	0.8	2.8
Instruments:						
MVK	13.5	49.3	62.8	30.8	6.4	37.2
MVK (retest)	9.4	80.1	89.5	2.8	7.7	10.5
Telebinocular	15.6	26.6	42.2	56.5	1.3	57.8
Telebinocular (retest)	9.6	77.2	86.8	5.7	7.6	13.3
OSU (32):[j] n = 483 people						
MCT	16.1	81.1	97.2	1.4	1.4	2.8
RDE[k]	10.6	75.4	86.0	8.1	6.0	14.1
Snellen letter acuity§	6.2	81.8	88.0	1.7	10.4	12.1

[a] Correct referrals: people correctly categorized by the vision screening method, they can be identified as referrals or nonreferrals.

[b] Referrals: people correctly identified by the vision screening method as needing further visual attention by meeting the criteria established for passing the screening.

[c] Nonreferrals: people correctly identified by the vision screening method as needing no further visual attention by meeting the criteria established for passing the screening.

[d] Incorrect referrals: people *not* correctly categorized by the vision screening method; they could be identified as overreferrals or underreferrals.

[e] Overreferrals: people incorrectly identified by the vision screening method as needing further visual attention. ("Referring children without vision problems")[3]

[f] Underreferrals: people incorrectly identified by the vision screening method as needing no further visual attention. ("Missing children with vision problems")[3]

[g] n: number of individuals participating in the study

[h] MVK: Massachusetts Vision Kit, a technique in which visual acuity, plus-sphere test, and Maddox rod at distance and near constitute the vision screening test.

[i] MCT: Modified Clinical Technique, a technique in which visual acuity, refractive error, ocular coordination, and organic assessment constitute the vision screening test.

[j] OSU: The Ohio State University, refers to the study that compares the RDE to other vision screening methods.

[k] RDE: Random Dot E, a stereogram used in this study as a vision screening test.

* Clinical criteria refer to complete vision examinations.

† Criterion to pass screening was 20/20 or better monocularly at a distance of 6 m or 20 feet.

‡ Criteria for passing screening were 20/40 or better, either eye, and/or a difference or less than 2 lines between eyes.

§ 20/40 or better, each eye. Difference of 2 lines between eyes resulted in automatic retest of acuity as did poor correlation with retinoscopy. Careful light control and line isolation were also utilized, thereby accounting for a lower number of incorrect referrals.

(Reproduced from Schmidt PP: Effectiveness of vision screening with the modified clinical technique when preferential looking cards are used to measure visual acuity. Am J Optom Physiol Opt 63:108P, 1986.)

only 21 percent of children have their vision screened prior to entering school, so many vision problems (strabismus, amblyopia) go undetected (26).

REASONS FOR VISION SCREENING

The principal reasons for the vision screening of school and preschool children are to detect children who have vision problems (or potential vision problems) that may affect physiological or perceptual processes of vision, and to find those who have vision problems that interfere with performance in school (13).

Further, reasons for conducting vision screening programs vary with the purpose of the sponsoring organization. The objective may be to survey a general population to determine their visual characteristics; to educate the public about vision problems and the importance of early detection; to respond to federal entitlement programs serving children in poverty or in low income homes or who are crippled; to give counseling regarding the careers of young students; or to enhance professional visibility in a community.

The visual conditions to be identified in children remain those set forth by the interdisciplinary team in the Orinda Study: vision problems, organic problems, and visual-perceptual problems. The goal of vision screening, then, is to identify children who need professional attention so they can benefit from early intervention or to monitor conditions for later treatment.

At what age should children first have their vision screened? Since the whole point of conducting screening programs is to detect conditions early enough in the course of development to maximize the effectiveness of treatment and since clinical evidence indicates treatment for anomalies affecting binocular vision is most effective when completed prior to 24 months of age, a strong case can be made for screening children under 24 months of age. Since the incidence of some vision problems increases with age, preschool and school-aged children should be rescreened (13). Preschool populations are more collec-

tively accessible in daycare and preschool program settings than younger children and should remain target populations.

VISION SCREENING VERSUS CLINICAL EXAMINATION

Vision screening should not be confused with a vision examination. Each produces distinctly different data. Clinical data are collected under conditions in which physiological control can be exercised (e.g., control of illumination during visual acuity measurement, a cover test completed through the patient's final subjective refraction), whereas screening is conducted on an as is basis, that is, visual acuity is measured through spectacles even if lenses are badly scratched. Referrals resulting from a vision screening then require further visual attention. The screening should not be viewed as an indication for treatment, though treatment may indeed be necessary, but only a need for evaluation in a more thorough manner and in a more controlled environment than can be carried out in the course of a screening procedure. Blum, Peters, and Bettman pointed out in the Orinda Study,

> [Your child] is being referred for professional vision 'attention' because he/she did not perform satisfactorily on our school screening test at this time. Since these tests are nondiagnostic and only rough measures of visual performance, we believe that it is in the best interest of each such child to have his vision evaluated by a professional person especially qualified in vision care to see if treatment is necessary.

The fact that screening procedures are nondiagnostic and therefore in no way indicate treatment will be required is an illusory concept at best for the general public. Too often the limitations of screening are not communicated effectively by organizations who advocate such programs; this is a great disservice to the public. Most importantly, people may infer (incorrectly) that anyone who "passes" a screening program has no vision problem. The vision of persons screened may be compromised, especially if the screening mechanism is of questionable effectiveness. The limitations of vision screening programs must be recognized, and the effectiveness of methods merits close scrutiny.

THE NATURE AND PROBLEMS OF SCREENING

Every child should receive a thorough professional vision examination. Because this is not currently possible, screening programs fill the void. It is essential, then, that vision screening programs accurately identify children in need of further visual attention. Screening programs divide persons into two groups: those who fulfill or fail to fulfill established criteria. Since screening programs are nondiagnostic, however, there are limitations. Persons may pass who should have failed the screening and others fail when they should have passed. In any screening procedure there are four referral categories that may result: correct referrals (true positive result), nonreferrals (true negative), overreferrals (false positive), and underreferrals (false negative). An effective screening program is one that has a high proportion of true results (correct referrals and correct nonreferrals) and a small number of false ones (underreferrals and overreferrals).

The basic problem with screening programs has been the generation of incorrect referrals. The larger the number of incorrect referrals, the less accurate and more expensive the screening technique is. Any referral for professional visual attention not truly required (overreferral) costs the patient money and the vision care system time. Unhappy parents may pressure sponsoring agencies to discontinue vision screening programs that overrefer. Parents should be congratulated for choosing to ensure their child's vision is evaluated thoroughly. In reality the more serious problem of screening programs is underreferral. Ehrlich et al (26) point out that underreferral—failure to identify persons who need further visual attention—compromises the effectiveness and credibility of the screening effort and raises questions about

medicolegal liability when vision problems are found later. The incalculable hidden cost of underreferrals in screening programs is vision loss. Properly selected and administered vision screening programs should have low rates of overreferral and underreferral.

Any discussion of screening must address the reliability and validity of the procedures. Reliability refers to the consistency or repeatability of a result with the screening procedure; validity refers to the ability of the procedure to divide a screened population into two groups, those who *may* have and those who *probably do not* have vision problems. Validity may be further defined in terms of *sensitivity* and *specificity*. Sensitivity is the percentage of individuals with vision problems who will be identified (the percentage of true positive results or correct referrals), and specificity is the percentage of persons without vision problems who pass the test (true negatives or nonreferrals). These terms may be expressed mathematically as percentages:

$$\text{Sensitivity} = \frac{a}{a + c} \times 100$$

where a = correct referrals and c = underreferrals.

$$\text{Specificity} = \frac{d}{b + d} \times 100$$

where d = nonreferrals and b = overreferrals.

Instead of describing validity in terms of sensitivity and specificity it can be described as effectivity using the phi (ϕ) coefficient. The ϕ coefficient, a statistical method closely related to the chi square (χ^2) test, can be used to measure the validity of a vision screening technique (14, 31, 70). The formula is as follows:

$$\phi = \frac{ad - bc}{\sqrt{(a + b)(c + d)(a + c)(b + d)}}$$

where a indicates correct referrals; b, overreferrals; c, underreferrals; and d, nonreferrals. Values range from -1.00 to $+1.00$; the closer the value is to $+1.00$, the more valid the test.

METHODS OF VISION SCREENING

Methods of vision screening are indeed varied. The following list provides an update of the work of Peters published in 1959 (66).

Symptoms Inventory A series of characteristic behaviors which when observed (in the presence or absence of symptoms) are suggested as indicative of vision problems. Symptoms inventories may use children, teachers, or parents to report the symptoms (Fig. 20.1).

Observation Watching the behavior of children in situations involving the use of the eyes, where signs of difficulty may reveal vision problems (see Fig. 20.1).

School Achievement When it is not commensurate with intellectual ability, particularly in reading, school performance may indicate the presence of vision problems.

Paper and Pencil Tests These require no content knowledge, only visual recognition of forms.

Visual Acuity By using different-sized figures or targets that the child is asked to identify or look at, it is possible to assess the ability to see detail.

Plus Sphere Test The subject looks through a pair of plus-sphere lenses (+1.50 DS to +2.50 DS have been used). If the child

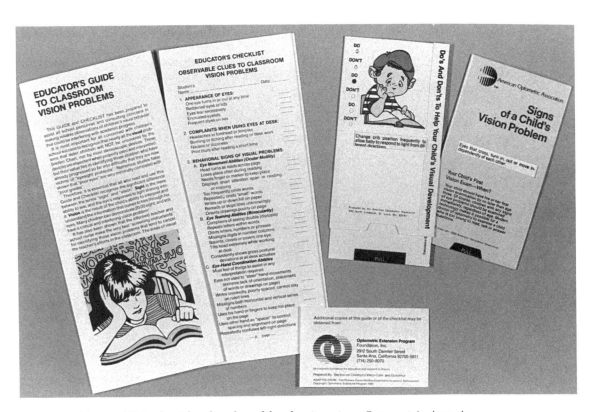

Figure 20.1 Two published guides distributed by the American Optometric Association and Optometric Extension Foundation, Inc. that list characteristic behaviors frequently associated with vision problems of children. (American Optometric Association, 243 North Lindbergh Blvd., St. Louis, MO 63141 and Optometric Extension Program Foundation, Inc., 2912 South Daimler St., Santa Ana, CA 92705-5811.)

can see the 20/20 row on the visual acuity chart he is considered to have a hyperopic refractive state equal to or greater than the correction in the lenses used in the test.

Cover Test A test to estimate the degree of coordination between the two eyes; it may be conducted at distance (20 feet or 6 m) or near point (16 inches or 40 cm) fixation.

Worth Four-Dot Test A bichrome test of fusion used to reveal coordination problems of the two eyes.

Maddox Rod Test This test determines the postural position of the eyes when fusion is interrupted; it detects coordination problems.

California State Recommended Procedure (CSRP) This combination method includes a visual acuity test, plus-sphere test, and an optional cover test.

Massachusetts Vision Test This combination method includes visual acuity, plus sphere, and Maddox rod tests at distance and near point fixation.

Telebinocular This stereoscope and a series of double-picture stereograms tests visual acuity, lateral imbalance (phoria), fusion, and stereopsis at optically projected far and near fixation points; it also includes a rudimentary color test.

Biopter Stereoscopes with pairs of slides similar in construction and test content to the Telebinocular.

Ortho-Rater Stereoscopes with pairs of slides similar in construction and test content to the Telebinocular.

Sight-Screener Stereoscopes with pairs of slides similar in construction and test content to the Telebinocular.

Vision Tester Stereoscopes with pairs of slides similar in construction and test content to the Telebinocular.

Modified Clinical Technique (MCT) A modification of clinical procedures used in screening that includes assessment of visual acuity, refractive state, ocular coordination at far and near point fixation, and inspection for pathology.

Random Dot Stereograms Random dot stereograms are stereoacuity screening tests used to identify persons who are suspected of having visual conditions that affect the desired functional outcome of vision, binocular performance, rather than a component of the process such as visual acuity, refractive state, or fusion. (See Fig. 20.2.)

New York State Optometric Association (NYSOA) This series of procedures includes the following tests: distance and near Snellen acuity; +1.50 sphere test; facility of accommodation; convergence ability; stereopsis; saccadic eye movements; vertical imbalance, lateral fusion at distance and near and color vision (measured on the Telebinocular); and visual motor integration, eye-hand coordination, visual organization, and form reproduction using the Winter Haven Copy Forms.

Modified Clinical Technique with Preferential Looking Acuity In this variation of the MCT preferential looking acuity cards are substituted for the Snellen acuity test to measure visual acuity in very young children.

Photorefraction A photographic retinoscopy procedure in which the retinal reflex, as seen in the pupil, is used to screen the refractive conditions and ocular alignment of young children.

Numerous variations and combinations of the aforementioned techniques are in use. The list is provided to give the reader some idea of the array of vision screening techniques and aspects of vision evaluated. It emphasizes that no uniform procedure is in use across the country and that there is no general agreement as to what aspects of vision should be included in a screening battery or what referral criteria should be. To be widely used a vision screening program must be

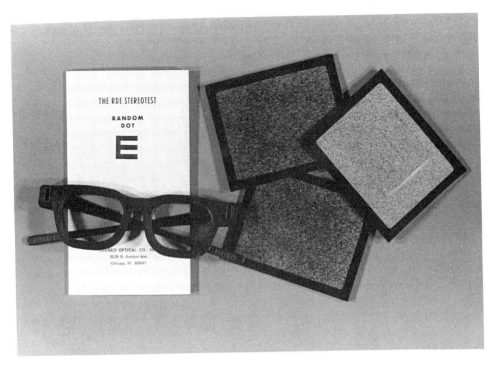

Figure 20.2   The Random Dot E (RDE) stereogram has been used for vision screening. It consists of three cards, one pair of polaroid glasses, and an instruction manual. The figure shows the front side of each of the 8 × 10 cm cards. Two have a polaroid surface and a random dot pattern. Only one of the two cards contains the stereographic E. The third card with nonpolarized random dot pattern contains a three-dimensional letter for purposes of demonstrating what should be seen on one of the other two cards. (Stereo Optical Co., Inc., 3539 N. Kenton Ave., Chicago, IL 60641.)

easy to administer, short, accurate, and cost effective.

VISUAL ACUITY

Snellen letter acuity testing alone has been promoted for detecting amblyopia and significant refractive error but not binocular vision problems. Acuity measurement with the Tumbling E chart has been shown to take an average of 2.0 minutes per child (79). At first glance Snellen acuity measurement would also appear to be an inexpensive screening method because large numbers of children can be screened in short periods. However, the relationship between visual acuity and refractive state is far from simple.

In the Orinda Study the relationship of refractive state and visual acuity was compared in 1920 eyes, with interesting results. Snellen letter or E acuity was measured using an isolated line presentation.* This study of children 6 to 13 years old without pathologic conditions demonstrates that significant refractive anomalies can be missed when visual acuity is the sole determinant for referral or nonreferral. In Figure 20.3, the shaded areas show a large range of significant refractive states that may not be detected by the Snellen letter acuity test (a visual acuity of 20/40 or better in each eye). Moderately high

---

* Peters HB: Personal communication.

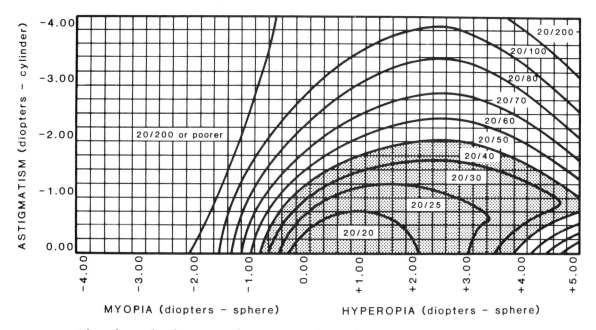

Figure 20.3 The relationship between refractive anomalies and Snellen visual acuity in 1920 eyes in the Orinda study. Mean acuity for each refractive anomaly is plotted with lines of isooxyopia. Shaded areas indicate uncorrected refractive anomalies with which 20/40 visual acuity could still be achieved, which, therefore, were not detected by Snellen acuity measurement. (From Blum H, Peters HB, Bettman JW: Vision Screening for Elementary Schools: The Orinda Study. Berkeley, CA, University of California Press, 1959.)

hyperopia, 3 to 5 D, with varying amounts of astigmatism, up to 2 D, still allows a Snellen acuity of 20/40 or better. For example, participants in the Orinda Study who exhibited an uncorrected refractive state of +4.00 DS with −1.00 D cylinder could still read the 20/30 row on the Snellen chart.

Methods for testing acuity range from symbol optotypes, such as those developed by Allen (1), to isolated letter optotypes, and isolated line as well as full chart presentations of letter optotypes. Among the various instruments used in screening programs the type of acuity measured also varies. Detection and resolution acuity have both been incorporated in one of the screening series on the Telebinocular (a widely used screening device).

The criteria for passing visual acuity screening procedures vary widely. There are

high standards at 20/20 or better monocularly, low standards of 20/40 or better for either eye or a difference of less than 2 lines between the eyes; age-related standards such as 20/40 or better for each eye for children 7 years of age or younger, 20/30 or better for each eye for children older than 7 years (20, 21, 25). Snellen acuity testing, even with high standards of 20/20 or better monocularly at a distance of 6 m or 20 feet, has been shown to yield a large number of incorrect referrals (6.3 percent overreferrals and 14.3 percent underreferrals). When lower standards such as 20/40 or better monocularly at 6 m or 20 feet are used, most studies of Snellen letter acuity testing show the overreferral rate is lowered; but, the underreferral rate becomes even higher, 21.3 percent (20, 21) (see Table 20.3).

Ehrlich, Reinecke, and Simons' studies

present conservative estimates of prevalence rates in amblyopia and strabismus as 2 and 4 percent, respectively (combined rate 5 percent). They conclude that the very low prevalence rates of amblyopia and strabismus reported by the NSPB are the result of the ineffectiveness of isolated symbol acuity testing for amblyopia detection and of the observation or cover test (when administered by nonprofessionals) for detection of strabismus.

The types of acuity measured, criteria for referral, and methods of testing appear to be as numerous as the investigators reporting the results of their studies.* There appears, therefore, to be little consistency in vision screening using visual acuity tests, and serious questions exist about their effectiveness. Nonetheless, visual acuity remains the most widely used vision screening method for children (26, 27, 29, 79, 83).

THE MODIFIED CLINICAL TECHNIQUE

The Orinda Study was an outstanding interdisciplinary approach to determine the effectiveness of procedures used on school-aged populations. It established a highly effective series of tests that were collectively named the Modified Clinical Technique (MCT, see above).

The test procedures and pass-fail criteria were agreed upon by a panel of optometrists from the faculty of the University of California, Berkeley, School of Optometry and ophthalmologists from the faculty of Stanford (California) University School of Medicine. The study showed that the MCT best determined which elementary school children needed further visual attention. When the results of the MCT were compared with clinical examinations conducted by both optometrists and ophthalmologists, 97.2 percent of the children screened were correctly identified: 17.2 percent referrals, 80.0 percent nonreferrals, and 2.8 percent incorrect referrals.

---

* References 11, 12, 15–18, 23, 25–28, 34, 35, 38, 49, 51, 52, 56, 58, 59, 62, 63, 65, 67, 72, 74, 81, 87, 89.

Effectiveness of the MCT established in the Orinda Study was $\phi = +0.91$. The relative accuracy of other vision screening techniques is shown in Table 20.3.

The American Optometric Association continues to favor the use of the MCT and a modification of the associated pass-fail criteria today, whereas the American Academy of Ophthalmology has recommended testing visual acuity and ocular alignment in school-aged children (26). The approach used in the Orinda Study was very successful in establishing screening procedures and referral criteria. These procedures and referral criteria were determined jointly by committees from the organizations sponsoring screenings and an interdisciplinary group of health care professionals (Table 20.4). The degree of effectiveness of the procedures and associated referral criteria was very high. Despite proven effectiveness, the MCT is not widely used as

Table 20.4   VISION SCREENING REFERRAL CRITERIA FOR USE WITH THE MODIFIED CLINICAL TECHNIQUE*

Procedures	Referral Criteria
Organic problems	Any
Visual acuity	20/40 or less either eye
Refractive error	
Hyperopia	+1.50 DS or more
Myopia	−0.50 DS or more
Astigmatism	±1.00 DC or more
Anisometropia	±1.00 DS or more
Coordination problems	
Distance	
Esophoria	5Δ or more
Exophoria	5Δ or more
Hyperphoria	2Δ or more
Tropia	Any
Near	
Esophoria	6Δ or more
Exophoria	10Δ or more
Hyperphoria	2Δ or more
Tropia	Any

* Established by optometrists and ophthalmologists in the Orinda Study (13).
(From Blum H, Peters HB, Bettman JW: Vision Screening for Elementary Schools: The Orinda Study. Berkeley, CA, University of California Press, 1959.)

a vision screening procedure because of the high degree of professional involvement required.

PHOTORETINOSCOPY

Photoretinoscopy and corneal fundus reflex photography have been proposed as vision screening procedures that are quick and require minimal cooperation of the subject. Photoretinoscopy is an optically based method for predicting refractive conditions from a retinal reflex photographed in the pupil (5–7). Corneal fundus reflex photography combines, for the detection of strabismus, photographic prediction of refractive state with the Hirschberg test and differences in color, intensity, or shape of the fundus reflex (45–48). Light reflected from the retina, except for the macular area, is said to appear brighter, so in a photograph the deviated eye shows a brighter fundus reflex than the nondeviated one. Photoretinoscopic techniques, then, have been proposed for the identification of refractive conditions predictive of amblyopia or strabismus (45).

In a study by Friedman and coworkers of 38,000 children between the ages of 1 and $2\frac{1}{2}$ years, 43 percent of those with esotropia (360 children) were emmetropic to hyperopic up to 2.00 D and would therefore have gone undetected by refractive screening (29). Another study in which Fulton and associates performed photorefraction with cycloplegia on infants using spherical equivalent hyperopia greater than 2.75 D as the cutoff point identified 67 percent of the esotropias and 78.5 percent of the amblyopias (30).

Although investigators such as Ingram and his colleagues have evaluated the suggestion by Kramer that refractive state could serve as a predictor for amblyopia and strabismus, they have concluded that the presence of either or both conditions does not appear to be highly correlated with refractive state (39–44, 53). Three reports by Ingram and coworkers have shown high underreferral rates in 1- to $3\frac{1}{2}$-year-old children (25 to 44 percent) (39, 40, 43). Altering the range of refractive states defined as normal simulta-

neously resulted in overreferrals (26). Therefore, as with visual acuity measurement, the underreferral rates have thus far proven unacceptable for predicting amblyopia and strabismus. Atkinson and associates have demonstrated photorefraction for screening infants with considerable success (4). Commercially available photoretinoscopy devices are also very expensive (61). Refinement in accuracy of the procedure and lower cost instrumentation will enhance the usefulness of this vision screening procedure.

RANDOM DOT STEREOGRAMS

A stereoscopic screening procedure appears to be the most effective vision screening procedure, as it assesses the desired functional result itself, normal binocular vision, rather than a single component of the binocular vision process such as acuity, refraction, or fusion. Reinecke and Simons, in separate and collaborative studies, have pointed out the potential of stereotests for identifying persons with abnormal binocular vision (69, 79, 80). They suggest that stereotests could be systems tests. Failing the screening procedure would result if any component of the binocular visual system is compromised (e.g., optical, motor, or neural components).

Reinecke and Simons reported that a random dot stereogram had proven effective in screening for strabismus and amblyopia where a 250 arc seconds disparity was used. None of the 70 strabismic and amblyopic patients with visual acuity worse than 20/30 in either eye and an interocular acuity difference greater than 1 line or with constant strabismus passed the test (69).

Rosner has also demonstrated the effectiveness of the Random Dot E (RDE) Stereogram in identifying all 10 children with binocular vision problems, including an intermittent strabismic condition in a screening of 60 preschool children (72). All 10 children failed to correctly identify the position of the stereoscopic target of 168-arc seconds disparity. These same 10 children failed a screening using the MCT.

Avilla and von Noorden have questioned

the effectiveness of a random dot stereogram for identifying amblyopia in five clinic patients with anisometropia or anisometropic amblyopia (9); however, the results were obtained from a single presentation of the TNO test stimulus; there was no effort to have any of the children repeat that performance. Other test conditions (e.g., the distance at which the test was conducted and the lighting used) were not enumerated, nor was it a masked investigation. So it is difficult to compare this report with those documenting random dot stereograms as effective in vision screening.

In a double-masked investigation, 483 school children (49.3 percent boys and 50.7 percent girls) with a mean age of 7.23 years had their vision screened using both the RDE Stereogram and the MCT. The validity of each technique was determined using the ϕ coefficient and was compared with results of similar reports in the literature for the MCT, Snellen letter acuity, and vision screening kits. Hammond and Schmidt found the effectivity to be +0.52 for the RDE and showed it was more effective than all procedures studied except the MCT (32). [Reevaluation of these results show the procedure (77) may be even more effective ($\phi = +0.70$).] In addition, screening with the RDE could be taught to nonprofessionals in 10 minutes or less, could be completed on each child in less than 2 minutes, and was inexpensive. According to multiple investigations it appears that random dot stereograms are effective for vision screening and that further investigation is warranted.

VISION SCREENING OF CHILDREN

The preceding information demonstrates that in the absence of mandatory vision examination vision screening continues to fill a need. A wide range of professional organizations are interested in vision screening procedures; however, the practice of vision screening today, as 30 years ago, is largely unchanged. Continued use of Snellen acuity testing has been shown to be ineffective by many investigators, yet it remains the most widely used vision screening procedure. If vision screening is to be a part of comprehensive vision conservation and vision health education activity in schools and preschools, only methods that have been proven effective in identifying children whose vision needs further attention should be employed. Screening methods are available that are effective, quick and easy to complete, and inexpensive and with further modification they may be made even more effective. Here, then, is the challenge: To prevent ineffective screening procedures from compromising the vision of developing systems, to clearly communicate the limitations of vision screening, to investigate and improve procedures that show promise of being effective, reliable, valid, inexpensive, easy, and universally and uniformly applicable.

REFERENCES

1. Allen HF: A new picture series for preschool vision testing. Am J Ophthalmol 44:38, 1957.

2. American Optometric Association Vision and School Health Committee: The American Optometric Association Guidelines on Vision Screening. St Louis, Optometric Development Enterprises, May, 1979.

3. Atkinson J, Anker S, Evans C, et al: The Cambridge Crowding Cards for preschool visual acuity testing. Trans Sixth Int Orthop Congress, UK, 482, 1987.

4. Atkinson J, Braddick O, Wattam-Bell J, Durden K, Bobier W, Pointer J: Photorefractive screening of infants and effects of refractive correction. Invest Ophthalmol 28:399, 1987.

5. Atkinson J, Braddick O: Assessment of vision in infants. Trans Ophthalmol Soc UK 99:338, 1979.

6. Atkinson J, Braddick O: The use of isotropic photorefraction for screening in infants. Acta Ophthalmol [Suppl] (Copenh) 157:36, 1982.

7. Atkinson J, Braddick O, Pimm-Smith E, et al: Refractive screening of infants. Am J Ophthalmol 93:372, 1982.

8. Austin C: Mass preschool vision screening. Children 6:58, 1959.

9. Avilla CW, von Noorden GK: Limitation of

the TNO random dot stereo test for visual screening. Am Orthoptic J 31:87, 1981.

10. Banks MS, Aslin RN: Sensitive period for the development of human binocular vision. Science 190:675, 1975.

11. Barker J, Barmatz H: Eye Function. Frankenburg WK, Camp BW (eds): Pediatric Screening Tests. Springfield IL, Charles C Thomas, 1975.

12. Blackhurst RT, Radke E: Vision screening procedures used with mentally retarded children. A second report. Sight Sav Rev 38:84, 1967.

13. Blum H, Peters HB, Bettman JW: Vision Screening for Elementary Schools: The Orinda Study. Berkeley CA, University of California Press, 1959.

14. Bruning JL, Kintz BL: Computational Handbook of Statistics. Glenview IL, Scott Foresman, 207, 1968.

15. Burman ML: Vision screening of pre-school children in Prince George's County, Maryland, nursery schools. J Natl Med Assoc 61:352, 1969.

16. Cohen AH, Lieberman S, Stolzberg M, et al: The NYSOA vision screening battery—A total approach. J Am Optom Assoc 54:979, 1983.

17. Colasuonno TM: Preschool vision screening study in Douglas County, Oregon. Sight Sav Rev 28:156, 1958.

18. Committee on Children with Handicaps: Vision screening of preschool children. Pediatrics 50:966, 1972.

19. Costenbader FD, O'Neill JF: Ocular examination before the age of four years. Sight Sav Rev 38:135, 1968.

20. Crane MM, Foote FM, Scobee RG, et al: Screening school children for visual defects. Washington DC, Government Printing Office, Children's Bureau Pub No 345, 1954.

21. Crane MM, Scobee RG, Foote FM, et al: Study of procedures for screening elementary school children for visual defects: Referrals by screening procedures vs ophthalmological findings. Sight Sav Rev 22:141, 1952.

22. Crewther DP, Crewther SG, Mitchell DE: The efficacy of brief periods of reverse occlusion in promoting recovery from the physiological effects of mononuclear deprivation in kittens. Invest Ophthalmol 21:357, 1981.

23. Cunningham F: Preschool vision screening. Sight Sav Rev 27:90, 1957.

24. Davens E: The nationwide alert to preschool screening. Sight Sav Rev 36:13, 1966.

25. Diskan SM: A new visual screening test for children. Am J Ophthalmol 39:369, 1955.

26. Ehrlich MI, Reinecke RD, Simons K: Preschool vision screening for amblyopia and strabismus: Programs, methods, guidelines. Surv Ophthalmol 28:145, 1983.

27. Fern KD, Manny RE: Visual acuity of the preschool child: A review. Am J Optom Physiol Opt 63:319, 1986.

28. Fink WH: Testing visual acuity of the preschool child. Minn Med 42:23, 1959.

29. Friedman Z, Neumann E, Hyams S, et al: Ophthalmic screening of 38,000 children, age 1 to $2\frac{1}{2}$ years in child welfare clinics. J Pediatr Ophthalmol Strabismus 17:261, 1980.

30. Fulton A, Dobson V, Salem D, et al: Cycloplegic refractions in infants and young children. Am J Ophthalmol 90:239, 1980.

31. Guilford JP: Fundamental Statistics in Psychology and Education. New York, McGraw-Hill 341, 1950.

32. Hammond RS, Schmidt PP: A random dot e stereogram for the vision-screening of children. Arch Ophthalmol 104:54, 1986.

33. Hatfield EM: A year's record. Sight Sav Rev 36:18, 1966.

34. Hatfield EM: Methods and standards for screening pre-school children. Sight Sav Rev 49:71, 1979.

35. Hilton AF, Stark DJ, Biggs AB, et al: Preschool vision screening—A pilot study. Aust J Ophthalmol 10:199, 1982.

36. Hohmann A, Creutzfeld OD: Squint and the development of binocularity in humans. Nature 254:613, 1975.

37. Hoyt CS: Photorefraction: A technique for preschool vision screening. Arch Ophthalmol 105:1497, 1987.

38. Hyams SW, Neumann E: Picture cube for vision screening of pre-school children. Br J Ophthalmol 56:572, 1972.

39. Ingram R, Barr A: Refraction of 1-year-old children after cycloplegia with 1% cyclopentolate: Comparison with finding after atropinization. Br J Ophthalmol 63:348, 1979.

40. Ingram R, Traynar M, Walker C, et al: Screening for refractive errors at age 1 year: A pilot study. Br J Ophthalmol 63:243, 1979.

41. Ingram R, Walker C: Refraction as a means of predicting squint or amblyopia in preschool siblings of children known to have these defects. Br J Ophthalmol 63:238, 1979.

42. Ingram RM: The problem of screening children for visual defects. Br J Ophthalmol 61:4, 1977.

43. Ingram RM: Refraction as a basis for screening children for squint and amblyopia. Br J Ophthalmol 61:8, 1977.

44. Ingram RM, Barr A: Changes in refraction between the ages of 1 and $3\frac{1}{2}$ years. Br J Ophthalmol 63:339, 1979.

45. Kaakinen K: A simple method for screening children with strabismus, anisometropia or ametropia by simultaneous photography of corneal and fundus reflexes. Acta Ophthalmol (Copenh) 57:161, 1979.

46. Kaakinen K: Photographic screening for strabismus and high refractive errors of children aged 1 to 4 years. Acta Ophthalmol (Copenh) 59:38, 1981.

47. Kaakinen K: Simultaneous two flash static photoskiascopy. Acta Ophthalmol (Copenh) 59.378, 1981.

48. Kaakinen K, Tommila V: A clinical study on the detection of strabismus, anisometropia or ametropia of children by simultaneous photography of corneal and fundus reflexes. Acta Ophthalmol (Copenh) 57:600, 1979.

49. Kaivonen M, Koskenoja M: Visual screening for children aged four years and preliminary experience from its application in practice (a preliminary report). Acta Ophthalmol (Copenh) 41:785, 1963.

50. Kelley CR: Visual screening and child development: The North Carolina study. Raleigh NC, North Carolina State College, 1957.

51. Kohler L, Stigman G: Vision screening of four-year-old children. Acta Paediatr Scand 62:17, 1973.

52. Kozaki M, Iwai H, Mikami C: Vision screening of three year old children. Jpn J Ophthalmol 17:60, 1973.

53. Kramar PO: The possibility of predicting the appearance of strabismus. Br Orthoptic J 30:66, 1973.

54. Leverett HM: A school vision health study in Danbury, Connecticut. Am J Ophthalmol 39:527, 1955.

55. Lieberman S, Cohen AH, Stolzberg M, et al: Validation study of the New York Optometric Association (NYSOA) screening battery. Am J Optom Physiol Opt 62:165, 1985.

56. Lin-Fu JS: Vision Screening of Children. Washington DC, US Maternal and Child Health Service, 1971.

57. Lippmann O: Vision screening of young children. Am J Public Health 61:1586, 1971.

58. LoCascio GP: Preschool-age vision screening. Am J Optom Arch Am Acad Optom 48:1044, 1971.

59. Morgan AL, Crawford JS, Pashby TJ, et al: A survey of methods used to reveal eye defects in school children. Can Med Assoc J 67:29, 1952.

60. Moran CT: Preschool vision screening in Louisville. Sight Sav Rev 28:92, 1958.

61. Morgan KS, Johnson WD: Clinical evaluation of a commercial photorefractor. Arch Ophthalmol 105:1528, 1987.

62. National Society to Prevent Blindness: Position Statement on HR 4092, the National Comprehensive Vision Care Act of 1975. New York, 1975.

63. Nordlow W, Joachimsson S: A screening test for visual acuity in four year old children. Acta Ophthalmol (Copenh) 40:453, 1962.

64. O'Shea JB: Optometric visual survey in schools of four Massachusetts towns. J Am Optom Assoc 17:253, 1946.

65. Patz A, Hoover RE: Protection of Vision in Children. Springfield IL, Charles C Thomas, 3, 1969.

66. Peters HB: Vision screening. In Hirsch MJ, Wick RE (eds): Vision of Children. Philadelphia, Chilton, 1963.

67. Pugmire GE, Sheridan MD: Revised vision screening chart for very young or retarded children. Med Officer 98:53, 1957.

68. Reinecke R: Current concepts in ophthalmology—Strabismus. N Engl J Med 300:1139, 1979.

69. Reinecke R, Simons K: A new stereoscopic test for amblyopia screening. Am J Ophthalmol 78:714, 1974.

70. Reynolds DC: Validity of a screening test. Am J Optom Physiol Opt 59:67, 1982.

71. Rosenbloom AA: A critical evaluation of visual diagnostic materials. Elementary School J 56(1):27, 1955.

72. Rosner J: The effectiveness of the Random Dot E Stereotest as a preschool vision screening instrument. J Am Opt Assoc 49:1121, 1977.

73. Russell EL, Kada JM, Hufhines DM: Orange County vision screening project. Part II. Ophthalmological evaluation. Sight Sav Rev 31:215, 1961.

74. Savitz RA, Reed RB, Valadian I: Testability of preschool children for vision screening. J Pediatr Ophthalmol 1:15, 1964.

75. Savitz RA, Reed RB, Valadian I: Vision Screening of the Pre-school Child: Report of a Study. Washington DC, U.S. Dept. HEW, Welfare Administration, Children's Bureau, 1964.

76. Schmidt PP: Effectiveness of vision screening with the modified clinical technique when preferential-looking cards are used to measure visual acuity. Am J Optom Physiol Opt 63:108P, 1986.

77. Schmidt PP: Sensitivity of RDE stereoacuity and Snellen acuity to optical blur. Invest Ophthalmol Vis Sci 30:303, 1989.

78. Shaffer TE: Study of vision testing procedure. Am J Publ Health 38:1141, 1948.

79. Simons K, Reinecke R: A reconsideration of amblyopia screening and stereopsis. Am J Ophthalmol 78:707, 1974.

80. Simons K, Reinecke R: Amblyopia screening and stereopsis. In: Symposium on Strabismus: Trans New Orleans Acad Ophthalmol. St Louis, CV Mosby, 15, 1978.

81. Sloane AE, Gallagher RJ: A vision test for pediatrician's use. J Pediatr 28:140, 1946.

82. Sloane AE, Gallagher JR: A comparison of vision screening tests with clinical examination results. Am J Ophthalmol 35:819, 1952.

83. Sloane AE, Rosenthal P: School vision testing. Arch Ophthalmol 64:763, 1960.

84. Stump NF: Report on Webster Study—The Modified Ortho-Rater Compared with the Massachusetts Vision Tests. Unpublished report. Rochester NY, Bausch and Lomb Optical, 1955.

85. Sulzman JH, Davis CJ: The New York school vision tester. NY State J Med 58:833, 1958.

86. Teller DY, Allen JL, Regal DM, et al: Astigmatism and acuity in two primate infants. Invest Ophthalmol 17:344, 1978.

87. Trotter RR, Phillips RM, Shaffer K: Measurement of visual acuity of preschool children by their parents. Sight Sav Rev 36:80, 1966.

88. Vellayappan K: Visual acuity in pre-school children. J Singapore Paediatr Soc 21:70, 1979.

89. Yasuna ER, Green LR: An evaluation of the Massachusetts vision test for visual screening of school children. Am J Ophthalmol 35:235, 1952.

Chapter 21

Learning Disabilities

Harold A. Solan

Optometrists, as a rule, do not treat learning or reading disabilities; they treat learning-disabled (LD) or dyslexic children who manifest some type of visual dysfunction. They treat visual and perceptual motor problems that impair the ability of an LD person to respond to specific instruction intended to mediate the disability. In some instances the visual problems may be primary in the development of the learning disability, but in many cases they are contributory, often making it profoundly difficult for the LD person to respond to educational intervention. The professional services rendered to a child who presents with a learning or reading disability depend to some extent upon how the clinician attending the child conceptualizes the problem.

Until recently it has been generally accepted that a learning-disabled child fails to respond to classroom instruction appropriately in spite of average or better than average intelligence, normal motivation, adequate (or even abundant) educational opportunities, normal sensory development (auditory and visual), normal culturation, no primary emotional disorder, and no frank brain damage. This definition of learning disabilities lends itself to the misinterpretation that persons with learning disabilities cannot be multiply handicapped or be from different cultural or linguistic backgrounds. The "definition by exclusion" is useful clinically, but it lacks the force of a positive statement. In 1981, The National Joint Committee on Learning Disabilities formulated a new definition of learning disabilities:

Learning disabilities is a generic term that refers to a heterogeneous group of disorders manifested by significant difficulties in the acquisition and use of listening, speaking, reading, writing, reasoning, or mathematical abilities. These disorders are intrinsic to the individual and presumed to be due to central nervous system dysfunction. Even though a learning disability may occur concomitantly with other handicapping conditions (e.g., sensory impairment, mental retardation, social and emotional disturbance) or environmental influences (e.g., cultural differences, insufficient or inappropriate instruction, psychogenic factors), it is not the direct result of those conditions or influences (94).

Optometrists recognize that learning and reading disabilities are multidisciplinary disorders that often require the services of a number of professional disciplines. For example, endocrinology, neurology, optometry, pediatrics, psychiatry, psychology, and speech and hearing specialists have all contributed to the common body of knowledge. Special educators and classroom teachers are the "primary care" practitioners for LD children, as it is they who must plan children's classroom experiences in such a way as to facilitate learning.

The purpose of this chapter is to summarize the potential role of optometry and those optometrists whose training, credentials, and personal interests have provided the motivation to treat this special group of children who have been identified as learning disabled.

CASE HISTORY AND ETIOLOGY

When evaluating an LD child, the case history provides the optometrist with visual, behavioral, developmental, environmental, and medical histories that may have contributed to the child's learning problems. The relationship of some of these factors to learning disabilities has been validated by clinical research, whereas the relationship of others is supported by clinical experience.

Establishing the chief complaint immediately is important to clear the air (Fig. 21.1). In the child's presence the parent should be asked "Why are you here?" Responses vary widely, from "John has been complaining that the print blurs when he reads" to "Charles seems bright enough, but he has been having reading and spelling problems for the past 2 years, since he was in second grade." Sometimes the child is referred by a reading or learning disabilities specialist who suspects a visual input or a visual perceptual disorder. The question often has additional value in that it provides an opportunity for the parent(s) to crystallize their own thinking about the child's problem, often for the first time. A child who is 2 years behind in reading *knows* he has a problem. It is equally important, however, that there be a mutual understanding and sharing of this problem, which very likely is affecting the homeostasis of the family system. The remaining questions in Figure 21.1 provide the customary baseline. The case history provides the optometrist with the information necessary to view the child's learning problems more comprehensively.

A knowledge of the child's developmental and behavioral abnormalities (and subnormalities) is valuable if the optometrist is to participate effectively as a member of the interdisciplinary team. Precursors of learning disabilities may have biologic, biosocial, gross and fine motor, neurologic, language, psychological, laterality, genetic, behavioral, and nutritional elements. Interlinking is the rule in this heterogeneous group of disorders. For example, although motor problems may be a subset of neurologic problems, a neurologic deficit can be a by-product of malnutrition. The areas listed in Case History 2 (Fig. 21.2) offer the optometrist the opportunity to weigh the cumulative effects of combinations of potentially harmful factors that may be present during successive developmental stages. Also included is a brief school history.

Although hyperactivity is often seen in LD children, it is not a universal sign. Hyperactivity implies an inability to control motor activity so that it is situationally and socially appropriate. A hyperactivity syndrome may be organic or psychogenic (secondary to the learning disability). Excessive extraneous movement, especially of the head and eyes,

VISUAL INFORMATION

1. Why are you here? _____

2. Is the child able to see things far away (like the chalkboard and street signs) clearly? _____ or are they blurry? _____

3. Is the child able to see the print in books clearly? _____ comfortably? _____ Does he/she ever complain of the print coming in and out of focus? _____

4. Does the child complain of his/her eyes causing discomfort—like burning _____ itching _____ tearing _____ pains in the eye _____ When _____

5. Does he/she report frequent headaches associated with reading or close work? _____ After how long? _____

6. Does the child show any unusual habits when reading: Such as holding the print very close _____ Far away _____ Squinting eyes _____

7. Does the child ever see double? (See two when there is really only one object) _____

8. When was the child's last thorough eye exam? _____ Were glasses ever prescribed? _____ When? _____ For near (reading) _____ For far (blackboard) _____ Other _____

9. Has the child ever had Vision Training? _____ How long? _____ At what age? _____ What were the goals in Vision Training?

10. Is there a history of crossed eyes (Strabismus)? _____

At what age _____ How treated _____

Eye patching _____ Eye surgery _____ Eye injuries _____

Eye medications _____

Additional remarks _____

Figure 21.1   Case history form 1.

may disrupt learning by interfering with accurate intake of information during crucial periods of learning (81). Distractibility, the sensory analog of hyperactivity, manifests itself as a short attention span and may be present with or without hyperactivity. Poor impulse control is frequently associated with this behavioral triad. The child's inability to inhibit the performance of an act long enough to become concerned about the immediate consequences of behavior results in "social impulsivity." Academically, Kagan (73) notes that these same children "select and report solution hypotheses quickly with minimal consideration for their probable accuracy. Other children of equal intelligence take more time to decide about the validity of solutions. The former group has been called impulsive, the latter reflective." Recognizing the futility of subdividing these mutually interacting and reciprocal behaviors, the recently revised Diagnostic and Statistical

NAME _____ AGE _____ GRADE _____ DATE _____

Prenatal history:

_____

Perinatal history: BW _____
Labor _____ (hrs) FT _____
Postnatal history:

_____

Motor Milestones:
Sucked/swallowed _____
Crept   _____
Walked   _____
Gross Motor   _____
  Skip, climb, run, etc.
Fine motor _____

Laterality:
          writes _____
Hand: right-left eats _____
          throws _____

Eye (mono) right-left reached with
   (bino) right-left _____ hand

Foot: right-left

Left-right discrimination:
a) on self (body parts):
b) on examiner (facing):
c) Using 3 coins:

Hyperactive _____

Distractible _____

Attention Span _____
Impulsivity _____

Language Milestones:
First words _____
First sentence _____
Articulation:
  Animal _____
  Hospital _____
  Spaghetti _____
Vocabulary _____
Syntax _____

Miscellaneous

Temper tantrums _____

Others in family with
learning difficulties _____

Color Vision _____

Remarks

_____
_____
_____

Brief School History:
1. Has child ever been placed in a special class, resource room, or received special testing in school?

_____
2. Has child ever been retained in grade? _____
3. Is child receiving any supplementary help? _____
Which subjects? _____
4. Do you feel child is not working up to his/her potential (full ability) at school? _____
5. Does the child have a behavior problem at school? _____
At home? _____

If the answer is *yes* to any of the above questions:

6. Has the child ever been evaluated by a psychologist, or a professional other than the pediatrician?

_____

Are reports available? _____

Figure 21.2 Case history form 2.

Manual (DSM III-R) (34) of the American Psychiatric Association has identified a single syndrome, attention-deficit hyperactivity disorder (ADHD), 314.01, which includes all of the essential features of the disorder: inappropriate degrees of inattention, impulsiveness, and hyperactivity.

Three decades have passed since Kawi and Pasamanick (80) published their paper that associated pre- and perinatal disorders with reading and learning. This retrospective study compared the hospital records of 205 poor readers with those of 205 good readers for whom hospital records were also available. The mothers of 16.5 percent of the children who were poor readers had experienced two or more maternal complications during pregnancy or delivery, usually related to a reduction of oxygen supply to the fetus or neonate. Only 1.5 percent of the good readers had such a history. While the prevalence of prematurity in the group with reading disorders was 11.6 percent, only 4.6 percent of the good readers were premature ($p < .05$). Toxemia, hypertension, and marked edema are other pregnancy complications that have been reported by Kaffman, Sivah-Sher, and Carel (71). Like Kawi and Pasamanick, they concluded from their controlled study that pregnancy and birth complications increase the risk of central nervous system (CNS) damage and minimal brain dysfunction (MBD). (See D. C. Creevy for excellent chapter on this subject [26].)

Low birth weight (LBW) is an important parameter, because it provides one of the few available objective measurements at birth. Defined as a birth weight less than 2500 g, it applies to both premature and full term infants. Birth weight may be appropriate for gestational age (AGA) or small for gestational age (SGA). Low birth weight has been associated with lower IQ scores (36, 131). Taub, Goldstein, and Caputo (127) observed that while WISC-R verbal IQ scores for children with a history of prematurity were not significantly different from those of children born at term, performance IQs were significantly lower. Performance subtests requiring visu-

ally mediated behavior were particularly affected. Poor visually mediated functioning and perceptual organization were similarly noted on the Visual-Motor Gestalt Test. It is of further interest that a double gradient exists: for a given birth weight (under 2000 g), the lower the socioeconomic status the lower the IQ; and for a given socioeconomic level (particularly below middle class) as the birth weight drops below 2000 g, the IQ also drops (36). Cohen (20) postulates that social factors are more important than biologic insult. Because early motor abnormalities may be an indication of problems of CNS integrity, it is significant that the LBW group typically score lower on motor development both in infancy and in preschool years than the control group (20). Not all children in the LBW group, however, are learning disabled.

Low birth weight has also been attributed to maternal cigarette smoking during pregnancy. Cigarette smoking during pregnancy has been associated with specific decrements in reading and arithmetic, reduced IQ, learning disorders, hyperactivity, impulsivity, and neurologic soft signs during childhood (17, 70).

Although the average optometrist is not likely to treat a dysmorphic, retarded child showing the pattern of growth characteristic of fetal alcohol syndrome, it is probable that she or he will see children whose maternal history includes moderate alcohol use. Although there are no controlled research studies of this group that reveal a definite cause-and-effect relationship with learning disabilities, "there is ample evidence of the adverse impacts of both alcohol and nicotine on the fetus to support the surgeon general's recommendation that women not drink and smoke during pregnancy" (123, 125). Discreet inquiries concerning these two risk factors should be made when completing the prenatal history.

Perinatal complications focus on conditions that may contribute to fetal hypoxia; they include prolonged labor, difficult delivery, and cyanosis. While 25 percent of Hoffman's (63) population of failing students were products of difficult deliveries, only 1.5 percent of the normally achieving students were so identified. Similarly, 11 percent of the LD students had a history of cyanosis, but only 0.5 percent of the better students. Prolonged labor was reported in 10 percent of the poorer students' births, compared to 0.5 percent of the academically normal children.

Postnatal conditions that appear more frequently in the LD population include convulsions, concussions, dehydration, prolonged high temperature, hypoxia, and chronic ear infections. Any medical episode involving hypoxia or cerebral trauma increases the risk for learning disability. Neonatal sucking and swallowing difficulties (27) sometimes produce psychological tensions between mother and child. In addition to the potential nutritional considerations, the problem may be a harbinger of a subsequent articulation problem.

In recording the case history, optometrists should always think of motor performance in terms of age-expected performance. That is, how do most children perform at a particular age? For example, if 95 percent of the children at a given age are able to creep spontaneously on all fours, then the small group who drag a leg or push themselves across the room in a sitting position is demonstrating behavior that deviates from the norm. Cross-gait creeping requires bilateral integration and cephalocaudal coordination. The exact age at which unaided walking begins is not always predictive of a motor maturational lag, provided the child took a few steps by 15 months and walked unassisted by 18 months (51). Most children walk at least a few steps by 13 months. Persistent delays in creeping and walking suggest the presence of a neurologic deficit. On the other hand, some children who are hyperactive in the primary grades began to walk (and run) at age 10 months. Comparing the case histories of 100 LD children with 200 children who did not exhibit learning problems, Hoffman (63) reported late, abnormal, or no creeping in 50 percent of the LD group but only in 1.7 percent of the normally achieving children.

While 26 percent of the LD children walked late (after 18 months), just 1 percent of those with satisfactory school performance were delayed.

Gross motor performance of children in kindergarten and grade one is of special interest to the optometrist, as children who are experiencing academic difficulties in grade two often report a history of delayed gross motor skills such as skipping, climbing, and running. Clumsiness and poor balance and coordination are also mentioned frequently. A lag in fine motor development is of great concern, because integrative skills that require the coordination of sensory and motor skills are involved. For example, a child who cannot button his coat, tie his shoelaces, or cut with a scissors is suspect, as these are tactile-visual and sensorimotor tasks that require visual feedback. When a child has persistent gross and fine motor difficulties that are not easily remediated, consultation with a pediatric neurologist experienced in examining LD children should be considered.

Although it is the unique functional qualities of the visual system that make reading possible, the definition of learning disabilities supports the hypothesis that the constituents of learning also involve a great deal of speech and language. It is not unexpected, therefore, that the prevalence of delayed speech (dyslalia) in studies of dyslexic and LD children has been reported to vary between 30 and 40 percent (83). The ability of the child to use two consecutive words to communicate, such as "baby ball" when asking for the ball, should be evident between 18 and 24 months. Sometimes, speech is delayed until 30 months, but if the child then speaks in paragraphs, the delay is acceptable. On the other hand, some children begin to speak at age 26 months but are difficult to understand until age 4 years.

The ability to be understood by others without undue effort requires normal articulation skills. Of the 499 subjects tested by Klasen (83), 22 percent showed speech defects. Hallgren (55) identified speech defects in 41 percent of the boys and 32 percent of the girls who were slow readers. Combining delayed and abnormal speech, Hoffman (63) found 70 percent of the failing students were affected, but only 4.5 percent of the passing students. Case History 2 (see Fig. 21.2) provides a simple test of echolalia using the words animal, hospital, and spaghetti (112) that is frequently helpful in evaluating children in kindergarten and the primary grades. Repeating each word several times may not only reveal articulation difficulties but also tests for speech blocking and overload. Animal may become *aminal,* hospital becomes *hopsibul,* and spaghetti after a few repetitions becomes *bisghetti.* DeHirsch (30, 31), Jansky (31), Langford (31), and Ingram (65) also observed that healthy children of average intelligence who showed delayed speech development would later have more difficulty learning to read and spell than a comparable group of children without delayed speech development.

Speaking vocabulary and syntactical development during the primary grades, respectively, often provide measures of the child's acquired and innate language development. A child's potential to learn to read must depend to some extent on the vocabulary he has learned to use (acquired) and brings to the task. In addition, superimposed on a child's innate language capacity is some amount of learned intrinsic structure of the grammatical system of the language (48). Although not all children who have good vocabularies and speak grammatically become excellent readers, the absence of these skills is a handicap and impairs the ability to learn to read. That is, good semantic and syntactical skills are necessary but not sufficient to learn how to read.

A complete case history should include some information about the development of laterality and lateral awareness. As it is customarily measured, laterality involves motor processes. Whether a child is left- or right-handed or mixed presumably is determined by which cerebral hemisphere is dominant. The results of research, however, are not conclusive. Belmont and Birch (5) report that boys who were retarded in reading did not

differ significantly in any type of mixed hand-eye dominance from normal readers of the same age. Further, within each group no consistent relationship between lateral preferences and level of reading performance was found. Lyle (88) also failed to find a relation between lateral dominance and mixed hand-eye dominance on the one hand and reading ability on the other. In discussing asymmetries in lateral preference, Hynd and Cohen (64) conclude, "Certainly, an argument can be made that deficient right-handed performance or lateralization to the left hand may reveal underlying damage to the cerebral cortex. Such a conclusion, however, cannot be made on the basis of handedness observation data or performance on a handedness questionnaire, as some would advocate" (p. 116). Ingram and Reid (66), on the other hand, reporting on their study of 65 boys, 6 to 15 years old, observed that 71 percent of the subjects and 30 percent of their parents were ambidexterous. Testing 9-year-olds, Harris (57) reported 8 percent of unselected school children and 25 percent of reading-disabled clinic children demonstrated mixed hand dominance ($p < .01$).

After establishing that there is no significant difference in hand dominance between normal and retarded readers, Belmont and Birch (5) investigated right-left discrimination and lateral awareness, which are sensory functions. Using Piaget's (100) protocol of right-left awareness (Fig. 21.3) they were able to test the child's ability to make left-right discriminations on his own body and on that of the examiner who was facing him. The last two of the six conditions in Figure 21.3 require an awareness of object relations in space. When 50 normal readers were compared with 150 retarded readers, the responses of the normal readers were superior to the retarded readers' on all six tasks. When comparing performance on the first four items (the items that they would have been expected to pass at their age), the achievement differences were statistically significant at the $p < .01$ level.

In summary, although mixed laterality did not consistently serve to distinguish be-

Directions: All responses are recorded and any numbered group is scored as correct only when all of its component parts are answered appropriately.

Right-Left Awareness Items

1. Show me your right hand. _____ Now show me your left hand. _____ Show me your right leg. _____ Now show me your left leg. _____

2. (E sits opposite S) Show me my right hand _____ Now my left _____ Show me my right leg. _____ Now my left leg _____

3. (Place coin on table left of a pencil in relation to S.) Is the pencil to the right or to the left? _____ And the penny, is it to the right or to the left? _____ (Have S go around to the opposite side of table and repeat questions.) Is the pencil to the right or to the left? _____ And the penny, is it to the right or to the left? _____

4. (S is opposite E; E has a coin in right hand and a bracelet (or watch) on left arm.) You see this penny. Have I got it in my right hand or in my left? _____ And the bracelet, is it on my right arm or my left? _____

5. (S is opposite three objects in a row: a pencil to the left, a key in the middle, and a coin to the right.) Is the pencil to the left or to the right of the key? _____ Is the key to the left or to the right of the penny? _____ Is the penny to the left or to the right of the pencil? _____ Is the penny to the left or to the right of the key? _____

6. (S is opposite three objects in a row: a key to the left, a piece of paper in the middle, and a pencil to the right. The following instructions are given to S: "Listen carefully, I am going to show you three things for a very little while. You must look at them very carefully, and then afterwards tell me from memory how the things are arranged." Ready. The three objects were presented to S for 30 seconds, and then covered, and he was then asked the following questions.) Is the key to the left or the right of the piece of paper? _____ Is the key to the left or the right of the pencil? _____ Is the paper to the left or the right of the key? _____ Is the paper to the left or the right of the pencil? _____ Is the pencil to the left or the right of the key? _____ Is the pencil to the left or the right of the paper? _____

Expected Responses:

Age	Items Passed
5	1
6	1
7	1 and 3
8	1, 2, 3, 4
9	1, 2, 3, 4
10	1, 2, 3, 4
11	1, 2, 3, 4, 5
12	1, 2, 3, 4, 5, 6

Figure 21.3 Right-left awareness items

tween good and poor readers in the studies reported, developmental expecteds do exist; most 6-year-olds have established handedness (52). When an 8-year-old fails to show consistent hand preference, a maturational lag in the development of lateral preference clearly exists. Left-right awareness and a good sense of directionality in space are apparently more important attributes of learning to read. Completing Case History 2 (see Fig. 21.2) provides the optometrist with an appreciation of the child's development in these areas.

LD children are continually frustrated by being asked to perform at a more advanced level than their current capabilities. Temper tantrums and other forms of compensatory acting out are not unusual. These demands are not only academic but also include developmental behavior (Sit still!), physical coordination (Don't be so clumsy!), and social grace (Look at a person when he talks to you!). The frustration emanates from the child's inability to answer: I would if I could.

In some instances the learning disability is the result of a hereditary predisposition (see below.). It is, therefore, proper to inquire whether other family members are learning disabled. Problems involving members of the immediate family are of special interest. Of course, such information could document either genetic or social transmission, since there are two possible explanations: (1) genetic transmission of an organic neurologic deficit and (2) transmission by common environmental influences such as social or educational values in the home that are not conducive to learning (128).

Color vision is included because many of the workbooks used by LD children are color coded. For example, consonants may be red, middle vowels blue, and final vowels (final *e* rule) yellow. An unrecognized deficit in color vision could impede the child's progress.

The brief case history forms enable the optometrist to complete a visual, behavioral, developmental, and educational profile in about 15 minutes. The clinical impressions developed from the information are helpful in establishing a preliminary estimate of the nature and severity of the child's problem based on numerous and valid causal factors. The optometrist should not rely on a single-deficit diagnosis. Most LD children exhibit a cluster of developmental and behavioral signs. Often reports from other professionals who have seen the child are available; they should be read carefully prior to arriving at a diagnosis and treating the child.

GENETICS

> What is inherited is not this or that phenotypic "trait" or "character," but a genotypic potentiality for an organism's developmental response to its environment. Given a certain genotype and a certain sequence of environmental situations, the development follows a certain path. . . . The observed phenotypic variance has both a genetic and an environmental component (35).

Learning disabilities comprise a group of disorders with both genetic and environmental determinants. Careful correlation between genetic data and clinical findings can help achieve a more precise delineation of specific learning disabilities. Precision in diagnosis and classification adds to our understanding of the learning deficits that ultimately will enable the clinician to develop more effective preventive and remedial techniques (93). Optometrists, for example, should be especially interested in knowing whether the efficacy of optometric intervention in genetic dyslexia or learning disability is similar to the results obtained when a disorder is acquired.

One of the prime issues facing the genetic studies of learning disabilities is that of phenotype definition. Presently, the resulting heterogeneous population of subjects hinders any research that intends to treat LD children as a homogeneous, undifferentiated group. Smith (113) concludes that such inability to determine the phenotype makes any effort to elucidate underlying genotypes futile. The ultimate goal of genetic studies, therefore, must be to refine the definition of the phenotypes to get closer to the actual genetic effects.

Family studies to elucidate the genetics of a disorder are further complicated by reduced penetrance (not everyone with genotype exhibits phenotype), age of onset of disorder, and developmental changes in the manifestations of the disorder. The ideal phenotype (marker phenotype) for family studies is one that is fully penetrant, manifests early in development, and persists in similar form throughout development (e.g., stuttering, dyslexia, and hyperactivity may show developmental remission).

An often cited early study by Hallgren (55) involved 112 families of dyslexic probands (affected subjects). Diagnosis of the 116 probands was preceded by educational, psychological, and neurologic evaluations. The results revealed a significant sex difference, 89 boys and 27 girls ($p < .001$). Personal histories, school records, and, for some, a simple word reading test were used to classify parents and siblings. Of the 391 parents and siblings, 160 were identified as dyslexic. In 90 families one parent was designated; both parents were identified in three families; and neither parent was affected in nineteen. The data suggest an autosomal dominant mode of inheritance. Since it is often the case that father and son are affected, X-linked transmission is precluded. The autosomal dominant mode of transmission also applies to dyslexia subgroups. For example, visual-predominant and auditory-predominant dyslexia were more evident in the families of the dyslexics who showed each of these characteristics (96). Poor reading parents who are either dysphonetic or dyseidetic are more likely to have children who are poor readers and make similar spelling errors (45). These findings suggest that there are also genetically distinct subgroups of dyslexia (93).

By taking advantage of the uniqueness of twins, the investigator has a natural experiment in which the degree of environmental similarity is equal and the degree of genetic similarity of the two types of co-twins can be reasonably estimated and compared. (An essential part of any twin research design is determining the zygosity of same-sex twin pairs.) If a genetic contribution exists, it may be expected that the correlation for the monozygotic pairs would be greater than the correlation for the dizygotic pairs and the dizygotic twins should be more alike than two subjects chosen at random. A crucial assumption of this twin model is the equality of the environmental covariance for both types of twin pairs (59).

A longitudinal study by Matheny, Dolan, and Wilson (89) confirmed that the likelihood of both twins in a pair being reported to have academic problems was markedly increased if the twins were identical than if they were fraternal ($p < .001$) or same-sex fraternal ($p < .01$). Furthermore, the identical twins were more concordant than same-sex fraternal twins for all of the preschool behaviors such as activity level, distractibility, and feeding and sleeping problems. While 76 percent of the monozygotic pairs were concordant for poor academic performance, the dizygotic twins showed a pairwise concordance rate of 20 percent (2 in 10). None of the opposite-sex dizygotic twin pairs were concordant. Wender (128) contended that other random biologic factors are operating in conjunction with the genetic predisposition of the children. For example, compared to singletons, twins are more liable to biologic insults in the prenatal and perinatal periods.

Harris' (58) study of 108 twin first- and second-graders lends further support to familialty for reading achievement ($r = 0.93$ for the composite reading test score) for the monozygotic pairs while still maintaining a significant genetic contribution for the dizygotic pairs ($r = 0.59$). The dizygotic pairs, however, showed greater within-pair variations than the monozygotic pairs.

The genetic transmission of visual and perceptual deficits that have been associated with learning disabilities and dyslexia should be investigated with similar twin research designs. The hereditary component of intelligence, the high correlation between intelligence and reading, and the probability that visual functional, perceptual, and attentional disorders may have their own genetic models all tend to contribute to the outcome of genetic studies. Equally important, the results could be helpful in refining the definition of the phenotype.

While the twin studies are impressive, not *all* the cotwins of learning-disabled monozygotic twin children are affected. In addition to genetic factors, environmental influences also impair the ability of the child to respond to academic teaching. We are still dealing with a heterogeneous disability whose phenotype remains to be refined (see Chapter 5.)

NUTRITION

For poorer children are not merely born *into* poverty; they are born *of* poverty, and are thus at risk of defective development even before their birth. . . . A child born of such circumstances is likely to be smaller at birth than his more fortunate contemporaries and is more likely to die at birth or before his second year of life. . . . Throughout the preschool and school years the survivors are more likely to be more poorly fed and cared for in their homes, overexposed to disease in their communities, and the recipient of little or no medical supervision. The failure of such children in school is not only not a mystery but is virtually foreordained. Hence a serious attack on school failure must be an attack on the life conditions which characterize poverty wherever it is found (11).

For maturation and growth to be maintained, nutrition must be adequate. Abundant research exists that supports the hypothesis that malnutrition interferes with the orderly development of the physiologic and neurologic systems essential for normal growth and development. Also affected are intelligence, perceptual maturation, and school learning. While many of the studies have been carried out in Central and South America and Africa, there is increasing evidence that severe malnutrition exists in many parts of the United States (133). Optometrists who are interested in treating the child who has been identified as learning disabled should be knowledgeable about the influence of undernutrition on the development of the brain.

Two principal strategies have been used to study the consequences of poor nutrition. One approach is to infer a history of malnutrition from deviations of height for age. That is, short children have been assumed to be at greater risk nutritionally than taller ones in communities where malnutrition is endemic. Winick (133) suggests that even in its milder forms malnutrition during the growing period may stunt growth. An alternate and perhaps more frequently used strategy is follow-up studies several years after infants have been hospitalized for malnutrition. The identified children are compared to siblings close in age, classmates, or neighbors who do not have a similar history of malnutrition but who reside in communities where the nonnu-

tritional social and economic variables are equally hostile.

A study conducted in Jamaica by Hertzig and associates (60) typifies this experimental design. They concluded that children who have experienced severe malnutrition in the first 2 years of life have statistically lower intelligence at school age than their siblings and classmates. No association between intellectual level and the ages at which the children were hospitalized for the treatment during the first 2 years of life was revealed by the study. Brain vulnerability, therefore, is not limited to the first year of life. Axonal branching, dendritic elaboration, and synaptic formation, other aspects of nervous system growth, have a developmental course that is not restricted to early infancy.

Cravioto and DeLicardie (24) cite a number of studies that revealed significant differences in performance between malnourished and matched controls involving intersensory development (19, 25). They also report that tall children (upper quartile of height) performed at a higher level of competence on tests of intersensory integration than stunted children (lower quartile). Of special interest to the optometrist is the implication that functional lags could result from mild to moderate degrees of protein-calorie malnutrition and may not be limited to the extremely severe cases. Serial studies of sensorimotor development have also shown that as recovery from malnutrition takes place developmental quotients, which are much lower than those obtained in nonmalnourished children of similar age and social class, increase in most patients. Champakam's malnourished subjects were also more retarded in perceptual skills and abstracting ability.

Winick (133) and other investigators remind us that if strict scientific standards are applied to many of the studies relating malnutrition to intelligence, language development, neurointegrative skills, perceptual development, and learning, many faults could be found. On the other hand, we are working with a population of persons for whom chronic malnutrition is the norm and survival in a poverty-stricken milieu few of us can imagine is the primary goal in life. Within this framework, the evidence that implicates malnutrition, either alone or in conjunction with a poor socioeconomic environment, appears to be overwhelming.

To what extent can the optometrist who includes nutritional counseling in his clinical practice profit from the experience of Winick, Cravioto, Birch, and others? Although there is no shortage of evidence of the impact of severe malnutrition on the developing brain and neurointegrative systems, there is, in fact, a dearth of systematic investigations relating visually related learning disorders to the typical case of undernutrition seen in an optometrist's office.

Practitioners of holistic optometry, such as Kavner (79), suggest that nutritional deficits may be the cause of blurring when reading, photophobia, and reduced visual skills such as tracking, accommodation, and ocular fusional reserves. Kappel (75) sums up the viewpoint of the optometrists engaged in nutritional counseling: "Nutrition blends very well with the behavioral vision philosophy. We must look at the whole person. . . . We should all be aware of how nutrition affects visual performance." Although the clinical reports are encouraging, controlled studies to validate the procedures are needed.

References to orthomolecular medicine are often cited in articles prepared by behavioral optometrists. According to Alan Cott (23), "In the orthomolecular approach, we are basically correcting an imbalance of brain chemistry that does not exist among other children." Sometimes referred to as a megavitamin regimen, the program includes high doses of vitamins and minerals and the elimination of starches, sugar, and artificial flavors and colors from the diet. Cott summarizes case histories of LD children whose school performances have improved dramatically as a result of his program.

The numerous case histories of LD children who have been helped by nutritional counseling lend support to the importance of treating the child as well as the problem. For example, Baker (2) investigated nutritional substances that were lacking as well as those present in excess in a dyslexic sixth-grade boy. Improvement of the boy's schoolwork followed the correction of the deficits and excesses in his diet. On a larger scale, Benton and Roberts (6) conducted a double blind study of 90 British school children aged 12 and 13 years. A multivitamin and mineral supplement or a placebo was administered for 8 months to 60 of the children. The supplement group, but not the placebo group or the remaining 30 who took no tablets, showed a significant increase in nonverbal intelligence.

Fifteen years has elapsed since Feingold (43) wrote a preliminary report suggesting the effect of salicylates, food colorings, and additives on hyperactivity and learning disabilities in children. The following year Feingold (44) postulated that hyperactive children can be helped without drugs. He estimated that 5 million children in the United States suffer from *hyperkinesis-learning disability* (H-LD). A diet was recommended that excluded salicylates and *all foods* and *all drugs* that are artificially flavored and colored. Feingold's initial presentations were criticized by physicians as being too anecdotal, but this did not discourage parents' groups across the country from forming chapters of the new Feingold Association. Feingold alleged that 48 percent of the children on his diet showed improvement, and in about two thirds of this group, the improvement was dramatic. This figure was about the same as that reported from the use of psychostimulant medication (see below).

Feingold was ambiguous on a number of points. For example, was he dealing with an allergic or a toxic reaction? How did he define the hyperkinetic syndrome? What was the role of salicylates, a substance whose importance Feingold was reconsidering?

A group of investigators headed by Conners (22) tested Feingold's hypothesis using a double-blind experimental design. Although they voiced certain reservation, they confirmed Feingold's hypothesis. Diets of the 68 children were carefully monitored. The Conners Ten-Item Parent Questionnaire of hyperactive behavior was used in this and subsequent studies (Fig. 21.4). The investigators' conclusions were as follows:

> The results of this study strongly suggest that a diet free of most natural salicylates, artificial flavors, and artificial colors reduces the perceived hyperactivity of some children suffering from hyperkinetic impulse disorder. Teachers who observed the children over a 12-week period without knowledge of when the child started his diet and without knowledge of the fact that there were two diets which were employed, rated the children as less hyperactive while the children were on

the diet recommended by Feingold ($p < .005$).

A second study was conducted by Williams and his associates (132), who investigated the relative effects of drugs and diet on hyperactive behavior. In this study stimulant medications (see below) were more effective than diet in reducing hyperactive behavior. As in the previous study the observations by teachers in school were more positive than observations by parents at home. When the children were receiving the challenge food, their behavior in the classroom was more hyperactive when they ate cookies with artificial colors than when they ate cookies with-

	Degree of Activity			
	None	Just a Little	Pretty Much	Very Much
1. Restless or overactive				
2. Excitable, impulsive				
3. Disturbs other children				
4. Fails to finish things (s)he starts; short attention span				
5. Constantly fidgeting				
6. Inattentive, easily distracted				
7. Demands must be met immediately; is easily frustrated				
8. Cries often and easily				
9. Mood changes quickly and drastically				
10. Temper outbursts, explosive and unpredictable behavior				
Scoring factor	0	1	2	3

Score: 15 or less: Normal
16–20: Suspected hyperactivity
21–25: Hyperactive
26–30: Serious problem

Figure 21.4 Conners' abbreviated symptom questionnaire.

out artificial colors. Concerning the K-P diet, the investigators concluded that a diet free of artificial flavors and colors reduces symptoms of *some* hyperactive children. The task is now to find ways to identify which hyperactive children are most likely to respond to diet and to have them participate in further clinical evaluation of the diet (132).

Harley and his coinvestigators (56) obtained teacher ratings, objective classroom and laboratory observational findings, and other psychological measures on 36 school-aged hyperactive boys under experimental and control diet conditions. Laboratory observations did not support the parents' behavioral ratings, which indicated a positive response to the experimental diet. The authors further noted,

> Nevertheless, objectivity and completeness in reporting our data require us to repeat our finding that ten of ten mothers and four of seven fathers of the preschool sample rated their children's behavior as improved on the experimental (K-P or Feingold) diet.

More recently Kavale and Forness (78) reviewed 23 studies of primary research investigating the Feingold hypothesis using the techniques of metaanalysis. They concluded that children placed on the Feingold K-P diet were better off than only 55 percent of control subjects at the end of treatment. The child placed on the Feingold K-P diet may exhibit slight improvement in hyperactivity, but attention and learning disability revealed no treatment effects.

If optometry is to continue to develop its role in nutritional counseling as an adjunct to correcting vision deficiencies, optometrists must also accept the responsibility of standardizing and validating their procedures. This research necessarily must be an interdisciplinary effort using controlled studies. Individual cases without controls can be misleading. We must become expert at understanding to what extent nutritional deficits interfere with visual behavior and divert physical energy and attention from educational pursuits. The optometrist should not only address the undernourished child whose visual system may be performing sub-

optimally but should also participate in community service activities that have as their goal the amelioration of nutrition deficiencies that lead to school failure.

VISUAL ACUITY, REFRACTION, AND BINOCULAR VISION

Visual acuity, hyperopia, myopia, astigmatism, and anisometropia are the most prominent areas of interest that have been addressed by investigators. (For a complete exposition of the topics discussed in this section, see Grisham and Simons [54] and Simons and Grisham [111]). Although some of the research relating refractive states to learning disabilities and reading disorders do not fulfill optimal scientific design criteria, a discussion that reviews a cross-section of the existing studies does provide students, clinicians, and researchers with a useful overview.

Visual Acuity

As might be expected, no significant differences in the mean level of distance visual acuity exist between normal and disabled readers. A number of investigators have found that normally achieving readers and those included in an unselected population show patterns of (single-eye) distance visual acuity similar to those of poor readers (1, 12, 37, 39, 67, 121). There is no intent to imply, however, that a child with a significant refractive state who is attending the primary grades, when considerable instruction takes place at the chalkboard, would not be handicapped in the classroom. Jackson and Schye (67) observe that children often learn to compensate with "normalizing" efforts such as changing seat position, copying from an adjacent classmate's paper, and squinting or straining. Therefore, one cannot always rely on subjective complaints from the child.

Refractive States

Although no consensus exists, there appears to be sufficient evidence to support the contention that there is a relationship between type of refractive state and academic performance, especially reading. Eames, for example, reported in his earlier study (37) of 114 reading-disabled students and 143 unselected subjects that 43 percent of the reading-disabled had hyperopia but only 26 percent of the unselected group. In a subsequent investigation (39) that included 1000 reading failures and 150 unselected subjects, hyperopia (1 D or more) was again present in 43 percent of the reading-disabled group but in just 13 percent of the unselected group. The higher prevalence of hyperopia obtained by Eames in the reading-disabled groups is indeed reasonable. Hyperopia is more difficult to detect with the Snellen test, which is used so frequently in schools as the sole method of vision screening. If the referral criterion is 20/30 or 20/40, it is possible that the child is compensating for 3 D or more of hyperopia, which may represent as much as 6 D of accommodation at the reading distance. As we shall see subsequently, this burden could translate binocularly into a significant amount of esophoria at near with depressed fusional divergence and a degraded accommodative-convergence relationship. These findings are likely to cause intermittent blurred vision, headaches, and fatigue during reading and close work, which may be mistaken for a short attention span. The child also becomes conditioned to put off studying and in some cases develops an aversion to reading and other near point activities. For LD children who are not especially motivated to learn to read, this symptom complex is a serious impediment.

Unlike hyperopia, myopia is usually not congenital, but strong hereditary tendencies do exist. Children with mild or moderate (up to −3.00 DS) myopia usually have no difficulty seeing at the reading distance, but they are handicapped without glasses when viewing the chalkboard or following a discussion that involves a visual aid. Developmental myopia may commence at about age 8 years and progress until age 15 or 16 years. Sometimes the progression begins after puberty and continues later. Whether or not myopia is

preventable or controllable once it is present is beyond the scope of this discussion.

Compared to hyperopia, the prevalence of myopia is quite different in reading-disabled students—3 percent in Eames' 1932 study and 4 percent in 1948 (37, 39). Young (136) reported statistically significantly higher reading scores ($p < .05$) for subjects with myopia than for those with hyperopia. It is of special interest that no significant difference was measured between the two groups on a parallel achievement test administered orally. This would seem to indicate that although myopic students often do better on tests requiring a visual input, they are not necessarily more intelligent, as there is no significant difference when a test is presented orally. Earlier Hirsch (62) also observed that differences of intelligence between hyperopia and myopia appeared to be a function of the mode of presentation, written or oral. Since most LD children, both hyperopic and myopic, have problems in reading, only individually administered oral intelligence tests are valid.

When comparing the difference between chronologic age and reading age of grade 4 and 5 failed readers and successful ones grouped according to refractive condition, Eames (40), in a controlled study, observed that there were practically no differences among the successful students, regardless of refractive state. Among the failed readers, however, the hyperopic ones were considerably farther behind the passing students than those with emmetropia or myopia. All of the subjects had a complete eye examination.

The evidence extant supports the contention that providing a LD child with the appropriate lens correction may indeed have a salutary effect on academic progress. Vision screening has its value in identifying children who should be referred for a complete eye examination (85); however, even a complete vision screening may not probe the affected functions among LD children. Robinson and Huelsman concluded, "When scores of high and low achievers were compared, only tests of binocular functions (e.g., *near phoria, divergence,* and *convergence*) not included in commercial batteries distinguished the two groups consistently" (102). That hyperopia and binocular incoordination are characteristic of poor readers was confirmed by Robinson in a subsequent study in 1968 (104).

Binocular Vision

Although it is not always possible to separate all of the parameters when performing research on LD children (a designation whose boundaries have not been accurately defined) the overall research picture supports the hypothesis that binocular anomalies are implicated in the reading and learning problems of children. Eames (39) reported 33 percent of 1000 reading failures measured 6 PD or more exophoria compared to 22 percent of the unselected group ($n = 150$). Fusion deficiencies were 22 percent greater among the reading failures. Similarly, 76 percent of the 41 poor readers compared to 62 percent of the 200 good readers in Bilka's (12) study were exophoric.

Robinson's noteworthy volume *Why Pupils Fail in Reading* (103) provides us with the results of a well-planned interdisciplinary study. Thirty children between the ages of 6 and 16 years whose mean reading retardation was 3.95 years were evaluated. Many of her findings are relevant to the present discussion: 74 percent of the 27 subjects tested had significant phorias at the reading distance, 12 with esophoria and eight with exophoria. Near convergence and divergence findings were reported to be inadequate in 52 percent of the cases. Twenty-four percent were unable to attain a near point of convergence of 4 inches or less. Overall visual anomalies were found in 73 percent of the 22 cases that were studied fully but were considered to be contributing causes of reading failure in only 50 percent of these cases. Significant binocular incoordinations were reported in 48 percent of the cases examined by the participating ophthalmologists.

Park and Burri (97, 98) selected 225 children in grades one through eight, at random in order to study the relationship between reading achievement and eye conditions and to analyze the effect of various eye abnormalities on reading. Initially (98) they reported that 69 percent of the group were exophoric, 34 percent were esophoric, and 44 percent had weak prism vergence (ductions). They concluded that abnormal peripheral ocular variations such as were considered in the study were invariably concomitants in direct ratio to abnormal reading skill or efficiency and were quite constant throughout the grade levels. In a follow-up study (97) they reported correlations between visual functions and reading scores that were based on mental age expectancies (MAE). Although total eye score (from 14 separate findings) showed a correlation of $r = 0.465$ with reading scores (MAE), the correlation was just $r = 0.161$ when using ordinary grade equivalents. Other MAE correlations were: reading and eye scores of those with exophoria, $r = 0.631$ and with esophoria, $r = 0.422$. The correlation between reading and total duction score was $r = 0.647$. The authors observed that the greater the reading ability, the fewer the abnormal eye conditions. It is not usually prudent, though, to consider the vision problem as the sole cause of a reading disorder; however, the impact of correcting for mental age is indeed significant.

Bettman and his associates (7) compared 47 dyslexic readers with 58 good readers of the same age and grade. Two important differences in visual functioning between the groups were reported: "Forty-two percent of the dyslexic children had foveal suppression detected by the 4 D prism test at distance or near point, compared to 9 percent of the controls. This difference is highly significant statistically ($\chi^2 > 14$). . . . Fifty-two percent of dyslexic children showed gross jerkiness of the eyes during attempts to follow a pencil tip moved along a diagonal line. Only 11 percent of the controls had such jerkiness. The difference between the two groups was readily apparent to the observer and is highly statistically significant ($\chi^2 = 6.9$). This may be another manifestation of defective fine motor coordination" (7).

Norn, Rindziunski, and Skydsgaard (95)

found significantly more dyslexics (15) than controls (3) who presented with latent strabismus. Most of their other findings were negative, except for the presence of exophoria greater than 6 PD. They concluded that, although the evidence in their study does not suggest that vision defects bear a causal relation to specific dyslexia, the condition may be intensified when vision anomalies are present, thereby rendering reading extremely difficult.

There is abundant evidence (38, 41, 107, 124) to support the existence of a disproportionate prevalence of hyperopia and binocular dysfunctions in children with learning and reading disorders. Although in some instances the vision problems may be primary in the development of the learning disability (e.g., 7 D uncorrected hyperopia), in many cases they are contributory, often making it profoundly difficult for LD persons to respond to educational intervention. The effort required to maintain clear, single binocular vision serves not as essential background in the organization of the visual system when reading but as a displacement stimulus resulting in the disorganization of the visual-cognitive response. Fortunately, ample research exists to support the efficacy of optometric vision therapy to improve specific visual functions such as convergence, accommodation, ocular motility, and the range and quality of ocular fusion (122).

Finally, much of the research reviewed attempts to equate reading and learning disorders with a single visual entity. For example, Rosenbloom (105) found that the degree of aniseikonia does not significantly correlate with poor reading, but within the same monograph (104), the presence of hyperopia and binocular dysfunction was significantly related to reading performance in grades one through eight. Even within a single sensory system such as vision, the problems are multifaceted. Experienced clinicians are aware of the additive nature of the true relationships between visual factors and learning. Future researchers should recognize that we are dealing with a multidimensional model which requires for its solution multivariate analysis.

PERCEPTUAL AND COGNITIVE DEVELOPMENT

Perception is the process of extracting and organizing information from the environment. The implication is that it is an *active process* of searching for, selecting, and organizing stimuli from the immediate surroundings and that these acts occur in relation to specific purposes or tasks (4). Perceptions, which are more complex than sensations, are the product of previous organization, experience, and elaboration of the nervous system (3). Forgus (49) reasoned that perception is the core process in the acquisition of cognition or knowledge. If we accept the premise that what one does about a problem depends on how the problem is conceptualized, then the theoretical rationales used in the treatment of LD children become very important.

Learning (and therefore learning disabilities) may occur at any or several of the following levels, according to Johnson and Myklebust (69): sensation, perception, imagery, symbolization and language, and conceptualization. Interruption of this hierarchy at any level may jeopardize functioning at more advanced levels. For example, an inability to perform at the visual perceptual level may affect visual memory (imagery), symbolization, and conceptualization. One can justifiably conceptualize perceptual-motor functioning as an active process amenable to therapy. The active searching movements of the eyes (86, 135) and the constant flow of afferent impulses to the brain during sensorimotor activities, as when writing or copying a geometric form, are just two examples. In writing, the child must recall each letter and must perform the task by executing a series of carefully but not too well-articulated motor movements. Visual feedback is required to guide the graphomotor activity. Good visual motor skills place a premium on the child's ability to perceive discrepancies and approximations in his own behavior in relation to a good model or plan. Gradually, with maturation and practice, writing becomes an automatic motor skill. It is important to differentiate between perceptual and perceptual motor functioning. Many children who lack the perceptual motor skills to reproduce the model correctly in a copy-form test are capable of selecting the failed items in a multiple choice situation. Visual perception of spatial position, spatial relations, and design forms is intact.

Visualization or imagery is another example of how a child depends on a different system of working zones (87) in the cerebral cortex than does an adolescent or adult. The young child thinks by recollecting, and his visualizations, memories, and perceptions are concrete. In adolescence, on the other hand, abstract thinking involves abstract visualization. That is, thinking by *recollecting* has developed into perceiving by *reflection*. Language, expressive and receptive, produces the formation of an auditory or visual image of an object or symbol represented by a word. Eidetic imagery enhances a child's retrieval capacity and is an important attribute in vocabulary development, mathematics, and spelling. LD children often experience deficits in imagery.

Symbolization and language form a bridge between perception and conception. Language facilitates logical thinking. Language is almost always involved in conceptualizing a task and in following directions. Children with learning disabilities often have greater difficulties naming pictured objects, which may suggest to the optometrist the presence of *dysnomia*, an expressive language disorder (33).

Conceptualization depends on the orderly maturation of perceptual skills, imagery, and symbolization and is the ultimate goal of thought and language. Concept formation may be impeded not only if there is a dysfunction at the level of conceptualization but also if one occurs at a prior level in the learning hierarchy. Although intervention is beyond the scope of this discussion, it should be stated that optometric therapy provides a viable therapeutic approach for the improvement of perceptual skills, visualization, and visual conceptualization (see Chapter 14).

Birch (8) postulated an orderly ontogenesis of sensory dominance from the proximoceptive input (gustatory, somatic, and tactual) of an infant and toddler to the teleoceptor control system (auditory and visual) of a 7-year-old child. He stated, "Reading disability may stem from the inadequate development of appropriate hierarchical organization of sensory systems and so, at least in part, be the product of the failure of visual system hierarchical dominance. . . . Failure for such dominance to occur will result in a pattern of functioning which is inappropriate for the development of reading skills" (8). Both the Divided Form Board test (119) and the tachistoscope (114) afford optometrists means of testing for the presence of visual dominance.

Another rationale stems from the analysis of intersensory processes that focus on auditory-visual integration. Sir Charles Sherrington (108) observed that, for sensory function, the principal strategy in the evolution of the central nervous system has not been the elaboration of new avenues of sense but rather the development of increased liaison among the existent major sensory input systems. The investigations of Birch and Belmont (9, 10) strongly suggested that the ability to treat auditory-visual patterned information as equivalent is one of the factors that differentiates good from poor readers. They postulated that reading involves not only the visual and auditory modalities but more importantly, the supramodal integration of the two. Solan and his colleagues (120) confirmed that the ability to equate a temporally distributed auditory stimulus to a spatially distributed visual response is, indeed, related to reading ability in the primary grades. Furthermore, there is a significant temporal-spatial relationship present within the visual modality: 58 percent of the variations in the cross-modal auditory-visual integration test (AVIT) may be explained by changes in temporal-spatial processing. One may also theorize that good temporal-spatial integration requires the degree of interhemispheric liaison that satisfies the cognitive demands of written and mental arithmetic. As we shall see, auditory-visual integration skills correlate significantly through grade five with reading and arithmetic.

If optometric vision therapy is to have a positive impact on learning, we must first understand how and why the developmental procedures of optometrists affect young patients in a way that results in improved academic response. Werner (130) distinguished between **growth** and **development.** While the former may represent merely the change one sees as a coral reef or stalagmite becomes larger, development implies an increased level of complexity. Sensory and motor development, according to Werner, progresses from a state of relative globality and lack of differentiation to a state of increased differentiation, articulation, and hierarchical integration.

Piaget (101) pursued the meaning of development one step further by introducing the concept of embryogenesis, which is concerned with the integration of the nervous system and mental functions. For Piaget, *development* means a total and spontaneous process in which each element of learning occurs as a function of total development. Development, therefore is **not** the sum of discrete learning experiences. Learning is a limited process, sometimes limited to a single structure, situation, or didactic point. Without the prior development of an operational framework, learning is achieved by external reinforcement and is more likely to be temporary. That is, learning in the absence of suitable developmental structures precludes assimilation and internalization, since the resulting associative learning does not result in generalization. After administering perceptual therapy, the optometrist asks, "What more complex behavior is this child now capable of performing?"

Jensen (68) also stressed the need to generalize when he defined readiness to learn (at any level) as the ability (1) to integrate subskills into a cognitive whole; (2) to generalize; (3) and to transfer previous learning to new learning. These three steps in perceptual therapy provide the LD child with an orderly therapeutic sequence applicable to improvement in classroom learning. Simultaneously, the child must learn to develop his own perception of his increasing mastery of the skills he is trying to acquire. Piaget suggested that this results in the reinforcement that produces *intrinsic motivation.* Procedures must also be included to teach the LD child to conceptualize the learning task and to grasp the aim of his efforts long before achieving mastery of the task.

Good reading requires both simultaneous and successive processing (29). Spatial perception has been identified with simultaneous processing and verbal skills with successive processing of information in serial order. In successive processing the stimuli are not totally surveyable or globally available at one point in time as they are in simultaneous processing. We most often think of reading comprehension as the ability to interpret successive elements of incoming information, and therefore we feel more comfortable with the substantial influence of verbal skills. On the other hand, the spatial skills provide a measure of the subject's ability to convert the consecutive presentation of the elements of a situation into a new quality of simultaneous perceptibility. Readers who lack this ability may have a good understanding of the meaning of individual words but may not grasp the meaning of the thought as a whole, such as the relationships in father's brother and brother's father (87).

Simultaneous and successive processing appear to be differentially related with respect to age-grade level in normally achieving students. In kindergarten and grade one, simultaneous processing skills are a necessary condition for learning whole words (119). By grade two, however, successive processing seems to be more important for the mastery of early decoding skills (28, 118). At higher levels when reading comprehension is more dependent upon conceptual-linguistic skills, simultaneous and successive processing are equally important. In grades four and five, 40 percent of the variations in reading vocabulary of normally achieving readers may be accounted for by variations in each, visual-spatial and verbal-successive factors (115). Other investigators have provided evidence that the two processing systems may also be differentially important with respect to achievement level: better readers tend to show higher levels of simultaneous processing than poor readers (28, 29).

The relative influences of simultaneous and successive processing are also evident when analyzing performance of normally achieving children in grades four and five in written and mental arithmetic. Spatial-simultaneous factors yield a statistically significantly higher positive correlation than verbal-successive skills with performance in written arithmetic. Sixty-seven percent of the variations in written arithmetic in these grades may be explained by variations in visual-spatial factors. On the other hand, successive skills appear to render a positive, but not statistically significantly higher, correlation with mental arithmetic than spatial skills (116).

Optometrists should be aware of the potential for treatment of visual and perceptual dysfunctions in children who are experiencing problems in reading and written and mental arithmetic. Both successive and simultaneous processing skills are amenable to training (76, 84). Furthermore, Krywaniuk's intervention encouraged the subjects to use the appropriate strategy, and they learned how to transfer the processing techniques to school achievement.

It is evident from this brief review that learning requires the development and application of many skills that are differentially important with respect to age-grade and achievement levels. For example, research involving multivariate analysis has revealed that variations in spatial perceptual skills account for more than 50 percent of the variations in learning readiness in kindergarten and reading vocabulary in grade one, but only 25 percent by the end of grade two (118, 119).

Perceptual therapy is a reasonable and viable approach to remediating perceptual deficits that have been shown to contribute to learning difficulties in children. Furthermore, studies demonstrate that the efficacy of a perceptual therapy program depends on a number of factors, including the following: (1) The subjects have identifiable perceptual deficits associated with their reading and learning disorders. (2) The perceptual therapy program is individualized. (3) The perceptual therapy must complement, not replace, reading instruction in a controlled study. (4) Therapists must be specially trained (117).

Optometrists in practice and in research are cautioned against conceptualizing and treating reading and learning problems in terms of a single-factor theory. Unidimensional conceptions of learning disabilities are narrow and incomplete and seem to reflect the professional backgrounds of the theorists (134). Problems of reading disabilities are so complex that no theory positing a unitary deficit hypothesis is acceptable (47). The interdisciplinary sample of studies discussed supports the hypothesis that both perceptual and verbal skills are correlated with early reading problems.

IMPULSIVITY AND REFLECTIVITY

Kephart (82) postulated that a closed system involving feedback control is operative in the perceptual process. Information from the output end of the system is oriented toward the input end and used for control (see Fig. 21.5). Such a system becomes its own control. In the perceptual process, this feedback output pattern becomes a part of the input. As the feedback reenters on the input end of the system, it alters the input pattern and thereby calls for a new cycle of the perceptual process. Thus, it is possible to generate an output pattern, drain most of it off in feedback for control purposes, and permit so little to continue to muscle response that no overt movement of the organism occurs. Input and output, therefore, should not be thought of as separate terms in an integrative system but rather as input-output, where input represents the perceptual process and output the motor response.

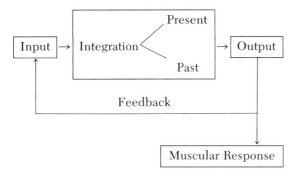

Figure 21.5   Diagram of feedback mechanisms in perception. (Reproduced from Kephart, NC: The Slow Learner in the Classroom. Columbus OH, Charles E Merrill, 1971)

When vision and perceptual therapy are administered patients who continue the perceptual process until a suitable perceptual-motor match has been made before a motor response occurs are identified as *reflective*. On the other hand, there are patients who have not developed the delay in response necessary for successful problem solving who are labeled *impulsive*. Impulsivity is especially evident among children who have been identified as learning disabled.

It is not surprising, therefore, that many LD children are characterized as having a tendency to act without forethought. Wender (128) defines the child's inability to inhibit the performance of an act long enough to become concerned about the immediate consequences of his behavior as *social impulsivity*. In discussing cognitive style, Kagan (73) notes that these children "select and report solution hypotheses quickly with minimal consideration for their probable accuracy. Other children, of equal intelligence, take more time to decide about the validity of solutions. The former group has been called impulsive, the latter reflective" (73). Reflectivity customarily improves with age and education in normally achieving children (14). They are constantly presented with situations involving response uncertainty and are required to make a response. The child must choose between answering quickly (quick

success) and the anxiety generated by the possibility of committing an error (not making a mistake). These two factors influence decision time and cognitive style. It is important that *anxiety over possible failure* be distinguished from *expectation of failure*, since they represent different mind sets. Children who repeatedly experience failure become habituated to failure and experience minimal anxiety from failure. On the contrary, they may answer rapidly without any expectation of success; this constitutes a special entity.

While there is general agreement about the meanings of the terms impulsivity and reflectivity, some questions have developed about the validity of the Matching Familiar Figures Test (13, 72, 73). (Further information concerning the Matching Familiar Figures test may be obtained by writing to: Jerome Kagan, Ph.D., Harvard University, Cambridge, MA 02138. For "misgivings" concerning the test, address: Jack Block, Ph.D., University of California, Berkeley, CA 94720.) In optometric terms, the MFFT is a form perception test that requires the subject to match a standard drawing of a familiar object to one of six similar variants, one of which is an exact reproduction. The test results are scored for errors and latency (time delay in responding). Impulsive children have short response times, with numerous errors, whereas reflective children have longer latency periods but fewer errors. When administered prior to and following training, this visual discrimination test provides a measure of any change in cognitive style that may be a result of the training. The therapist should observe the child's cognitive style whenever he is engaged in a testing or training situation.

Using three tests, the MFFT, a design recall test, and a haptic visual matching test, Kagan (72) found that first and second grade children with rapid response times and high error scores on visual matching problems made more errors reading English words than those with longer response latencies and low error scores. Messer (92) tested the stability of the cognitive disposition of primary-grade children to be impulsive or reflective over a $2\frac{1}{2}$-year period. The results revealed moderate but significant correlations ($r = 0.25$ to $r = 0.43$). Children who had failed a grade were found to possess verbal skills comparable to those of their peers but were considerably more impulsive at the start of grade one and again $2\frac{1}{2}$ years later. Cathcart and Liedke (18) cautioned teachers of mathematics not to require immediate and automatic responses from children who are learning number facts. Their data suggested that the children who achieve best are those who are more reflective and take longer to consider their responses. Reflective subjects, however, are not always superior performers. When the stimuli requires global as opposed to detailed processing, impulsive children were not only as accurate, but also faster, and consequently more efficient (137). When successful solutions could be reached employing either strategy, performance of impulsive children using a global strategy was equal to that of the reflective children using a detail strategy. The more frequent superiority of reflective children may be attributed to the fact that, in most instances of learning, detail analysis rather than global analysis is required.

There are certain obvious and significant implications for the optometrist who engages in visual and perceptual training. A number of studies support the hypothesis that cognitive tempo is modifiable. That is, processing strategies can be developed to modify the speed and accuracy of problem solving. Kagan, Pearson, and Welch (74) were successful in increasing response latencies by emphasizing inhibition of impulsive responses for 15 seconds without introducing other problem-solving strategies. Although the training produced response latencies that matched those of normal reflectives, the effect on error scores was minimal. This author's experience has been that the child adapts to delay training by delaying his or her response to the examiner after arriving at an instantaneous decision.

In a controlled study, Egeland (42) trained impulsive children not only to delay their responses but to use more efficient scanning techniques. Learning several detail-processing strategies, such as comparing the standard to all the variants and breaking the alternatives down into component parts, significantly reduced the number of errors on immediate and delayed post-tests.

Training impulsive children to talk to themselves, a program of self-verbalization, is an effective method of modifying behavior. Meichenbaum and Goodman (91) demonstrated the efficacy of cognitive self-instructional training in altering the behavior of children who have been labeled impulsive. The goals of the training procedures are "to develop for the impulsive child a cognitive style or learning set in which the child could 'size up' the demands of a task, cognitively rehearse, and then guide his performance by means of self-instructions, and when appropriate reinforce himself" (91). While appropriate "modeling" by the examiner was helpful in increasing the decision time, the combination of modeling plus self-instruction was most effective in altering the decision time and reducing the number of errors significantly on Kagan's MFF test. These procedures are of special interest to optometrists who treat children identified as LD. Vision and perceptual training tasks customarily do not include cognition (knowledge *that*), but developing metacognitive strategies of solving problems provides the learning-disabled child with an improved learning style, increased attention to detail, and a means by which the child manages his own thinking (90). Although "academic reflectivity" has been stressed, the effects of the training may be generalized and contribute to a reduction in asocial behavior.

PSYCHOLOGICAL FACTORS

The multidisciplinary nature of the treatment of learning disabilities was stressed in the introductory statement of this chapter. In most disciplines, the boundaries of the different professions are immediately evident. For example, the role of the endocrinologist or pediatric neurologist in providing medical guidance for an LD child is unambiguous.

This is not necessarily the case with the psychologists (clinical, neuro-, or experimental) and psychiatrists. Some diagnostic tests used by optometrists to evaluate visual dysfunctions are the same as or are parallel to the tests used by some psychologists and psychiatrists. Typical examples include: gross and fine motor development, sensorimotor integration, form perception and visual discrimination, visual memory, laterality and directionality, and visual reasoning. It is not unusual, however, for the psychological interpretation of the results to stress patient behaviors that are different from those probed by the optometrist. It would not be reasonable to suggest that a comprehensive psychological evaluation be performed prior to initiating optometric treatment with each LD child. Many children, however, have been "worked-up" either privately or in school prior to visiting the optometrist. Every effort should be made to secure the reports, and they should be reviewed carefully.

It has been stated that optometrists do not treat learning disabilities. Their therapeutic goal is to ameliorate visual and perceptual dysfunctions in children who have been identified as learning disabled. That is, the purpose of the therapy is to make the child more responsive to the educational efforts that are being provided, and in many cases the child does become more ready for learning. Unfortunately, some children do not make suitable progress in school although the child's educational program seems to be appropriate; and it is the responsibility of the optometrist to review the possible reasons. Assuming that the student is participating and cooperating in the office phase of the program, the child's teacher can be very helpful in providing additional information. Is the school providing the expected **individual** supplementary instruction in subjects where learning difficulties exist (e.g., reading, math, spelling)? Does the child reveal evidence of aberrant behavior in school? If the answer to the first question is no, arrangements should be made for private instruction to complement the optometric therapy until the school fulfills its obligations.

Often a consultation with the school psychologist is very helpful. A positive response to the second question suggests the potential for more complex problems. At this juncture, the optometrist should be concerned about whether the behavior is secondary to the learning disability because the child is failing and frustrated or whether there is a primary emotional disorder. In either case, the child should see a psychologist or psychiatrist. Gardner (50) recommends, "In my opinion, the treatment of these children involves four approaches: (1) medication, (2) education, (3) parental guidance, and (4) psychotherapy (in that order)." The critical question, according to Silver (110), is whether emotional, social, or family problems are *causing* the academic difficulty or are the *consequence* of the frustrations and failures brought on by academic difficulty. If the emotional, social, or family problems persist after dealing with issues 1, 2, and 3 above, then some form of psychotherapy may be needed.

The optometrist should be familiar with at least a few of the adaptive behaviors that children with learning disabilities develop.

Withdrawal Reaction By not participating in situations that can lead to failure or frustration, the child learns to avoid life experiences (such as reading and math) that are stressful. Sometimes the child reverts to inner fantasy. In either case, the withdrawn child is not available for learning.

Regressive Reaction To avoid the potential embarrassment of not being able to perform at an acceptable level, the child regresses to a less mature level of social and emotional development. Behaviors such as enuresis, baby talk, and silliness reappear. This adaptation helps to rationalize a decreased level of school performance.

Clowning Reaction When a mother describes symptoms that suggest that the child is clowning in school, the optometrist is probably dealing with a serious problem. Here, the child can rationalize that he is not learning because he chooses not to learn. Peer reinforcement is always available, as the lesson is disrupted. Teacher reinforcement may also be present if the child is asked to leave the room, especially if he or she will miss a turn to read. (For a more complete discussion of adaptive reactions, both acute and chronic, of LD children and their parents and siblings, the reader is referred to Gardner and Silver (50, 109, 120).

This brief review reinforces the concept that treating an LD child is a complex undertaking that often requires interdisciplinary cooperation. On the other hand, there are ways in which the optometrist can provide guidance to parents when minimal problems seem to exist. One such example is to provide parents with Wender's four simple rules for dealing with their child (128):

1. Establish a hierarchy of importance, distinguishing between misdemeanors and felonies. Parents must decide what is trivial, what is important, what is essential.
2. Decide in advance upon a plan for rewards and punishment. The rewards and punishment must be commensurate with the behavior. Also, it should be remembered that either provides attention; thus punishment is more rewarding than ignoring.
3. The one-time principle: By proscribing and prescribing behavior only once before punishing, the child is provided with a predictable environment.
4. Both parents must abide by a prescribed course of action.

Psychotherapy has a salutary effect on a child's performance in school and during training. Therapy that provides the child with additional ego strength counteracts some of the failure and frustration that have been experienced by the child. The optometrist can be helpful by sensitizing the child during perceptual and/or visual training to recognize his increasing mastery of the skills he is trying to acquire, providing reinforcement which can lead to intrinsic motivation. On the other hand, compliments that are not based on concrete accomplishments can be ego debasing. Visual and perceptual training programs, therefore, should be planned to be success oriented.

PSYCHOSTIMULANTS

What are psychostimulants? When should they be prescribed for children who have been identified as learning disabled? The psychostimulants that are prescribed most frequently include methylphenidate (Ritalin), dextroamphetamine (Dexedrine), and to a lesser extent pemoline (Cylert). While specific doses are beyond the scope of this discussion, it should be emphasized that compliance is important if the child is to benefit from the medication. The action of the drugs has been described as paradoxical, because of the salutary effects of a stimulant on hyperactivity, distractibility, and impulsivity. While the explanation remains unclear, when effective, the medication inhibits motor activity, improves attention and concentration, and reduces impulsivity. More acceptable social behavior, increased sensitivity to reward and punishment, and improved goal-directed behavior are also reported.

Occasionally there are side effects. Loss of appetite is sometimes experienced initially, but normal eating habits tend to return within a few weeks. Some children have difficulty falling asleep at first, but this problem also usually disappears. If the insomnia persists at bedtime, the parents should discuss the situation with the prescribing physician. Mild stomachaches, headaches, and tension-releasing behavior such as blinking and nail biting may be observed.

During the past 20 years, the goals of the research in this area have become much more differentiated. There is abundant evidence that positive changes in behavior take place while a hyperactive child is receiving the appropriate psychostimulant (15, 77). Kavale performed a metaanalysis of 135 controlled studies which revealed an 85 percent positive response to drug intervention for hyperactivity.

ADHD, previously described, is not just a school problem; it is a life problem (61,

110). Children so identified often manifest symptoms at home, in the playground with friends, and in food markets and restaurants in addition to their aberrant behavior in school. Psychostimulants have been effective in modulating the behavior of many ADHD children, *but only as long as they are being medicated.* For this reason, Denckla (32) proposes, ". . . Stimulants are less than one quarter of the treatment program and until the other three quarters are in progress in home and school it will not even be possible to perceive and/or report the benefits of that one quarter treatment. Such a perspective on stimulants is a middle-of-the-road position: stimulants are useful adjuncts but not decisive or exclusive cures" (32). Denckla's position is supported by the American Academy of Pediatrics Council on Children with Disabilities (21), which recommended that medication for children with attention deficit disorder should never be used as an isolated treatment.

In discussing psychostimulants, Silver (110) notes that one of the advantages of the treatment is that the child becomes "more available" for learning. Another school of thought holds that the medications themselves, or in conjunction with an adjunct therapy (e.g., cognitive or metacognitive therapy) should improve academic performance, even after medication has been discontinued. In one double-blind controlled study (16), three broad areas of functioning were assessed prior to and following intervention: cognitive performance in the laboratory, academic achievement, and behavior at home and at school. Treatment included the administration of methylphenidate (Ritalin), cognitive behavioral self-control training, and attention-control therapy which differed from cognitive training in that problem-solving strategies were not taught. The post-testing was completed a few days after medication was discontinued. The investigators failed to obtain significant cognitive, academic, and behavioral improvements over the 22-week training program on the immediate and the 3-month delayed post-tests. Brown and his colleagues concluded, "Follow-up studies of

these children have not provided any real evidence to suggest that ADHD children maintained on stimulants fare any better in the long haul than their ADHD peers who have not been treated with medication. This is probably due to the fact that the effects of stimulant medications dissipate rapidly, if not immediately, upon discontinuation" (16).

This and other studies (53) do not support the value of stimulant medication in improving academic skills, especially pure reading disorders, per se. The results, however, should not detract from the potential for hyperactive children to become more available for instruction with improved behavior control. Unfortunately, research studies do not lend themselves to matching intervention strategies to the cognitive and behavioral strengths and weaknesses of individual children.

Summary Although some uncertainty exists concerning the physiologic mediators activated by psychostimulants, the efficacy of their use in the treatment of hyperactive children has been thoroughly documented. When taking medication, hyperactive children are less distractible and exhibit enhanced attention and concentration. Undirected motor activity is reduced. Fewer episodes of impulsive behavior are evident, and socialization skills improve. These and other positive effects more than compensate for the few and occasional problems that have been reported, such as depressed appetite and sleep disturbances. It is reasonable to expect improvement in the academic performance of children who are hyperactive and taking psychostimulants, but only when the medication represents part of a total program. Specific academic instruction in reading, arithmetic, and spelling, as needed, should accompany drug therapy. Metacognitive and cognitive reinforcement should provide improved learning style and problem-solving techniques.

On the other hand, the results of controlled investigations have been less encouraging regarding school achievement. In addition, follow-up studies have yielded disappointing data, consistently finding a re-emergence of symptoms upon cessation of pharmacotherapy (16). A brief review of the potential reasons for the equivocal results seems to point to methodologic problems. That we are dealing with a multivariate problem further complicates the outcome. Samples often are not homogeneous. Brown and coworkers (16) used a sample that included 24 percent ADD and 76 percent ADHD subjects. Sixteen percent had conduct disorders. When using a heterogeneous sample, the average level of performance for a total group composed of diverse subtypes will conceal the diversity and misleadingly suggest that "this technique" is ineffective for everyone (106). Drug dosage requires further verification. The range varies from 0.3 mg/kg of body weight to 1.0 mg/kg, the lower dose being used to facilitate learning and the upper level to improve classroom behavior (though it had an adverse effect on short-term memory). Compliance should also be monitored more carefully. The nature and amount of concurrent interventions need to be clarified. Cognitive, metacognitive, and instructional (academic) variables need to be balanced for maximum classroom improvement (99).

In order to respond to parent inquiries and understand reports received from other professionals relating to individual patients, the optometrist must be familiar with the clinical effects of psychostimulants. Prevalence estimates indicate that about 500,000 children receive stimulant drugs. As a member of the interdisciplinary team treating the LD child, the optometrist should recognize when a child could be helped by psychostimulants and, equally important, communicate with the prescribing physician when the dosage may need to be monitored, perhaps as the result of perceptual therapy.

CONCLUSIONS

In this age of specialization and subspecialization it would not be realistic to expect all optometrists to become knowledgeable in all of the nuances of learning disabilities.

Sooner or later, however, optometrists are confronted with the task of examining a person who has been identified as learning disabled. Several manifestations of this affliction often are evident in the course of a routine examination. Poor visual tracking when reading the Snellen chart, inability to follow directions, inadequate directionality during phoria measurements, and the need to repeat questions because of poor auditory acuity or listening comprehension are some signs the primary care optometrist may recognize.

At the other extreme of the professional continuum are optometrists who serve a significant number of LD patients. It is the responsibility of this group of practitioners to have detailed knowledge of all aspects of this complex discipline. They must be prepared to provide the highest quality of care and to be confident of the validity of their diagnoses and treatment regimens.

It is the purpose of this chapter to provide both groups of optometrists with the information necessary to understand the problems of children who are learning disabled. While the relevance of visual acuity, refraction, binocular vision, and perception is evident, understanding the causes of learning disabilities, distinguishing between hereditary and environmental influences, and the extent to which nutrition and malnutrition affect growth, neural maturation, and learning are areas of knowledge that also affect the outcome of optometric treatment. The inclusion of impulsivity and reflectivity adds another dimension to vision and perceptual therapy. The modification of the LD child's behavior that takes place during the course of treatment can provide the child with an improved cognitive style that enhances learning efficiency.

As with any pathologic condition, it is better to err on the side of overreferring children for psychological consultation. Sometimes optometrists are unaware of family problems that contribute to or result from the learning disability. When it appears that the appropriate optometric therapy is being provided and the LD child is not making a normal and customary response, referral to a psychologist or psychiatrist should be considered.

Although psychostimulants have been prescribed for hyperactive children for 50 years, there is still a great deal of controversy concerning the value of their use for a particular child. As a member of the interdisciplinary team, the optometrist should leave the final decision to a child psychiatrist or a pediatric neurologist who is experienced in treating hyperactive LD children who show signs of attention deficit disorder. It is of professional interest, however, to monitor changes in behavior that may occur as a result of the medication.

Overall, this chapter presents rationales and essential information for optometrists who treat LD children. They should feel comfortable communicating with educators and other members of the interdisciplinary team. Of equal value are the opportunities to participate in community programs intended to ameliorate the social, economic, and educational problems that contribute to the growing number of LD children.

Acknowledgment

The author thanks the staff of the Harold Kohn Visual Science Library at the State College of Optometry/SUNY for their valued assistance in securing many of the references cited in this chapter.

REFERENCES

1. Aasved H: Ophthalmological status of school children with dyslexia. Eye 1:61, 1987.

2. Baker SM: A biochemical approach to the problem of dyslexia. J Learn Disabilities 18:581, 1985.

3. Bartley SH: Principles of Perception. New York, Harper & Row, 1958.

4. Belmont I: Perceptual organization and minimal brain dysfunctions. In Rie HG, Rie ED (eds): Handbook of Minimal Brain Dysfunction. New York, Wiley-Interscience, 253, 1980.

5. Belmont L, Birch HG: Lateral dominance, lateral awareness and reading disability. Child Dev 36:57, 1965.

6. Benton D, Roberts G: Effects of vitamin and mineral supplementation on intelligence of a sample of school children. Lancet Jan 23:140, 1988.

7. Bettman Jr JW, Stern EL, Whitsell LJ, et al: Cerebral dominance in developmental dyslexia: Role of ophthalmology. Arch Ophthalmol 78:722, 1967.

8. Birch HG: Dyslexia and the maturation of visual function. In Money J (ed): Reading Disabilities. Baltimore, Johns Hopkins University, 164, 1962.

9. Birch HG, Belmont L: Auditory-visual integration in normal and retarded readers. Am J Orthopsychiatry 34:852, 1964.

10. Birch HG, Belmont L: Auditory-visual integration, intelligence and reading ability in school children. Percept Mot Skills 20:295, 1965.

11. Birch HG, Gussow JD: Disadvantaged children: Health, nutrition and school failure. New York, Grune & Stratton, 1970.

12. Blika S: Ophthalmological findings in pupils of a primary school with particular reference to reading difficulties. Acta Ophthalmol (Copenh) 60:927, 1982.

13. Block J, Block JH, Harrington DM: Some misgivings about the matching familiar figures test as a measure of reflection-impulsivity. Dev Psychol 10:611, 1974.

14. Brown RT: A developmental analysis of visual and auditory sustained attention and reflection-impulsivity in hyperactive and normal children. J Learn Disabilities 15:614, 1982.

15. Brown R, Sleator E: Methylphenidate in hyperkinetic children: Difference in dose effects on impulsive behavior. Pediatrics 64:408, 1979.

16. Brown RT, Wynne ME, Borden KA, et al: Methylphenidate and cognitive therapy in children with attention deficit disorder: A double blind trial. Dev Behav Pediatr 7:163, 1986.

17. Butler NR, Goldstein H: Smoking in pregnancy and subsequent child development. Br Med J 2:127, 1973.

18. Cathcart WG, Liedthe W: Reflectiveness/impulsiveness and mathematics achievement. Arithmetic Teacher 16:563, 1969.

19. Champakam S, Srikantia SG, Gopolan C: Kwashiorkor and mental development. Am J Clin Nutr 21:844, 1968.

20. Cohen SE: The low-birthweight infant and learning disabilities. In Lewis M (ed): Learning Disabilities and Prenatal Risk. Urbana, University of Illinois, 153, 1986.

21. Committee on Children with Disabilities, Committee on Drugs, American Academy of Pediatrics: Medication for children with attention deficit disorder. Pediatrics 80:758, 1987.

22. Connors CK, Goyette CH, Southwick DA, et al: Food additives and hyperkinesis: A controlled double blind experiment. Pediatrics 58:154, 1976.

23. Cott A: Dr. Cott's help for your learning disabled child. New York, Time Books, 1985.

24. Cravioto J, DeLicardie ER: Nutrition, mental development and learning. In Falkner F, Tannen J (eds): Human Growth 3: Neurobiology and Nutrition. New York, Plenum, 481, 1979.

25. Cravioto J, Gaono-Espinosa C, Birch HG: Early malnutrition and auditory-visual integration in school age children. J Spec Ed 2:75, 1967.

26. Creevy DC: The relationship of obstetrical trauma to learning disabilities: An obstetrician's view. In Lewis M (ed): Learning Disabilities and Prenatal Risk. Urbana, University of Illinois, 91, 1986.

27. Cruickshank WM: Learning disabilities in home, school, and community. Syracuse, Syracuse University Press, 14, 1977.

28. Cummins J, Das JP: Cognitive processing and reading difficulties: A frame work for research. Alberta J Ed 67:245, 1977.

29. Das JP, Kirby JR, Jarman RF: Simultaneous and successive processes. New York, Academic Press, 1979.

30. de Hirsch K: Gestalt psychology as applied to language disturbances. J Nerv Ment Dis 120:257, 1954.

31. de Hirsch K, Jansky JJ, Lanford WS: Predicting Reading Failure. New York, Harper & Row, 1966.

32. Denckla MB: Minimal brain dysfunction. In Chall JS, Hirsky AF (eds): Education and the Brain: The 77th Yearbook of the National Society for the Study of Education, part 11. Chicago, University of Chicago Press, 223, 1978.

33. Denckla MB, Rudel R: Rapid "automatized" naming of pictured objects, colors, letters and numbers by normal children. Cortex 10:186, 1974.

34. Diagnostic and Statistical Manual of Mental Disorders, 3rd Ed, Revised (DSM III-R). Washington DC, American Psychiatric Association, 1987.

35. Dobzhansky T: On genetics, sociology, and politics. In Solan HA (ed): The Psychology of Learning and Reading Difficulties. New York, Simon & Schuster, 430, 1973.

36. Drillien CM, Thomas AJM, Burgoyne K: Low birth weight children at early school age: A longitudinal study. Dev Med Child Neurol 22:26, 1980.

37. Eames TH: A comparison of the ocular characteristicis of unselected and reading disability groups. J Ed Res 25:211, 1932.

38. Eames TH: Improvements of reading following the correction of the eye defects of non-readers. Am J Ophthalmol 27:324, 1935.

39. Eames TH: Comparison of eye conditions among 1,000 reading failures, 500 ophthalmic patients and 150 unselected children. Am J Ophthalmol 31:713, 1948.

40. Eames TH: The influence of hypertropia and myopia on reading achievement. Am J Ophthalmol 39:375, 1955.

41. Eames TH: The effect of anisometropia on reading achievement. Am J Optom Arch Am Acad Optom 41:700, 1964.

42. Egeland B: Training impulsive children in the more efficient use of scanning techniques. Child Dev 45:165, 1974.

43. Feingold BF: Food additives and child development, editorial. Hosp Pract Oct: 11, 1973.

44. Feingold BF: Why Your Child Is Hyperactive. New York, Random House, 1974.

45. Finucci JM, Childs BA: Dyslexia family studies. In Ludlow C, Cooper G (eds): Genetic Aspects of Speech and Language Disorders. New York, Academic Press, 1983.

46. Finucci JM, Guthrie J, Childs A, et al: The genetics of specific reading disability. Ann Hum Genet 40:1, 1976.

47. Fletcher JM, Satz C: Unitary deficit hypothesis of reading disabilities. Has Vellutino led us astray? J Learn Disabilities 12:155, 1979.

48. Fodor JA: How to learn to talk: Some simple ways. In Smith F, Miller GA (eds): The Genesis of Language. Cambridge MA, MIT Press, 105, 1966.

49. Forgus RN: Perception. New York, McGraw-Hill, 1966.

50. Gardner RA: MBD: The Family Book about Minimal Brain Dysfunction. New York, Jason Kronson, 1973.

51. Gesell A, Amatruda CS: Developmental Diagnosis. New York, Harper & Row, 59, 1946.

52. Gesell A, Ilg FL: The Child from Five to Ten. New York, Harper & Brothers, 73, 1946.

53. Gittelman R, Klein DF, Feingold I: Children with reading disorders-II. Effects of methylphenidate in combination with reading remediation. J Child Psychol Psychiatry 24:193, 1983.

54. Grisham JD, Simons HD: Refractive error and the reading process: A literature analysis. J Am Opt Assoc 57:44, 1986.

55. Hallgren B: Specific dyslexia (congenital word blindness). Acta Psychiatr Scand [Suppl] 65:1, 1950.

56. Harley JP, Ray RS, Tomasi L, et al: Hyperkinesis and food additives: Testing the Feingold hypothesis. Pediatrics 61:818, 1978.

57. Harris AJ: How to Increase Reading Ability. New York, David McKay, 231, 1970.

58. Harris EL: Genetic and environmental influences on reading achievement. A study of first- and second-grade twin children. Acta Genet Med Gemellol (Roma) 31:64, 1982.

59. Harris EL: The contribution of twin research to the study of the etiology of reading disability. In Smith SD (ed): Genetics and Learning Disabilities. San Diego CA, College-Hill, 1986.

60. Hertzig ME, Birch HG, Richardson SA, et al: Intellectual levels of school age children severely malnourished during the first two years of life. Pediatrics 49:814, 1972.

61. Hesterly SO: Clinical management of children with hyperactivity. Postgrad Med 79:299, 1986.

62. Hirsch MJ: The relationship between refractive state of the eye and intelligence test scores. Am J Optom Arch Am Acad Optom 36:12, 1959.

63. Hoffman MS: Early indications of learning problems. Academic Therapy 7:23, 1971.

64. Hynd GW, Cohen M: Dyslexia: Neuropsychological Theory, Research and Clinical Differentiation. New York, Grune & Stratton, 1983.

65. Ingram TTS: The nature of dyslexia. Bull Orton Soc 19:18, 1969.

66. Ingram TTS, Reid JF: Developmental aphasia observed in a department of child psychiatry. Arch Disabilities Child 31:161, 1956.

67. Jackson T, Schye V: A comparison of vision with reading scores of ninth grade pupils. Elemen Sch J 46:33, 1945.

68. Jensen AR: Understanding readiness. In Solan HA (ed): The Psychology of Learning and Reading Difficulties. New York, Simon & Schuster, 1973.

69. Johnson DJ, Myklebust HR: Learning Disabilities, Educational Principles and Practices. New York, Grune & Stratton, 26, 1967.

70. Johnston C: Cigarette smoking and the outcome of human pregnancies: A status report on the consequences. Clin Toxicol 18:189, 1981.

71. Kaffman M, Sivah-Sher A, Carel C: Obstetric history of kibbutz children with minimal brain dysfunction. Isr J Psychiatry Related Sci 18:69, 1981.

72. Kagan J: Reflection-impulsivity and reading ability in primary grade children. Child Dev 36:609, 1965.

73. Kagan J: Reflection-impulsivity: The generality and dynamics of conceptual tempo. J Abnorm Psychol 71:17, 1966.

74. Kagan J, Pearson L, Welch L: Modifiability of an impulsive tempo. J Ed Psychol 57:359, 1966.

75. Kappel GD: Vision and nutrition. Curriculum II, Optometric Extension Program. 56; Oct 1983–Sept 1984.

76. Kaufman D: The relation of academic performance to strategy training and remedial technique: An informational processing approach. Unpublished doctoral dissertation. Edmonton, University of Alberta, 1978.

77. Kavale KA: The efficacy of stimulant drug treatment for hyperactivity: A meta-analysis. J Learn Disabilities 15:280, 1982.

78. Kavale KA, Forness SR: Hyperactivity and diet treatment: A meta-analysis of the Feingold Hypothesis. J Learn Disabilities 16:324, 1983.

79. Kavner RS: Your child's vision. New York, Simon & Schuster, 1985.

80. Kawi AA, Pasamanick B: Association of factors of pregnancy with reading disorders in children. JAMA 166:1420, 1958.

81. Keogh B: Hyperactivity and learning disorders: Review and speculations. Except Chil 38:101, 1971.

82. Kephart NC: The Slow Learner in the Classroom. Columbus OH, Charles E Merrill, 107, 1971.

83. Klasen E: The Syndrome of Specific Dyslexia. Baltimore, University Park, 1972.

84. Krywaniuk LW: Patterns of cognitive abilities of high and low achieving school children. Unpublished doctoral dissertation. Department of Educational Psychology. Edmonton, University of Alberta, 1974.

85. Lieberman S, Cohen AH, Stolzberg M, et al: Validation study of the New York State Optometric Association (NYSOA) vision screening battery. Am J Optom Physiol Opt 62:165, 1985.

86. Ludlam W: Review of the psycho-physiological factors in visual information processing as they relate to learning. In Greenstein TN (ed): Vision and Learning Disability. St Louis, American Optometric Association 179, 1976.

87. Luria AR: The Working Brain. New York, Basic Books, 1973.

88. Lyle JG: Reading retardation and reversal tendency: A factorial study. Child Dev 40:833, 1969.

89. Matheny Jr AP, Dolan AB, Wilson RS: Twins with academic learning problems: Antecedent characteristics. Am J Orthopsychiatry 46:464, 1976.

90. Meichenbaum D: Cognitive-functional approach to cognitive factors as determinants of learning disabilities. In Knights RM, Bakker DJ (eds): The Neuropsychology of Learning Disorders. Baltimore, University Park, 432, 1976.

91. Meichenbaum DH, Goodman J: Training impulsive children to talk to themselves: A means of developing self-control. J Abnorm Psychol 77:115, 1971.

92. Messer S: Reflection-impulsivity: Stability and school failure. J Ed Psychol 61:487, 1970.

93. Moser HW: Genetic aspects of learning disabilities. In Lewis M (ed): Learning Disabilities and Prenatal Risk. Urbana, University of Illinois, 228, 1986.

94. National Joint Committee For Learning Disabilities: Definition of Learning Disabilities. In Learning Disabilities: A Report to the U.S. Congress. Interagency Committee for Learning Disabilities, NIH. Bethesda, MD, 219, 1987.

95. Norn MS, Rindziunski E, Skydsgaard H: Ophthalmologic and orthoptic examinations of dyslectics. Acta Ophthalmologica (Copenh) 47:147, 1969.

96. Omen GS, Weber BA: Dyslexia: Search for phenotypic and genetic heterogeneity. Am J Med Genet 1:333, 1978.

97. Park GE, Burri C: The effect of eye abnormalities on reading difficulty. J Ed Psychol 34:420, 1943.

98. Park GE, Burri C: The relationship of various eye conditions and reading achievement. J Ed Psychol 34:290, 1943.

99. Pelham Jr WE: The effects of psychostimulant drugs on learning and academic achievement in children with attention-deficit disorders and learning disabilities. In Torgesen JK, Wong BYL (eds): Psychological and Educational Perspectives on Learning Disabilities. New York, Academic Press, 259, 1986.

100. Piaget J: Judgment and Reasoning in the Child. London, Kegan Paul, 1928.

101. Piaget J: Development and learning. In Ripple R, Rockcastle V (eds): Piaget Rediscovered. New York, Cornell University, 7, 1964.

102. Robinson HM, Huelsman Jr CB: Visual effi-

ciency and progress in learning to read. In Robinson HM (ed): Clinical Studies in Reading II: Supplementary Educational Monographs #77. Chicago, University of Chicago, 31, 1953.

103. Robinson HM: Why Pupils Fail in Reading. Chicago, University of Chicago, 1946.

104. Robinson HM: Visual efficiency and reading status in the elementary school. In Robinson HM, Smith HK (eds): Clinical Studies in Reading III: Supplementary Educational Monograph #97. Chicago, University of Chicago, 49, 1968.

105. Rosenbloom Jr AA: The relationship between aniseikonia and achievement in reading. In Robinson HM, Smith HK (eds): Clinical Studies in Reading III: Supplementary Educational Monograph #97. Chicago, University of Chicago, 109, 1968.

106. Rourke BP: Outstanding issues in research on learning disabilities. In Rutter M (ed): Developmental Neuropsychiatry. New York, Guilford, 564, 1983.

107. Seiderman AS: Optometric vision therapy—Results of a demonstration project with a learning disabled population. J Am Optom Assoc 51:489, 1980.

108. Sherrington C: Man and His Nature. Cambridge, Cambridge University, 175, 1951.

109. Silver LB: The child psychiatrist's role. In Solan HA (ed): The treatment and management of children with learning disabilities. Springfield IL, Charles C Thomas, 88, 1982.

110. Silver LB: The Misunderstood Child: A Guide for Parents of Learning Disabled Children. New York, McGraw-Hill, 1984.

111. Simons HD, Grisham JD: Binocular anomalies and reading problems. J Am Optom Assoc 58:578, 1987.

112. Slingerland B: Screening Tests for Identifying Children with Specific Language Disabilities. Cambridge, MA, Educators Publishing Service, 1964.

113. Smith SD: Review and recommendations for the future. In Smith SD (ed): Genetics and Learning Disabilities. San Diego CA, College-Hill, 205, 1986.

114. Solan HA: Visual processing training with the tachistoscope: A rationale and grade one norms. J Learn Disabilities 2:32, 1969.

115. Solan HA: A comparison of the influences of verbal-successive and spatial-simultaneous factors on achieving readers in fourth and fifth grade: A multivariate correlational study. J Learn Disabilities 20:237, 1987.

116. Solan HA: The effects of visual-spatial and verbal skills on written and mental arithmetic. J Am Optom Assoc 58:88, 1987.

117. Solan HA, Ciner EB: Visual perception: Issues and answers. J Am Optom Assoc. In Press.

118. Solan HA, Mozlin R: The correlations of perceptual-motor maturation to readiness and reading in kindergarten and the primary grades. J Am Optom Assoc 57:28, 1986.

119. Solan HA, Mozlin R, Rumpf D: The relationship of perceptual-motor development to learning readiness in kindergarten: A multivariate analysis. J Learn Disabilities 18:337, 1985.

120. Solan HA, Usprich C, Mozlin R, et al: The auditory-visual integration test: Intersensory or temporal-spatial? J Am Optom Assoc 54:607, 1983.

121. Spache G: Eye preference, visual acuity and reading ability. Elemen Sch J 43:539, 1943.

122. Special Report: The efficacy of optometric vision therapy. J Am Optom Assoc 59:95, 1988.

123. Streissguth AP: Smoking and drinking during pregnancy and offspring learning disabilities: A review of the literature and development of a research strategy. In Lewis M (ed): Learning Disabilities and Prenatal Risk. Urbana, University of Illinois, 28, 1986.

124. Suchoff IB: Research on the relationship between reading and vision—What does it mean? J Learn Disabilities 14:573, 1981.

125. Surgeon General's Advisory on Alcohol and Pregnancy: FDA Drug Bull 2, 1981.

126. Surgeon General's Advisory on the Health Consequences of Smoking for Women: US Department of Health and Human Services, 1980.

127. Taub HB, Goldstein KM, Caputo DV: Indices of prematurity as discriminators of development in early childhood. Child Dev 48:797, 1977.

128. Wender P: Minimal Brain Dysfunction in

Children. New York, Wiley-Interscience, 40, 1971.

129. Wender EH: Food additives and hyperkinesis. Am J Disabled Child 131:1204, 1977.

130. Werner H: Comparative Psychology of Mental Development. New York, Science Editions, 1948.

131. Wiener G, Rider RV, Oppel WC, et al: Correlates of low birth weight: Psychological status at six to seven years of age. Pediatrics 52:434, 1965.

132. Williams JI, Cram DM, Tausig FT, et al: Relative effects of drugs and diet on hyperactive behaviors: An experimental study. Pediatrics 61:811, 1978.

133. Winick M: Malnutrition and Brain Development. New York, Oxford Press, 1976.

134. Wong B: The role of theory in learning disabilities research, Part 1: An analysis of problems. J Learn Disabilities 12:585, 1979.

135. Yarbus A: Eye Movements and Vision. New York, Plenum, 1967.

136. Young FA: Reading, measures of intelligence and refracture errors. Am J Optom Arch Am Acad Optom 49:237, 1963.

137. Zelniker T, Jeffrey WE: Reflective and impulsive children: Strategies of information processing underlying differences in problem solving. Child Dev Mono ser no 168, 41:1976.

Chapter 22

Perspectives on Reading Disabilities

David Grisham

Herbert Simons

Many school children fail to learn to read, for a variety of reasons. The factors that influence reading progress are complex and interwoven, but when teachers and parents first notice a child struggling with reading, they often consider the possibility of a vision disorder and refer the child for an optometric examination. The teacher may have observed behaviors that suggest vision deficiencies, such as holding a book too close or at an odd angle, using a finger to keep one's place, rubbing the eyes while reading, or squinting when looking at the chalkboard. Besides diagnosing vision anomalies and dysfunctions, the optometrist is confronted with the task of making a differential diagnosis of the causes of the reading difficulty. The optometrist must decide to what extent a particular vision anomaly affects the child's reading. The optometrist must also discuss the expected impact of the recommended therapy (e.g., corrective lenses, orthoptics) on the child's reading problem. As a primary care practitioner, the optometrist should be aware of the many possible factors that influence school performance and direct the parents and patient to other professionals who may be of service.

Although all optometrists are expected to diagnose and treat vision anomalies, many are ill-prepared to discuss the impact of specific vision disorders on reading. A fundamental understanding of the reading process itself is important in making a differential diagnosis. The present chapter introduces three different yet complementary perspectives on reading problems: the view of a reading specialist, and the clinical approach and knowledge of an optometrist and of a scientist engaged in reading eye movement research. An educator's view of the reading process, the nature of various reading problems, and some of the unresolved issues relevant to a vision care specialist are presented first (see Chap. 21). Then follows an analysis of the relationships between common vision anomalies and reading difficulties. Special attention is given to the impact of glasses and vision therapy on reading performance. Some optometrists record and evaluate reading eye movements as part of their assessment of deficient readers, and there has been renewed scientific interest in this topic. In the final sections we demonstrate how a detailed analysis of reading eye movements may yield information relevant to both optometrists and educators. The overall purpose of this chapter is to provide the optometrist with pertinent information about vision disorders, eye movements, and their relationships to the reading process. It is hoped this review will translate into a higher standard of optometric care and will facilitate communication with teachers, school administrators, nurses, and parents about children who have reading difficulties. This discussion is framed within a series of questions that various parties might ask.

What Are the Categories of Poor Readers?

There is a great deal of research on children who have difficulty learning to read, but unfortunately the terminology for labeling these children varies widely. A particular problem appears to be the indiscriminate use of the labels *reading disability* and *dyslexia*. We will attempt to clarify current terminology.

The categorization of poor reading is based on the relationship between a child's expected reading level and actual reading level as measured by a standardized reading test. Expected performance is most often assessed by IQ testing. Children are expected to read at grade level if their IQ is average.

Grade level reading is defined as reading performance equivalent to the average performance of students in any grade in school.

There are two general categories of poor reading performance. *Slow learners in reading* (backward readers, in England), are children who are reading below grade level and whose IQ is below average (Table 22.1). This group reads below grade level but the reading level is consistent with lower capacity. They are, in effect, reading as well as can be expected of them. The choice of the IQ test must be appropriate to make this distinction. If the test is weighted toward reading items, children who have difficulty reading may appear retarded. Slow learners may or may not have adequate word recognition skills, but they almost always have lowered reading comprehension. They are also usually below grade level in all subjects and may or may not be assigned to special education, depending on the severity of the intellectual deficit.

The second major category is the *underachiever in reading*. These students are called underachievers because there is a discrepancy between their actual reading performance and their expected reading performance as predicted by IQ scores. They have grade-equivalent scores that are below that predicted by their IQ. Given this definition, a student with a high IQ who reads at or even above grade level could be an underachiever.

Underachievers in reading are further subdivided on the basis of presumed cause of the underachievement. One group is called *remedial readers* or said to have *reading problems*, or *reading difficulties*. It includes students whose underachievement can be attributed to an identifiable cause such as economic and social disadvantage, lack of adequate instruction, emotional problems, or vision or hearing disorders. The students in this category are generally reading below grade level and may be doing poorly in other subjects, as these factors can have generalized effects. Affected students can exhibit word recognition or comprehension problems. Remediation of this group involves compensating for the instructional deficiencies through school-based remedial instruc-

Table 22.1 CATEGORIES OF POOR READING PERFORMANCE

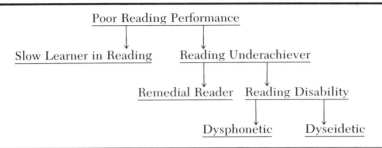

Slow Learner in Reading:
  Causes: Low general IQ
  Reading deficiency: Comprehension, decoding to a lesser degree
  Remediation: Intensive skills instruction in deficit areas

Reading Underachievement:
  Average or above average general IQ; reading level is below that predicted by IQ.

Remedial Reader (reading problem or reading difficulty):
  Causes: Inadequate instruction, primary emotional problems, insufficient motivation, economic or
    social disadvantage, hearing and language disorders, vision disorders
  Reading deficiency: Primarily decoding
  Remediation: Elimination of specific blockage, intensive instruction in reading deficiencies

Reading Disability (dyslexia):
  Causes: Absence of instructional, emotional, motivational, social, auditory and visual etiologies;
    central nervous system dysfunction; large difference between verbal and performance IQ.
    (Wechsler Intelligence Scale for Children—Revised)
  Reading deficiency: Decoding, spelling
  Remediation: Intensive multisensory reading instruction (Determine the strongest modality and
    teach to it.)

Dysphonetic (auditory-linguistic dyslexia):
  Causes: CNS dysfunction resulting in auditory perceptual problems and a higher performance IQ
    than verbal IQ.
  Reading deficiency: Poor decoding, phonetic spelling errors, adequate sight vocabulary

Dyseidetic (visual-spatial dyslexia):
  Causes: CNS dysfunction resulting in visual-perceptual problems and a higher verbal IQ than
    performance IQ
  Reading deficiency: Poor sight vocabulary, nonphonetic spelling errors, adequate phonetic de-
    coding

tion and, where possible, the removal or amelioration of the primary cause.

The problem of the other group of underachievers also has several names: *reading disability, primary or specific reading disability, dyslexia, developmental dyslexia,* and *specific reading retardation* (England). As in the remedial reading group there is a discrepancy between expected reading achievement and actual reading performance; however, this category uses an exclusionary definition. It is defined by the absence of the previously mentioned causes. Thus, by definition underachievement among this group is not caused by economic and social disadvantage, lack of adequate instruction, emotional problems, or vision or hearing disorders. Such factors may be present, but they are assumed to be secondary to the reading disability. The actual cause of the problem is assumed to be an intrinsic dysfunction of the central nervous system; however, the nature of the neurologic dysfunction need not be positively identified for a student to be labeled reading disabled. In effect a student can be labeled as reading disabled when there is no obvious cause for the underachievement, and this frequently happens. Reading disability is a subgroup of the general category of learning disability in which the problem is limited to reading. In point of fact, the vast majority of learning-disabled children are reading disabled. Poor word recognition is the major skill deficit of reading-disabled persons. Comprehension may be normal or it may be impaired as a secondary effect of the word recognition problem. Reading-disabled students usually manifest severe and persistent spelling difficulty, laboriously slow reading, and an unusually high number of letter reversals in reading and spelling. The discrepancy between predicted and actual reading level is usually much greater than that among remedial readers. A minimum of 2 years below grade level is often used as a cut-off point. These students often received traditional remediation in school without success, so they are thought to require special instruction. Finally, there are often perceptual, memory, language, or speech problems of some type.

Some investigators distinguish between two subtypes of dyslexia that can be characterized generally as auditory and visual (7, 44, 49, 59). Boder (7) has called the auditory disability *dysphonesia* and the visual reading disability *dyseidesia*. The two subtypes exhibit different types of reading and spelling behavior. Dysphonetic readers have an auditory-linguistic dysfunction that makes it difficult to learn to decode words. Dyseidetic readers are considered to have a visual-spatial processing deficiency that makes it difficult to remember the visual forms of words and results in very poor spelling. The problems of the dysphonetic and the dyseidetic

are not attributed to peripheral sensory anomalies of hearing or vision but are assumed to be caused by a central neurologic deficiency. There is some anatomic evidence that dyslexia is associated with neurologic disorganization in the association cortex supporting one or the other sensory system or in language integrative centers such as Wernicke's area or the angular gyrus of the left temporal lobe (30–32).

Distinguishing reading disabilities from other reading problems has been the subject of much controversy and confusion among educators, health care professionals, and researchers. Reading disability is distinguished from reading problems on the basis of ruling out potential causes. A reading disability is assumed if the reading problem remains unexplained. This use of exclusionary criteria has been criticized because it defines a disability by what it is not rather than by what it is. In actual practice the task of ruling out every potential cause of poor reading progress is very difficult. Have speech, hearing, and vision been evaluated thoroughly? Is there any evidence of nervous system dysfunction and has a causal relationship to reading been established? Which factors are primary and which secondary? In practice, reading-disabled persons are identified on the basis of a large degree of underachievement, the failure of previous remediation, and the absence of any obvious extrinsic cause.

There are also social and political forces that encourage labeling an underachiever as reading-disabled rather than a remedial reader. Sleeter (97) has argued that the category of learning disability was created to explain the failure of white, middle class children in a manner that distinguished them from lower class and minority children. The influence of white, middle class parents can be seen in federal money that is available for treating learning disabilities, especially reading disabilities. National and local parent groups like the California Association for Neurologically Handicapped Children (CANHC) put pressure on schools and state legislatures to provide special help for reading-disabled children. Dyslexic students are allowed extra time on tests such as the Scholastic Aptitude Test by many educational institutions and national testing agencies. There are also some psychological advantages to being labeled dyslexic. Parents' sense of guilt over the problem is often relieved and the student is provided an acceptable explanation for the poor performance that is beyond control and blame. Neurologic explanations are afforded higher status among educators and lay people than educational and environmental causes. These pressures, combined with the problems in making categorical distinctions, inflate the number of students labeled reading disabled. Mislabeling remedial reading students as reading disabled also affects the research literature. The distinctions in Table 22.1 are not rigorously observed in most studies and confound their interpretation, as will be seen in the section on visual conditions and reading difficulties.

It must be emphasized that the basic distinction between remedial readers and reading-disabled students does not have solid scientific support. The research evidence is highly contradictory: some studies demonstrate a basic distinction whereas others offer little support. One obvious problem is that the categories are not mutually exclusive. A dyslexic reader, with a constitutional disability, is just as likely to have poor teaching, economic and social disadvantages, or vision problems as any other student. Political and social factors also cloud the distinction.

WHAT IS THE READING PROCESS AND HOW IS IT LEARNED?

Optometrists who examine children with reading difficulties should have some basic understanding of the reading process. This knowledge can be useful when communicating with the schools and in determining the significance of vision disorders in a child's progress. The reading process involves getting the meaning from the printed page. Two basic aspects are involved in the process, as this riddle demonstrates (51):

A man received a letter in a foreign language that he spoke fluently but could not read. He had a friend who could make the sounds indicated by the writing, but who understood nary a word. The man who received the letter took it to his friend who pronounced the words which allowed the recipient of the message to understand the letter. Which one was reading?

The friend had knowledge of one of the major aspects of reading, *decoding*. He knew the relationship between the printed symbols and the sounds they represent. Decoding involves several component skills. It requires the knowledge that spoken words are composed of separate sounds (phonologic awareness), the ability to discriminate and identify the printed letters, a knowledge of letter-sound correspondences, and the ability to rapidly and automatically combine sounds into words. Decoding skills allowed the friend to pronounce the words. They also make it possible for a reader to pronounce a nonsense word like 'glurck' that has never been encountered before.

The recipient of the letter possesses the second aspect of the reading process, *comprehension*. He can interpret the meaning of the message once it is decoded. Comprehension involves knowledge of the syntax and grammar of the language, the meanings of words, the underlying semantic relations, text structure, and world knowledge. World knowledge is an important but often overlooked part of the comprehension process. World knowledge enables a reader to understand that in the sentence *She wore alligator shoes* a woman wore shoes made of alligator skin, not shoes made for alligators. Readers make the right interpretation because they know from their experiences living in the world that alligators normally do not wear shoes and their skins are in demand by shoemakers.

The answer to the riddle is that neither one by himself is reading but together they are. Reading involves *decoding* and *comprehension* combined. What is the process by which decoding and comprehension work together to produce an understanding of print?

The process works in two ways: top-down and bottom-up. Top-down processing goes from the reader's mind, where the meaning resides, to the print; bottom-up processing goes from the print to the meaning in the mind.

Top-down and bottom-up processing can be understood by examining the following sentences:

1. The boy swung his bat at the *ball.*
2. The girl looked down at the ground and saw a *ball.*

Assume that each sentence has been processed up to the word "ball." The question is: How is the word "ball" recognized and comprehended? In sentence 1 a top-down process can be employed: the reader uses syntactic, semantic, and world knowledge to predict what word will follow. The reader knows from syntax (rules of phrase and sentence structure) that the word will be a noun or an adjective. The underlying semantics of the sentence tell the reader that an actor (boy) acted (swung) at an object (ball) with an instrument (bat). Vocabulary and world knowledge inform the reader that bats are typically swung at balls by boys playing baseball or a similar sport. All of this knowledge predicts that the last word in sentence 1 is *ball.* The reader then needs only to use the print to confirm this prediction and needs only to process the letter *b* to confirm it. Readers can fill in text from their knowledge and do not have to do a full analysis of the print. In fact it has been shown that words can be left out of text and the text is still understood. Children's oral reading errors can show the effects of top-down processing. The substitution of *a* for *one* in sentence 3 or the substitution of *small* for *little* in sentence 4 are examples of top-down errors.

(a)
3. There was one dinosaur.
    (small)
4. You're too little.

In top-down processing the direction of processing goes from the meaning to the print. All the information to make a predic-

tion exists in the reader's mind before he or she begins to read. Smith (98) calls this nonvisual information. Visual information is the print that exists on the page and disappears when the lights go out. Nonvisual information is still there when the lights go out. Visual information plays a much smaller role in top-down processing than nonvisual information.

Visual information plays a much more prominent role in bottom-up processing, which can be seen in sentence 2. The reader's previous processing and nonvisual knowledge provide very little information about the last word in the sentence beyond that it is a noun. The reader must use bottom-up processing to identify the word ball. The processing goes from print to meaning. One must decode the word ball; that is, identify all the letters, match them to their sounds, and retrieve the word ball from memory. An alternative route would involve going from the letters directly to the word ball in memory without first translating them into sounds. By either route the processing starts with the print. There is a close analysis of the visual stimulus, and nonvisual information plays a much smaller role here than in top-down processing.

Reading is a combination of bottom-up and top-down processing. The degree of each varies with the individual reader, the type of reading material, and the place in the text. More top-down reading processing is employed on easy material and more bottom-up processing is required for difficult material. Both top-down and bottom-up processing are used at all stages of learning to read, but the relative proportions change as skill develops. In general, children in the beginning stages of reading use more bottom-up processing and mature, skilled readers use more top-down processing.

The first major task in learning to read is learning to decode using bottom-up processing. Learning to decode involves learning the alphabetic principle that letters in words map onto sound in English rather than to the meaning directly. It involves learning that words, in fact, are composed of separate sounds, learning to discriminate the letters, learning the names of the letters and the sounds associated with them, and learning to combine the sounds associated with letters to form words. When readers encounter new words they must proceed bottom-up through this process; however, in subsequent exposure to the same words the process is accelerated. With enough exposures a point is reached at which the words are decoded and recognized quickly and automatically as whole units. In the *automatic* stage, word recognition takes place by a direct route that bypasses the process of translating the letters into sounds.

As reading skill develops, children need to acquire a large number of words that are recognized automatically. This entails repeated exposures to the same word. It is through wide and sustained reading that automaticity is developed. In addition to the development of automaticity, wide reading helps students acquire a large knowledge base, which in turn improves comprehension. A nonvisual knowledge base is also increased by exposure to oral language and simply collecting experiences by living in the world, but reading plays a central role.

If a student has a reading problem or reading disability, what aspect of the acquisition process has been disrupted? The two major aspects that can be deficient are, of course, decoding and comprehension. Any subskill deficits in these processes can also result in reading difficulty. Failure in learning to decode will cause the most severe disruption, because comprehension requires decoding. A student with a decoding problem has trouble recognizing words so reading is slow and laborious. Spelling is also poor. The majority of remedial and learning-disabled readers have decoding problems.

With primary comprehension problems decoding skills are intact. Comprehension can be limited by inadequate vocabulary and world knowledge or ineffective strategies for organizing and applying this knowledge (i.e., semantic and syntactic structures). Much of this knowledge comes from varied life experiences and exposure to oral language in the home. Decoding skills and automaticity are more dependent on what happens in the classroom. Thus a student can have adequate decoding skills and automatic word recognition and still have primary comprehension problems.

Reading disabled students almost always have profound decoding problems, which helps to explain the severity of the reading lag. Remedial readers, on the other hand, can have decoding or comprehension difficulties of any severity (see Table 22.1).

HOW DO SCHOOLS REMEDIATE READING PROBLEMS AND DISABILITIES?

Remediation of reading problems is usually directed toward the specific deficient reading skill, decoding or comprehension. Individualized or small-group instruction is implemented as a supplement to the regular classroom curriculum. In general, remediation is similar in content to the original curriculum, only it's more intensive and individualized. Like the regular classroom, there is usually a heavy emphasis on phonics instruction (letter-sound correspondence) using workbooks and reading exercises.

On the other hand, the remediation of reading-disabled (dyslexic) students is widely thought to require special instruction. Standard reading or remedial instruction on a more intensive basis is thought to be inadequate for their problems. Since a reading disability is believed by many to be a neurologically based deficiency in language processing related to a particular sensory modality (visual-spatial or auditory-linguistic), remediation methods have been developed that employ more than one channel. These are called multisensory or multimodal methods, some of which are combined with intensive phonics instruction. Several modalities are used in the belief that reading-disabled students require the extra reinforcement. These methods are often referred to as VAKT methods, indicating the use of visual, auditory, kinesthetic, and tactile modes of learning. One widely used multisensory method is

Fernald's method, which initially requires the student to trace the written word with a finger as it is pronounced. Copying and writing of words is also emphasized. Variations on this method include tracing words in sand (Cooper's method) or tracing words on the student's back (modality blocking). These methods focus on the whole word and deemphasize phonics.

Other popular multisensory methods that emphasize phonics are those of Gillingham-Stillman, Slingerland, and Hegge-Kirk-Kirk. These methods focus on letter-sound correspondences and learning new words by simultaneously seeing, saying, and writing them (Table 22.2).

Another remediation method that is relatively new and gaining in influence and that contrasts sharply with the traditional methods is the holistic, or whole language, approach. This method, which focuses on comprehension, involves reading a lot of stories. It deemphasizes phonics and concentrates on the meaning of stories. One of the basic assumptions of the holistic method is that reading-disabled students suffer from too much emphasis on phonics and word recognition and do not progress beyond that level to understand content. The whole language approach is often used with remedial readers and reading-disabled students without acknowledging the possibility that there is a need to differentiate the two groups.

There is no conclusive evidence that one method is superior to any of the others. Each has its dedicated adherents and undoubtedly works for some students. Which method is used should depend on the type of reading difficulty the student has as indicated by psychoeducational testing. However, the method most frequently employed usually depends on the personal biases, preferences, and experiences of the remedial teacher.

Another set of remedial training methods is more familiar to optometrists, owing largely to the influence of the Optometric Extension Program (OEP) and the College of Optometrists in Vision Development

Table 22.2   REMEDIAL READING APPROACHES FOR LEARNING-DISABLED STUDENTS

Name of Educator	Type/Concept	Example Procedures
Grace Fernald	Multisensory and language experience approach; teaches whole words with tactile reinforcement.	Tracing whole words with fingers Writing words as units from memory Vocally using words in context No copying or phonics allowed
G.T. Hegge, Samuel Kirk, Winifred Kirk	Structured phonetics approach; simple units to complex; much oral repetition.	Starts by teaching letter sounds Oral sound-blending drills Repetitive sound family drills (hat, bat) Writing words while saying sounds
Anna Gillingham, Bessie Stillman	Multisensory phonetics, alphabetic method, based on Orton's model of incomplete cerebral dominance	Drill cards of letter names and sounds Phoneme sound-writing association Reading words as syllables Syllable blending into words Memorization of spelling rules
Beth Slingerland	Multisensory phonetics and visualization approach; extensive modification of Gillingham and Stillman	Oral repetition of sound rules Sound blending while writing Cursive writing in air from memory Rote memorization of phonics rules

(See Myers and Hammill for a detailed description)
Myers PI, Hammill DD: Learning Disabilities: Basic Concepts, Assessment Practices, and Instructional Strategies. Austin, TX, Pro-ed, 207, 1982.

Table 22.3 PERCEPTUAL AND MOTOR APPROACHES TO LEARNING-DISABLED STUDENTS

Name of Author, Profession, Groups Most Often Associated with Therapy Approach	Type/Concept	Example Procedures
Marianne Frostig Psychologist Special educators	Vision perception program: Fine motor coordination, figure-ground, size, and shape constancy, spatial relationships	Drawing lines within guidelines Tracing figures in complex background Choosing like and difference patterns Copying dot-to-dot patterns
Jean Ayres Psychologist Occupational Therapist	Sensory-integration program: Functional interdependence of vestibular-sensory-motor systems with language	Tactile stimulation of body with brush Swinging or spinning in a net hammock Riding a scooter board Sitting or standing on a balance board
Delacato and Dolman Physical educators Special educators	Perceptual-motor program: Normal neurologic development requires the orderly acquisition of PM skills, uses patterning exercises	Patterned swimming movements Cross-pattern crawling and walking Ocular smooth pursuit activities Hand, eye, and foot dominance activities Auditory and visual perceptual discrimination
Brian Cratty Physical educator Special educators	Perceptual-motor program: Physical education approach to motor development—strength, agility, and balance	Balance in many different positions Crawling, skipping, hopping activities Simon says game for directionality Throwing, catching, and batting games
Newell Kephart Psychologist Special educators Developmental OD's	Perceptual-motor program: Develop perceptual motor matches, eye motor control, form perception, general motor coordination	Chalkboard activities in directionality Drawing circles and other forms Angel-in-the-snow movement training Marsden ball hand-eye coordination Rhythmical clapping, balance
Gerald Getman Optometrist Developmental OD's	Developmental vision program: Body and eye movements, memory and form perception are the foundations of reading skill	Angel-in-the-snow movement patterns Vision exercise while on walking beam Chalkboard bimanual drawing of circles Tracing the visualization of a word

Table 22.3 *(Continued)*

Name of Author, Profession, Groups Most Often Associated with Therapy Approach	Type/Concept	Example Procedures
Jerome Rosner Optometrist Optometrists Special educators	Perceptual skills program: Early academic performance is correlated with visual and auditory analysis skills	Copying forms onto geoboards and dot maps Solving parquetry block puzzles Reproducing pegboard patterns Vocal deletion of phonemes in words

(See Myers and Hammill for a detailed description)
Myers PI, Hammill DD: Learning Disabilities: Basic Concepts, Assessment Practices, and Instructional Strategies. Austin, TX, Pro-ed, 342, 1982.

(COVD). These are the visual-perceptual-motor and gross motor training methods, which are intended to improve various visual-perceptual skills, perceptual-motor integration, and gross motor coordination. Advocates of the programs often claim that this training establishes reading readiness skills that are prerequisite to normal reading progress. The training does not teach children to read, but it prepares them to learn to read more efficiently. The training programs of Frostig and Rosner emphasize perceptual discrimination and visual-motor integration (copy form) activities (Table 22.3). The programs of Ayers, Delacato, Cratty, Kephart, and Getman place more emphasis on gross motor learning, balance, and hand-eye coordination. Children who complete these programs are usually considered to show more vigilant visual attention, better perceptual discriminations, improved coordination, and a positive self-image (see Myers and Hammill for a detailed description of these programs) (65). It is through these programs and their variations that optometrists often become involved in treating children with reading difficulties. There is a great deal of controversy among special educators, health care professionals, and optometrists about the effectiveness of these programs in helping reading-disabled children.

WHAT ARE THE RELATIONSHIPS BETWEEN VISION DISORDERS AND READING DIFFICULTY?

A joint policy statement from the American Academy of Pediatrics and the American Academy of Ophthalmology, renewed every few years, states that children with dyslexia and associated learning disabilities have the same incidence of visual disorders (refractive anomaly, muscle imbalance, fusional deficiencies) as children without learning difficulties. Unfortunately the term *dyslexia* means different things to different people. Most medical sources refer to dyslexia as a severe reading disability of neurologic origin, which is the sense intended in this review. However, this statement has been incorrectly interpreted by many school officials to mean that children having any reading difficulty require no special vision screening program beyond the distance Snellen acuity test. On the other hand, many practicing optometrists note that children who have reading difficulties frequently manifest some primary vision disorder that could be a significant contributing factor to reading comfort, efficiency, and endurance. The medical policy statement has been critiqued by Flax (27), who impugns its strong political and weak academic character. It is important that optometrists be aware of the evidence for the relationship between primary vision disorders and reading achievement so they may give accurate and credible information to parents and school personnel. This review includes only studies that adhered to the rudiments of scientific investigation, present data, and include control groups when appropriate. The literature on the question of relationships between visual disorders and reading performance was subjected to two forms of analysis: a literature review evaluating the results and relative significance of studies (38, 96) and a metaanalysis of studies, a quantitative technique for combining the results of multiple studies that reduces the subjectivity of literature reviews. This metaanalysis included 34 studies that met the criteria for inclusion (95).

Visual Acuity

The Snellen distance visual acuity test has served as the national standard for vision screening for several decades, but it is largely ineffective in identifying visual conditions that affect reading performance. Despite the common-sense association of blurred vision and inefficient reading, a higher prevalence of reduced distance or near point acuity among poor readers has not been demonstrated in the literature. Reduced distance acuity appears more frequent among poor readers only in the early elementary school grades, second and third grades specifically (26, 68), where reading material is often presented on the blackboard, but this relationship vanishes in the higher grades, as one might expect.

More surprising is the lack of a consistent relationship between low near point acuity and reading performance. Most studies investigating this question utilized the near point acuity test on a Brewster type stereoscope, which has doubtful validity and reliability for vision screening (5). The one study that used near point charts in free space did report a significantly higher incidence of low visual acuity among the second and third grade poor reader group (26). Except in ex-

treme cases, poor near vision in the early grades should not present much of a handicap, as most elementary school books are printed in large type and children naturally tend to hold reading material close. However, for reading rate and efficiency to be maximal, the print size should be much larger than a reader's resolution threshold, at least three times the minimum angle of resolution for adults (3). There is a need to better define the near visual acuity requirements and skills of elementary school children, to ensure that they are resolving print at their optimal level for reading efficiency and comfort.

Refractive Anomaly

One would not expect simple bilateral myopia of low to moderate degree to impede reading near point material. Indeed, all studies, except one (21) found either no difference in the incidence of myopia when comparing normal and poor readers or a higher incidence among the better readers. The metaanalysis indicated a statistically significant positive association between reading skill and myopia. There is no information in these reports, however, about the causal relationship. Do myopic children become better readers because near point material is easier to read? Does reading itself contribute to the development of myopia? Do other intervening factors such as genetic predisposition account for the association? These questions have not yet been answered in a coherent and convincing way. In any event, the distance acuity test, which is a valid and efficient method for screening for myopia, also tends to identify the better readers in the class.

The refractive state most often cited as being related to reading problems is hyperopia. There are compelling reasons to suspect that it might influence reading comfort and efficiency. Even moderate hyperopia (2 to 4 D) rarely causes constant blur at distance or near point, but the extra accommodative effort produces bothersome asthenopic symptoms of intermittent blur, headaches, fatigue, and lapses of concentration in some patients. Uncorrected hyperopia is frequently associated with esophoria at near point, which can stress the fusional vergence system that holds the eyes in correct alignment. If the hyperopia and esophoria are excessive, an accommodative esotropia can result. Even though most of the studies that investigate refractive state and reading can be criticized on methodologic grounds, there is a strong pattern of relationship between hyperopia and lower reading performance (Table 22.4). Two studies that found no such association can be faulted for not using a valid quantitative test of refractive state (101, 102). The refractive state was inferred by subjects' re-

Table 22.4 HYPEROPIA AND READING

Name of Investigator	Year	Groups	Results and Comments
1. Eames (17)	1932	114 PR; 143 U No age matching	**43% poor readers vs 27% control** (clinical sample; no reading test)
2. Eames (18)	1935	100 PR; 143 U Age matched	**53% poor readers vs 28% control** (no reading test mentioned)
3. Farris (25)	1936	78 H; 78 E 7th grade Matched IQ, age	**Emmetropes gained more in reading than hyperopes over 1 year**
4. Swanson & Tiffin (102)	1936	70 PR; 63 GR; 94 U College students No matching	No significant difference in hyperopia (Keystone testing for refractive state)
5. Stromberg (101)	1938	71 PR; 71 GR College students Matched for IQ	No significant difference in hyperopia (Keystone testing for refractive error)
6. Eames (19)	1948	1000 PR; 150 N Median age 9 vs 10	**43% poor readers vs 13% control** (clinical sample)
7. Eames (21)	1955	64 PR; 57 GR 3rd–4th Grade	**RE not related to reading in GR; in PR, hyperopes made less gains than myopes or emmetropes**
8. Morgan (63)	1960	111 5th grade, U	**Hyperopia related to low bookishness in females**
9. Young (113)	1963	36 H; 29 M; 93 E Matched IQ	**Hyperopes lower in reading skill than myopes and emmetropes**
10. Robinson (84)	1968	60 PR; 63 GR 1st–8th grade No matching	**More hyperopes in PR** (vision screening test for hyperopia)
11. Norn et al. (67)	1969	117 Dyslexics 117 Normals Ages 9–14 Matched IQ, age	**32% dyslexics were hyperopic vs 26% control** (cycloplegic refraction done, all Danish)

Key: PR, poor readers; GR, good readers; U, unselected readers; RE, refractive error; H, hyperopes; M, myopes, E, emmetropes. Statistically significant results are indicated by bold type.

sponses on the Keystone Telebinocular, a screening instrument, using Betts' blue filter test.

Norn and coworkers (67) also found no significant difference in the incidence of hyperopia between groups, but the poor readers were well-diagnosed dyslexics. The cause of the profoundly poor reading performance was presumably neurologic. When the poor reading group is widely based to include subjects with a variety of reading problems, as in the remaining eight studies, a significantly higher incidence of uncorrected hyperopia is found among poor readers. When the results of these studies are pooled for metaanalysis the inverse relationship between hyperopia and reading achieves statistical significance. Hyperopia contributes to poor reading.

Astigmatism, both hyperopic and myopic, was found to have no statistically significant relation to reading skill; however, clinical experience suggests that astigmatism over −1.50 D can often cause severe eye strain and interferes with reading. Even lesser degrees can be significant in some patients. In addition, the effects of against-the-rule astigmatism tend to be more severe than those of with-the-rule astigmatism. The studies reviewed in the metaanalysis did not provide enough information about the magnitude or type of astigmatism. Thus, the finding of no association between astigmatism and reading performance may reflect methodologic problems with the studies.

Anisometropia and aniseikonia are both associated with below-average reading performance by metaanalysis (95). This literature analysis yielded four studies of the relation of anisometropia and reading and two of aniseikonia. These results should be accepted with caution because the best controlled study of those reviewed (87) did not demonstrate a significant difference in prevalence between the experimental and the control groups (25 and 17.5 percent, respectively). Anisometropia or aniseikonia can potentially disrupt binocular functioning and cause visual discomfort, which, in turn, could make reading difficult. In the presence of unresolved visual symptoms 1 D or more of an-

isometropia or 1 percent aniseikonia is generally considered clinically significant.

Binocular Vision

Clinical experience teaches that many minor problems of binocular vision (heterophoria, deficient vergence ranges, convergence insufficiency, accommodative dysfunctions) can cause or contribute to reading discomfort and inefficiency in adults. Often patients with severe developmental disorders of binocular vision such as constant strabismus, amblyopia, and deep suppression read normally because there is no longer stress on binocular physiologic mechanisms. It can be argued that young children have lower vision requirements, or possibly greater adaptability, which would reduce the impact of binocular vision deficiencies on reading performance. Consequently, there would be less need to screen for these disorders in the schools. An analysis of the literature does not support this idea. Most investigators have reported on the association of isolated binocular vision conditions and reading performance. A pattern of relationships emerges from a detailed inspection of these studies (Table 22.5). The binocular conditions most frequently associated with lower reading performance in school-aged children are near point exophoria, deficient fusional reserves, excessive fixation disparity, hyperphoria, and convergence insufficiency. These associations were confirmed by metaanalysis. There is also some weak evidence for esophoria at near point and reduced stereopsis, but these associations did not prove statistically significant.

A troublesome aspect of the literature has been the many conflicting findings. For a given binocular anomaly, some studies find a relationship and others do not. Besides the usual difficulties in evaluating different studies with dissimilar population characteristics and sampling criteria, many studies use testing techniques of questionable validity and use nonstandard referral criteria. As can be seen from an inspection of Table 22.6, 9 of 13 negative studies can be criticized on this ba-

Table 22.5   STUDIES FINDING A RELATIONSHIP BETWEEN BINOCULAR ANOMALIES AND READING

Name of Investigator[a]	Year	Groups	Results (Comments)
1. Eames	1932	114 PR, 143 N Clinical sample	**Near exophoria, vergence** (Professional vision testing)
2. Eames	1934	88 PR, 52 N Clinical sample	**Vergence** (Professional vision testing)
3. Farris	1934	78 PR, 78 N Grade 7 Matched age, IQ	**Strabismus,** phoria NS (Professional vision testing)
4. Eames	1935	100 PR, 143 N Clinical sample	**Near exophoria, vergence** (Professional vision testing)
5. Clark	1936	6 HXP, 11 OP Ages 16–35	**High exophoria was associated with poorer reading eye movements** (Professional vision testing)
6. Whitty, Kopel	1936	100 PR, 100 N Grades 3–6	**High phoria and poor fusion** (Telebinocular testing)
7. Good	1939	25 PR, 25 N Matched age, IQ	**High phoria, vergences** (Professional vision testing)
8. Parks, Burri	1943	225 N Grades 1–8 Adjusted for IQ	**Correlation with eye score, exophoria, vergence ranges, and recovery** (Professional vision testing)
9. Eames	1948	1000 PR, 150 N Clinical sample	**Near exophoria, near esophoria, vergence** (Professional vision testing)
10. Robinson	1968	60 PR, 63 GR Grades 1–8 Adjusted for IQ	**High phoria and vergences** (Professional vision testing)
11. Silbiger, Woolf	1968	25 PR, 38 GR College students	**Fixation disparity,** phoria N.S. (Professional vision testing)
12. Dunlop, Banks	1973	15 PR, 15 GR H.S. students Matched for age	**Convergence, distance, esophoria and near exophoria, stereopsis** (Professional vision testing)
13. Wilson, Wold	1973	79 PR, 81 GR Grades 2 and 3	**Motilities,** phoria and convergence N.S. (Professional vision testing)
14. Bedwell et al.	1980	25 PR, 15 GR Age 13 and 14	**Convergence and divergence stereopsis, diplopia, motilities** (Professional vision testing)
15. Hoffman	1980	107 PR, 25 N Children, clinical sample	**Binocular coordination, motilities, accommodation** (Professional vision testing)
16. O'Grady	1984	227 N Grade 2	**Near phoria, convergence, fixation disparity** (Professional vision testing)

Key: PR, poor reader; GR, good reader; N, unselected readers; NS, not significant; HXP, high exophoria; OP, orthophoria. Statistically significant results for PR indicated by bold type.
[a] See reference listing of Reference 96 for complete information.

Table 22.6 STUDIES NOT FINDING A RELATIONSHIP BETWEEN BINOCULAR ANOMALIES AND READING

Name of Investigator[a]	Year	Groups	Results (Comments)
1. Farris	1934	78 PR, 78 NR Grade 7 Matched age and IQ	Phoria not related to reading (Professional vision testing, appears to be distance phoria)
2. Fendrick	1935	49 PR, 50 GR Grades 2 and 3 Matched age and IQ	Phoria NS (Professional vision testing)
3. Swanson, Tiffin	1936	70 PR, 63 GR College students	Phoria, fusion NS (Telebinocular testing)
4. Stromberg	1937	71 PR, 71 GR College students	Phoria, Fusion NS (Telebinocular testing)
5. Dalton	1943	1000 N Grades 3–8	NS correlation of reading with sum of distance and near phoria (Telebinocular testing)
6. Edson et al.	1953	188 N Grade 4	No difference in reading for failures on phoria and fusion tests (Telebinocular testing, no data presented)
7. Spache, Tillman	1962	114 PR, 114 NR College students	Vertical and horizontal phoria NS (Stereoscope testing)
8. Norn	1969	117 Dyslexics 117 NR children Matched age and IQ	NS trend for exophoria and hyperphoria vergences NS (Severe dyslexic sample, professional vision testing, Denmark)
9. Parks	1969	100 PR, 50 NR Children	Phoria NS (Professional vision testing, criteria unclear for vision disorder)
10. Wilson, Wold	1972	79 PR, 81 GR Grades 2 and 3	Distance and near phoria, convergence NS (Professional vision testing, high criteria)
11. Fitzpatrick	1973	65 N, Grade 3 Two test times	NS correlation of reading and phoria in morning, but trend in afternoon (Telebinocular testing)
12. Blika	1982	41 PR, 200 GR Grades 1–6	NS phoria, vergence, and stereopsis (Professional vision testing, Norway)
13. Helveston et al.	1985	1,910 N Grades 1 and 3	NS phoria, vergence, and stereopsis (Amblyoscope phoria and vergence testing)

Key: PR, poor reader; GR, good reader; NR, normal readers; N, unselected readers; NS, not significant.
[a] See reference listing of Reference 96 for complete information.

sis and one study used severely dyslexic children the cause of whose reading failure was well-documented (67). Generally the studies that found a significant association between poor reading and some binocular dysfunction were better designed and utilized professional testing procedures (see Robinson and O'Grady in Table 22.5) (68, 84). The meta-analysis of studies generally confirmed that several single condition associations exist, but in the future studies should be designed that look at several findings or conditions taken together. In one example of this type of analysis, Dunlop (16) found that a combination of esophoria, defective stereopsis, and crossed dominance distinguished between good and poor readers. It seems reasonable to assume that any binocular condition that clinicians have found to affect near point performance in adults may also significantly impair reading performance in some school-aged children. Screening programs should be designed that take this possibility into account.

HOW DO VISION ANOMALIES AFFECT THE READING PROCESS?

Vision anomalies can have complex relationships to reading problems and disabilities. There are at least two major ways that vision anomalies interfere with reading. Some vision anomalies can cause direct misperception of the print. If a patient's symptoms include constant or intermittent blur, diplopia, jumping, or distortion, misreading of symbols, a decoding error, can occur. The anomaly disrupts the first stage of bottom-up processing, the discrimination and identification of symbols, and all subsequent higher stages of processing are affected. Second, nearly all vision anomalies that affect reading at all affect it indirectly by slowing or limiting reading performance through some neurophysiologic stress response—eye strain, headache, fatigue, inflammation, or a vague sense of discomfort. The reader must exert more effort to decode and comprehend the meaning of the passage. Both direct misperception and indirect asthenopic symptoms can also contribute to conscious or unconscious avoidance behavior commonly seen as inattention, distractibility, restlessness or hyperactivity, boredom, fatigue, and a general dislike of reading tasks.

Asthenopic symptoms most often appear after sustained near work of 15 to 20 minutes and rarely have an immediate onset. During the early grades, learning to decode involves looking at the chalkboard as the teacher explains concepts and reading word lists and brief selections of text. Thus, learning to decode does not involve much sustained near work and would not be as subject to asthenopic interference as other aspects of reading training. However, when a child attempts sustained reading to develop automaticity of word recognition and ultimately comprehension, asthenopic symptoms might become a more limiting factor. Reading would be slow and stressful and could produce inattention and avoidance of reading altogether (86). The net result is less exposure to print, which would retard growth of automatic word recognition and comprehension. In summary, direct interference of blur, distortion, or diplopia could interfere with the entire reading process, decoding through comprehension, while asthenopic symptoms that increase in severity over time might interfere more at the level of automaticity and comprehension.

WHAT ARE THE VISION SCREENING NEEDS OF STUDENTS WHO ARE EXPERIENCING READING DIFFICULTIES?

The literature is quite clear in pointing to the inadequacy of the distance Snellen acuity test for vision screening purposes (Chap. 20). Only about one third of patients who need referral as identified by the Modified Clinical Technique (MCT) referral criteria are properly identified by the Snellen test (5). The Snellen test used alone fails to identify most visual conditions associated with reading difficulties—low to moderate hyperopia, hyperopic anisometropia, heterophoria, fusional deficiency, among others. Myopia and moderate to high astigmatism reduce distance acuity and can be adequately identified by Snellen testing in most grades, with the possible exception of kindergarten; however, we have seen that these conditions are not usually associated with reading difficulties. The virtues of the Snellen test include its low overreferral rate and cost effectiveness (school personnel can administer the test). These factors have been the primary considerations in its national acceptance as the standard school vision screening technique. A successful vision screening technique and protocol certainly must be cost effective, but the cost of identification must be proportional to the extent and severity of the conditions under investigation. This review of the literature documents significant associations between several visual disorders and reading difficulties. It is also apparent that screening programs that rely on Snellen acuity testing are ineffective in identifying most visual conditions affecting reading and the real costs of this policy in terms of human suffering have not been properly assessed.

The MCT, an alternative vision screening program to the Snellen test, is conducted by a vision care doctor and includes the essential techniques used to identify most visual conditions associated with reading problems. Five procedures are usually included: Snellen distance acuity, retinoscopy, cover test at distance and near, ocular health observations, and a color vision test. MCT screening programs are often sponsored by local optometric societies and need not impose a severe financial burden on school districts. The procedure has been accepted by many school districts across the nation and represents a much higher and better standard of vision care.

Unfortunately, certain visual efficiency conditions that appear to be associated with impaired reading performance are not identified by MCT procedures. In an investigation of binocular vision conditions in reading-deficient junior high students and their normally achieving peers (37), three conditions not identifiable by MCT screening were found to be statistically more prevalent among the poor readers: accommodative infacility, fusional vergence deficiency, and gross convergence insufficiency (Table 22.7). These conditions were found to be two or three times more prevalent among students in remedial reading classes than in their normally achieving age peers in the same school. These three conditions can all compromise visual efficiency and comfort, but once identified they can usually be managed successfully with a short vision therapy program that involves training for one half hour per day over a 4- to 6-week period.

Considering the high prevalence of vision disorders and visual efficiency dysfunctions among children in remedial reading programs or special education (see Tables 22.4 to 22.6), it seems appropriate that a com-

Table 22.7 SUNNYVALE JUNIOR HIGH SPECIAL EDUCATION STUDY, 1986, VISUAL EFFICIENCY AND READING DIFFICULTIES

	Incidence		Chi Square Analysis	
	(No.)	(%)	Normal	Deficiency
Analysis of focusing deficiency				
Normal readers	7/37	19	30	7
Disabled readers	47/115	41	68	47
			$x = 5.89$	$p < .02$
Analysis of fusion deficiency				
Normal readers	3/34	9	31	3
Disabled readers	38/112	34	74	38
			$x = 8.14$	$p < .005$
Analysis of gross convergence				
Normal readers	2/36	6	34	2
Disabled readers	24/113	21	89	24
			$x = 4.66$	$p < .03$

(Reproduced from Grisham JD: Computerized Vision Training: First Year Report. Palo Alto CA, American Institutes for Research, 1985)

plete optometric examination by a doctor skilled in children's vision problems should be required for entry into any special education program. Rosenbloom (86) asserts that a preschool vision examination for all new students should be as routine as inoculations against childhood diseases. The responsibility of the schools for vision screening would be satisfied, but it is important that the vision examination include a comprehensive investigation of acuity, refractive state, binocular vision, visual efficiency, and ocular health. A school report form could include a list of the visual functions known to be related to reading difficulties, which the examining doctor would complete and return to school officials. If requiring a comprehensive vision examination for reading underachievers is not a feasible policy for a particular school or district, the next best solution for proper identification would be employing an optometrist or ophthalmologist to conduct a MCT screening that includes tests of visual efficiency.

Standards for MCT referral are described in the Orinda study (5) and elsewhere in this text, but since visual efficiency screening is a relatively new concept, some guidelines are included here. Normative data for monocular accommodative facility have been determined for children aged 8 through 14 years (Table 22.8). Using ±2 D flipper lenses with a 20/30 acuity target placed 33 cm from the child, a mean time of 52 seconds was found for 10 cycles (SD 24 seconds). Using the low tail of the first standard deviation as an arbitrary standard, a referral would be considered if the test required 75 seconds or more to complete with the full cooperation of the child. Many children who have accommodative deficiencies cannot complete the 10 cycles and blur out at some point during the test. Norms could not be determined for younger children because their subjective responses proved to be unreliable by objective evaluation on an optometer (56).

Vergence deficiencies can be identified with an objective technique, the reflex fusion stress test. The compensating vergence system for the heterophoria at near point is tested—convergence or base-out prism for

Table 22.8   UNIVERSITY OF CALIFORNIA SCHOOL OF OPTOMETRY CLINICAL NORMS FOR MONOCULAR ACCOMMODATIVE FACILITY OF DOMINANT SIGHTING EYE

Children (ages 8–14 years; N = 105):
±2.00-D flippers; 10 cycles; @33 cm:
Mean = 52 sec ± 24 (SD)
Low tail = ≥75 sec
Rate = 7.5 sec/cycle

Adults (N = 211):
±1.50-D flippers; 20 cycles; @40 cm:
Mean = 64 seconds ± 26 (SD)
Low tail = ≥90 sec
Rate = 4.5 sec/cycle

Children's norms. From Mah MM, Pope RS, Wong JH, et al: Adult norms. From Optometry Laboratory Exercises. Berkeley, CA, 1980.

exophoria and divergence or base-in prism for esophoria. A 6-PD loose prism is inserted in front of the sighting dominant eye for 10 cycles, and the elapsed time is recorded. Clinical norms indicate a deficiency may be present if the response time for 10 cycles of either base-in or base-out prism is 25 seconds or longer. The base-in test has a mean of 21 ± 4 seconds, and the base-out test has a mean of 22 ± 3 seconds. A fusional vergence deficiency is suggested by a long response time or the inability to complete the task due to diplopia.

Near point of convergence is measured at least three times. If a break point of 10 cm or further away is found with repetition, a gross convergence insufficiency is indicated. Some patients who have visual stress do not see diplopia at the near point of convergence, and this observation would confirm the diagnosis.

WHAT EFFECT DOES OPTOMETRIC VISION THERAPY HAVE ON READING PROGRESS?

Much controversy surrounds the use of optometric vision therapy when there is the expectation, implicit or explicit, of improving

reading performance. The professional literature from reading research, learning disabilities, medicine, and optometry frequently addresses this question, with contradictory
conclusions. Some noted reading researchers
strongly oppose the use of saccadic eye
movement training as a means to improving
reading efficiency (81, 106) whereas some educators and optometrists recommend it (99).
The position statement of the American
Academy of Ophthalmology also claims there
is no scientific evidence to support the use of
eye exercises in the management of dyslexia
and associated learning disabilities. The
meaning of this statement again hinges on
how dyslexia is defined. Many optometric
writers, on the other hand, extol the virtues of
various forms of optometric vision therapy.
They often see dramatic changes in a patient's symptoms and reading performance
following treatment.

In their literature review of the efficacy
of optometric vision therapy, Barbara Keogh
and Pelland (48) noted that the issues are
confusing and the evidence contradictory.
The literature is plagued with methodologic
errors and lack of rigor in defining the categories of reading difficulties. Another difficulty
arises from not clearly identifying the type of
vision therapy concerned. Rather than treating vision therapy as a single treatment entity, which it certainly is not, this review describes the record of specific types of vision
therapy. Is there evidence that correcting refractive anomalies, in and of itself, improves
reading performance? If a student has a binocular vision dysfunction, can one expect increased comfort and reading skill after completion of an orthoptics program? Do
oculomotor or binocular enhancement procedures have some beneficial effects on reading? Does developmental vision and perceptual skills training have sufficient evidence to
support its claim of improving the reading
capability of learning-disabled children?
This last issue is too complex to answer adequately within the scope of this review, but
for the sake of completeness it needs to be
raised.

Correcting Refractive Anomalies

It seems obvious that a moderate or large uncorrected refractive anomaly could cause or
contribute to reading difficulty. What is often
surprising to many clinicians is how much
change in comfort and reading efficiency
comes from correcting even small amounts of
hyperopia, astigmatism, and anisometropia.
Clinicians commonly examine patients who
complain of asthenopic symptoms while
reading caused by an uncorrected refractive
anomaly, but surprisingly few studies document the influence of correcting a refractive
anomaly on reading tasks other than reading
acuity charts.

One of the first and best studies was that
of Farris in 1936 (25). Two large groups of
seventh grade students were matched for
type of refractive anomaly, age, and IQ. One
group received the needed glasses, the other
group did not. Reading progress over a 1-year
period was tested. Students wearing lenses
generally made greater gains in reading, but
when the data were analyzed relative to type
of refractive anomaly, dramatic differences
were found. The students whose hyperopia
and hyperopic astigmatism were corrected
made substantial gains in reading compared
to students with similar disorders that were
not corrected, but those with uncorrected
myopia improved more than myopic students
who faithfully wore their glasses.

The benefit of glasses for hyperopia was
also demonstrated in a study by Eames (20).
He tested word recognition speed in 100 students wearing prescription glasses. The
speed of recognition was measured with and
without spectacles at near point by tachistoscope. All hyperopic subjects wearing 2 D or
more showed faster word perception with the
glasses than without. The majority of hyperopic students with as little as 1 D correction
also read better with their glasses. As would
be expected, those with myopia over 3 D
showed increased speed with their correction, but 20 percent of those with low myopia
could read faster without their glasses. This
report and that of Farris (25) are consistent

with the idea that strain on the accommodative system contributes to visual comfort and efficiency during reading.

Some recent evidence that correcting significant hyperopia early in life can have a positive effect on academic skills development comes from the Rosner (89). A retrospective analysis of 500 pediatric clinic records revealed 48 cases of hyperopia of +2.50 D or greater. The copy form scores (visual analysis skills) for this group were compared with those of a group of peers without significant refractive anomaly. The young hyperopic students, aged 6 to 13.4 years, were more likely to show substandard visual analysis skills than their peers, but those whose condition was corrected before age 4 years had better copy form skills than those who received spectacles after age 4 ($p < 0.001$). This study suggests there may be developmental advantages to correcting moderate hyperopia during the preschool years.

Another interesting investigation by Eames (22) suggested that uncorrected anisometropia can have an even greater effect on reading performance than an uncorrected refractive anomaly of equal amount in each eye. Two groups of uncorrected patients, one group with anisometropia and another with equal refractive anomalies, were matched in age, sex, and IQ. The subjects with uncorrected anisometropia were found to be reading at a level 1 year behind the control group. Six months after correction of both groups, the reading performance had equalized. Uncorrected anisometropia compromises the integration of images in the cerebral cortex and so can be considered a problem of binocular vision.

Vision Therapy and Reading Performance

Vision therapy is defined as the art and science of developing visual abilities to achieve optimal visual performance and comfort (Policy Manual AOA 1966). When vision therapy is directed toward developing or improving oculomotor and binocular skills, the term becomes synonymous with the medical term *orthoptics*. Orthoptics has a long history, dating from at least the middle of the nineteenth century. Although it was developed as a nonsurgical alternative or adjunct to the treatment of strabismus, orthoptics' best successes have been with functional deficiencies of binocular vision and the accompanying asthenopic symptoms. There are many fine review articles on the efficacy of vision therapy, but only a few report the effect on reading skills. This issue is the focus of the next section.

Training of Ocular Motility

The optometric literature indicates that the control characteristics of fixations, pursuits, and saccades can be trained to a high degree in many patients (41) and even improved in cases of cerebral palsy (15). Several case reports of oculomotor-deficient patients also demonstrate improved reading skills following therapy (11, 79). If a child presents with reading difficulties and demonstrates deficient ocular motility on both reading and nonreading tasks, an ocular motor training program may improve fixation control during reading.

A more general question can be asked: Would children benefit from the training of eye movement control independent of oculomotor deficiencies? Would the use of oculomotor techniques enhance reading performance independent of specific signs and symptoms of dysfunction? There are a few controlled studies (41, 105) that suggest that reading might be improved by such training. The study by Heath and associates (41) is important, because, besides two different oculomotor training groups of second- and third-grade students, the experiment included Hawthorne and no-intervention control groups. The Bender proprioceptive feedback oculomotor training group showed significant gains in pursuits, convergence, Metropolitan Reading Test scores, and eye track measurements superior to the no-intervention control group. The Bender group also showed a strong trend in reading score improvement and eye track results compared to the Hawthorne control group ($p = 0.07$ and 0.08, respectively). On the other hand, in their influential literature reviews, Tinker (106) and Rayner (81) have adopted a skeptical attitude toward this approach to improving reading skills, for reasons cited below.

Rhythmic Reading   One oculomotor technique is to teach readers to move their eyes across print in a regular, prescribed pattern. When readers show approximately the same eye movement pattern from line to line they are said to employ a rhythmic pattern of eye movements. Some current speed reading programs teach students to rapidly fixate equally spaced dots to build a rhythmic pattern (58). This notion of rhythmic reading is not only useless but harmful. Many studies indicate that central factors of comprehension and assimilation, rather than peripheral ones like mechanical factors, are dominant in determining reading proficiency (81, 106). The two important determinants of regularity in eye movements are difficulty of material read and purpose of reading.

Controlled Reader Training   Another popular method for training reading eye movements over the years has been the use of a controlled reader. Reading material is presented at a controlled rate, forcing readers to move their eyes more rapidly and form new habits. It is probable that more skills than just eye movements are being trained with this technique (e.g., perceptual span, memory, scanning). Many investigations without adequate controls have consistently shown substantial improvement in reading efficiency (50, 99), but several controlled studies have indicated that controlled reader training is not better than either motivated library reading or simply reading with the intent to improve (34, 110). Tinker (106) believes that controlled reader techniques might well be used to supplement a program in which reading comprehension is emphasized, but training eye movements per se does not increase reading ability. Controlled reading techniques have

lost their appeal among remedial reading teachers and are rarely used today.

In summary, it can be said that since there is little evidence to support rhythmic eye movement training for improving reading skills, it seems prudent not to recommend its general application in the classroom or in an optometric practice. Controlled reader training is not currently in vogue, but it may be a useful adjunct in a comprehensive remedial reading program. There remains the open question of the efficacy of oculomotor enhancement training, such as the Bender proprioceptive feedback method. Few studies isolate oculomotor training; it is often included with other procedures in a general vision therapy program. On the other hand, if a patient has an eye movement control deficiency, as seen in some cases of idiopathic nystagmus, remedial therapy seems appropriate and may be undertaken with the expectation that some improvement in reading skills may result.

Training of Accommodation and Fusional Convergence

Optometrists and ophthalmologists are aware of the negative influence accommodative deficiencies have upon near point comfort and performance (10, 90). Clinicians routinely prescribe presbyopic and nonpresbyopic reading glasses to affected patients, and in some cases recommend vision training for functional accommodative deficiencies. The efficacy of training accommodation in cases of accommodative insufficiency, infacility, and fatigue is now well-established (6, 52, 90). It is therefore surprising to find so few studies that have looked at the influence of accommodative therapy on near point performance other than visual acuity measurements. Utilizing a controlled experimental design and studying school children who have deficient accommodation, Weisz (109) showed that accuracy in a pencil-and-paper task improved after accommodative training. Hoffman (43) also investigated the transfer effects of accommodative training in accommodation-deficient children. He found a significant improvement in visual attention and in the perceptual skills of visual discrimination and visuomotor integration among children in the 5- to 8-year-old accommodative training group. Control group children in all age categories and the older experimental group children failed to show significant improvement. Probably the best study to date was that of Cooper and coworkers (13), who used each adult accommodative training subject as their own control in a crossover design. Concurrent with only the automated accommodative training phase was a marked increase in accommodative amplitude and a decrease in asthenopic symptoms. Decreases of blur and increases of reading time were the most frequently reported changes. Unfortunately, only five subjects were studied. With these encouraging reports and the literature implicating accommodative disorders in poor readers, it is imperative that investigators continue to look for direct effects of accommodative therapy on reading performance.

There has been considerably more interest in the transfer effects on reading of vision therapy emphasizing vergence procedures. Essentially two subject groups have been investigated: (1) students who have both vergence dysfunctions and reading problems and (2) college students who experience reading difficulties without reference to their binocular vision status. Several detailed case reports (54, 55) and large patient series have been reported in which the presenting complaint was poor reading performance and a vergence dysfunction was identified (2, 29, 39, 112). Various vision therapy procedures for fusional vergence and other binocular functions were applied successfully over a period of time. Improvements in reading performance were noted in each report. Of particular interest is the report from Haddad and associates (39), an ophthalmology patient series, which helps to clarify the relationships between dyslexia and fusional disorders. This series consists of 73 children referred for vision examinations because of reading difficulty. Fifty-eight percent of the total

group were considered to have dyslexia, but it isn't clear how dyslexia was determined; 25 percent had overt refractive anomalies; and 51 percent, including over half of the dyslexic children had deficient fusional amplitudes. The authors noted that merely wearing the glasses ameliorated the reading difficulty in students who needed them. A therapy program designed to increase fusional amplitudes, improve the near point of convergence, and break suppression was initiated in cases of fusional deficiency. Improvements in attention and reading performance (length of time of uninterrupted reading) were found following resolution of the fusional deficiency in both the dyslexic and nondyslexic children. The authors concluded that the training did not cure dyslexic students' perceptual problems but did enhance reading performance. Dyslexia and fusional deficiencies are considered to be largely independent disorders. Hammerberg and Norn (40), in another ophthalmology patient series, found that 27 percent of their dyslexic population had some disorder of accommodation or convergence and found that orthoptics training was indicated and beneficial, although dyslexic complaints persisted. These reports document a high rate of fusional deficiency among students referred for reading difficulty and demonstrate the value of vision therapy in these cases, dyslexic or nondyslexic.

Since accommodative and fusional vergence deficiencies appear to be quite prevalent among poor readers and can usually be corrected with a short therapy program, it would be desirable if these deficiencies could be managed in the classroom. One controlled study on the efficacy of computer-based vision training indicated there may be some potential in this approach. Grisham (37) matched three groups of remedial readers in seventh grade on the bases of type of binocular vision deficiency, reading level, and IQ. One group received computer vision therapy for a half hour per day for 10 weeks at the school. A second group received remedial reading instruction for the same time interval, and a third group served as a Hawthorne control by practicing computer games unrelated to reading or vision training. Only the computer group showed significant gains in their binocular vision skills of accommodative facility, fusional vergence, and near point of convergence (Fig. 22.1). The computer-based vision therapy program was considered successful in training binocular vision skills and was administered by trained teaching assistants under the supervision of a consulting optometrist. All groups increased equally in their reading skills during the 3-month project.

Orthoptics training has also been used as a general remedial strategy, regardless of any identified binocular vision deficiency. Using college freshmen enrolled in a remedial reading class, Peters (76) compared the reading improvement associated with remedial reading instruction and orthoptics therapy. He found equal improvement by either strategy, and the better students seemed to benefit the most from the vision training. Binocular skills increase significantly in the orthoptics training group, and there was relatively no change in visual functions accompanying remedial reading instruction alone. That is a fascinating finding: enhancement vision training yields the same increase in reading performance as educational instruction, but the design and result of the study do not allow strong conclusions to be drawn.

A similar experiment was conducted by Olson and coworkers (72). In this well-designed study, there were controls for the placebo effect. One matched group of college students received vision therapy only; a second group had vision therapy and psychological counseling for their problems; a third group participated in counseling alone; and the fourth group was merely retested without any form of therapy as a baseline control. Analysis of variance indicated statistically significant gains in silent reading rates only in the two groups undergoing vision therapy. There was no significant increase in comprehension or mental ability in any group. Taken together, these two studies suggest that there may be some beneficial effects for reading

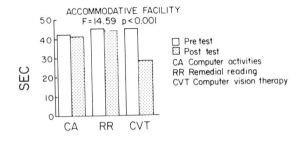

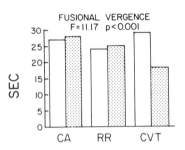

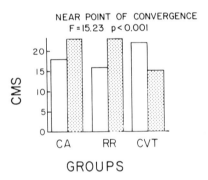

Figure 22.1 Results of the Computerized Vision Training Project. Matched junior high and high school remedial reading students with binocular deficiencies were distributed between three groups of 20 subjects each: (1) Computer activities (CA), a Hawthorne control; (2) remedial reading (RR); and (3) computerized vision therapy (CVT) for accommodation and vergences. Each group was followed for 10 weeks; only the CVT group showed significant improvement in binocular vision functions. (Reproduced with permission from Grisham JD: Computerized Vision Training: First Year Report. Palo Alto CA, American Institutes for Research Publication, 1985.)

performance from binocular vision enhancement therapy for remedial reading students. Currently it is not clear what accounts for the gains, but the assumption is greater comfort and efficiency of binocular vision. This also appears to be a fertile area for investigation.

Developmental Vision Therapy

Developmental optometry has not yet found a secure place in the mainstream of optometric thought and practice, but it has been very influential in extending optometric vision therapy beyond the scope of orthoptics training. Nurtured primarily by the Optometric Extension Program (OEP) and the College of Optometrists in Vision Development (COVD), most developmental optometrists view vision and vision dysfunctions from a psychological-educational perspective of empiricism. They generally believe most vision disorders and learning problems arise from environmental and learned behavioral factors that can be corrected by appropriate vision therapy. These optometrists frequently integrate binocular vision training into a varied program of perceptual-motor and gross coordination activities and the use of small amounts of plus lens power in bifocal form. The glasses are sometimes called *learning lenses*. It is difficult to generalize about the content of these training programs because they vary so greatly from one practitioner to another. The developmental optometry literature supporting vision therapy activities includes many inspiring clinical reports of children who improved their self-image, concentration, visual and general body coordination, and school performance, but developmental vision therapy approaches will not be generally accepted by optometrists and other professionals until their merits are demonstrated by more controlled clinical trials.

The efficacy and validity of perceptual, or process, training programs for improving reading performance have been the subject of much research and heated debate among eye care professionals, educators, and psychologists for many years, and still there are deep divisions of opinion. While there is strong evidence of a correlation between visual perceptual skills and reading achievement (85), particularly visual memory, closure, and discrimination (46), and a number of studies demonstrate positive results with selected programs (64, 93, 103), the results of the preponderance of controlled studies in the research literature have been negative or inconclusive (65). Traditional methods of remediation more often produced reading progress superior or equal to that of perceptual remedial programs. Using metaanalysis that evaluates trends in multiple studies, Kavale and Mattson (47) found no significant effect of perceptual motor training programs on reading performance. They analyzed 180 studies, including those using the methods of Delacato, Frostig, Getman, and Kephart. The numerous negative studies and the current belief among educators that reading is more of a linguistic process than a visual-perceptual one has led educators to be generally skeptical of perceptual training programs for reading-disabled persons. Much more discriminating research is needed before the issue is settled. Large-scale studies of groups should address the possibility that certain subgroups of underachievers with particular clinical signs might benefit more from perceptual or process training than from traditional approaches alone. There is some evidence that perceptual skills deficits may have an impact on the reading process only during beginning educational stages, preschool through third grade (24, 61, 89). Even if further research shows that perceptual training provides little direct benefit toward resolving the reading difficulty per se, children may learn other valuable skills that would be helpful in and out of the classroom. Improved attention, perceptual discrimination, and physical coordination may be its own reward. Only time and continuing research will tell.

One noteworthy and well-designed study of perceptual training known as the Cambrian Project (92) was not included in Kavale and Mattson's metaanalysis (47). This 3-year, multidisciplinary, controlled study compared the reading progress of reading disabled elementary school students in response to one of two remedial approaches, visual, auditory, and motor perceptual therapy or superintensive remedial reading instruction. The Cambrian Project demonstrated that remediation of perceptual disabilities resulted in reading gains superior to those achieved in a remedial reading program. It is interesting to note that vision therapy and perceptual motor therapy alone were necessary but not sufficient to produce the superior results. The best reading results accrued after auditory perceptual training was incorporated into the experimental group's remedial program. These results argue for a multidisciplinary approach to testing, training, and research in reading disabilities.

In summary, optometric vision therapy includes a wide range of therapeutic approaches for a large number of vision conditions. A serious evaluation of the effect of vision therapy procedures on reading performance must take into account this diversity. There is evidence that for persons who suffer from certain refractive conditions and nonstrabismic deficiencies of ocular motility, accommodation, and fusional vergence, optometric vision therapy may have the added benefit of improving reading comfort and efficiency. Clinical evidence suggests that even dyslexics who have fusional deficiencies can benefit from binocular vision therapy without the expectation of their perceptual confusion being resolved. It is less clear, however, that ocular motor and binocular vision enhancement training should be generally employed in the hope of improving reading performance. Despite a few positive reports (69, 76), it seems appropriate to wait for more definitive research to support these practices. The efficacy of perceptual motor training programs or optometric vision therapy for children with severe reading problems or dyslexia is still much disputed and no early resolution appears imminent. Further research is needed to target specific types of reading and perceptual deficiencies with specific techniques. Multidisciplinary evaluation and cooperation could reduce the confusion and suspicion between all concerned

professionals. It seems prudent that optometrists who specialize in treating children with reading difficulties should pursue graduate (postdoctoral) training in child development, neuropsychology, remedial reading, and special education, thereby expanding their optometric expertise.

One growing area of research that has direct relevance to an optometric perspective toward reading difficulties is the clinical evaluation of reading eye movements. In recent years there is increased interest in looking at the fine structure of these eye movements to gain insight into the reading process. Armed with proper instrumentation and training, optometrists may be able to make clinical judgments that are important to the educational and optometric management of persons experiencing reading problems of unknown origin. In the remainder of this chapter we explore these possibilities.

WHAT ARE THE CHARACTERISTICS OF NORMAL READING EYE MOVEMENTS?

Saccades and Ocular Motility

The eye movements involved in reading attracted the attention of scientists during the last century. In 1878, Professor Lewis Emile Javal made a significant discovery by simply watching the eyes of a school child in the act of reading. His predecessors had assumed that the eyes sweep along a line of print in a smooth pursuit movement. Javal observed not a steady sweep but a series of small jumps (saccadic movements) with intervening fixation pauses. The fixation pauses (duration of fixation) are the periods of clear vision when perception occurs. Thus, the input of visual information resulting in perception during the act of reading is not continuous but is interrupted several times each second by eye jumps. The material is thus naturally divided into chunks or packages that are reassembled by the brain into a spatiotemporally continuous visual experience (35).

The principal components of reading eye movement patterns are saccades and fixational pauses (Fig. 22.2). The eyes are stationary, resting in a fixational pause, about 90 percent of the time during a reading task (82). Rapid saccadic eye movements take about 20 msec for a 3-degree jump. Reading eye movements form a stereotyped pattern consisting, in large part, of a series of small (2- to 4-degree) rightward progressive saccades, jumping from word to word and often skipping common small words. When the end of the line is reached, a larger leftward saccade jumps about 10 degrees to the beginning of the next line. These return sweep saccades are often followed by smaller corrective saccades that readjust eye position to the beginning of the next line. About 5 to 20 percent of the time, regressive saccades occur moving leftward or backward. These saccades probably serve a grammatical or syntactical function. On each fixation the fovea processes high-resolution linguistic information and other details while the retinal periphery directs saccadic eye movements.

Other eye movements besides saccades often occur during reading. Small vergence adjustments are needed as the eyes move from line to line or when the reading material is rotated or moved fore and aft. Head and general body movements during reading inevitably occur in children and adults alike, and these movements activate vestibular ocular reflexes. Residual position and velocity errors must then be corrected by the saccadic and smooth pursuit systems in the attempt to maintain precise fixation. The accommodative system maintains accurate near point focus and adjusts focus for changes in distance to the printed word. Thus, all ocular motor systems are interacting constantly in everyday reading situations.

Perceptual Span and Fixation Pauses

The perceptual span of recognition is defined as the area within which visual information is processed for each fixation. This region extends from three or four character positions to the left of fixation to approximately 15 characters to the right of fixation. Furthermore, within the perceptual span, different types of information are utilized. Information used for word and letter identification is obtained from a smaller region than is information used to determine where to look next. Spatial information out to 14 or 15 character spaces is used to direct subsequent fixations (60), whereas letter information may be processed only up to 8 characters from fixation (107). This means that mature readers identify the semantic content of words falling on and immediately to the right of the fovea. Beyond that area, however, readers are processing word shape and length information. Research indicates that word length information affects reading farther into the periphery than does word shape information or specific letter information. Word shape may be used in the semantic analysis, whereas word length in-

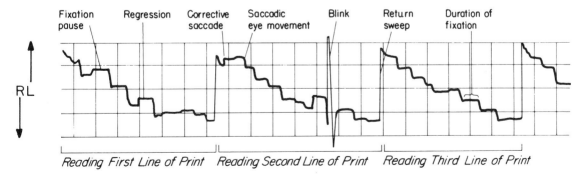

Figure 22.2 Strip chart record of reading eye movements taken on a photoelectric Eye Trac. This record illustrates the characteristic features of reading eye movement behavior.

formation helps guide the eyes to the location of the next fixation. If a word is longer, the eyes tend to jump farther.

What process controls the pause duration of fixation? The cognitive lag hypothesis holds that the eye movements are so rapid and the durations of fixation so short that the semantic processing of the text must necessarily lag behind the perceptual input. A second position, which is referred to as the process-monitoring hypothesis, holds that fixation durations are affected by the cognitive processing that occurs during the time of the specific fixation. Thus, more difficult words and passages should lead to longer fixation durations. Research data indicate that fixation durations on unfamiliar words are longer than fixations on known words, such as the word *the*. Also, a regression occurs immediately after a fixation falls upon a pronoun that has an ambiguous antecedent. Rayner (81) and others have demonstrated that the cognitive content of a word does affect the fixation duration, so the process-monitoring position seems to be supported by most current experimental data.

In general, the fixational pause duration for skilled adult readers fluctuates around 250 msec. The pause includes perception time, thinking time, and some level of comprehension. In reading simple material, pause duration is relatively constant, but with more complex materials it can be highly variable.

Regressions

It is believed that regressive eye movements are a necessary part of the reading process. These leftward or backward saccades make up about 5 to 20 percent of all reading eye movements among skilled readers. Regressive eye movements are executed for a variety of purposes, most of which involve the cognitive process of decoding and comprehending of text. They occur to correct misreading of words or phrases, to glance back at interesting details, to verify meanings of words, and to correct for oculomotor inaccuracies. The number of regressions normally increases with text difficulty, owing to the increased cognitive requirements of understanding the text.

Integration Across Saccades

As previously discussed, a current approach is to consider mature reading primarily a top-down pattern-recognition (guessing) process. Top-down processing implies that a reader makes a guess a priori from context and then quickly checks word shape for confirmation. Some form of a prediction and confirmation process is involved at all levels of reading skill. Top-down processing probably accounts for the high reading rates of superior readers.

A blurred vision image would occur during the saccadic eye movement from one position to another on a page if it were not for suppression of vision during the movement. Besides suppression or masking of vision during each saccade, there appears to be suppression 50 msec before and after the eye movement. At a higher level of processing there apparently is integration of information across saccades from the fixation pauses. Some investigators have suggested that during an eye fixation readers obtain visual information from parafoveal and peripheral vision and store this information in a temporary visual buffer, which they call the integrative visual buffer (60). The implication is that this information buffer is used for confirmation of word recognition guesses on subsequent fixations. The reader has to be actively constructing the scene as the eyes search, and the construction is based in part on visual information and in part on the expectations developed by the reader about what he will see as he moves his eyes. Much more knowledge about the integration of information across saccades is needed and the study of eye movements seems to be a promising powerful technique for investigating this issue (82).

Reading Rate

The reading rate is defined simply as the number of words per minute (wpm) read and serves as an important index of reading efficiency. This index is affected by all the components of reading eye movements but particularly by fixation duration, perceptual span, and number of regressions. Even with easy material, 500 wpm is very fast reading. Most skilled adult readers read at rates between 200 and 400 wpm. Tinker (106) believes that speed reading programs usually teach students not to read in the usual sense of the word but to scan or skim text. Taylor (104) found that when speed readers move their eyes down the middle of a page, the average fixation duration is normal, but they skip a number of lines per saccade. The eye movement patterns of speed readers closely resembled eye movement patterns produced during skimming or scanning activities. As one might expect, comprehension of details suffers.

WHAT ARE THE DEVELOPMENTAL CHARACTERISTICS OF READING EYE MOVEMENTS?

Throughout the elementary school years, as reading fluency increases reading eye movements also show a steady progression of skills. The number of fixations and regressions decreases. The span of recognition and reading rate with comprehension increases with grade level. After the fourth grade the average duration of fixation (i.e., the amount of time the eye pauses during each fixation) decreases very little (Table 22.9). Adult reading appears to be affected much more by the loss of spatial cues such as spacing between words than that of third grade students. It seems that young readers are not as aware of syntactic and semantic constraints as more mature readers. Young children do not have the cognitive control over their eye movements that older children do, and they do not use their peripheral vision as effectively for oculomotor guidance or prediction of upcoming text. Also, young children are not sure where the distinguishing features of letters are located. There is probably concurrent development of eye movement patterns and perceptual skills.

WHAT ARE THE SOURCES OF VARIATION IN READING EYE MOVEMENTS?

When one considers the variation of eye movement patterns in the general population, it is apparent that genetic factors exert a large influence. Morgan (62) reported that correlations for eye movement patterns are low for random pairs of readers (.24) as one might expect, but they are higher for fraternal twins (.53) and highest for identical twins (.72). It is noteworthy that duration of fixation shows the highest correlations for twins and is least susceptible to training. IQ is also a behavioral index that has a strong genetic basis, and studies have shown IQ and reading performance to be strongly associated. Consequently, it is reasonable to expect significant concordance of eye movement patterns in identical twins.

The characteristics of the eye movement patterns (e.g., fixations, regressions, duration of fixation pauses) do not vary significantly from one language to another or when a native speaker of one language learns to read well in another language. A study of the eye movement records of mature readers in 14 different languages indicated that the general nature of the reading act is essentially the same among all mature readers (106). As mature readers seek the meaning of the passage, they follow along the lines with alternating saccades and pauses. At each fixation pause they recognize words as wholes, often two or three at a time, by means of their configuration and striking characteristics.

The major sources of variation among individuals originate from basic cognitive-linguistic abilities, developmental level, and reading experience. For efficient readers, the eye movement pattern changes most dramatically with the level of text difficulty or a change of reading strategy, such as switching from careful reading to skimming. Reading performance of mature readers does not appear to deteriorate much over time. Studies have revealed little or no deterioration due to fatigue after 4 to 6 hours of continuous reading (9, 42). The time course of reading fatigue

Table 22.9 DEVELOPMENTAL CHANGES IN READING EYE MOVEMENTS

Grade	1	2	3	4	5	6	7	8	9	10	11	12	Col.
Fixations (including regressions) per 100 words	224	174	155	139	129	120	114	109	105	101	96	94	90
Regressions per 100 words	52	40	35	31	28	25	23	21	20	19	18	17	15
Average span of recognition (in words)	0.45	0.57	0.65	0.72	0.78	0.83	0.88	0.92	0.95	0.99	1.04	1.06	1.11
Average duration of fixation (in seconds)	0.33	0.30	0.28	0.27	0.27	0.27	0.27	0.27	0.27	0.26	0.26	0.25	0.24
Rate with comprehension (in WPM)	80	115	138	158	173	185	195	204	214	224	237	250	280

(This table is reproduced with permission from Taylor SE, Franckenpohl H, Pettee JL: Grade Level Norms for the Components of the Fundamental Reading Skill. EDL Research and Information Bulletin No. 3, Educational Developmental Laboratories, New York, 1960. WPM = words per minute.)

in persons who have oculomotor, accommodative, or binocular vision dysfunctions has not been reported, but visual fatigue is a common clinical complaint from these patients and one would expect to find a significant detrimental influence upon reading performance. Studies of variation in heterophoric, vergence, fixation disparity, and accommodative functions during prolonged reading (four hours) reveal considerable individual variation in these visual functions which may be the source of asthenopic symptoms in some individuals (94).

WHAT ARE THE CHARACTERISTICS OF THE EYE MOVEMENTS OF POOR READERS?

It is now well-established that oculomotor reactions are exceedingly flexible and quickly reflect any variation in the central processes of perception, judgment, and comprehension. In other words, eye movement patterns primarily reflect ease or difficulty of reading, efficient or poor reading performance, and degree of comprehension, rather than cause good or poor reading in themselves. Poor readers typically make more fixations and regressions than skilled readers (91). Their duration of fixation is long, so, consequently, the reading rate is slow (33). Fast readers have short mean fixation durations and longer mean saccade lengths. Gilbert found that wpm scores correlate highly (.89) with both mean fixation duration and mean saccade length. Also, poor readers typically do not vary their eye movement pattern with the difficulty of reading material. They maintain a stereotyped pattern with easy or difficult text.

Physiologic oculomotor skill is a small but significant contributing factor in the complex interactions that support reading performance. In a study designed to determine the relation between oculomotor functions and reading ability in fourth- and sixth-grade children, oculomotor functions were collectively related to reading ability ($r = .45$), accounting for 20 percent of the variance (78). When ocular motility functions are examined independently, only marginally significant relations to reading ability appear. Of the four oculomotor functions studied, fixation frequency and lag of accommodation had the strongest influence. The authors proposed a reciprocal causation model of oculomotor functions and reading ability. Deficient language skills result in poor reading, a lack of interest in reading, and untrained ocular motor skills. It is also possible that language skills are adequate and an oculomotor functional deficiency could interfere with the reading process. A third possibility is that causation might operate simultaneously in both directions. Other studies have shown differences in the prevalence of oculomotor deficiencies between poor and normal readers using upper and lower quartile reading ability scores (33, 66, 111). While oculomotor skills generally are not the limiting factor in reading performance, it should be remembered that some persons have neurologic eye movement control disorders that do interfere with the reading process, but these are the exceptions rather than the rule.

There is no doubt that several oculomotor control disorders can interfere with the reading process. Several cases are well-documented in the eye movement literature. Disruption of the normal reading eye movement patterns has been described in patients suffering from intermittent exotropia, nystagmus, saccadic intrusions, and oscillopsia. One very well-documented patient presented with oscillopsia and saccadic intrusions (12). The patient showed repetitive regressive saccades present during all types of eye movements and was not able to read for more than a few minutes without experiencing discomfort, confusion, and frustration as words appeared to jump on the page. There were also periods of prolonged fixation (500 to 4000 msec), during which the patient was unable to move the eyes (oculomotor apraxia). Early multiple sclerosis was suspected. This patient received some symptomatic relief and extended her comfortable reading time to an hour by using a typoscope or a low-power magnifier and taking frequent breaks.

WHAT ARE THE CHARACTERISTICS OF DYSLEXIC EYE MOVEMENTS?

Dyslexics have long been noted for their erratic eye movement patterns while reading. The patterns are characterized by the excessive number of regressions, which often occur two or more times in succession. Unlike normal regressions, those of dyslexics are sometimes larger than the preceding forward eye movement. Fixations also show greater variability in size and duration. The overall pattern lacks consistency from line to line.

Although investigators agree that dyslexics exhibit erratic eye movements, they disagree on the extent and nature of the relationship between the eye movements and the disability itself. The most widely held position claims that dyslexia is primarily a language-based disability (108). The erratic eye movements merely reflect frustrated attempts to extract meaning from the text. Saccades are completely normal except when the reader attempts to decode and comprehend language symbols. A second theory views dyslexia as a perceptual problem. The erratic eye movement pattern reflects a more basic spatial processing deficiency that renders forms difficult to recognize and affects spatial sequencing of eye movement control. This perceptual problem contributes to reading failure and is evident using nonreading visual stimuli. It is important to evaluate the evidence for each theory carefully before jumping to a conclusion. The following evaluation suggests there may be a satisfactory reconciliation of these opposing views based on subtypes of dyslexia.

Dyslexics Eye Movements Are Abnormal

One of the first dyslexic cases reported where eye movement control appeared to be a primary factor in limiting reading performance came from Zangwill and Blakemore (114). They described a 23-year-old dyslexic college student who showed many regressions and had a strong tendency to scan from right to left rather than in the usual direction. He could read with normal accuracy isolated words, letters, or digits presented in a tachistoscope, which obviated eye movements. They concluded that the reading difficulty was one of directional scanning characterized by an irrepressible tendency to move the eyes from right to left.

As this case illustrates, some eye movement anomalies can cause or contribute to a reading problem, but a few investigators have suggested that eye movement disorders are characteristic of dyslexic students as a group. Griffin and associates (35) reported a controlled study of normal and disabled readers and found that the disabled readers had less efficient eye movements (more regressions and larger variability) even for nonlanguage targets like dot and picture cards. There is no indication that the groups were equated for general IQ, as in subsequent studies. It is possible that the disabled readers were less skilled at following instructions in both reading and nonreading tasks. In a recent controlled study of fixational stability in dyslexic and normal readers, aged 9 to 13 years, the dyslexics, all of whom showed the soft neurologic signs of mild ataxia and impaired tandem walking, also had greater fixational instability independent of visual attention (80). In these two studies, the reading-disabled students demonstrated reduced oculomotor control independent of reading material, and the authors suggested that this deficiency was a factor in their reading problems.

The most compelling evidence, although controversial, for ocular guidance factors limiting reading performance in dyslexics comes from reports by Pavlidis (73, 75). He compared 12 dyslexics with normal readers, advanced readers, and readers whose skill was retarded by school absenteeism and socioeconomic factors. The groups were matched for general IQ. Their eye movements were recorded as they fixated five equidistant lights that were illuminated sequentially for 1- or 2-second intervals. The dyslexics made significantly more foreword and regressive fixations than all other matched groups. There was little overlap between dyslexics and other readers in the number of their regressions. The dyslexics also made a similar percentage of regressions following the lights as they did while reading text. By way of contrast, the percentage of regressions dropped significantly from reading to lights in the other groups. A discriminant analysis was used to reclassify children as dyslexic or nondyslexic based on the results of the light-tracking task. There was 93 percent agreement with the original psychoeducational criterion used in subject selection. Pavlidis drew several conclusions "(1) Dyslexics' erratic eye movements found during reading are not solely caused by the problems they have with reading. In fact, they are relatively independent of the reading material. (2) The results of the nonreading tasks demonstrate that the dyslexics' erratic eye movements are due to a brain malfunction(s) yet to be determined. (3) The nonreading lights test can differentiate dyslexics from these groups of readers" (74). An etiologic implication of his results is that the dyslexic "brain malfunction" may involve the spatial-temporal saccadic guidance control of the eyes. Pavlidis views dyslexia as a condition of disturbed sequencing function in many parallel systems—language, memory, and eye movement control. This view also has some support from work on simultaneous and successive processing in poor readers (14). A clinical implication is that eye movement records of reading and nonreading visual stimuli can provide an accessible, objective, and unambiguous marker of dyslexia, a long-sought goal of many investigators. If the relationship can be verified, it may be possible to identify preschool children who are prone to dyslexia before they experience reading failure. Educational and perceptual techniques to help students cope with dyslexia could be introduced early. Currently many dyslexic students fail in reading for a year or two before their problem is identified and they are referred for remedial services.

Support for the existence of ocular motor sequencing deficiencies in at least some dyslexics has been forthcoming from case reports by Elterman and colleagues (23) and a detailed study by Jones and Stark (45). In several cases, Jones and Stark demonstrated reverse staircase eye movements during reading which did not appear to be related to information processing (Fig. 22.3). Dyslexic subjects made their return sweeps using a series of small backward saccades rather than a single eye movement. Also, some dyslexic subjects showed episodic tracking inaccuracies to sequentially presented spot targets.

Dyslexic Eye Movements Are Normal

Standing in direct contradiction to the conclusions of Pavlidis and others, several studies of dyslexic eye movement patterns found no primary saccadic tracking deficiency independent of reading material (1, 4, 8, 72). They conclude that saccadic control is normal when nonreading visual stimuli are used and that the erratic eye movement pattern of dyslexics reflects deficiencies in language information processing. The study by Brown and associates (8) was particularly well-designed and had a well-matched control group for the dyslexic subjects. Judging from the dyslexic selection criteria, though, it appears that the dyslexias were all of the dysphonetic type. In response, Pavlidis (74) claimed that these studies are not comparable because they did not replicate his experiments. He attributed the differing results to four factors: (1) subject selection criteria, which is critical for filtering out nondyslexic persons; (2) experimental procedures; (3) data analysis procedures; and (4) temporospatial characteristics of the sequentially illuminated lights. His critics suggest that Pavlidis might have attracted a rare subgroup of dyslexic subjects who have eye movement control deficiencies, but their research indicates that the vast majority of dyslexic persons manifest no primary eye movement control problem.

Eye Movements Depend on the Subgroup of Dyslexia

One intriguing possibility is that oculomotor sequential deficiencies are associated with a

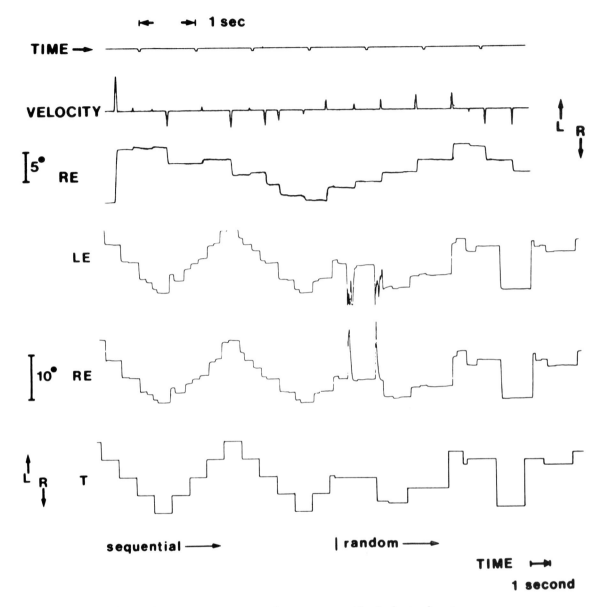

Figure 22.3 (A) The reading eye movements of a young specific dyslexic showing an occurrence of a complete reverse staircase. Note the prolonged fixation pauses within the reverse pattern. (B) The eye movement record of a young specific dyslexic boy who tracked sequential target displacements followed 2 seconds later by a random tracking task. Prediction is evidenced by short, zero, or positive saccadic latencies that dominate the sequential tracking record. A short episode of accurate sequential tracking can be noted at the beginning of the record. (Reproduced with permission from: Jones A, Stark L: Abnormal patterns of normal eye movements in specific dyslexia. In Rayner K (ed): Eye Movements in Reading: Perceptual and Language Processes. NY, Academic Press, 1983. Figures 27.1 and 27.5.)

visual-spatial subgroup of dyslexia and not with the more prevalent auditory-linguistic subgroup (Table 22.1). Those with auditory-linguistic dyslexia tend to have a lower verbal IQ relative to performance IQ, developmentally delayed language skills, reading errors mainly involving the phonologic aspects of language, a letter-by-letter decoding strategy, and relatively intact visual-spatial skills. Contrasting characteristics of the visual-spatial type include lower performance IQ compared to verbal, right-left and other spatial disorientation, reading errors involving visual aspects of text, many reversals and omissions of words and letters, use of phonetic decoding strategy, and relatively normal oral language abilities (77). In a study of saccadic latency and reading eye movements among dyslexic subtypes and normal subjects, Pirozzolo found that those with visual-spatial dyslexia had shorter latencies for leftward saccades whereas those with auditory-linguistic dyslexia and normal readers had shorter latencies for rightward saccades. Furthermore, the visual-spatial subtypes were distinguishable by return sweep inaccuracies, the frequency of which was independent of text difficulty. They also showed evidence of frequent right-to-left scanning, suggesting the irrepressible tendency to scan text from right to left that was first reported by Zangwell and Blackmore in 1972 (114). Pirozzolo concluded that the visual-spatial subgroup of dyslexics can be distinguished by their eye movement pattern and that the differences probably result from poor visual-spatial programming of saccadic eye movements. If these results are confirmed by further research, a clinical evaluation of reading eye movements could be an important part of dyslexia screening and classification.

WHAT ARE THE CLINICAL METHODS OF EVALUATING OCULAR MOTILITY AND READING EYE MOVEMENTS?

One precipitant of optometric referral from the schools is that a teacher or nurse observes a student making what appear to be wild eye movements. The erratic eye movements are noticed as the child reads or attempts to track some visual target. As a routine screening procedure, and particularly in cases of school referral, fixation skill and motilities should be assessed carefully. Direct observation is the technique most often used to assess the physiologic capabilities of oculomotor systems—position maintenance (fixations), pursuits, and saccades. The assessment is directed toward answering the following questions: Is there a physiologic immaturity, a pathologic disorder, or an abnormality of ocular motor functions? If there is an observed dysfunction, does inattention, a lack of interest or cooperation, or some other psychological state explain or contribute to the deficient oculomotor responses?

Confrontation Testing

Steadiness of fixation (position maintenance) can be observed directly with or without lens magnification as a student attempts to hold binocular fixation on a small discreet target for about 10 seconds. School-aged children free of neurologic deficits should be able to maintain a steady response with no observable movement of the eyes. The micromovements of fixation are usually subclinical by direct observation. A precise evaluation of each eye's centricity and steadiness of fixation can best be accomplished by using a reticule pattern on direct ophthalmoscopy. Small-amplitude nystagmus, eccentric fixation, and fixation inaccuracy can easily be seen if the foveal light reflex and reticule are visible. A dilated fundus examination may be necessary for some children.

The clinically important characteristics of pursuit eye movements which the clinician should observe directly are smoothness, accuracy, and perseverance. A small discreet target or penlight can be used as a stimulus. The patient is instructed to keep the eyes on the moving target as accurately as possible. The optometrist moves the target across the patient's midline several times while carefully observing the response. The target should be moved into all cardinal fields of gaze in the standard H pattern. Also, it can be moved slowly in a figure-eight pattern to inspect tracking along diagonals and rotations. School age children should have the physiologic eye movement skill to complete this task accurately with only a few lapses into corrective saccadic movements. There are clinical reports of "midline hesitations" among developmentally immature students, but the optometrist must take care not to misinterpret those occasions when an anxious child makes eye contact with the tester. The most common cause of a lag or overshoot during a pursuit test is a lapse of attention. For this reason, children should be reminded frequently to track accurately. If a penlight is used, asking the patient to report any blinking of the light typically increases the interest of the procedure. The child tracks the light intently watching for blinks and indicates when one is observed. Clinically relevant questions are: With full cooperation and interest, can the patient track accurately in a sustained task of 30 seconds or more? Are the pursuit eye movements accompanied by head movements or are they independent?

Saccadic eye movements are assessed clinically in several ways—direct observation, timed testing, and eye movement recordings. Several direct observation techniques and rating systems have been advocated by various authors, but the following straightforward method seems as useful as any other. Two letter targets of approximately 20/80 acuity level are separated approximately 25 cm and held 40 cm away from the patient. The patient is instructed to move the eyes back and forth to each target 10 times (36). It seems appropriate that observations also be taken for target separation of about 10 cm, as this distance would approximate the return sweep made during reading. Short saccades require a higher level of guidance control. The examiner notes the number of inaccuracies, velocity, and conjugacy. If a school-aged child shows more than two inaccuracies on either test, physiologic immaturity is suspected. Care must be taken in evaluating any observed inaccuracies, as, again, psychological factors easily influence these

results. One might expect that the reliability of gross observations of pursuits and saccades might present a serious problem, but a recent study of interrater and test-retest reliability indicated acceptable reliability using a rating scale recommended by Northeastern State University College of Optometry (57).

Timed Tests of Saccades

Two clinical tests that are currently used to assess saccadic eye movements are the Pierce and King-Devick saccadic tests. Following the presentation of a demonstration card, the patient reads aloud random numbers placed in sequence on three separate test pages. The response times and number of errors are then compared to normative data. Since both tests require number reading as a response indicator, it seems inappropriate to use this method with a child who is suspected of having a reading disability. An abnormally low score might very well reflect difficulty with naming symbols or maintaining the required attention to task rather than a deficiency in saccadic eye movement control per se. These tests do not discriminate saccadic control factors from cognitive factors (83). Two studies have also called into question their test-retest reliability (28, 71).

Eye Trac and Visagraph Recording

Two clinical photoelectric eye movement recording systems, the Eye Trac and the Visagraph, are currently used by optometrists, special educators, and other professionals interested in evaluating reading eye movements (Fig. 22.4). The older one, Eye Trac, is a portable, self-contained, monitor and strip chart recording unit. The newly introduced Visagraph is a computerized monitor and recording unit designed to run with an Apple II series computer. These systems have several advantages over other saccadic assessment techniques. Each provides a permanent objective eye movement record for further analysis and longitudinal documentation. Reading eye movements are analyzed into specific components and more general indices. The

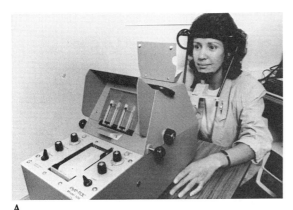

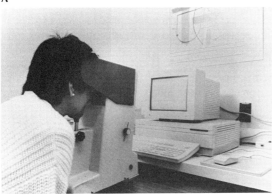

Figure 22.4 (**A**) Eye-Trac, Model 106: Photoelectric sensors register reading eye movements by monitoring the limbal reflection as the subject reads test paragraphs printed on 3 × 5-inch cards. The output is a strip chart recording of the eye movements, which must be analyzed by inspection. (**B**) Visagraph: Reading eye movements are monitored by a photoelectric limbal reflection method as the test paragraphs are presented on a computer monitor. The output is a hard copy report of the analyzed eye movements and/or a strip chart record of the unanalyzed eye movements.

analysis delineates the number of fixations and regressions, the duration of fixation, the span of perception (recognition), reading rate, relative efficiency, and grade equivalency. These components and indexes are then compared against established norms for elementary school children through adults (see Table 22.9). These instruments can also be used to evaluate saccadic eye movements independent of information processing. A test card can be designed with dots, asterisks, or other simple fixation targets. Patients are asked to accurately and quickly move their eyes to each target in sequence. Five lines of five equally spaced dots can be used for this purpose. Saccadic control independent of reading is judged by comparing the accuracy and number of fixation responses with the stimulus pattern.

The Visagraph, in particular, holds great promise as a diagnostic instrument. The computer program objectively analyzes the reading eye movement record relative to all the standard components and presents a summary report. This has been a laborious and subjective process done by hand using the Eye Trac strip chart record. The Visagraph printout of the actual unanalyzed eye movement record is also available for inspection if desired. A recent study of concurrent validity between the Visagraph and Eye Trac indicated that the two instruments yield comparable data for subjects who are properly aligned. The reading eye movement records of 30 young adults were analyzed and concurrent validity was found to be acceptable ($r \geq +0.6$) for measures of fixations, span of perception, reading rate, relative efficiency, and grade equivalency. Test-retest reliability of the Visagraph proved acceptable ($r \geq +0.8$) for measures of span of perception, relative efficiency, and number of fixations (53). The Visagraph appears to have acceptable concurrent validity and reliability for use in clinical practice. Optometrists with special interest and training in vision and reading problems will find these assessment techniques a useful addition to their standard optometric examination.

SUMMARY

The field of remedial reading and reading disabilities is complex, multidisciplinary, and important to the welfare of any modern society. The optometrist has significant services to contribute because the factors leading to underachievement in reading certainly include several visual conditions. When a broadly drawn sample of poor readers is compared to normal achieving peers, the research literature indicates a higher prevalence of hyperopia, anisometropia, aniseikonia, hyperphoria, exophoria, and fusional vergence and accommodative deficiencies. Optometric intervention in many of these cases has helped to improved reading performance. The correction of significant hyperopia and training of fusional vergence can increase the ease and comfort of reading in visually dysfunctional individuals. Primary vision disorders may not cause neurologically based dyslexia per se, but if a dyslexic child has a vision disorder, then optometric treatment can produce an incremental improvement in reading performance, as for anyone else. For these reasons it is important that any child who is experiencing reading difficulties receives a complete optometric examination.

It is also important that optometrists maintain proper perspective about reading difficulties and recognize the many possible causal factors. From an educational perspective, most underachieving students have problems with decoding or comprehension, or both. Decoding skills are taught first—letter discriminations, symbol-sound correspondences, sound blending, and automatic word recognition, among other skills. Comprehension of print starts with decoding, a bottom-up process, but mature reading is characterized by top-down processing where the meaning is anticipated from syntax, semantics, world knowledge, and previous reading and language experience. Difficulty in learning to read can occur from inadequate learning at any stage in the reading process. One of the causes of underachievement is a learning disability in reading, dyslexia, which is presumed to have a neurologic basis. Reading-disabled students almost always have profound decoding problems, and special educational techniques involving multisensory instruction might be required before reading skill can develop. Although managing a child's vision disorder is certainly necessary in many cases, it does not substitute for appropriate remedial reading or other special instruction.

Properly equipped and trained, the optometrist is one professional in a position to help make some important and difficult distinctions about the factors that contribute to reading problems. First, as previously discussed, is the presence of contributing visual factors—refractive, binocular, oculomotor, or visual-perceptual. Beyond this obvious responsibility is the possibility of helping educators make a perplexing distinction, the distinction between a remedial reading student and a reading-disabled student. Not withstanding much controversy, there is some evidence that certain types of dyslexic children have peculiar reading eye movement patterns that students whose reading failure stems from other causes do not manifest. Some show an inordinate number of regressions, reverse staircase saccades, return sweep inaccuracies, longer latencies on rightward saccades, and saccadic inaccuracies with and without language symbols. Armed with a thorough optometric examination and a reading eye movement analysis, the optometrist can help to properly identify learning-disabled readers with a contributing vision problem. The optometrist should also know the vocabulary and perspective of the reading teacher, for this will facilitate communication and interprofessional cooperation for the sake of students who are suffering from reading difficulties. In the hope of furthering these goals, this review was written.

REFERENCES

1. Adler-Grinberg D, Stark L: Eye movements, scanpaths, and dyslexia. Am J Optom Physiol Opt 55:557, 1978.

2. Atzmon D: Positive effect of improving relative fusional vergence on reading and learning disabilities. Binocular Vision 1:39, 1985.

3. Bailey I: Night Vision: Current Research and Future Directions. NAS-NRC Committee on Vision monograph. Washington DC, National Academy Press, 1987.

4. Black JL, Collins DWK, DeRoach JN, et al: A detailed study of sequential saccadic eye movements for normal and poor reading children. Percept Mot Skills 51:423, 1984.

5. Blum HL, Peters HB, Bettman JW: The Orinda Study: Vision Screening in the Schools. Berkeley, University Press, 1959.

6. Bobier WR, Sivak JG: Orthoptic treatment of subjects showing slow accommodative response. Am J Optom Physiol Opt 60:678, 1982.

7. Boder E: Developmental dyslexia: A diagnostic approach based on three atypical reading patterns. Dev Med Child Neurol 15:663, 1973.

8. Brown B, Haegerstrom-Portnoy G, Yingling CD, et al: Tracking eye movements are normal in dyslexic children. Am J Optom Physiol Opt 60:376, 1983.

9. Carmichael L, Dearborn WF: Reading and Visual Fatigue. Boston, Houghton-Mifflin, 1947.

10. Chrousos GA, O'Neill JF, Lueth BD, et al: Accommodation deficiency in healthy young individuals. J Pediatr Ophthalmol Strabismus 25:176, 1988.

11. Ciuffreda KJ, Bahill AT, Kenyon RV, et al: Eye movements during reading. Am J Optom Physiol Opt 53:389, 1976.

12. Ciuffreda KJ, Kenyon RV, Stark L: Saccadic intrusions contributing to reading disability: A case report. Am J Optom Physiol Opt 60:242, 1983.

13. Cooper J, Feldman J, Selenow A, et al: Reduction of asthenopia after accommodative facility training. Am J Optom Physiol Opt 64:430, 1987.

14. Das JP, Kirby J, Jarman RF: Simultaneous and successive synthesis. Psychol Bull 82, 1975.

15. Duckman RH: Vision therapy for the child with cerebral palsy. J Am Optom Assoc 58:28, 1987.

16. Dunlop P: The changing role of orthoptics in dyslexia. Br Orthoptics J 33:22, 1976.

17. Eames TH: A comparison of the ocular characteristics of unselected and reading disability groups. J Educ Res 25:1932.

18. Eames TH: A frequency study of physical handicaps in reading disability and unselected groups. J Educ Res 29:1935.

19. Eames TH: Comparison of eye conditions among 1000 reading failures, 500 ophthalmic patients, and 150 unselected children. Am J Ophthalmol 31:713, 1948.

20. Eames TH: The effect of glasses for the correction of hypermetropia and myopia on the speed of visual perception of objects and words. J Educ Res 42:534, 1949.

21. Eames TH: The influence of hyperometropia and myopia on reading achievement. Am J Ophthalmol 39:375, 1955.

22. Eames TH: The effect of anisometropia on reading achievement. Am J Optom Arch Acad Optom 41:700, 1964.

23. Elterman RD, Abel LA, Daroff RB, et al: Eye movement patterns in dyslexic children. J Learning Disab 13:16, 1980.

24. Farr JA, Leibowitz HW: An experimental study of the efficacy of perceptual-motor training. Am J Optom Physiol Opt 53:451, 1976.

25. Farris LP: Visual defects as factors influencing achievement in reading. Ph.D. Thesis. Berkeley, University of California, 1936.

26. Fendrick P: Visual characteristics of poor readers. Teachers College Contributions to Educ. No. 656. NY, Columbia University, 1935.

27. Flax N: The eye and learning disabilities. J Learning Disab 6:60, 1973.

28. Fleming JC, Barney P: A reliability study of tests measuring saccadic ability. Senior Research Project, MB Ketchum Library, S.C.C.O. Fullerton CA, 1984.

29. Friedman N: Specific visula fixation stress and motor-learning difficulty—Part II. J Am Optom Assoc 43:166, 1972.

30. Galaburda AM, Kemper TL: Cytoarchitectonic abnormalities in developmental dyslexia: A case study. Ann Neurol 6:94, 1979.

31. Geschwind N: Disorders of higher cortical function in children. In Geschwind N (ed): Selected Papers on Language and the Brain. Dordrecht Holland, D Reidel, 1974.

32. Geschwind N, Galaburda AM: Cerebral Lateralization: Biological Mechanisms, Associations, and Pathology. Cambridge MA, MIT Press, 1987.

33. Gilbert LC: Functional motor efficiency of the eyes and its relation to reading. University California Public Education. 11:159, 1953.

34. Glock MD: Effect upon eye movements and reading rate at the college level of three methods of training. J Educ Psychol 40:93, 1949.

35. Griffin DC, Walton HN, Ives V: Saccades as related to reading disorders. J Learning Disabl 7:310, 1974.

36. Griffin JR: Binocular Anomalies: Procedures for Vision Therapy. Chicago IL, Professional Press, 1982.

37. Grisham JD: Computerized Vision Training: First Year Report. Palo Alto CA, American Institutes for Research Publication, 1985.

38. Grisham JD, Simons HD: Refractive error and the reading process: A literature analysis. J Am Optom Assoc 57:44, 1986.

39. Haddad HM, Isaacs NS, Onghena K, et al: The use of orthoptics in dyslexia. J Learning Disabl 142, 1984.

40. Hammerberg E, Norn MS: Defective dissociation of accommodation and convergence in dyslexic children. Acta Ophthalmol (Copenh) 50:651, 1972.

41. Heath EJ, Cook P, O'Dell N: Eye exercises and reading efficiency. J Academic Therapy 11:435, 1976.

42. Hoffman AC: Eye movements during prolonged reading. J Exp Psychol 36:95, 1946.

43. Hoffman LG: The effect of accommodative deficiencies on the developmental level of perceptual skills. Am J Optom Physiol Opt 59:254, 1982.

44. Ingram TS, Mason A, Blackburn I: A retrospective study of 82 children with reading disability. Dev Med Child Neurol 12:271, 1970.

45. Jones A, Stark L: Abnormal patterns of normal eye movements in specific dyslexia. In Rayner K (ed): Eye Movements in Reading: Perceptual and Language Processes. New York, Academic Press, 481, 1983.

46. Kavale K: Meta-analysis of the relationship between visual perceptual skills and reading achievement. J Learning Disabl 1:1982.

47. Kavale K, Mattson D: "One jumped off the balance beam": Meta-analysis of perceptual-motor training. J Learning Disabl 3:1983.

48. Keogh DD, Pelland BA: Vision training revisited. J Learning Disabl 18:228, 1985.

49. Kinsbourne M, Warrington E: Developmental factors in reading and writing backwardness. Br J Psychol 54:145, 1963.

50. Leeds JP: Speed reading and visual training. Am J Optom Arch Am Acad Optom 5:254, 1960.

51. Levin H: Reading research: What, why and for whom? Elementary English 41:138, 1950.

52. Liu JL, Lee M, Jang J, et al: Objective assessment of accommodative orthoptics. 1. Dynamic insufficiency. Am J Optom Physiol Opt 56:285, 1979.

53. Low LR, Scolaro DL, Greenwood BR: Concurrent validity and reliability of the Visagraph reading eye movement system. Grisham JD (advisor): OD project. Berkeley CA, School of Optometry Library, 1988.

54. Ludlam WM: Visual training, the alpha activation cycle and reading. J Am Optom Assoc 50:111, 1979.

55. Ludlam WM, Twaroski C, Ludlam DP: Optometric visual training for reading disability—A case report. Am J Optom Arch Am Acad Optom 50:58, 1973.

56. Mah MM, Pope RS, Wong JH: Testing of accommodative facility in elementary school age children. Grisham D, Stark L (advisors): OD thesis. Berkeley CA, School of Optometry Library, 1981.

57. Maples WC, Fickin TW: Interrater and test-retest reliability of pursuits and saccades. J Am Optom Assoc 59:549, 1988.

58. Marron J: Smart Eyes: Program Manual, A Software Learning Program. Menlo Park CA, Addison-Wesley, 1985.

59. Mattis S, French JH, Rapin I: Dyslexia in children and young adults: Three independent neuropsychological syndromes. Dev Med Child Neurol 17:150, 1975.

60. McConkie GW, Rayner K: Identifying the span of the effective stimulus in reading: Literature review and theories of reading. In Singer H, Rudell R (eds): Theoretical Models and Processes of Reading. Newark DE, International Reading Assoc, 1976.

61. Miller JW, McKenna MC: Disabled readers: Their intellectual and perceptual capacities at differing ages. Percept Mot Skills 52:467, 1981.

62. Morgan DH: Twin similarities in photographic measures of eye movements while reading prose. J Educ Psychol 30:572, 1939.

63. Morgan MW: Relationship of refractive error to bookishness and androgyny. Am J Optom Arch Am Acad Optom 37:171, 1960.

64. Morgan MW: The effect of visual perceptual training upon subsequent scholastic progress of children with specific visual disabilities. MA thesis. Reno NV, University of Nevada, 1966.

65. Myers PI, Hammill DD: Learning Disabilities: Basic Concepts, Assessment Practices, and Instructional Strategies. Austin TX, Pro-ed, 1982.

66. Nedrow JL: A comparative study of accommodative performance in a selected group of good and poor readers. MS dissertation. Forest Grove OR, Pacific University, 1970.

67. Norm MS, Rindziunski E, Skydsgaard H: Ophthalmologic and orthoptic examinations of dyslexics. Acta Ophthalmol (Copenh) 47:147, 1969.

68. O'Grady J: The relationship between vision and educational performance: A study of year 2 children in Tasmania. Aust J Optom 67:126, 1984.

69. Olson HC, Mitchell CC, Westberg WC: The relationship between visual training and reading and academic improvement. Am J Opt Arch Am Acad Optom 30:3, 1953.

70. Olson RK, Kliegl R, Davidson BJ: Dyslexic and normal readers' eye movements. J Exp Psychol [Hum Percept] 9:816, 1983.

71. Oride MKH, Marutani JK, Rouse MW, et al: Reliability study of the Pierce and King-Devick saccade tests. Am J Optom Physiol Opt 63:419, 1986.

72. Oslon HC, Mitchell CC, Westberg WC: The relationship between visual training and reading and academic improvement. Am J Optom Arch Am Acad Optom 30:3, 1953.

73. Pavlidis GT: Do eye movements hold the key to dyslexia? Neuropsychologia 19:57, 1981.

74. Pavlidis GT: Erratic eye movements and dyslexia: Factors determining their relationship. Percept Mot Skills 60:319, 1985.

75. Pavlidis GT: Eye movements: the diagnostic key to dyslexia? Contemp Optom 5:7, 1986.

76. Peters HB: The influence of orthoptic training on reading ability, Part II: The problem, study and conclusions. Am J Optom Arch Am Acad Optom 19:152, 1942.

77. Pirozzolo FJ: Eye movements and reading disability. In Rayner K (ed): Eye Movements in Reading: Perceptual and Language Processes. NY, Academic Press, 499, 1983.

78. Poynter HL, Schor C, Haynes HM, et al: Oculomotor Functions in Reading Disability. Am J Optom Physiol Opt 59:116, 1982.

79. Punnett AF, Steinhauer GD: Relationship between reinforcement and eye movements during ocular motor training with learning disabled children. J Learning Disabl 17:16, 1984.

80. Raymond JE, Ogden NA, Fagan JE, et al: Fixational instability in dyslexic children. Am J Optom Physiol Opt 65:174, 1988.

81. Rayner K: Eye movements in reading and information processing, Psychol Bull 85:618, 1978.

82. Rayner K: Eye movements in Reading: Perceptual and Language Processes. NY, Academic Press, 1983.

83. Richman JE, Walker AJ, Garzia RP: The impact of automatic digit naming ability on a clinical test of eye movement functioning. J Am Optom Assoc 54:617, 1983.

84. Robinson HM: Visual efficiency and reading status in the elementary school. In Robinson HM, Smith AC (eds): Clinical Studies in Reading. Chicago, University of Chicago Press, Suppl Educ Monographs 97:49, 1968.

85. Robinson HM, Mozzi L, Wittick ML, et al: Children's perceptual achievement forms: A

558 *Specific Conditions in Diagnosis and Management*

three year study. Am J Opt Arch Am Acad Optom 37:223, 1960.

86. Rosenbloom AA: Promoting visual readiness for reading. In Figurel, JA (ed): Changing Concepts of Reading Instruction. NY, Inter Reading Assoc Conf Proceedings 6:89, 1961.

87. Rosenbloom AA: The relationship between aniseikonia and achievement. In Robinson HM, Smith AC (eds): Clinical Studies in Reading III. Chicago, University of Chicago Press, Suppl Educ Monographs 97:109, 1968.

88. Rosner J, Rosner J: The clinical management of perceptual skills disorders in a primary care practice. J Am Optom Assoc 57:56, 1986.

89. Rosner J, Rosner J: Visual perceptual skills development of young hyperopes and age of first lens correction. Clin Exp Optom 69:166, 1986.

90. Rouse MW: Management of Binocular Anomalies: Efficacy of vision therapy in the treatment of accommodative deficiencies. Am J Optom Physiol Opt 64:415, 1987.

91. Rubino CA, Minden HA: An analysis of eye-movements in children with a reading disability. Cortex 9:217, 1973.

92. Ryan PJ: The Cambrian Project: An experiment in the remediation of reading retardation of first through sixth graders by means of auditory, visual and/or motoric perceptual therapy, final report. Project #43-69384-35-26424, Research and Teacher Education, Bureau of Prof Devel Division of Compensatory Education, Calif State Dept of Education. Also Berkeley CA, Optometry Library, 1973.

93. Seiderman AS: Optometric vision therapy: Results of a demonstration project with a learning disabled population. J Am Optom Assoc 51:489, 1980.

94. Shadid PD, Sturgis MD: Variability of oculomotor functions with reading. O.D. thesis. Grisham JD (Advisor): U.C., Berkeley CA, School of Optometry Library, 1984.

95. Simons HD, Gassler PA: Vision anomalies and reading skill: A meta-analysis of the literature. Am J Optom Physiol Opt 65:893, 1988.

96. Simons HD, Grisham JD: Binocular anoma-

lies and reading problems. J Am Optom Assoc 58:578, 1987.

97. Sleeter CE: Learning Disabilities: The social construction of a special education category. Except Child 53:46, 1986.

98. Smith F: Understanding Reading. NY, Holt, Rinehart & Winston, 1982.

99. Solan HA: Eye movement problems in achieving readers: An update. Am J Optom Physiol Opt 62:812, 1985.

100. Stanley G, Smith G, Howell EA: Eye movements and sequential tracking in dyslexic and control children. Br J Psychol 74:181, 1983.

101. Stromberg EL: The relationship of measures of visual acuity and ametropia to reading speed. J Appl Psychol 22:70, 1938.

102. Swanson DE, Tiffin J: Betts' physiological approach to the analysis of reading disabilities as applied to the college level. J Educ Res 29:433, 1936.

103. Swanson WL: Optometric vision therapy: How successful is it in the treatment of learning disorders? J Learning Disabl 5:37, 1972.

104. Taylor SE: Eye movements while reading: facts and fallacies. Am Educ Res J 2:187, 1965.

105. Tillson MW: Changes in eye movement pattern. J Higher Educ 26:442, 1955.

106. Tinker MA: Recent studies of eye movements in reading. Psychol Bull 55:215, 1957.

107. Underwood NR, McConkie GW: The effect of encountering errors at different retinal locations during reading. Unpublished manuscript. Available from McConkie GW: Center for the Study of Reading, 51 Gentry Dr, Champaign IL 61820, 1981.

108. Vellutino, FR: Dyslexia: Theory and Research. Cambridge MA, MIT Press, 1979.

109. Weisz CL: Clinical therapy for accommodative responses: Transfer effects upon performance. J Am Optom Assoc 50:209, 1979.

110. Westover FL: Controlled eye movements versus practice exercises in reading: A comparison of methods of improving reading speed and comprehension. Teach Coll Contr Educ 917:1946.

111. Wilson K, Wold R: A report of vision screening in the schools. Academic Therapy 8:155, 1972.

112. Wold RM, Pierce JR, Keddington J: Effectiveness of optometric vision therapy. J Am Optom Assoc 49:1047, 1978.

113. Young FA: Reading measures in intelligence and refractive error. Am J Optom 49:237, 1963.

114. Zangwill OL, Blakemore C: Dyslexia: Reversal of eye movements during reading. Neuropsychologia 10:371, 1972.

Chapter 23

Optometrists on the Team: Holistic Care and the Patient-Parent-Educator Interface

Alana M. Zambone

The purpose of this chapter is to present optometrists with an overview of the larger intervention system in which they must operate when serving a child with a visual anomaly. The team approach to intervention and strategies for participating as a member of the team are explored, as is the idea that professionals can and should develop mutually beneficial ways to combine their skills with those of other professionals and of informal helpers, in providing a system of care for children in need (5).

The chapter includes summaries of legislation and practice that impact on the child and the team, descriptions of the other team members and their roles, responsibilities, and areas of expertise, and techniques for team participation and communication. The chapter discusses the role of the optometrist in the management of children's visual needs in the context of the full scope of children's developmental and maturational needs.

HOLISTIC ASSESSMENT AND INTERVENTION—BEYOND MEDICAL MANAGEMENT

Because a variety of forces influence a child's function, behavior, and learning, a holistic approach that utilizes multiple skills and various orientations is necessary to identify a child's needs and to develop strategies to meet those needs. For the child with severe vision dysfunction, the issues in providing vision care extend beyond those of identifying optimal treatment and correction, to encompass such areas as self-image, function in the classroom and at home, and vision-directed skill development such as writing and reading, to name a few. According to Gearhart, DeRuiter, and Sileo (6), the holistic approach is based on a developmental perspective that "recognizes a functional relationship between parts in a whole rather than a view that focuses on discrete behaviors," or characteristics.

The optometrist provides diagnosis and treatment in the context of the child's functional vision needs and in the context of the resources of the larger system in which the child participates. Such variables as the vision demands placed on the child during school, the degree of active participation in recreational activities, family financial resources, and cosmetic considerations all influence the prescription of corrective lenses. The optometrist must therefore work with others to ensure that the vision services provided are appropriate and effective.

OVERVIEW OF THE SOCIAL, HEALTH, AND EDUCATIONAL SERVICE DELIVERY SYSTEMS

The term service delivery system refers to three broad categories or subsystems of public and private human services: social, health, and education services. Typically, most children require services from all three categories simultaneously, but at varying levels of intensity. There are numerous types of services and service settings within each service category. The requirements of children with vision problems increase in direct relation to the degree of dysfunction. Primary responsibility for providing services passes among the three categories as the child's age changes or depending on the availability of services, income level, health- and disability-related needs, and a multitude of other factors related to the needs of the child and the needs and resources of the family and community (9).

The service delivery system is vast, complex, and, to varying degrees, has interrelated functions. In essence, while it is called a system, services are, in fact, more representative of a collection of separate efforts to address single needs.

If the child has a disability or a condition that may interfere with development, the educational subsystem may begin to assume responsibility as the primary provider early in the child's life. As the child moves through the education system, referrals to the health and social subsystems will occur as the school or family deems necessary.

The education system for the child with a special need such as a vision loss is a highly complex range of program options, that represent a variety of settings and models, from the public school classrooms to highly specialized residential centers. Special education programs are generally categorized by the amount of special services children receive and the amount of time they spend away from a regular classroom with peers whose needs are similar to their own. Educational services available to children with special needs from the ages of 6 through 21 years are presented in Table 23.1.

With the passage of a variety of laws guaranteeing education and other civil rights for children with special needs and their families, by 1990 educational services will be provided in all states from birth to age 21 and will be guaranteed for this population from 3 years of age through 21 years. The two predominant models for services to children from birth through 3 years of age are home- and center-based. Essentially, the majority of early childhood services reflect one of these two models or a combination.

Home-Based Services are provided to children and the primary caretaker by one or more specialists. The specialist visits the home and works predominantly with the caretaker, providing information and referral, liaison between other services providers, and guidance in ways to enhance the child's development. The specialist may work directly with the child, but in the context of demonstrating strategies for the caretaker. Visitation can vary from several times a week to once a month or less. This is usually the approach of choice for children under age 3 years.

Table 23.1 RANGE OF EDUCATIONAL SERVICE SETTINGS FOR EXCEPTIONAL CHILDREN

Regular Classroom: Children with and without special needs participate with little outside assistance. Modifications may be made in the environment, materials, or type of instruction provided.

Consultant Teacher Model: Specialist provides assistance to the teacher and provides assistance in procuring special materials or equipment. The consultant teacher also serves as liaison between the classroom and other relevant resources, such as the optometrist.

Itinerant Teacher Model: Specialist travels from school to school and works directly with the student on skills related to the student's disability. This teacher also fulfills the responsibilities of the consultant teacher.

Resource Room Model: Majority of education occurs in the regular classroom. Special services are received in a separate room with other children who have similar needs.

Specialized or Segregated Classrooms: Differs from the resource room in that students receive the majority of their education in the specialized setting.

Specialized or Segregated Day School: Children reside in their own communities and attend a special public or private school.

Residential Schools: Similar to specialized day schools in that they serve children with similar needs. Children reside at the school, returning home on weekends and holidays. All special education services are provided at the school. Primary focus is education.

Institutional Models: Primary focus is long-term total care, including education.

Homebound and Hospital: Provided to children who cannot attend school because of special health care requirements. Educator provides one-to-one instruction.

Center-Based In this model, the child attends a center or classroom program, often accompanied by the caretaker, one or more times per week. The child works on developmental and functional skills such as language and eating independently. The teacher coordinates other specialized services within the center and the larger community, such as physical therapy and optometric care, and helps the family gain access to them.

An important component of all of the educational services described above is team coordination, including case management demands. There is, however, no mandate for a team approach for regular education, so children who do not receive special education services do not have a case manager or formal team services.

THE TEAM APPROACH TO INTERVENTION

The team approach as a model for provision of special education services is mandated by the passage of P.L. 94-142, the Education for All Handicapped Children Act of 1975, and, more recently, by amendments to that law, P.L. 99-457. A team is described as a group of professionals from various disciplines, the parents, and the exceptional child. This group makes decisions together about the child's educational needs, placement, and program (8).

The Team Approach to Treatment of All Children

Because a variety of forces influence the child's behavior and learning, multiple skills and various orientations are necessary to identify the child's needs and to tailor a program to the nature and severity of the vision problem. Each behavior a child exhibits or task a child performs involves several complementary functions. For example, walking down a crowded hallway demands that, at minimum, gross motor skills, balance, motor planning, visual scanning, and visual perception be applied to the task simultaneously. A deficit in any one of these areas, such as vision, requires compensation or adjustment in the integration of another area for performance to take place.

If a plan is to be developed that reflects a complete and integrated picture of the child's strengths and weaknesses a team must function from an interdisciplinary, rather than a multidisciplinary approach. The team decision-making process is labeled *multidisciplinary* when each member interacts separately with the child and the aggregate of their findings and recommendations then becomes the plan. A team is labeled *interdisciplinary* when each discipline's representative shares and integrates impressions and recommendations rather than simply aggregating them into a plan.

Legislation Regulating Educational Intervention

The primary laws dictating a team approach to intervention are those in education (for an overview of this legislation see Chapter 1). *P.L. 94-142: The Education for All Handicapped Children Act of 1975:* This law mandates that all children aged 6 through 21 years with special needs have the right to a free, appropriate public education, and it provides a series of procedural and administrative guidelines for implementation. While the law is comprehensive, some basic components that define the intent beyond the law and shape the nature of services provided as a result of the law have implications for all practitioners. Table 23.2 describes the major programmatic requirements of this law.

P.L. 99-457: The 1986 Amendments to the Education for All Handicapped Children Act: Although this law addresses a variety of areas relevant to education of children with disabilities, some components represent significant changes to the earlier law, P.L. 94-142. The major components of P.L. 94-142, including the seven areas listed above, were maintained within the amendments. What P.L. 99-457 most notably accomplished was extension of the mandate for educational services for children 6 years old down to 3 years

old through 21 years and provision of strong incentives for service delivery to children from birth (referred to in the law as Part H). Services to children from age 3 must meet the same requirements as those outlined in P.L. 94-142 (see Table 23.2) except that the children do not have to be counted as a member of a specific disability group. Table 23.3 outlines the major requirements under Part H.

As of July, 1987, all 50 states, the District of Columbia, and the five trusts and territories agreed to participate in Part H, referred to as the Early Intervention State Grant Fund. Thus, the above described provisions will be applicable nationwide by 1990.

An important provision in P.L. 99-457 is the requirement for interagency collaboration. Any state that agrees to participate in Part H is required to appoint a State Interagency Coordinating Council consisting of 15 members representing all provider agencies, the State Legislature, Personnel Preparation Programs, and parents themselves. Each state may appoint a lead agency to administer the program, coordinate resources, monitor program and activities, resolve disputes, and develop interagency agreements. The Council may also be appointed to fulfill this function.

An Overview of Members of the Team: Roles and Responsibilities

In each phase of the development of an Individualized Education Program (IEP) for a child with special needs, as described in P.L. 94-142, the team membership changes, depending on the information required at that stage, the resources available in the system, and the unique needs of the individual child and family. The major phases and decision points in the educational process are: (1) identification; (2) assessment; (3) determination of eligibility; (4) determination of strengths and needs, and of the educational program required to address them; (5) placement in an educational setting; and (6) implementation of the educational program. The educational program—and consequently placement and eligibility decisions—are reviewed and revised at least annually, so these

Table 23.2 MAJOR PROGRAM COMPONENTS OF P.L. 94-142 AND THEIR RELATIONSHIP TO THE OPTOMETRIST

Requirement	Optometrist's Role
Child Find and Early Identification	
Requires each state to implement a system for identifying children in need of special services and to count them as members of a special disability group according to criteria described in the law.	May provide first documented indication of a visual condition that places the child at risk for delay or identifies the child as disabled according to the criteria outlined in the law.
Free Appropriate Public Education	
Each child must receive an education based on an individualized education plan (IEP), developed by a team of specialists and the family, at no cost to the family. The IEP includes (1) current level of functioning; (2) strengths and weaknesses; (3) goals and objectives for the school year; (4) procedures for meeting goals and evaluating progress; (5) identification of the person responsible for seeing the plan is carried out; and (6) settings in which the program is provided and the degree of integration with nondisabled peers.	Contribute to the design of the child's program, including recommendations for environmental modifications, specialized equipment and materials. The optometrist's information about the child's vision is critical to the decision-making process, including the potential impact of the child's visual condition on functionality.
Multidisciplinary Unbiased Assessment and Programming	
Each child's program is based on a culture-free, accessible, multiple-source assessment conducted by a multidisciplinary team.	Along with the information stated above, the optometrist's information would be critical to ensuring that the child was assessed in an accessible medium (e.g., with magnification).
Placement in the Least Restrictive Environment	
Each child's education is to be provided in the setting that is as close to the regular classroom (see Table 23.1) as is beneficial for that child. Placement is determined individually, based on the range of needs the child exhibits and is reviewed annually as part of the IEP review process.	
Provision of Related Services	
Each child's IEP must include those related services necessary for the child to benefit from the educational program, including but not limited to physical and occupational therapy; speech and language therapy; audiology and vision assessment; and psychological and behavioral services.	Functional vision assessment, vision therapy, etc., could all be considered as a related service, depending on the child's needs.
Protection of Due Process and Confidentiality	
The law stipulates a series of procedures to protect the child's and family's rights and provide for correction of violation of those rights, including dispute resolution through due process hearings. These procedures are to be followed throughout identification, assessment, IEP development, placement, and evaluation process. The law also stipulates regulations protecting confidentiality of records and other information with parental or guardian determination of information distribution.	These regulations also apply to optometrists' records.

Table 23.2 *(Continued)*

Requirement	Optometrist's Role
Parent Rights and Involvement	
Parent involvement in educational decisions is mandated. They are full participants on the team and have full protection of due process, including participating fully in all decisions about their child's program.	

decision points recur in the course of the child's education, and team membership changes accordingly. The range of potential roles that could be represented on the team is, however, consistent across settings and children and could include:

The Caregiver The natural parents, legally determined parental representative, or parent surrogate is the person who persists on the team over time and contributes valuable information about the child's functioning, learning style, preferences, personality characteristics, functional needs, performance, and so forth.

The Educator(s) The regular classroom teacher, if the child is mainstreamed, is responsible for modification of teaching strategies, equipment and materials, criteria for performance, and environment within the context of teaching the regular curriculum content to the child. Special educators are responsible for all of the above and also determine what modifications may be required, teaching specialized skills, remediating skill deficits, and procuring or adapting equipment and material as needed.

Related Services Specialists Generally, physical and occupational therapists, speech

Table 23.3 BASIC PROVISIONS OF P.L. 99-457, PART H: SERVICES FROM BIRTH TO 3 YEARS

1. Provides financial and regulatory incentives to states to provide services to children from birth to 3 years, according to the following criteria:
   A. Children with developmental delay
   B. At risk for developmental delay
   C. Diagnosed physical or mental condition with a high probability of resulting in developmental delay.
   "At risk" and "developmental delay" are to be defined by each state.

2. Provides for early identification, screening, and assessment by a multidisciplinary team.

3. Services are provided according to a team-developed individualized family service plan (IFSP) that includes:
   A. Child's present developmental level
   B. Family's strengths and needs as they relate to assisting the child
   C. Specific services to be provided
   D. Anticipated outcomes
   E. Progress evaluation provisions
   F. Designation of a case manager
   G. Protection of due process

and language specialists, orientation and mobility specialists, low vision specialists, psychologists, nurses, administrators, and social workers may participate in the assessment process and provide consultative or direct services as needed.

The nature and level of participation required of each member varies from role to role and situation to situation for each child's team. Some team procedures are mandated by law, others reflect good team practice. The critical components of team procedures, however, are communication among members and integration of information received. Certain procedures, however, are mandated by law and, so, are consistent across teams and setting. Others are recommended to ensure interdisciplinary team function and effective service.

Formal and Legally Mandated Procedures The regulations attached to P.L. 94-142 and P.L. 99-457 spell out specific timelines and procedures for informing parents of their rights, involving parents in the decision-making process, and ensuring that assessment and IEP development are representative of the input of multiple disciplines and perspectives. Each team must generate a document (the IEP) that reflects team input and consensus. Beyond these guidelines there are no specific regulations that address such issues as number and length of meetings, number and nature of participants, and so forth.

Recommended Procedures for Optimal Team Function Procedures that ensure optimal team function are those that facilitate sharing of information and cooperative decision-making in the context of resource, time, and personality constraints. Unidirectional transmission of information, communication of assessment results and recommendations based on independent action, and withholding information about perspective, bias, and approach that influence assessment results and recommendations sabotage team process. Thus, for a team to function effectively, procedures that enable collaborative effort must be agreed upon by all members. These

procedures can be as elaborate or as simple as the individual members and their time and resources allow. The critical variables are that, by the end of the team process everyone understands the other's perspective and everyone has the same knowledge about the child's strengths and needs.

While we have been discussing the team model as mandated by the laws discussed above, every child who is receiving services from two or more sources, as from a teacher and an optometrist, can be considered to have a team, although its members may not perceive themselves as such. Thus, team functions should prevail for all children.

THE OPTOMETRIST ON THE TEAM

Two legislative mandates are described above that have direct relationship to the optometrist providing care for children with vision dysfunction—identification and eligibility determination. These are particularly critical because of the importance of early vision stimulation and developmental intervention for young children with vision anomalies.

The optometrist's contribution, however, extends beyond that of documenting eligibility to receive specialized services, or providing correction or other treatment to the child with vision dysfunction. From the perspective of the family and the other professionals serving the child, the optometrist is seen as the source of information about the child's eye condition, prognosis, and functional vision. This information is critical for determining environmental modifications, instructional strategies, and long-range educational goals and objectives. For example, families and educators often have difficulty knowing which of the child's behaviors are related to the vision needs, where to present materials within the child's field of vision, and whether to recommend caution in certain playground activities. The optometrist's role is therefore one of diagnosis, management, and information exchange.

The optometrist can become involved with the team at a variety of levels, depending on time, resources, degree of contact with the child, and personal style of interaction. At a minimum, she or he submits the vision report to the parent or the school for inclusion in the child's file; most intense involvement can include observing the child in a variety of settings, such as the classroom, and attending team meetings.

Essentially, four elements require coordination for integrated service delivery: individuals involved; resources; information; and programs (1, 7). When considering integrated programming and planning, linkages are forged at the service delivery or case management level. Baumheimer (2) describes service delivery or case management level linkages as interactions that are designed to improve services to the individual—case conferences, team meetings, case management, and case consultation.

Coordination can occur at the levels of agency interaction, program articulation, or individual relationships and should focus on the child, the family, and the unique characteristics of the community (3, 4). Elder goes on to describe the key elements in coordination as: creating a base of knowledge; individualizing the coordination process for patient characteristics; and communicating. As these form the basis for team participation, it is this level that will be expanded below. Depending on the scope of the optometrist's practice, additional interaction can occur at the agency level in the form of in-service training for teachers and low vision services for students, vision screening for school systems, and similar services.

Because the pediatrician is usually the first professional to see the child and family, it is important for optometrists to work together with pediatricians in the treatment of young children, to share the optometrist's knowledge and perspective on vision. Often, subtle functional vision indicators are overlooked during the traditional pediatric examination. Palfrey, Singer, Walker, and Butler (12) reported that the mean age of identification of vision dysfunction (including blindness) by a physician was 54.9 months in their study of five metropolitan communities. With the increased survival rates of low–birth weight and premature infants, whose limitations in functional and perceptual visual skills are extensively documented (10, 11, 13), many more young children are at risk today for developmental delays, reading problems, and other conditions resulting from inadequate vision care during early childhood.

COMMUNICATING WITH PROFESSIONALS IN HEALTH, EDUCATION, AND RELATED SERVICES

Team participation and decision making generally follow a four-step process: (1) information sharing and exchange; (2) information analysis and synthesis; (3) decision making; and (4) summarization. Information sharing and exchange is necessary. The sources of information are multiple and range from the results of evaluations to subjective information based on observation. Information analysis and synthesis involves comparing the different sources of information for agreement, conflict, or inconsistency. This process should result in clarification and prioritization of the information most critical to decision making.

Given that the foundation of team participation is creating a common base of knowledge so that communication can occur, the first component of team participation is educational and thus broad in scope. Once this base of knowledge is established, the focus can be brought to bear on the individual child and family of concern to the team.

Sharing Information

Information required by nonoptometric professionals who work with children who have vision problems goes beyond acknowledging the need for correction. In essence, the optometrist should inform the health, education, and related services professionals about: terminology; dimensions of optometric services; other nonschool resources and services; implications of common eye conditions; the nature and purpose of correction; and information typically contained in a vision report. Of these areas, terminology, dimensions or scope of optometric services, and other services are the most critical in assuring that other professionals know what to expect from the optometrist.

The type of information required by educators and other personnel should be designed to clarify the level of accessibility to, and relationship with, the optometrist. Specifically:

1. What is the optometrist's philosophy and perspective on vision and vision care?
2. Is the optometrist available by phone to answer questions?
3. Does the optometrist provide visual efficiency training and other types of low-vision care?
4. Does the optometrist provide optical corrections, vision therapy, and comprehensive vision care?
5. Is the optometrist available to consult with the school on such variables as lighting, seating position in the classroom, contrast and other characteristics of materials, and use of low-vision devices?
6. Is the optometrist available to attend IEP meetings and other planning meetings?
7. Is the optometrist willing to serve as an intermediary between the school and the family if needed?
8. Is the optometrist willing to review therapeutic and educational goals and programs and provide feedback on their relationship to the child's vision needs?
9. Does the optometrist provide assistance in finding financial resources and other services for purchase of corrective devices and access to other needed care?

Once optometrists begin to serve a child, they can append a glossary of terms and a description of their services and the scope of their role to the eye report. More personal contact may include a letter or a phone call to a key team member such as the classroom teacher outlining the level of participation in team efforts and the strategies they would prefer for further contact such as answering

questions or developing joint visual efficiency goals to be pursued at school, at home, and during the child's low-vision therapy, if appropriate. The goal is to ensure that team members clearly understand the scope of the optometrist's services and the level of involvement in the educational process.

Provision of background information on the child's vision condition and its implications and prognosis should also be provided to educators. For example, nystagmus is often regarded with great concern by those who are not vision professionals, as they assume that the child is unable to focus during the eye movement. Many educators may not realize the strain and exhaustion that reading imposes on a child with moderate amounts of uncorrected hyperopia. Educators may not be aware that an aphakic child may have perceptual difficulties and acuity limitations, even with corrective lenses. Again, when ensuring that all professionals concerned with a child's development and learning share a common base of knowledge, the rule of thumb is to err on the side of more than enough information rather than too little. Whenever possible, functional translation of vision problems should be furnished.

Gathering Information

There are a multitude of variables beyond the eye condition itself that can affect how a child functions visually. Chapter 1 provides an overview of the various disabilities children may experience. Gathering this information can also serve to educate others concerned with the child about vision. Table 23.4 lists the types of information available from education-related professionals that may be of benefit to the optometric evaluation.

This information can be gathered by talking on the telephone or face to face, mailing questionnaires and other requests for information to the team members, or submitting questionnaires and other requests for information to the education professional serving the child. If there is some confusion over who

Table 23.4 INFORMATION FROM THE EDUCATIONAL TEAM, THAT IS RELEVANT TO THE OPTOMETRIC EXAMINATION

Type of Information	Education Team Members
General concerns and questions about the child's vision	Parents and all professionals
Optimal position and handling (i.e., head position, reducing tone)	Physical and/or occupational therapist
Sensitivity or aversion to light or touch	Teachers, parents
Attention span	Teachers, parents
Visual stimuli preferences (i.e., colors, objects)	Teachers, parents
Ability to understand and follow directions	Speech and language therapist
Response to sound and touch vs. vision	Teachers, therapists
Reinforcer preferences (i.e., food, pats or hugs, praise)	Teachers, parents
Response to new persons	Teachers, parents
Type of skills child needs to participate in examination (i.e., can indicate direction on the Snellen *E*; can answer questions; other behaviors exhibited by the child to indicate when something is seen such as an increase or cessation of sounds, breathing changes)	Teachers, parents
Type of activities in the classroom and at home that place vision demands on the child (i.e., the teacher uses a lot of visual media like films)	Teachers, parents
Types of activities at which the child does well or poorly that require vision	Teachers, parents

is functioning as the team coordinator, the optometrist can contact the parent or other person who made the referral.

The optometrist may also want to record the child's behavior during the optometric examination and share it with the team. This information is helpful in determining what vision the child has and how it is used when typical responses are not demonstrated.

When decisions must be made about a child's degree of vision and treatment needs, a team effort ensures attention to the full range of variables, such as the nature of the task; adapting the environment to increase contrast and reduce glare; providing additional support, such as a notetaker or copies of whatever is placed on the chalkboard at school; determining an appropriate reading medium, such as print or large print; and correction, such as glasses and low-vision devices. The optometrist should provide information that enables other professionals and the family to interpret the child's behavior in relation to his or her use of vision and to address vision needs that extend beyond corrective lenses.

Recommendations by the optometrist should be supported in the results and interpretation of the evaluation. The usefulness of the optometric report is further enhanced by the earlier efforts to educate team members about vision and the optometrist's services and to outline procedures for interaction between them.

Table 23.5   EDUCATIONALLY RELEVANT INFORMATION

Information	Role
Recommendations on environmental variables such as: lighting, contrast, space, distance, time, size, color, and position	Optometrist
Optical devices: their use, care, etc.	Optometrist
Visual skills to be addressed in the school program	Optometrist
Care of eyes and prognosis for condition	Optometrist
Modification of environment, materials, or task	Teacher/parent
Follow-through of optometric recommendations	Teacher/parent
Training in how to care for optical devices	Teacher/parent
Visual demands in the classroom and the home	Teacher parent
Functional vision assessment data	Teacher/optometrist
Teaching children about their vision problems and visual abilities	Optometrist/teacher/parent
Health status	Pediatrician/optometrist/ teacher/parent

The Optometrist and the Teacher: Communication Needs and Processes

One of the most important relationships for the optometrist as a team member is with the child's teacher. Beyond a shared understanding of each profession's concerns, priorities, and language, the optometrist and the teacher together address treatment and remediation of the vision problems, vision deficits, and visual function. The teacher can be the link between the optometrist and the family and other service providers. The teacher cannot, however, perform these functions without information about the child's ocular condition and the nature and justification for correction and other intervention measures. Table 23.5 presents an overview of how teacher and optometrist interact on behalf of the child.

COMMUNICATING WITH THE FAMILY AND CHILD

The family is part of the team and the most important and consistent presence in the child's life. It is also affected most by the child's ocular condition and most informed about how the child functions and uses his or her vision. All of this has implications for how the optometrist interacts with the family.

Strategies for Gathering and Providing Information

Interacting with families, including the child who is the patient, requires special consideration of a variety of factors to ensure that families respond correctly to the optometrist's recommendations (Table 23.6).

The family's ability to work with the optometrist and respond to the child's needs is highly dependent on the type of information it receives and the way that information is presented. Without reiterating the stages of grief and adjustment to loss and disability, it is important for the optometrist to be aware that families whose child suffers a severe vision loss experience those stages. Furthermore, for the family, the stages are neither sequential nor discrete, as is indicated in the literature on adjustment to a death.

A disability is a chronic condition, fre-

Table 23.6   FACTORS AFFECTING HOW THE OPTOMETRIST MUST WORK WITH THE FAMILY

Current reaction to the diagnosis of vision dysfunction

Life issues, such as financial concerns or disagreements between members

Priorities and values

Knowledge base and experience with the service system and with vision loss

Confusion about how the system works

Lack of awareness of resources

A sense of being overwhelmed by other problems and thus less concern about the vision dysfunction than the optometrist might expect.

---

quently manifesting itself in relation to loss or change in expectations throughout life. Family members and the child may feel anger or sadness or deny the condition at different points in time. Conversely, many professionals interpret behavior that departs from their expectations as a manifestation of one of the adjustment stages, when, in fact, it may simply reflect disagreement or frustration with services on the part of the family or child.

Families need concrete information in understandable language. That information should include justification for the diagnosis and treatment options and an explanation of their implications. Equally important is the way the information is provided. The fact that someone has heard information does not ensure that they have comprehended it. The following are a series of considerations and techniques that the optometrist can employ to facilitate communication.

- Provide information clearly and in nontechnical language. Tell them only as much as they are ready to hear. Use their questions to determine how much information they may require at the time.
- Plan a time and strategy for following up or gathering additional information. For example, leave the room, or set up a follow-up appointment, or give them a phone number and a specific time to call.
- Provide the information in at least two forms. Give them a summary of what is discussed in writing or suggest that they take notes or tape any conferences with you. Provide all recommendations in writing with a brief justification and an explanation for each. Give clear and detailed solutions for solving problems.
- Allow caregivers time to act on recommendations. Make specific referrals and include a contact person, guidelines on how to approach the referral, and a list of questions to ask. If the resource is unfamiliar to you, contact him or her first, to make sure that it is appropriate and to determine to whom the family should speak and how the family should make contact.
- Be sensitive to families' feelings and reactions. Do not personalize anger or disagreements. Work from their bias and values. Allow families to express the range of concerns they may have, even if they are not directly within your capacity to address. Recognize that their concerns may be different from yours.
- Be very clear about what you can and cannot do and when and how you will respond. Provide suggestions or referrals for issues you cannot resolve directly. Remember that for many families you are the only contact and information source about their child's vision needs. Help them to access other resources.
- Be positive yet honest. As much as possible, share the positive before the negative and describe abilities and needs of the child from the perspective of what he or she can do. Caregivers will understand the limitations implied in the description of what is possible. Remember that if families came to you about their child, they are aware there is a problem. It is the confirmation, not the description, that is painful for them.

Just as there are a variety of family constellations, each of these groups represents a myriad of cultures. (The reader is referred to Chapter 1 for a discussion of the variations related to different cultural backgrounds.) People of different cultures often have different goals, attitudes toward disability, assumptions of responsibility for a particular problem, senses of protectionism of cultural identity, and a resulting mistrust of the dominant culture's providers and systems.

For families who are not members of a community's dominant culture, particularly those for whom there is a language barrier, special consideration must be taken to ensure that they (1) understand the optometrist, (2) are able to talk to the optometrist about their concerns, (3) can get access to appropriate services and act on recommendations, and (4) believe their particular perspectives and priorities are taken into consideration during the treatment process. Many families who are members of a culture other than that which is dominant may not follow through on recommendations or act on referrals out of a sense of responsibility for meeting needs within the family, lack of experience with intermediaries and other indirect service providers, values about acceptance of a disability, or values that oppose or are not supportive of certain treatment measures. The optometrist must respect and address these issues in the treatment process to ensure maximum benefit for the child.

For all families, treatment must take into consideration the family's needs, styles of interaction and care, daily schedules, and other characteristics. Unless intervention is prescribed within the context of the family and recognizes the needs, beliefs, and styles of the family, follow-through will be limited, at best, and at worst the sense of alienation from potential sources of assistance will increase.

PUTTING IT ALL TOGETHER: EDUCATIONAL SERVICES AND DECISIONS, AND THE OPTOMETRIST'S ROLE

The role of the optometrist as a primary vision care practitioner in patient management is extensive. Just as the growth and develop-

ment of children are affected directly by vision, so are they affected by the type of care provided for their vision. For the child with mild to severe vision dysfunction and the child with dysfunctions in other systems, that care can have an impact on how these children progress perceptually, cognitively, physically, emotionally, and socially. Simultaneously, vision and vision care are affected by a myriad of other interpersonal and intrapersonal variables in the young patient's life.

The pediatric optometrist can have an effect on the self-esteem of the child with low vision, the reading progress of the highly hyperopic child, the sports participation of the myopic child, and the day-to-day functionality of the child with a hearing loss or mental retardation, to cite but a few examples. To ensure that care is maximally efficient and effective requires more than clinical skills and a basic knowledge of growth and development, reading and reading problems, and other disabilities, including vision loss. It requires applying that knowledge, in conjunction with the other professionals available, within the context of the larger service system in which children and their families participate.

To this end, in this chapter—and in this book as a whole—we have endeavored to present the concept of the pediatric optometrist's "patient" as the child, the family, and other primary providers such as the pediatrician and teacher simultaneously. As is so thoroughly explained in Chapter 1, the processes of growth, development, and learning, and the presence of disabling conditions result in a demand for input from many persons with diverse skills and perspectives for care or intervention to be effective. As the chapters on vision development, eye and brain function, and care and treatment indicate, within that complexity the optometrist has a critical role in, and contribution to, the developmental process.

Whether advising a family on how to care for a child's glasses or administer medication, attempting to evaluate visual function in a child with cerebral palsy, or monitoring development of acuity and accommodation in an infant, the optometrist is a member of a larger team, to and from which he or she both contributes and receives information and effort necessary for optimal care and treatment. The foundation of team participation, whether formally (as is mandated in the special education laws), or informally, is two-way communication of information.

In summary, this means (1) gathering information that will be helpful in diagnosis and treatment from persons who are familiar with the child, the visual function, and the visual demands placed on it and (2) sharing information about optometric services, resources, and strategies for enhancing the care and function of vision through environmental and material adaptation, visual efficiency training, and planning for continuing comprehensive visual care services.

The family and other professionals may participate in the examination, managing the child's behavior or providing feedback on how to communicate with the child and the treatment, encouraging children to wear their glasses or use their low-vision devices. More important, the many contributions the optometrist can make expand the role beyond attention to the child. The optometrist can educate others about vision and can consult on optimal environmental conditions, activities to stimulate vision, and techniques for screening. He or she can expand the perspective of the medical professional beyond that of the health status of the eye to an awareness of the complexity of vision and the visual process. The optometrist can help educators and parents understand the impact of visual anomalies on development, learning, and function. Conversely, educators and families can provide practical insight into the scope of resources beyond the medical arena, strategies for eliciting maximum information about a child's vision and visual function, and the day-to-day impact of a child's vision on his or her ability to learn, grow, and function in the environment.

For teamwork to occur, the optometrist should reach out beyond the clinical setting to establish linkages with others at the patient level and the agency or service level.

Patients, resources, information, and programs all must be coordinated among the many persons concerned with the child. Just as this book is an example of gathering and sharing information from many people, representing a variety of perspectives and areas of expertise, so should the optometrist ensure that part of the primary care of their young patients reflects a coming together of many people for optimal care to occur.

Case 1

Background
The patient is a 16-month-old boy, with mild cerebral palsy (hypotonia in trunk and extremities), and no evidence of mental retardation.

He was referred to an ophthalmologist by the pediatrician when he was 9 months old because of comments from the mother about lack of attention to visual stimuli within 12 to 18 inches. The mother and the early childhood teacher reported that the child would not reach for objects and seemed to "lose objects" as they came close to him, although he would fixate and respond to objects beyond about 24 inches. He would attempt to cross the room to get objects as small as 2 inches, but as he neared them, would no longer see them and would abandon the effort.

The teacher and parent were concerned because reach and grasp were not developing as expected, even when the cerebral palsy was taken into account.

The ophthalmologist said that the child was too young to be evaluated fully, although light response and examination of the ocular structure indicated that the visual system was intact. He also reported that the child demonstrated visual motor skills appropriate for his age level at far point. He suggested he return around his fourth birthday.

The child was referred to an optometrist after the optometrist conducted a workshop for all of the early education teachers in the area on vision and the role of the optometrist.

Teamwork
The teacher and the mother provided careful descriptions of the child's visual behaviors. The teacher met briefly with the optometrist to discuss the impact of the cerebral palsy on the child's ability to participate in the examination (particularly head control and fatigue and difficulty at midline) and the child's behaviors, likes, and dislikes. She asked the optometrist what sort of preparation the

child and the mother should have for the examination. He described the examination and made suggestions for getting the child used to having his face touched and sitting alone. The teacher met with the mother and they worked out some games and motions to play with the child that would simulate situations in the examination. The mother remained with the child during the examination and brought some of his favorite toys and food.

Diagnosis and Treatment
Binocular corrective lenses were prescribed to correct high hyperopia.

Outcomes and Team Intervention
The optometrist, after reviewing the information provided by the mother and teacher and questioning the mother further, conducted an examination that was in part functional and in part more clinical. He determined that the child had significant hyperopia, coupled with difficulty controlling the eye muscles, problems similar to those seen in other parts of the body and probably, in part, because of the cerebral palsy. He also noted somewhat sluggish pupil response to light and inconsistent performance of ocular motor tasks such as tracking. He prescribed corrective lenses and made suggestions about color and contrast variables and lighting, particularly in relation to changing light conditions.

The child responded immediately to the glasses, so there was no need to develop a program to keep them on him. The teacher sent a report to the optometrist on the child's response and performance with the glasses and the increase in contrast. As a result, the optometrist made a slight change in the child's correction. The optometrist and the teacher then developed a program to further encourage functional vision development, particularly oculomotor skills, which was shared with the parent and the child's physical therapist. The child remained under the care of the optometrist, providing the teacher and parent with periodic lists of questions and guidelines for updating the child's functional vision assessment to facilitate future examinations.

Case 2

Background
A 7-year-old girl attended school in a regular classroom setting and had no identified disabilities. She was born 10 weeks prematurely and weighed approximately 3 pounds at birth.

The child was referred by her mother after the teacher discussed the possibility of a learning disability. The teacher reported that the child was not learning to read as expected, was irritable and distracted, particularly as the school day progressed, and had difficulty staying in her seat and attending to classroom tasks.

Diagnosis and Treatment
Corrective lenses were prescribed to correct high myopia.

Teamwork
Initially, the child was seen by the optometrist, who prescribed correction for a myopic condition. The child wore the glasses but continued to avoid tasks at school and to act out. She spent a lot of time sitting in the hall as punishment. She also began to color in the pictures on the classroom bulletin boards and draw on the blackboard, creating more conflict with the teacher.

The mother returned to the optometrist and asked whether he thought there could be other vision problems and if the optometrist would be willing to meet with the teacher and discuss the child. The optometrist set up an appointment and wrote the teacher asking her to come to the office after school.

The optometrist described for the teacher how things must have looked to the child and how her vision problem would have affected her ability to attend to far point tasks. He mentioned that the child may not have well-developed perceptual and oculomotor skills or might simply have developed an aversion to school tasks because of the difficulty she had been experiencing. He stated that her sudden interest in the details of the pictures in her classroom indicated that the glasses were helping her. He suggested ways for her to make things more comfortable for the child visually—controlling glare, giving her periodic breaks—and suggested some activities that would be enjoyable to the child and would enhance visual function and visual perception. The teacher redesigned the child's reading program, began to focus on giving her opportunities to succeed at academic tasks, and arranged for remedial instruction. The teacher shared what she learned from the optometrist with the remedial reading teacher.

The child began to improve, and testing for a learning disability was deferred. The principal also contacted the optometrist for suggestions on how to revise the school's vision screening, which currently consisted of a Snellen test only.

Case 3

Background
The patient was a 5-year-old boy with a diagnosis of ocular albinism who had just entered a kinder-

garten in a mainstream setting. He had received services from the optometrist since the age of 14 months, after a referral from the pediatrician, who had been a guest speaker at the local optometric association meeting that the optometrist attended. The optometrist's report documented that the child qualified for the clinical designation "partially sighted." When the parents enrolled the child in school they submitted the report, and the child was determined to be eligible for special education services.

The optometrist was contacted by the child's itinerant vision teacher, who asked to participate in the team meeting to develop his IEP.

Diagnosis and Correction
The diagnosis was ocular albinism. Glasses were prescribed with tinted lenses. Plans were made for later use of additional optical devices.

Teamwork
The optometrist was unable to attend the team meeting. The kindergarten teacher was very apprehensive about having a low-vision student in her class. The itinerant vision teacher was newly graduated and uncertain about how the child's visual condition might affect his performance. He also found the child's medical records quite confusing.

The optometrist suggested that the teachers and the parents write down their questions and concerns. She also suggested that they send some examples of the kinds of print materials used in the classroom. After receiving these, the optometrist responded to the questions, made some general suggestions for environmental adaptations and material adaptations, and sent a glossary and a fact sheet on albinism. Before the next session with the child, the optometrist arranged a phone conference with the teachers and gave them a list of questions to answer prior to the examination.

Because the child's father was laid off from his job and lost all insurance benefits they did not appear for the appointment. The optometrist called the teacher, after not hearing from the parents for quite a while. The teacher met with the parents to discuss why they did not keep the appointment. He agreed to explore funding sources and contacted the staff at the optometry office, who informed him of resources for Medicaid applications and other financial aid. The optometrist agreed to attend the next IEP meeting, during which planning for first grade would occur, and to visit the classroom. Although the parents found financial resources, the optometrist decided to wait to see the child again until after the IEP meeting so that she would have a better idea of the

kinds of visual demands that would be placed on the child. She then adjusted the child's correction and recommended low-vision therapy. She also provided recommendations on seating arrangements, lighting, and material adaptations to reduce glare and increase contrast. A physical therapist also evaluated the child and attended the meeting because the child was exhibiting some motor delays. It was determined that, along with the low-vision therapy, the child would be placed in a resource room to remediate some gaps in motor and concept development. The child had not received early intervention, although, even with correction, he still had a serious visual impairment.

The teacher also provided the optometrist with some sources for early intervention so that she could refer other parents of children with vision loss at a much younger age.

The optometrist, teacher, and the parent then developed a schedule for regular contact so that the low-vision therapy would be reinforced in the home and the school and additional aids or other vision services could be provided as appropriate in a timely manner as the child progressed through elementary school.

REFERENCES

1. Aiken M, Dewar R, DiTomaso N, Hage J, Zeitz G: Coordinating Human Services. San Francisco, Josey-Bass, 1975.

2. Baumheimer E: The cause and consequences of interagency conflict. Social Inquiry 33:31–33, 1979.

3. Bensen JK, Kunce J, Thompson C, Allen D: Coordinating Human Services. Columbia, MO, University of Missouri Press, 1973.

4. Elder J: Essential components in development of interagency coordination. In McGrab P, Elder J (eds): Planning Services to Handicapped Persons: Community, Education, Health. Baltimore, Paul Brooks, 1979.

5. Froland C, Pancoast D, Chapman N, Kimboko P: Helping Networks and Human Services. Beverly Hills, Sage Publications, 1981.

6. Gearhart B, DeRuiter J, Sileo, T: Teaching Mildly and Moderately Handicapped Students. Englewood Cliffs, NJ, Prentice-Hall, 1986.

7. Levine S, White P: Exchange as a conceptual framework for the study of interorganizational

relationships. Admin Sci Quart 5:583–601, 1961.

8. Losen S, Losen J: The Special Education Team. Boston, Allyn and Bacon, 1985.

9. McGrab P, Elder J: Planning Services to Handicapped Persons: Community, Education, Health. Baltimore, Paul Brooks, 1979.

10. Morante A, Dubowitz LM, Levene M, Dubowitz V: The development of visual function in normal and neurologically preterm and full-term infants. Develop Med Child Neurol 24:771–784, 1982.

11. Paine PA, Pasquali L, Spegiorin C: Appearance of visually directed prehension related to gestational age and intrauterine growth. J Genet Psychol 142:53–60.

12. Palfrey JS, Singer JD, Walker DK, Butler JA: Early identification of children's special needs: A study of five metropolitan communities. J Pediatr 111:651–659, 1987.

13. Ruff HA, Lawson KR, Kurtzberg D, McCarton-Daum C, Vaughn HG: Visual following of moving objects by full-term and pre-term infants. J Pediatr Psychol 7:375–386, 1982.

Index

Note: Page numbers followed by *f* or *t* indicate figure or table, respectively.

ISBN 0-397-50917-0

90000

9 780397 509171